10 0293182 5

D1439094

DATE DUE FOR RETURN

UNIVERSITY LIBRARY

2 4 MAR 2003

8WL GML 01

UNIVERSITY LIBRARY

1 2 JUL 2004

8WL GML 07

UNIVERSITY LIBRARY

1 8 JUL 2003

8WL GML 13

UNIVERSITY LIBRARY

- 7 DEC 2004

8WL GML 07

UNIVERSITY LIBRARY

2 8 AUG 2003

8WL GML 13

UNIVERSITY LIBRARY

0 2 FEB 2005

8WL GML 13

UNIVERSITY LIBRARY

1 5 DEC 2003

8WL GML 07

UNIVERSITY LIBRARY

2 9 APR 2005

8WL GML 07

UNIVERSITY LIBRARY

2 0 APR 2004

8WL GML 07

UNIVERSITY LIBRARY

0 4 SEP 2012

GML 02

e recalled before the above date.

This comprehensive compilation, written by an authoritative team of international contributors, surveys the role of *Escherichia coli* in health and disease. The potential of *E. coli* as a pathogen has increasingly been recognised in recent years and its mechanisms of virulence have been extensively investigated. This valuable and timely account brings the subject fully up to date. First the diseases due to *E. coli* in humans and animals and the part it plays in the normal flora are described in general terms. Then chapters are devoted to each of the recognised virulence factors and mechanisms, including capsules, adhesins, haemolysins, endotoxins, exotoxins and iron scavenging. The third section deals in detail with various diseases and their mechanisms. Finally, the host responses to infection and the design of vaccines are considered.

This book will be of value to all scientists and clinicians with an interest in microbial pathogenicity.

ESCHERICHIA COLI:
MECHANISMS OF VIRULENCE

ESCHERICHIA COLI: MECHANISMS OF VIRULENCE

Edited by

MAX SUSSMAN

Department of Microbiology, Medical School,
Newcastle upon Tyne

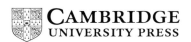
CAMBRIDGE
UNIVERSITY PRESS

MEDICAL LIBRARY
QUEEN'S MEDICAL CENTRE

PUBLISHED BY THE PRESS SYNDICATE OF THE UNIVERSITY OF CAMBRIDGE
The Pitt Building, Trumpington Street, Cambridge CB2 1RP

CAMBRIDGE UNIVERSITY PRESS
The Edinburgh Building, Cambridge CB2 2RU, United Kingdom
40 West 20th Street, New York, NY 10011-4211, USA
10 Stamford Road, Oakleigh, Melbourne 3166, Australia

© Cambridge University Press 1997

This book is in copyright. Subject to statutory exception
and to the provisions of relevant collective licensing agreements,
no reproduction of any part may take place without
the written permission of Cambridge University Press.

First published 1997

Printed in the United Kingdom at the University Press, Cambridge

Typeset in Linotron Times 10/13pt

A catalogue record of this book is available from the British Library

Library of Congress Cataloguing in Publication data

Escherichia coli: mechanisms of virulence/edited by Max Sussman.
  p. cm.
  ISBN 0 521 45361 5 (hardback)
  1. Escherichia coli. 2. Virulence (Microbiology) I. Sussman, Max.
QR82.E6835 1997
616′.0145–dc20   96-20969 CIP

ISBN 0 521 45361 5   hardback

1002931825

RO

For
Jonathan and Judith
With love

Contents

Contributors

S. N. Abraham
Department of Pathology, Jewish Hospital of St. Louis and Departments of Pathology and Molecular Microbiology, Washington University School of Medicine, St. Louis, Missouri 63110, USA

T. J. Baldwin
Microbial Pathogenicity Research Group, Department of Microbiology, University Hospital, Queens Medical Centre, Nottingham NG7 2UH, UK

K. A. Bettelheim
Biomedical Reference Laboratory, Victorian Infectious Diseases Reference Laboratory, Fairfield Hospital, Fairfield, Victoria 3078, Australia

K. W. Dodson
Department of Molecular Microbiology, Washington University School of Medicine, Washington University Medical Center, St. Louis, Missouri 63110-1093, USA

C. J. Dorman
Department of Microbiology, Moyne Institute, University of Dublin, Trinity College, Dublin 2, Republic of Ireland

P. Echeverria
Department of Bacteriology, Immunology and Molecular Genetics, Armed Forces Research Institute of Medical Sciences, RajVithi Road, Bangkok, Thailand

W. Gaastra
Department of Bacteriology, Institute of Infectious Disease and Immunology, University of Utrecht, Yalelaan 1, 3508 Utrecht, The Netherlands

W. Goebel
Theodor-Boveri-Institut für Biowissenschaften, Universität Würzburg, Würzburg, Germany

F. K. de Graaf
Department of Molecular Microbiology, Institute of Molecular and Cellular Biology, Vreije Universiteit, de Boelelaan 1087, 1081HV Amsterdam, The Netherlands

J. W. Gray
Department of Microbiology, Birmingham Children's Hospital, Ladywood Middleway, Ladywood, Birmingham B16 8ET, UK

E. Griffiths
Biologicals, World Health Organisation, CH 1211-Geneva, 27 Switzerland

T. L. Hale
Department of Enteric Infections, Walter Reed Army Hospital Institute of Research, Washington D.C. 20307, USA

J. Holmgren
Department of Medical Microbiology and Immunology, University of Göteborg, Guldhedsgatan 10, S-41346 Göteborg, Sweden

S. Hull
Department of Microbiology and Immunology, Baylor College of Medicine, One Baylor Plaza, Houston, Texas 77030, USA

S. J. Hultgren
Department of Molecular Microbiology, Washington University School of Medicine, Washington University Medical Center, St. Louis, Missouri 63110-1093, USA

F. Jacob-Dubuisson
Department of Molecular Microbiology, Washington University School of Medicine, Washington University Medical Center, St. Louis, Missouri 63110-1093, USA

S. Jaiswal
Department of Pathology, Jewish Hospital of St. Louis and Departments of Pathology and Molecular Microbiology, Washington University School of Medicine, St. Louis, Missouri 63110, USA

B. Jann
Max-Planck-Institut für Immunbiologie, Stübeweg 51, D-79108 Freiburg, Germany

K. Jann
Max-Planck-Institut für Immunbiologie, Stübeweg 51, D-79108 Freiburg, Germany

J. R. Johnson
Department of Medicine, Division of Infectious Diseases, University of Minnesota, Medical School, 516 Delaware Street S.E., Minneapolis, Minnesota 55455, USA

S. Knutton
Institute of Child Health, University of Birmingham, Birmingham B16 8ET, UK

A. Ludwig
Theodor-Boveri-Institut für Biowissenschaften, Universität Würzburg, Würzburg, Germany

D. M. MacLaren
Klinische Microbiologie en Ziekenhuishygiene, Academisch Ziekenhuis, Vreije Universiteit, Amsterdam, The Netherlands. Present address: Moidart House, Chapel Lane, Bodicote, Banbury, Oxfordshire OX15 4DA, UK

G. B. Nair
National Institute of Cholera and Enteric Diseases, Calcutta, India

J. P. Nataro
Department of Pediatrics, Division of Infectious Diseases and Tropical Pediatrics, University of Maryland School of Medicine, 10 South Pine Street, Baltimore, Maryland 21201, USA

N. Ní Bhriain
Department of Microbiology, Moyne Institute, University of Dublin, Trinity College, Dublin 2, Republic of Ireland

B. Rowe
Laboratory of Enteric Pathogens, Central Public Health Laboratory, 61 Colindale Avenue, London NW9 5HT, UK

S. M. Scotland
Laboratory of Enteric Pathogens, Central Public Health Laboratory, 61 Colindale Avenue, London NW9 5HT, UK

H. R. Smith
Laboratory of Enteric Pathogens, Central Public Health Laboratory, 61 Colindale Avenue, London NW9 5HT, UK

R. Steadman
Institute of Nephrology, University of Wales College of Medicine, Cardiff Royal Infirmary, Newport Road, Cardiff CF2 1SZ, UK

R. T. Striker
Department of Molecular Microbiology, Washington University School of Medicine, Washington University Medical Center, St. Louis, Missouri 63110-1093, USA

M. Sussman
Department of Microbiology, Medical School, Newcastle upon Tyne NE2 4HH, UK

A.-M. Svennerholm
Department of Medical Microbiology and Immunology, University of Göteborg, Guldhedsgatan 10, S-41346 Göteborg, Sweden

Y. Takeda
Research Institute, International Medical Center of Japan, 1-21-1 Toyama, Shinjuku-ku, Tokyo 162, Japan

N. Topley
Institute of Nephrology, University of Wales College of Medicine, Cardiff Royal Infirmary, Newport Road, Cardiff CF2 1SZ, UK

P. H. Williams
Department of Microbiology, University of Leicester, Leicester LE1 7RH, UK

G. A. Willshaw
Laboratory of Enteric Pathogens, Central Public Health Laboratory, 61 Colindale Avenue, London NW9 5HT, UK

M. J. Woodward
Bacteriology Department, Central Veterinary Laboratory, New Haw, Addlestone, Surrey KT15 3NB, UK

C. Wray
Bacteriology Department, Central Veterinary Laboratory, New Haw, Addlestone, Surrey KT15 3NB, UK

Preface

It is more than 40 years since I first met *Escherichia coli* in a practical classroom in the Institute of Pathology at Leeds. This short Gram-negative bacillus soon distinguished itself from many of the other bacteria in my early experience by the ease with which it could be handled. At the time we were told that, although *E. coli* could cause disease, its virulence was low. At this time, unbeknown to me as a junior undergraduate, *E. coli* was the subject of groundbreaking work with bacteriophage that was to lay the foundations of virology and molecular biology. So little was then known about *E. coli* in medical circles that it was often still called *Bacillus coli*, more than 30 years after it had been named by Castellani and Chalmers for its discoverer, Dr Theodor Escherich.

Knowledge about the biochemistry, physiology and genetics of *E. coli* has grown continuously since the 1940s. At the same time our understanding of the nature and behaviour of the pathogenic types of *E. coli* has greatly increased. The Society for General Microbiology Symposium *The Virulence of Escherichia coli* in Newcastle upon Tyne in January 1983 and its proceedings, later published (London: Academic Press, 1985) in a well-received expanded version, marked the state of knowledge at that time.

The purpose of this monograph is to bring up to date that account of *E. coli* as a pathogen of humans, but also though only briefly of animals. The latter are subject to *E. coli* infections that result to some extent from current practices in animal husbandry and are of economic importance. Cattle are carriers of serogroup O157 strains that are increasingly seen as a potentially serious threat to human health; control of these strains is increasingly exercising public health authorities. In some respects this represents a 'replay' of the recognition, study and control of the great bacterial pathogens first recognised at about the turn of the century. Who knows what secrets *E. coli* may yet hold; the next decade promises to be as exciting as the last.

On account of its broad spectrum of pathogenic potential *E. coli* is a paradigm of pathogenic bacteria in general. I hope that this book will be a useful summary for those with an interest in this fascinating organism and also for those whose primary interest is in other areas of microbiology. Many students of microbiology now take modules that deal with pathogens and the mechanisms of pathogenesis. They will find many of the chapters helpful in their studies. I imagine that this book could be used as a text for more advanced courses on microbial pathogenesis.

My children Jonathan and Judith have both met *E. coli* in their studies. I suspect that for the good of their patients they would rather not meet it again! This book is dedicated to them with admiration and love.

Max Sussman

Newcastle upon Tyne, February 1996

Part one

Introduction

1

Escherichia coli and human disease

M. SUSSMAN

For more than half a century after its discovery *E. coli* was thought of as the major commensal in faeces and it was regarded as having only low virulence. This view changed progressively with recognition of the complexity of the faecal flora and the variety of superficially similar intestinal infections due to *E. coli*. The identification of a wide range of specific virulence factors followed and the individual basis of the diseases could be defined. In this way *E. coli* ultimately found its way into the pantheon of virulent pathogens that had been discovered before the turn of the century.

The genus *Escherichia*

The genus *Escherichia* is a typical member of the Enterobacteriaceae that have their principal habitat in the bowel of humans and animals. The genus is closely related to a number of others in the family, most particularly *Shigella*, to the extent that the two genera should be combined (Brenner, 1984). The distinction is maintained because of the separate clinical and epidemiological importance of the various species.

Several less frequently isolated species have also been described. The aerobic flora of the hind-gut of the cockroach *Blatta orientalis* includes *E. blattae* (Burgess *et al.*, 1973) but this has not been isolated elsewhere. *Escherichia fergusonii* has been found in the faeces of humans and domestic animals, and in clinical material, particularly urine and blood (Farmer *et al.*, 1985b). A yellow pigmented organism has been isolated from faeces, wounds, blood and cerebrospinal fluid, and named *E. hermanii* (Brenner *et al.*, 1982a). An organism related to *E. coli* (DNA relatedness 25–39 per cent) and *Enterobacter* (DNA relatedness 24–35 per cent) has been found in faeces and wounds, and given the name

3

E. vulneris (Brenner *et al.*, 1982b). The detailed characteristics of these species have been described by Farmer *et al.* (1985a). The species originally described as *E. adecarboxylata* has been transferred to the genus *Leclercia* (Tamura *et al.*, 1986).

The characteristics of *Escherichia coli*

Escherichia coli is a short, straight Gram-negative bacillus that is non-sporing, usually motile with peritrichous flagella, often fimbriate and occurs singly, or in pairs in rapidly growing liquid cultures. A capsule or microcapsule is often present and a few strains produce a profuse polysaccharide slime.

Biochemical and culture characteristics

Escherichia coli is a facultative anaerobe capable of fermentative and respiratory metabolism. Its optimum temperature is 37°C and it grows readily on a wide range of simple culture media and on simple synthetic media. Under anaerobic growth conditions there is an absolute require-ment for fermentable carbohydrate. Glucose is fermented to pyruvate, which is converted into lactic, acetic and formic acids. Part of the latter is converted into hydrogen and carbon dioxide by formic hydrogenlyase but some strains do not produce gas (anaerogenic). Some important physio-logical and biochemical characteristics of *E. coli* are summarised in Table 1.1.

On solid media colonies are non-pigmented and may be smooth (S) or rough (R). Colonies are usually circular and smooth with an entire edge; some strains, particularly those isolated from patients with cystic fibrosis, produce mucoid colonies (Macone *et al.*, 1981).

A soluble α-haemolysin can be demonstrated in erythrocyte-containing media and some strains possess a cell-associated β-haemolysin that may be released when the cells are lysed (Smith, 1963; and see Chapter 11).

Serological characteristics

The serological classification of *E. coli* depends on a number of antigens, somatic lipopolysaccharide O-antigens, capsular K-antigens, flagellar H-antigens and fimbrial F-antigens. The first three of these form the basis of the typing scheme introduced by Kauffmann (1944), which has since

Table 1.1. *Principal characteristics and reactions of* Escherichia coli *(after Brenner, 1984)*

Mole % G+C	48–52
Optimum growth temperature	37°C
Indole production	+
Methyl red reaction	+
Voges Proskauer reaction	−
Citrate utilisation	−

90–100 per cent positive:
 Glucose (mixed acid + gas); lactose; D-mannitol; D-mannose; D-sorbitol; L-arabinose; maltose; D-xylose; trehalose; mucate; nitrate → nitrate reduction; β-galactosidase

76–89 per cent positive:
 Lysine decarboxylase; motility; L-rhamnose; melibiose

26–75 per cent positive:
 Ornithine decarboxylase; sucrose; dulcitol; salicin; raffinose; aesculin hydrolysis

11–25 per cent positive:
 Arginine dihydrolase

0–11 per cent positive:
 H_2S; urease; phenylalanine deaminase; gelatine liquefaction; growth in CN^-; malonate utilisation; D-adonitol; *myo*-inositol; cellobiose; α-methyl-D-glucoside; D-arabitol; lipase; DNase; oxidase; pigment

then been greatly expanded (Gross & Rowe, 1985) to include the analysis of fimbriae (Parry *et al.*, 1982; Ørskov & Ørskov, 1983), but it has not yet become conventional to include the fimbrial serotype in the serological formula.

 Chemical analysis of the sugars of lipopolysaccharides has allowed the definition of *E. coli* chemotypes that frequently correspond to serological cross-reactions between different O-serogroups and *Salmonella* (Ørskov *et al.*, 1967).

Distribution

Normal flora, colonisation and persistence

Escherichia coli is a member of the normal commensal bowel flora of humans and colonisation takes place soon after birth (Escherich, 1885; Bettelheim *et al.*, 1974). The source is to be found in the mother and the inanimate environment (O'Farrell *et al.*, 1976) (see Chapter 3). It appears rapidly in the saliva (Russell & Melville, 1978) but does not appear to colonise the normal mouth or pharynx.

The function of *E. coli* in the faecal flora is difficult to assess. It has been suggested that it has a nutritional significance by providing a source of vitamins in some animals. The normal flora of the alimentary tract has been extensively reviewed (Drasar & Hill, 1974; Skinner & Carr, 1974; Clarke & Bauchop, 1977; Siitonen, 1992). In nature it is also found in soil, water or at any other site it can reach from its primary habitat, usually by faecal contamination.

The prevalence of certain serogroups in the human faecal flora is greater than that of others (Siitonen, 1992; Table 1.2) and this may in some way be due to their capacity to persist in the bowel (Ewing & Davies, 1961; Guinee, 1963). In healthy adults over 20 per cent of faecal *E. coli* have virulence-associated determinants and in seven per cent more than one is present (Siitonen, 1992).

Dubos *et al.* (1963) suggested that in mice, which they studied in some detail, *E. coli is* not a normal member of the flora but should rather be regarded as a potential pathogen. The possibility that the same applies to humans cannot be avoided.

Virulence characteristics

A number of virulence factors have been identified in *E. coli* and others probably remain to be discovered. The pathogenetic processes that operate in a given infection always involve more than one virulence factor. These usually interact in so complex a manner that the precise mechanisms still remain to be defined, but attempts to do so have been made by means of complex statistical analysis (*e.g.* Siitonen *et al.*, 1993).

Colonisation factors

Mucous surfaces have efficient clearance mechanisms to remove particles and bacteria, and to overcome these clearance mechanisms specific adhesion mechanisms have been evolved.

Table 1.2. *O-serogroups of* Escherichia coli *associated with the normal faeces and various infections of humans*[a]

Normal faeces	EPEC Outbreaks	EPEC Sporadic	ETEC	EIEC	VTEC	Neonatal meningitis	Urinary tract infection	Septicaemia
O1	O18	O1	O1	O28	O157[b]	O1	O1	O1
O2	O20	O2	O6	O29		O6	O2	O2
O4	O26	O4	O7	O112		O7	O4	O4
O5	O44	O6	O8	O115		O16	O6	O6
O6	O55	O8	O9	O121		O18	O7	O7
O7	O86	O15	O15	O124		O83	O8	O8
O8	O111	O21	O20	O135			O9	O9
O18	O112	O51	O25	O136			O11	O11
O20	O114	O75	O27	O143			O22	O18
O25	O119	O85	O60	O144			O25	O22
O45	O124		O78	O147			O62	O25
O81	O126		O80	O152			O75	O75
	O127		O85	O164				
	O128		O88	O167				
	O142		O89	O173				
	O158		O99					
	O159		O101					
			O109					
			O114					
			O115					
			O126					
			O128					
			O142					
			O148					
			O153					
			O159					

[a] The table was assembled from a variety of sources including: Ewing & Davies, 1961; Ørskov *et al.*, 1977; Rowe, 1979; Dupont, 1982. It should be noted that occasional strains may be found that do not fall into the above groups of pathogen types.

[b] A number of other less important serogroups, collectively termed non-O157 VTEC, have also been identified (see Chapter 15).

EPEC, enteropathogenic *E. coli*; ETEC, enterotoxigenic *E. coli*; EIEC, enteroinvasive *E. coli*; VTEC, Vero cytotoxigenic *E. coli*.

The fimbrial adhesins of *E. coli* are discussed briefly below and in detail in Chapters 6–8. Some non-fimbriate strains of *E. coli* are also capable of attaching to surfaces (Ip *et al.*, 1981; Sussman *et al.*, 1982a).

An unusual 'curly' type of structure has been identified on some non-haemagglutinating strains of enterotoxigenic *E. coli* (Knutton *et al.*, 1987) and rare strains of other types. They have been termed 'curli' (Olsen *et al.*, 1989). They bind to soluble fibronectin and their receptors may be the fibronectin that is a common constituent of cell membranes. Curli-bearing strains of *E. coli* have been isolated from bovine infections (see Chapter 2) but their significance in human disease remains uncertain.

Invasiveness

Certain strains of *E. coli* are able to invade colonic mucosal cells in a manner similar to *Shigella* spp. and to produce a dysentery-like disease in humans. The ability of these strains to invade colonic cells is paralleled by their ability to invade and multiply in HeLa cells (Dupont *et al.*, 1971) and HEp-2 cells (Mehlman *et al.*, 1977) (see also Chapter 16). Instillation of such strains into the eyes of guinea-pigs leads to keratoconjunctivitis (Sérény test; Sérény, 1955).

Lipopolysaccharides (endotoxins)

The lipopolysaccharides of Gram-negative organisms are integral components of the cell envelope and the molecule consists of three parts. *Lipid A* (i) is inserted into the outer membrane of the cell and this is attached to (ii) the *core oligosaccharide*. Attached to the latter and exposed to the environment is the outermost part of the molecule, (iii) the *polysaccharide side chains*. The latter endow organisms with their O-serogroup specificity (Ørskov *et al.*, 1977), while lipid A endows the lipopolysaccharide with its toxicity. Endotoxicity is expressed when lipopolysaccharide is released in the body by the death and breakdown of infecting bacterial cells; the effects can be reproduced in experimental animals by parenteral administration of purified lipopolysaccharide or lipid A.

Organisms in which the lipopolysaccharide, particularly the side chain structure, is complete are termed smooth (S) on account of their colonial morphology, and these tend to be virulent. Mutational loss of the O-antigenic polysaccharide side chains causes a reduction in virulence, which is due to the greater ease of opsonisation of such strains (Van Dijk *et al.*, 1981).

Endotoxins are directly involved in the genesis of disease symptoms that range from fever at one extreme to the potentially fatal endotoxic shock of septicaemia at the other (Morrison & Ryan, 1992; Levin *et al.*, 1993; see Chapter 5).

Exotoxins

Escherichia coli associated with intestinal infections may produce one or more toxins (see Chapter 9).

Heat-labile enterotoxin (LT) is related to *Vibrio cholerae* enterotoxin (choleragen). It is a subunit toxin that consists of an A subunit and five identical B subunits. The A fragment is an ADP-ribosyltransferase, while the B subunits are a binding protein that attaches to the GM_1 gangliosides in the intestinal mucosal cell (enterocyte) membrane, where they create a functional pore through which the A fragment enters the cell. The effect of LT on the intact intestinal mucosa is to induce a net secretion of water, sodium, chloride and bicarbonate ions.

The heat-stable enterotoxin (ST) is a poorly antigenic polypeptide, unrelated to choleragen and acts by stimulating the guanylate cyclase system of mucosal epithelial cells. The resulting increase in the production of guanosine 3′, 5′-cyclicmonophosphate (cGMP) also leads to net secretion of water and electrolytes. Two types of ST, STa and STb, can be distinguished. They differ in that STa is methanol-soluble and enterotoxic for the infant mouse intestine, while STb is methanol-insoluble and inactive in the infant mouse intestine, but it is enterotoxic in weaned pigs (Burgess *et al.*, 1978).

The secretion of water and electrolytes induced by LT and ST gives rise to a watery diarrhoea of small bowel origin that is characteristic of the toxin-induced disease of intestinal infection due to bacteria (Powell, 1991).

Filtrates of certain strains of *E. coli* contain a heat-labile protein that is cytotoxic for Vero cells (Konowalchuk *et al.*, 1977). This Vero cytotoxin (VT) is distinct from LT and ST in having no effect on Y1 adrenal or Chinese hamster ovary (CHO) cell lines. VT, which is also a subunit toxin and related to the cytotoxin of *Shigella dysenteriae* type 1 (Shiga) (O'Brien & Holmes, 1987), has also been termed shiga-like toxin (SLT). A number of different VTs have been identified (see Chapter 10).

Some strains of *E. coli* that cause septicaemic disease in cattle and sheep produce a plasmid-determined toxin that is lethal for rabbits, mice and chickens and is generally associated with the presence of a specific bacterial surface antigen (Smith, 1974; Smith & Huggins, 1976), termed Vir, that appears to be fimbrial (Lopez-Alvarez *et al.*, 1980). It is cytotoxic for HeLa cells and causes multinucleate giant cell formation, but it is not known to be involved human disease.

A cytotoxic necrotising factor (CNF), which causes multinucleate cell formation in HeLa and Vero cells, has been found in *E. coli* that cause diarrhoea in animals and humans (Caprioli *et al.*, 1987). It is closely related to Vir (De Rycke *et al.*, 1990) and its production is frequently associated with that of P-fimbriae and haemolysin (Blanco *et al.*, 1990; Jacobsen *et al.*, 1990). Filtrates of some strains of *E. coli* contain a heat-labile cytotoxin that causes the swelling of HeLa, Vero, HEp-2 and CHO cells and it has been termed cytolethal distending toxin (Johnson & Lior, 1988). The significance of these two toxins in human disease remains unclear.

Some pathogenic strains of *E. coli* produce haemolysins and such strains are said to be more common in animals than humans (Smith, 1963). The best studied haemolysin is the secreted α-haemolysin, which is centrally involved in the pathogenesis of invasive disease in humans.

Haemolysins are important virulence factors, probably because they function in bacterial iron scavenging. The haemolysins of *E. coli* and their significance for virulence are discussed elsewhere in this volume (see Chapters 11 and 12).

Human diseases due to *Escherichia coli*

The diseases that result from infection with *E. coli* may be classified into two groups, *specific* infections and *non-specific* infections.

Specific infections are those in which colonisation of a mucosal surface is an essential preliminary event and in which the principal signs and symptoms of disease are related to the site of colonisation; examples are intestinal and urinary tract infections. In such infections colonisation alone is not sufficient to cause the disease, which results from the subsequent action of other virulence factors and mechanisms.

Non-specific infections differ from the former in that the main signs and symptoms are not related to a site of mucosal colonisation, and mucosal colonisation is not an essential preliminary event. Thus, non-specific infections may result from the direct contamination of wounds or the peritoneal space during surgery, or they may result from secondary spread from a specific infection. A common example is septicaemia following a urinary tract infection. Septicaemia may also occur when the host is compromised by renal failure or alcoholism, and then colonisation factors are less important for *E. coli* virulence (Maslow *et al.*, 1993).

Escherichia coli is a multipotent pathogen that has evolved the ability to cause disease in several body systems and, at least in the bowel, there are several different mechanisms of pathogenesis. Moreover, the causative role of *E. coli* in a number of diseases may not as yet have been recognised, but it appears that only a limited range of serogroups is associated with each type of infection. The similarity of the serogroup distribution in urinary tract infection and septicaemia (Table 1.2) is accounted for by the fact that the latter often derives from the infected urinary tract.

Mucosal colonisation is a necessary preliminary for most of the diseases considered below. What then results may be due to local exotoxin production or mucosal cell invasion followed by intracellular multiplication. In some cases the precise mechanisms are not fully understood. Systemic invasive disease due to *E. coli* is unusual in humans. When it occurs the septicaemia that results may be accompanied by a distinct organotropism, as in neonatal meningitis. It is well to remember that mucosal colonisation of the intestine and the urinary tract may be asymptomatic. This may be because the host is immune to the virulence factors of the infecting strain or because the infecting strain does not possess the complete complement of virulence factors necessary to cause symptomatic disease. In the urinary tract, however, the situation is different in that asymptomatic infection may be a more or less extended interlude between episodes of symptomatic infection (Sussman *et al.*, 1969).

Gastro-intestinal infections

The commonest site of human infections due to *E. coli* is the gastro-intestinal tract, on account of the ease of access of pathogens ingested with food and drink. The incidence of such infections depends on a variety of factors, including personal and food hygiene, and environmental temperature. The part played by *E. coli* in gastro-intestinal infections was suspected long ago by Escherich and later by others (Rowe, 1979). These suspicions could not reliably be confirmed until the work of Kauffmann (1944) established and systematised the serology of *E. coli*, and it became possible to define and compare strains accurately.

Contemporary knowledge about the part that *E. coli* plays in gastro-enteritis began with the work of Bray (1945), who studied a hospital outbreak of infant diarrhoea and discovered that the strains isolated were serologically similar. A few years later several similar outbreaks were reported in which the serotype of the causative strain was defined (Giles & Sangster, 1948; Giles *et al.*, 1949; Taylor *et al.*, 1949). Later the serology of *E. coli* was refined and accurate serological identification of strains was greatly facilitated (Kauffmann, 1954, 1966). The first indication that a specific virulence factor might be associated with *E. coli* was provided by Taylor *et al.* (1961), who observed that certain *E. coli* strains associated with childhood diarrhoea induced fluid and electrolyte secretion in isolated rabbit ileal loops.

A strain of *E. coli* O148 associated with diarrhoea in British troops posted to Aden in 1969 was later shown to produce an enterotoxin (Rowe *et al.*, 1970) and, at about the same time, two enterotoxins were identified in porcine strains (Smith & Gyles, 1970). It was also shown that, to cause disease, enterotoxigenic and enteropathogenic *E. coli* strains had first to colonise the small bowel (Thomson, 1955; Gorbach *et al.*, 1971). Fimbrial colonisation factors of enterotoxigenic strains were then identified (Evans *et al.*, 1977). An unusual type of *E. coli* infection in Japan that closely resembled dysentery due to *Shigella* spp. was identified by Ogawa *et al.* (1968). More recently, epidemic outbreaks and sporadic cases of haemorrhagic colitis and haemolytic-uraemic syndrome (HUS) have been shown to be associated with strains of *E. coli* that produce VT (Konowalchuk *et al.*, 1977) and several types of this toxin have been identified.

The strains of *E. coli* associated with the infections described above fall into four groups. Strains that produce enterotoxins and are associated with diarrhoea in travellers, infants and children in developing countries are termed enterotoxigenic *E. coli* (ETEC). Strains that do not produce enterotoxins and are usually associated with infantile gastro-enteritis in the developed world are termed enteropathogenic *E. coli* (EPEC). *Escherichia coli* associated with dysentery-like disease are termed entero-invasive (EIEC), while those associated with haemorrhagic colitis and HUS are termed Vero-cytotoxin-producing *E. coli* (VTEC) or entero-haemorrhagic *E. coli* (EHEC). In addition, non-toxigenic *E. coli* associated with diarrhoea, but which do not fall into the EPEC serogroups, have been characterised by the appearance of their adherence to cells in tissue culture, as localised adherence, enteroaggregative adherence (enteroaggregative *E. coli*; EAggEC) and diffuse adherence (diffusely adherent *E. coli*; DAEC) (Nataro *et al.*, 1987).

Enteropathogenic Escherichia coli

Diarrhoeal disease, particularly associated with the warm seasons, has been recognised for many years and was at one time given evocative names, such as '*cholera infantum*', '*cholera nostras*', conditions now known as infantile gastro-enteritis. In the past this type of diarrhoea affected mostly infants and very young children, had a very high mortality, a high incidence among the underprivileged and an apparent association with artificial feeding. Though these characteristics suggested that an infective agent was involved, none was identified until modern times. Between the 1920s and the 1950s, for unknown reasons, summer diarrhoea declined in Britain. The history of EPEC infections has been reviewed by Rowe (1979).

The breakthrough to the understanding of EPEC infections was the observation that outbreaks of gastro-enteritis in Aberdeen and London were due to serotypes O55:B5 and O111:B4 (Giles *et al.*, 1949; Giles & Sangster, 1948; Taylor *et al.*, 1949). A number of other EPEC serogroups have since been identified (Taylor, 1961) (Table 1.2). Since the decline of community-acquired 'summer diarrhoea', infantile gastro-enteritis has occurred mainly as outbreaks in hospitals and day nurseries, but occasional sporadic and community infections have been observed. In developing countries community infections are not uncommon.

Recognition of the serogroups of *E. coli* responsible for hospital outbreaks of infantile gastro-enteritis made it possible to elucidate the epidemiology of EPEC infection. Community-acquired infection often preceded hospital outbreaks, which were due to admission to the hospital of a baby with established disease (Thomson *et al.*, 1956) or a carrier excreting the pathogenic strain.

Oral challenge experiments suggest that 10^5 to 10^{10} organisms are necessary to produce diarrhoea (Ferguson & June, 1952; Levine *et al.*, 1978). Ease of acquisition of such high doses can be accounted for by intense dispersal from the liquid stool and the rapid growth of *E. coli* in contaminated food. Bottle-feeding is a known risk factor and, in developing countries, accounts for the high incidence of infection at the time of weaning.

EPEC induce secretion of fluid into perfused segments of rat jejunum (Klipstein *et al.*, 1978) but they do not produce enterotoxins. Autopsy studies have shown that EPEC proliferate in the upper small bowel. Substantial advances have recently been made in understanding the mechanisms of EPEC pathogenicity (see Chapter 14).

Enterotoxigenic Escherichia coli

Diarrhoea due to ETEC is watery and of small bowel origin. It is mainly associated with tropical and developing countries and affects susceptible travellers to these places. The significance of ETEC in travellers' diarrhoea began to be clarified with the report that a single serotype (O148:H28), later shown to be enterotoxigenic, was responsible in 54 per cent of diarrhoea in soldiers posted from the United Kingdom to Aden (Rowe *et al.*, 1970). Similar observations were made of United States Army troops from whom the same serotype was isolated in the Far East (Dupont *et al.*, 1971).

Enterotoxigenic *E. coli* have been shown to be responsible for a substantial proportion of diarrhoea in travellers to a number of developing countries (Shore *et al.*, 1974; Gorbach *et al.*, 1975; Merson *et al.*, 1976; Sack *et al.*, 1977a). They have also been isolated from diarrhoea outbreaks on cruise liners, where food was shown to be the source (e.g. Hobbs *et al.*, 1976), and from staff and visitors to a national park in the United States of America, where contaminated water was the source (Rosenberg *et al.*, 1977). Apart from common-source food or water outbreaks, ETEC are probably spread directly from person-to-person by contact. The subject has been reviewed by Nye (1979).

The prevalence of ETEC is particularly high in tropical and developing countries and their acquisition by susceptible travellers from developed countries accounts for the association between infection and travel. The high risk is due to the indigenous high prevalence of ETEC diarrhoea at all ages in these countries, but more particularly in infants and children (Guerrant *et al.*, 1975; Nalin *et al.*, 1975: Wadström *et al.*, 1976; Sack *et al.*, 1977b). Where standards of hygiene are high, ETEC infections are not important as a cause of diarrhoea.

Human volunteer oral challenge has shown that, to establish ETEC infection and diarrhoea, 10^8 to 10^{10} organisms are necessary. The incubation period and severity of the infection are, to some extent, dose dependent (Dupont *et al.*, 1971; Levine *et al.*, 1977). Though ETEC produce LT or ST (e.g. Gross *et al.*, 1976) or both (e.g. Rosenberg *et al.*, 1977), enterotoxin production alone is not sufficient to allow the ETEC to colonise the bowel and render it pathogenic. Thus, a fimbrial colonisation factor, CFA/I, was shown to be present on an ETEC strain of serotype O78:H11 (Evans *et al.*, 1975). Other ETEC colonisation factors have been identified, including CFA/II (Evans & Evans, 1978), CFA/III and PCF8775 (CFA/IV) and several others (Smyth *et al.*, 1994). These colonisation factors allow ETEC to adhere to the bowel mucosa, where the enterotoxins are then secreted in close proximity to their target enterocytes (see Chapter 7).

Vero-cytotoxin-producing Escherichia coli

A type of kidney failure associated with intravascular haemolysis, known as haemolytic-uraemic syndrome (HUS) was described by Gasser *et al.* (1955). It is predominantly but not exclusively a disease of children with a peak incidence in infancy, at which age it is the commonest cause of renal failure. Typically it follows an attack of gastro-enteritis with bloody stools but without fever and it commonly occurs in late summer or early autumn in small outbreaks but cases may be sporadic.

Haemorrhagic colitis was defined in the early 1970s and distinguished from the bloody diarrhoea due to *Shigella*, *Campylobacter* and *Clostridium difficile* (pseudomembranous colitis) by a progression from watery to bloody diarrhoea, the absence of fever and pus cells in the stool (Sack, 1987). An association between haemorrhagic colitis and the consumption of hamburgers was observed in the United States of America (Riley *et al.*, 1983). Two food-related outbreaks occurred in Oregon and Michigan in which patients had sudden severe abdominal colic and grossly bloody diarrhoea, and in both outbreaks *E. coli* O157:H7 was isolated from the stools of affected individuals. Since then most outbreaks have been associated with the consumption of ground beef but a wide variety of other foods, including cold sandwiches, raw milk, and even apple cider, have also been involved. Outbreaks have often been associated with restaurants and institutions, and person-to-person spread has been observed. In institutional outbreaks involving children, the elderly or compromised individuals mortality rates may reach ten per cent, though in one outbreak a much higher mortality was observed (Carter *et al.*, 1987). In view of the haemorrhagic nature of the stool the strains responsible were called enterohaemorrhagic *E. coli* (EHEC).

Strains of the *E. coli* O157:H7 responsible for haemorrhagic colitis were shown by O'Brien *et al.* (1983) to produce Vero cytotoxin (VT) and were termed Vero-cytotoxin-producing *E. coli* (VTEC). Some of these strains belong to serotypes other than O157:H7 and are known as non-O157 VTEC. The term EHEC has a narrower connotation than VTEC, which is now the preferred term. Karmali *et al.* (1983) reported that 73 per cent of sporadic cases of HUS in Canada were due to VTEC.

It is clear that VTEC are responsible for a spectrum of diseases, including simple diarrhoea, haemorrhagic colitis and HUS and, as a result, they are important pathogens that have become the cause of serious concern (see Chapter 15). The common association between VTEC infection and consumption of meat and meat products indicates that the source of these organisms is to be found in animals eaten for meat. VTEC are the cause of disease in animals but they can also be found in healthy animals. The significance of VTEC as a food-borne pathogen in the United Kingdom has recently been assessed in detail (Advisory Committee on the Microbiological Safety of Foods, 1995) and guidelines have been published for the prevention of human transmission of VTEC (Public Health Laboratory Service, 1995). Some unexpected vehicles of *E. coli* O157:H7 transmission, including acidic foods and water, and the emergence of variants that may interfere with laboratory diagnostic methods have been described (Feng, 1995).

Enteroinvasive Escherichia coli

The close relationship between the genera *Escherichia* and *Shigella* is particularly in evidence with EIEC. As *E. coli* they are atypical, but they are similar to *Shigella* in that they are usually non-motile, late or non-lactose fermenting and anaerogenic, though frequently not all these characteristics are present. In addition, certain EIEC O-serogroups are antigenically related to *Shigella* (Edwards & Ewing, 1972; Ørskov *et al.*, 1977). The syndrome they produce is clinically similar to or indistinguishable from *Shigella* infection, in that the site of infection is predominantly in the colon and the diarrhoea tends to contain mucus and blood.

The pathogenesis of EIEC-induced dysentery has been studied by oral challenge of guinea-pigs and in rabbit ileal loops, and epithelial cell invasion was shown to be an essential feature (Dupont *et al.*, 1971). After oral challenge human volunteers develop the characteristic features of mild dysentery; as for *Shigella* dysentery (Levine *et al.*, 1973), the challenge dose for human volunteers is very low (Hobbs *et al.*, 1949).

The enteroinvasive characteristics of EIEC are associated with the presence of a large plasmid (Sansonetti *et al.*, 1982; Silva *et al.*, 1982). Disease due to EIEC is uncommon but its prevalence may be underestimated because of its marked similarity to shigellosis (see Chapter 16). A large outbreak in the United States of America was traced to imported French cheese (Marier *et al.*, 1973; Tulloch *et al.*, 1973) and water-borne epidemics are well known. The mechanism and route of transmission of EIEC are almost certainly similar to those of *Shigella*.

Enteroaggregative Escherichia coli

In some developing countries EAggEC appear to be associated with persistent diarrhoea (Bhan *et al.*, 1989; Cravioto *et al.*, 1991) but this is not always the case (Baqui *et al.*, 1992). In the United Kingdom they have been isolated from sporadic cases of diarrhoea (Scotland *et al.*, 1993).

The typical pattern of aggregative adhesion occurs *in vitro* on cultured human colon (Knutton *et al.*, 1992). In experimental animals infection with EAggEC produces small intestinal villus oedema and necrosis with leucocyte infiltration (Tzipori *et al.*, 1992). In an *in vitro* rabbit intestinal model, EAggEC have been shown to produce a low-molecular-weight enterotoxin (enteroaggregative heat-stable enterotoxin, EAST1), which may have a mode of action similar to other ST enterotoxins. Experiments with volunteers suggest that, in terms of their virulence, EAggEC represent a heterogeneous group of enteropathogens (Nataro *et al.*, 1995).

Diffusely adherent Escherichia coli

The relative risk of childhood diarrhoea due to diffusely adherent *E. coli* (DAEC) appears to increase with age (Levine *et al.*, 1993). This may account for conflicting reports, in which some observers found an association between DAEC and diarrhoea (Baqui *et al.*, 1992), while others did not (Bhan *et al.*, 1989; Cravioto *et al.*, 1991).

An attempt to transmit DAEC diarrhoea to volunteers failed (Tacket *et al.*, 1990) but a fimbrial adhesin (Bilge *et al.*, 1989) and a non-fimbrial adhesin (Benz & Schmidt, 1993) have been identified. The significance of DAEC as enteropathogens remains to be determined.

Urinary tract infection

Urinary tract infections are common, ranking in prevalence with gastro-intestinal and respiratory infections. Apart from their clinical significance, they are also a fascinating paradigm of mucosal colonisation and infection. Their importance lies in the fact that the normal urinary tract is sterile and easily accessible for direct and indirect observation.

Urine flows from the kidneys into the bladder and is voided through the urethra. This flow helps to prevent entry of bacteria and is also a highly effective wash out mechanism (O'Grady *et al.*, 1968). Functional valves between the bladder and the ureters normally prevent the backflow of urine but, if the valves are incompetent, urine may, under the influence of the pressure set up in the bladder during micturition, return (reflux) into the kidney. The pressure may be sufficient for the reflux to extend into the collecting ducts of the kidney (intrarenal reflux) (Rolleston *et al.*, 1974). The female urethra is short, and turbulence during micturition may cause backward flow along the urethra. Nevertheless, the normal urinary tract is best seen as a 'closed' system protected against the entry of micro-organisms.

In the light of the mechanisms that tend to prevent colonisation of the urinary tract, it is surprising that urinary tract infections are so common. In the absence of anatomical abnormalities, which may, for hydro-dynamic reasons, encourage infection and its persistence, a range of specific bacterial virulence factors accounts for uropathogenicity.

Incidence and prevalence

The incidence of urinary tract infections increases with age in both sexes and they are most common in females at all ages. An account of clinical urinary tract infection is given by Sussman & Gower (1996).

Urinary tract infection is frequently unaccompanied by symptoms, a condition known as covert or asymptomatic bacteriuria. An important advance in the diagnosis and study of the colonisation of the urinary tract was made by Kass (1956), who defined the diagnostic criteria for covert urinary tract infection. He showed that more than 10^5 colony-forming units/ml in a carefully collected specimen of urine is evidence, with a probability of greater than 80 per cent, for the presence of infection in the bladder rather than contamination during voiding and three such counts in separate specimens bring the probability close to 100 per cent. Covert urinary tract infections are probably the silent phase of an infection punctuated by symptomatic episodes (Sussman *et al.*, 1969).

Acute symptomatic infection may be limited to the bladder (acute cystitis) with mainly local symptoms or it may affect the kidney with bacterial invasion (acute pyelonephritis) and with more or less severe constitutional symptoms. Infection of the urinary tract may lead to septicaemia, and most septicaemia can be traced to an origin in the urinary tract. Chronic pyelonephritis, in which scarring of the kidney occurs, is usually a late result of kidney infection very early in life, especially before the age of five years. Chronic pyelonephritis may in time destroy sufficient of the kidney substance to cause chronic renal failure.

Escherichia coli *and urinary tract infection*

The most common cause of all types of urinary tract infection is *E. coli* (Kunin *et al.*, 1964; Sussman *et al.*, 1969; McAllister *et al.*, 1971; Newcastle Asymptomatic Bacteriuria Research Group, 1975). The strains responsible belong to a restricted range of serogroups (Kunin, 1966; Gruneberg *et al.*, 1968; Table 1.2) and their prevalence is similar to that in the faeces of normal individuals (Turck *et al.*, 1962; Gruneberg *et al.*, 1968; Gruneberg & Bettelheim, 1969; Roberts *et al.*, 1975). These observations led to the *prevalence theory* of *E. coli* uropathogenicity, which postulated that the strains responsible are merely those present in the faeces. The implication was that specific pathogenicity factors were not involved.

There are, however, distinct differences not only between the strains in faeces and those responsible for urinary tract infection, but also between the strains responsible for different types of urinary tract infection. This has given rise to the *special pathogenicity theory*, which is now generally accepted and is supported by the recognition of a variety of specific virulence factors associated with uropathogenic *E. coli*. These are considered briefly below and are discussed in detail in Chapter 18.

Virulence factors in urinary tract infection

Capsular antigens (k-antigens) These are antiphagocytic acidic polysaccharides and may be of considerable significance in relation to tissue invasion. Supportive evidence comes from the observation that in experimental pyelonephritis anti-K antibodies are more protective than anti-O antibodies (Kaijser *et al.*, 1978).

Only a limited range of K-antigens is found with significant frequency in urinary tract infection (Mabeck *et al.*, 1971; Kaijser *et al.*, 1977). Though there appears to be no difference in the frequency with which K-antigens are found in cystitis and pyelonephritis, in a mouse model the presence of K-antigens favours kidney invasion (Kalmanson *et al.*, 1975). Similarly, strains that cause acute pyelonephritis appear to contain more K-antigen than those responsible for cystitis (Glynn *et al.*, 1971; Kaijser, 1973; McCabe *et al.*, 1975).

Somatic antigens (O-antigens) The usual concordance between the O-serogroup of the predominant faecal strain and that responsible for urinary tract infection may be absent in covert bacteriuria (Roberts *et al.*,

1975) and it was suggested that in long-standing covert bacteriuria the O-serogroup of the faecal strain may have changed. Similarly, Lindberg *et al.* (1975) found that the eight most common faecal O-serogroups were more prevalent in symptomatic infection than in covert bacteriuria. It may be, therefore, that symptomatic infection occurs when a 'new' strain of *E. coli* first colonises the urinary tract. Rough strains of E. *coli* are more common in covert bacteriuria, in which colonisation is prolonged, than in symptomatic infection (Hanson *et al.*, 1975). Such strains tend to be more serum sensitive, which suggests that during prolonged colonisation strains with altered cell envelopes are selected. These strains are also less immunogenic than those from patients with acute urinary tract infection (Sohl-Akerlund *et al.*, 1977). This suggests that intact O-antigens are virulence factors of *E. coli* in urinary tract infection, and this is supported by evidence that when covert bacteriuria has been eliminated by antimicrobial therapy, reinfection with a strain of different O-serotype frequently gives rise to acute symptoms (Asscher *et al.*, 1969).

Haemolysin production Haemolytic *E. coli* were first observed in normal faeces, urinary tract infection and extra-intestinal infections (Dudgeon *et al.*, 1921, 1923). Such strains are more common in urinary tract infection and other extra-intestinal infections than in normal faeces (Cooke & Ewins, 1975; Minshew *et al.*, 1978a,b). Half of the strains isolated from urinary tract infection produce α- and β-haemolysins but they are uncommon in normal faeces (Cooke & Ewins, 1975). The main significance of haemolysin production for virulence is in relation to tissue, including kidney, invasion (O'Hanley *et al.*, 1991).

Adherence The capacity of *E. coli* to adhere to uroepithelial cells correlates with the severity of urinary tract infection from which they are isolated (Svanborg Eden *et al.*, 1976; Svanborg Eden, 1978). The properties of the various adhesion and colonisation factors of *E. coli* involved in urinary tract infections are considered elsewhere (see Chapters 6, 8 and 18) and this account will deal only briefly with the part they play in the pathogenesis of urinary tract infection and its consequences.

Some 70 per cent of *E. coli* isolated from patients with acute pyelonephritis adhere to uroepithelial cells but only a small proportion of faecal strains do so (Svanborg Eden *et al.*, 1978). The predominant faecal strain of patients with urinary tract infection has adherence properties similar to those of the urinary strain isolated early in the infection (Svanborg Eden *et al.*, 1979b), but strains that colonise the distal urethra and introitus of normal women are often non-adhesive (Sussman *et al.*, 1982a). Moreover, *E. coli* adheres preferentially to periurethral and vaginal cells from women and girls who are prone to urinary tract infection (Fowler & Stamey, 1977; Kallenius & Winberg, 1978). This is highly significant because colonisation of the periurethral area and introitus is seen as a prelude to urinary tract infection.

The adhesive properties of *E. coli* are accounted for by the presence of fimbriae, and haemagglutination is a valuable model for the analytical study of fimbrial adhesins. In this and other ways several types of fimbrial adhesin have been recognised. These are the mannose-sensitive haemagglutinins, which agglutinate guinea-pig erythrocytes and are inhibited by D-mannose, and the mannose-resistant haemagglutinins that agglutinate human erythrocytes but are not inhibited by D-mannose. Mannose-sensitive and mannose-resistant fimbriae adhere to uroepithelial cells (Parry *et al.*, 1982) but mannose-resistant fimbriae are particularly associated with strains from patients with urinary tract infection (Sussman *et al.*, 1982a; Parry *et al.*, 1983). Mannose-sensitive fimbriae attach to mannose groups and to uromucoid (Tamm–Horsfall glycoprotein), which contains mannose (Ørskov *et al.*, 1980; Parry *et al.*, 1982).

Whether adhesins are produced in the urinary tract is of importance in formulating convincing models for the function of virulence factors in the pathogenesis of urinary tract infection. Direct examination of *E. coli* in urine without subculture suggests that mannose-specific adhesins are not produced *in vivo*, while mannose-resistant adhesins are produced (Sharon *et al.*, 1981). Production of P-fimbriae *in vivo* has been confirmed (Kiselius *et al.*, 1989). The report by Harber *et al.* (1982) that demonstrated the absence of adherence to uroepithelial cells by freshly isolated urinary *E. coli* is, therefore, problematic and the methods used have been the subject of criticism (Sussman *et al.*, 1982b; Parry & Rooke, 1985). Nevertheless, the production of type-1 fimbriae is so common that their possible function in urinary tract infection cannot easily be excluded. If they have such a function, the differential attachment of type-1 fimbriae and P-fimbriae to young and mature cells of human ureter (Fujita *et al.*, 1991) may be of significance in the evolution of upper urinary tract infection.

A two-phase hypothetical model for colonisation of the urinary tract has been formulated by Ørskov *et al.* (1980), who proposed that type-1 fimbriae act as colonisation factors in the colon, where large amounts of mucus are produced. At other sites where mucus is produced and where there is a tendency to wash out, as in the urinary tract, mucus may have a dual role. Organisms are captured by free mucus and are removed during micturition or, if additional adhesins such as mannose-resistant fimbriae are produced, their expression, presumably after a phase switch (Eisenstein, 1981), may determine colonisation of the urinary tract. At least some adhesins of significance in urinary tract infection are co-regulated, so that the pathogen may be able to adjust their expression to best advantage (Morschhäuser et al., 1994; Ritter et al., 1995).

Indirect consequences of urinary tract infection

Several still obscure and indirect results of urinary tract infection have been described. Their effects may be far-reaching and they deserve careful attention.

In several surveys a relationship has been observed between covert bacteriuria and raised blood pressure (Kass et al., 1965, 1978; Freedman et al., 1965; Sussman et al., 1969) but the significance of the small increase has not been established (Kunin, 1979; Stamey, 1980). In pregnancy, covert bacteriuria is associated with a significant risk of acute pyelonephritis (Kass, 1960), some of which may be related to changes in the urinary tract associated with pregnancy (Williams et al., 1968; Gruneberg et al., 1969). The properties of urine in pregnancy that enhance its qualities as a bacterial growth medium may also play a marginal role in these phenomena (Asscher et al., 1966). Covert bacteriuria in pregnancy is associated with an excess risk of toxaemia of pregnancy, prematurity, low birth weight and stillbirth (Beard & Roberts, 1968; Norden & Kass, 1968; Kass, 1960) but it seems unlikely that covert bacteriuria alone is responsible (Asscher, 1980). However, in an experimental model, E. coli has a profound effect on fetal development in mice (Coid et al., 1978).

The suggestion that covert bacteriuria reduces life expectancy in old age (Dontas et al., 1981; Dontas, 1983) and at other ages (Evans et al., 1982) seems not to have been confirmed.

Wound infection

Surgical wound infections due to E. coli have long been recognised to follow operations in which the bowel has been opened (Keighley & Burdon, 1979). Such infections are usually prevented with antimicrobial prophylaxis.

Experimental wound infection with E. coli is difficult to establish (Quick & Brogan, 1968), because in clinical practice such infections are due to synergy between E. coli and non-sporing anaerobes, particularly

Bacteroides fragilis, both of which are present in the faeces (Onderdonk *et al.*, 1976). In a rat fibrin clot model inoculated with these organisms, *B. fragilis* first decline in numbers and then increase, while *E. coli* increase rapidly and only mixed infections result in abscesses (Verweij *et al.*, 1991). In guinea-pigs, sub-infective doses of *E. coli* and *B. fragilis*, inoculated together into surgical incisions, lead to infection with pus formation (Kelly, 1978). The amounts and ratios of inoculum are critical, and interference with neutrophil phagocytosis by the anaerobe is a possible mechanism by which *E. coli* infection becomes established (Ingham *et al.*, 1977). This mechanism is supported by the observation that metronidazole, which is active against anaerobes, prevents experimental *E. coli* sepsis (Onderdonk *et al.*, 1979). There is also evidence that the synergy is due to the use by *B. fragilis* of haem- or iron-binding proteins produced by *E. coli* (Verweij, 1993).

Little is known directly of the *E. coli* virulence factors operative in wound infection but antiphagocytic K-antigens and iron-uptake mechanisms play a significant role in its maintenance.

Septicaemia

For septicaemia to result, organisms must enter the circulation in large numbers. The source may be a discrete lesion, such as a collection of pus, or a more diffuse infected tissue lesion or, most commonly, a urinary tract infection. The organisms that enter the circulation in septicaemia are more or less rapidly removed, but endotoxin released by dying bacteria leads to the release of tumour necrosis factor (TNF-α) and interleukin 1 (IL-1). These bring about the severe physiological symptoms of septicaemia (see Chapter 5). Except when the function of the phagocytes is depressed or their circulating number is greatly reduced or in the agonal state, bacteria do not remain long enough in the bloodstream to multiply there. There is, however, a continuum between bacteraemia and septicaemia and it is the symptoms that are the hallmark of the latter.

Little is known of the virulence factors, other than endotoxin, associated with the capacity of *E. coli* to cause septicaemia in humans. However, iron-uptake mechanisms play a significant role in allowing organisms to survive in tissues, from which they enter the circulation. In neonates capsular antigen K1 is thought to be important in producing invasion and meningitis. In the light of the circumstances in which septicaemia occurs in patients, namely as a complication of common infections, and then usually in compromised individuals, host factors as well as microbial virulence factors are the determining features. *Escherichia coli* is the most frequent Gram-negative organism to cause septicaemia, probably because infections due to it are so common (McCabe, 1981).

Endocarditis

A wide range of micro-organisms, but only rarely *E. coli*, may colonise the internal lining of the heart (endocardium), if they enter the circulation. This is most common when the endocardium is already damaged. Part of the explanation for the rarity of *E. coli* endocarditis appears to be that it adheres to endocardium far less efficiently than many other organisms (Gould *et al.*, 1975). Thus, though *E. coli* septicaemia is common, it rarely causes endocarditis (Gransden *et al.*, 1990). Occasionally, however, such cases have been reported, and the strains responsible are serum resistant (Raymond *et al.*, 1992; Watanakunakorn & Kim, 1992).

Serum-resistant *E. coli* regularly cause endocarditis in rabbit experimental models, while serum-sensitive strains lodge on the endocardium and survive for only a short time, except in the presence of a deficiency of complement component C6, when endocarditis results. Capsular bacterial antigens appear not to be involved. These observations may explain the rarity of *E. coli* endocarditis (Durack & Beeson, 1977).

Meningitis

Meningitis due to *E. coli* is common in the newborn (McCracken, 1984) but it is not unimportant in adults.

About 80 per cent of the strains responsible for neonatal meningitis carry the K1 antigen (McCracken *et al.*, 1974) and they may be responsible for epidemic outbreaks of meningitis in hospitals (Headings & Overall, 1977). Such strains are carried in the faeces by up to 35 per cent of normal adults, who may yield an almost pure culture of K1-bearing *E. coli* and frequently they represent the majority of the strains isolated (Sarff *et al.*, 1975; Schiffer *et al.*, 1976). Up to 38 per cent of the newborn may carry these organisms in their stool (Schiffer *et al.*, 1976) and in the majority their origin is to be found in the stool of the mother (Sarff *et al.*, 1975). Some two-thirds of the strains responsible for meningitis belong to serogroups O1, O7, O16 and O18ac (Schiffer *et al.*, 1976). Grados & Ewing (1970) found that the *E. coli* isolated from the cerebrospinal fluid of a newborn infant with meningitis was agglutinated by antiserum specific for *Neisseria meningitidis* group B and Kasper *et al.* (1973) showed that the capsules of the two organisms shared antigenic specificity. The acidic K1 polysaccharide is a polymer of *N*-acetylneuraminic acid (Barry & Goebel, 1957; Barry, 1958) and is probably structurally identical with the meningococcal group B polysaccharide (Liu *et al.*, 1971).

A high proportion of *E. coli* isolated from neonatal sepsis and meningitis carry S-fimbriae and belong to a restricted range of serotypes (Korhonen *et al.*, 1985). Organisms that carry these fimbriae and the purified fimbriae attach to epithelium that lines the choroid plexus, cerebral ventricles and vascular endothelium of rats (Parkinnen *et al.*, 1988).

Serum antibody protects against blood-borne organisms that cause meningitis, but K1 antibodies are infrequently found in normal adults (Schiffer *et al.*, 1976). Even adult patients recovering from infections with group B meningococci may have only low levels of antibody (Brandt *et al.*, 1972) and children after recovery from urinary tract infection with *E. coli* K1 do not produce serum antibody against this antigen (Kaijser *et al.*, 1973). The poor immunogenicity of K1 antigen is probably due to similar host antigens (antigenic mimicry). Antibody produced in animals by injection of whole organisms is, however, protective (Wolberg & DeWitt, 1969). Human colostrum contains anti-K1 secretory immunoglobulin A (sIgA) (Schiffer *et al.*, 1976), which may be the usual protection for the newborn infant.

Only some 40 per cent of infants with *E. coli* septicaemia in the absence of meningitis are infected with K1-positive organisms (Schiffer *et al.*, 1976), that is about half their prevalence in meningitis. It is, therefore, possible that K1-positive organisms are particularly invasive and that they have the potential to give rise to septicaemia. The nature of the special tendency to attack the meninges is unknown but it may be that *E. coli* K1 in the bloodstream has an organotropism for the meninges similar to that described by Buddingh & Polk (1939). The first lines of defence against invasion are probably colostral and milk sIgA, but once invasion has taken place infants are unprotected in the absence of maternal circulating anti-K1 IgG (Wilfert, 1978).

Escherichia coli is also a common cause of spontaneous meningitis in adults (Cherubin *et al.*, 1981). Sequels to meningitis in infants and adults include infective complications, cranial and spinal subdural empyema and thrombosis of the cranial venous sinuses.

Clonality

The demonstration that *E. coli* is a specific pathogen was difficult before the introduction of serology. After its introduction an almost unmanageable range of serotypes appeared to be responsible for various types of infection. Attempts to establish correlations between serology and type of disease led to a better knowledge of the epidemiology of *E. coli* diseases and it became clear that only a limited number of O:H-serotypes within an O-serogroup were associated with outbreaks of diarrhoea but such findings were of limited value in understanding the pathogenesis of these diseases. The beginnings of a solution came into sight with the recognition of the important part that colonisation factors play in endowing strains with virulence but this did little to explain the apparent antigenic diversity of pathogenic *E. coli*. Approaches to this problem based on taxonomic principles are now pointing to some answers.

The first suggestion that particular clones of *E. coli* might be responsible for disease came from the recognition that ETEC isolated worldwide have specific combinations of serotype and biotype (Ørskov *et al.*, 1976). Examination of *E. coli* strains by starch gel electrophoresis of their cytoplasmic isoenzymes also suggested that the populations may consist of a number of clones (Ochman *et al.*, 1983). Achtman *et al.* (1983) selected a group of strains of *E. coli* isolated from extra-intestinal infections that had the K1 antigen in common but were otherwise serologically diverse and examined their outer-membrane proteins by sodium dodecyl sulphate (SDS) polyacrylamide gel electrophoresis. They were able to assign the strains to a series of stable clones that were geographically widespread, and no clonal difference was found between strains isolated from healthy individuals and those isolated from those with disease. Since it was likely that virulence is as stable a clonal property as other characteristics, it was suggested that recognition of clones might simplify the search for virulence determinants.

A detailed clonal analysis of *E. coli* O2:K1 isolates from human chicken and bovine infections showed that the human strains could be assigned to two clones, which respectively corresponded to the poultry and the bovine isolates. The best clonal distinguishing features were outer-membrane protein and electrophoretic enzyme patterns, and individual O:K-serotypes may contain different clonal groups with little genetic relatedness (Achtman *et al.*, 1986). In a similar study of EPEC belonging to different serogroups, two genetically closely related clusters were identified (Ørskov *et al.*, 1990), which differed only in their

O-antigen. This might be accounted for by horizontal transfer of the genetic background for the biosynthesis of the lipopolysaccharide side chains.

Unfortunately, virulence properties may not be uniform within a given clonal group (Achtman *et al.*, 1986), and this has reduced earlier hopes that the identification of clones might lead to the discovery of new virulence determinants (Achtman & Pluschke, 1986).

Immunity to *Escherichia coli*

Natural, non-specific immunity

In the absence of antibodies and complement, the result of the encounter between *E. coli* and phagocytes depends on the composition of the bacterial cell surface; phagocytosis under these conditions is described as non-opsonic.

Type-1-fimbriate *E. coli* bind to the surface of phagocytic cells through mannose-containing receptors, phagocytosis and killing then follow (Ofek & Doyle, 1994). This type of non-opsonic phagocytosis is less efficient than antibody-mediated opsonic phagocytosis and depends on the structure of the exposed bacterial surface. Thus, while rough lipopolysaccharide is hydrophobic and facilitates phagocytosis, smooth lipopolysaccharide is hydrophilic and anti phagocytic (Lock *et al.*, 1990). In comparison with type-1 fimbriae, P-fimbriae tend to bind poorly to human polymorph granulocytes (Blumenstock & Jann, 1982; Sussman *et al.*, 1982a; Svanborg-Eden *et al.*, 1984) but once binding has occurred, phagocytosis and killing take place. However, Prs-fimbriate *E. coli* associated with porcine septicaemia bind normally to phagocytes, but the fimbriae inhibit intracellular killing (Negeleka *et al.*, 1994). The non-fimbrial adhesins of *E. coli*, which appear to be represented on the bacterial surface as a 'capsule-like' layer, also mediate binding to phago-cytic cells (Grunberg *et al.*, 1994). Non-opsonic phagocytosis has been reviewed by Ofek *et al.* (1995). It seems clear that phagocytosis and intracellular killing of *E. coli* are crucially determined by the surface of the bacterial cell.

Natural antibodies

Antibodies unrelated to previous exposure to antigen have long been recognised (Boyden, 1965). Views have differed as to whether they are truly 'pre-formed' and unrelated to previous exposure to antigenic stimulation, or are produced in response to cross-reacting antigens (see Chapter 20). It has been suggested, for example, that anti-A and anti-B blood group isoantibodies are due to immunisation with bacteria including *E. coli* (Springer, 1970). However, serum antibodies against *E. coli* are present in germ-free animals (Ikari, 1964).

Most natural, or normal, antibodies are non-specific (polyreactive) IgM, though some may be IgG or IgA. Most of these natural antibodies are produced by lymphocytes that are common in the neonate (CD5+ B-cells) (Casali & Schettino, 1996). On account of their broad reactivity, these antibodies may be an early defence against infections.

Immune responses to Escherichia coli

Immunogenic components of Escherichia coli

Infection with *E. coli* gives rise to immune responses against the individual antigenic structural components exposed on the bacterial surface and depends on their immunogenicity.

Flagellins, the subunit constituents of flagella, are markedly immunogenic proteins that give rise to IgG antibody responses generally characteristic of protein immunogens. Fimbriae, too, consist of protein subunits (pilins) and can be expected to be strong immunogens, but little is known about fimbrial synthesis during the course of tissue infection and immune responses under these conditions have been little studied.

The immunogenicity of K-antigens depends on their chemical structure. While some K-antigens give rise to good immune responses, others like K1 and K5 are poorly immunogenic (see Chapter 4).

O-antigens are poorly immunogenic. The IgM antibodies directed against their exposed polysaccharide side chains are produced by a macrophage- and T-cell-independent mechanism in which B-cells are stimulated directly. At low concentrations B lymphocyte activation appears to be specific, while at higher concentrations polyclonal activation takes place. The thymus-independent immunogenicity of O-antigens is due to their repeating epitopic oligosaccharide groups. Though the antibody response is generally limited to IgM production, long-term or chronic stimulation leads to IgG production.

Response to mucosal colonisation

Passively acquired maternal serum IgG antibody to *E. coli* is present in the infant circulation at birth, but mucosal surfaces are unprotected. This depends on passive protection by maternal colostrum and milk-derived secretory IgA; sIgA formation is the latest of the specific immunity mechanisms to develop (Burgio *et al.*, 1980; Hanson *et al.*, 1983). The sIgA produced by infants and children appears only rarely to include anti-fimbrial antibody (Hanson *et al.*, 1983) but such antibodies are present in breast milk (Svanborg Eden *et al.*, 1979a) as are anti-K1 antibody (Carlsson *et al.*, 1982) and anti-O antibodies (Gindrat *et al.*, 1972). Milk anti-fimbrial antibody is probably responsible for preventing neonatal colonisation with *E. coli*, since neither anti-O antibody (Carlsson *et al.*, 1976) nor anti-K antibody (Carlsson *et al.*, 1982) are able to do so. In infants intestinal colonisation induces production of serum antibodies (Lodinova *et al.*, 1973).

Normal urine contains IgG and IgA, both of which appear to originate from the glomerular filtrate and from tissue fluid (Burdon, 1973b), and their concentration increases in urinary tract infection (Burdon, 1970). Some of these antibodies are specific for *E. coli* (Tourville *et al.*, 1968) but probably play little, if any, part in local antibacterial defence in the urinary tract. Such a role is reserved for sIgA (Burdon, 1973b, 1976). The local immune response in the urinary tract has been reviewed by Holmgren and Smith (1975).

The response to tissue infection

Systemic infections can be separated into those in which infection is limited to the tissues and those in which organisms enter the bloodstream. In either case serum IgM and IgG are sequentially produced. In terms of its immune response, kidney-invasive urinary tract infection may be regarded as typical of tissue-invasive *E. coli* infections in general. Thus, in lower urinary tract infection, which is usually superficial, sIgA is produced locally in the bladder and can be found in the urine. In acute pyelonephritis the kidney parenchyma is invaded and this is at first accompanied by the appearance of IgM in the circulation (Needell *et al.*, 1955; Percival *et al.*, 1964), while in recurrent or chronic infection IgG appears (Hanson & Winberg, 1966; Hanson *et al.*, 1969). Other aspects of the immune response to urinary tract infection have been reviewed by Holmgren & Smith (1975).

The immune response to *E. coli* in septicaemia is similar to that of tissue invasion, since the latter almost always follows the former. The nature of the response to septicaemia without previous tissue invasion, as may follow instrumentation of the infected urinary tract, has not been recorded but can be expected to be similar. An analogous situation may be the chronic leakage of bacterial antigens into the circulation in cirrhosis of the liver, in which the detoxication functions of the liver are depressed and there is a marked increase in anti-*E. coli* antibodies (Wright, 1982).

Protective mechanisms

Secretory IgA acts at mucosal surfaces by inhibiting adhesion of the infecting organism (Svanborg Eden *et al.*, 1976) and by neutralising toxins (Rowley, 1983); it may also be bactericidal (Burdon, 1973a).

It is difficult, because of their inaccessibility, to analyse the sequence of events during tissue infections. The peritoneum is more easily accessible and provides a useful model that may have more general relevance. The first event in experimental intraperitoneal *E. coli* infection is immigration of phagocytic cells. Under these conditions both anti-O and anti-K antibodies are protective but the effect of the latter is greater (Ahlstedt, 1983). The same seems to apply in experimental model pyelonephritis in the rabbit (Kaijser *et al.*, 1983) and the mouse (Kaijser & Ahlstedt, 1977). Anti-O antibodies are bactericidal but the greater effectiveness of anti-K antibodies is probably related to their opsonic effect (Van Dijk *et al.*, 1977); polyclonal IgM is not protective, probably because of its low specificity. Another mechanism in immunity against *E. coli* is antibody-dependent cell-mediated cytotoxicity, which also has the potential to cause tissue damage (Hagberg *et al.*, 1982).

Autoimmunity

Primary biliary cirrhosis

Primary biliary cirrhosis is a chronic autoimmune liver disease in which the intra-hepatic bile ducts are progressively destroyed by an inflammatory process that ends in cirrhosis and liver failure. The serum of patients with this condition contains antibodies against certain mitochondrial enzymes, some of which are antigenically cross-reactive with components of *E. coli* (Stemerowicz *et al.*, 1988; Burroughs *et al.*, 1992).

A unique association has been proposed between *E. coli* urinary tract infection and primary biliary cirrhosis. Burroughs *et al.* (1984) observed a

19 per cent prevalence and a 35 per cent incidence of urinary infection in patients with primary biliary cirrhosis, as compared with a far lower incidence in controls with other liver diseases or rheumatoid arthritis. This association did not, however, correlate with the adhesive properties of the *E. coli* strains isolated or the blood group of the patients (Rosenstein *et al.*, 1984) as might have been expected in ordinary urinary tract infection. Others have been unable to confirm this association between primary biliary cirrhosis and urinary tract infection (Floreani *et al.*, 1989).

Rough strains of *Salmonella minnesota*, injected into rabbits, induce antibodies that cross-react with mitochondria (Stemerowicz *et al.*, 1988) and rough strains of *E. coli* are common in the faeces of patients with primary biliary cirrhosis (Hopf *et al.*, 1989). Similarly, rough strains of *E. coli* appear to be common in the urine of such patients (Butler *et al.*, 1993).

It may be that, in response to an *E. coli* infection, T-cells recognise certain bacterial antigens and because of molecular mimicry they then also recognise a cross-reacting peptide on biliary epithelial cells, with a resulting autoimmune reaction (Burroughs *et al.*, 1992). The structure of the similar biliary and bacterial enzymes is, however, strikingly homologous and it is equally possible that primary biliary cirrhosis is an autoimmune disease, unrelated to an infection, in which the antibodies fortuitously cross-react with *E. coli*; the matter remains to be resolved.

Protective immunisation

The mechanisms of immunity against *E. coli* infections immediately suggest a number of ways in which immunisation against them may be achieved, depending on their pathogenesis. In surface infections specific local sIgA production would be protective but means for achieving this are only now being defined. The use of purified fimbrial vaccines for this purpose was reviewed by Korhonen & Rhen (1982) and the use of a variety of oral toxoid and toxin subunit vaccines for the prophylaxis of diseases due to toxin-dependent pathogenicity mechanisms is discussed in Chapter 21.

A human monoclonal IgM antibody (HA-1A) that binds to the lipid A region of lipopolysaccharide has been described (Teng *et al.*, 1985), and it has been suggested that it is safe and effective in the treatment of patients with Gram-negative septicaemia (Ziegler *et al.*, 1991). Nevertheless, animal experiments indicate that HA-1A does not inhibit the interaction between lipopolysaccharide and its target cells (Baumgartner *et al.*,

1990). Since it is necessary to treat patients early, the antibody would in practice also sometimes be given to patients in whom the diagnosis of septicaemia is in doubt and not ultimately confirmed. Unfortunately, the HA-1A monoclonal antibody appears to increase mortality when given to patients who do not have Gram-negative septicaemia and this has led to its withdrawal from clinical use (Horton, 1993). Much effort continues to be applied to the search for new approaches to the treatment of Gram-negative septicaemia (Morrison & Ryan, 1996).

References

Achtman, M., Heuzenroeder, M., Kusecek, B., Ochman, H., Caugant, D., Selander, R. K., Väisanen-Rhen, V., Korhonen, T. K., Stuart, S., Ørskov, F. & Ørskov, I. (1986). Clonal analysis of *Escherichia coli* O2:K1 isolated from diseased humans and animals. *Infection and Immunity*, **51**, 268–76.

Achtman, M., Kusecek, B., Heuzenroeder, M., Aaronson, W., Sutton, A. & Silver, R. P. (1983). Six widespread bacterial clones among *Escherichia coli* K1 isolates. *Infection and Immunity*, **39**, 315–35.

Achtman, M. & Pluschke, G. (1986). Clonal analysis of descent and virulence among selected *Escherichia coli*. *Annual Review of Microbiology*, **40**, 185–210.

Advisory Committee on the Microbiological Safety of Food (1995). *Report on Verocytotoxin-Producing Escherichia coli*. ISBN 0–11-321909–1. London: HMSO.

Ahlstedt, S. (1983). Host defence against intraperitoneal *Escherichia coli* infection in mice. *Progress in Allergy*, **33**, 236–46.

Asscher, A. W. (1980). *The Challenge of Urinary Tract Infection*. London: Academic Press.

Asscher, A. W., Sussman, M., Waters, W. E., Davis, R. H. & Chick, S. (1966). Urine as a medium for bacterial growth. *Lancet*, **2**, 1037–41.

Asscher, A. W., Sussman, M., Waters, W. E., Evans, J. A. S., Campbell, H., Evans, K. T. & Williams, J. E. (1969). Asymptomatic significant bacteriuria in the non-pregnant woman. II. Response to treatment and follow-up. *British Medical Journal*, **1**, 804–6.

Baqui, A. H., Sack, R. B., Black, R. E., Heider, K., Houssain, A., Abdul Alim, A. R. M., Yunus, M., Chowdhury, H. R. & Siddique, A. K. (1992). Enteropathogens associated with acute and persistent diarrhea in Bangladeshi children <5 years of age. *Journal of Infectious Diseases*, **166**, 792–6.

Barry, G. T. (1958). Coliminic acid, a polymer of N-acetylneuraminic acid. *Journal of Experimental Medicine*, **107**, 507–21.

Barry, G. T. & Goebel, W. F. (1957). Coliminic acid, a substance of bacterial origin related to sialic acid. *Nature*, **179**, 206–8.

Baumgartner, J. D., Heumann, D., Gerain, J., Weinbreck, P., Grau, G. E. & Glauser, M. P. (1990). Association between protective efficacy of anti-lipopolysaccharide (LPS) antibodies and suppression of LPS-induced tumor necrosis factor α and interleukin 6: comparison of O-side chain specific antibodies with core LPS antibodies. *Journal of Experimental Medicine*, **171**, 889–96.

Beard, R. W. & Roberts, A. P. (1968). Asymptomatic bacteriuria during pregnancy. *British Medical Bulletin*, **24**, 44–9.

Benz, I. & Schmidt, M. A. (1993). Diffuse adherence of enteropathogenic *Escherichia coli* strains–processing of AIDA-I. *International Journal of Medical Microbiology, Virology, Parasitology and Infectious Diseases*, **278**, 197–208.

Bettelheim, K. A., Breadon, A., Faiers, M. C., O'Farrell, S. M. & Shooter, R. A. (1974). The origin of O-serotypes of *Escherichia coli* in babies after normal delivery. *Journal of Hygiene*, **72**, 67–78.

Bhan, M. K., Raj, P., Levine, M. M., Kaper, J. B., Bhandari, N., Srivastava, R., Kumar, R. & Sazawal, S. (1989). Enteroaggregative *Escherichia coli* associated with persistent diarrhea in a cohort of rural children in India. *Journal of Infectious Diseases*, **159**, 1061–4.

Bilge, S. S., Clausen, C. R., Lau, W. & Moseley, S. L. (1989). Molecular characteristics of a fimbrial adhesin F1845, mediating diffuse adherence of diarrhea-associated *Escherichia coli* to HEp-2 cells. *Journal of Bacteriology*, **171**, 4281–9.

Blanco, J., Alonso, M. P., Gonzalez, E. A., Blanco, M. & Garabal, J. I. (1990). Virulence factors of bacteraemic *Escherichia coli* with particlar reference to production of cytotoxic necrotising factor (CNF) by P-fimbriate strains. *Journal of Medical Microbiology*, **31**, 175–83.

Blumenstock, E. & Jann, K. (1982). Adhesion of piliated *Escherichia coli* strains to phagocytes: differences between bacteria with mannose-sensitive pili and those with mannose-resistant pili. *Infection and Immunity*, **35**, 264–9.

Boyden, S. (1965). Natural antibodies and the immune response. *Advances in Immunology*, **5**, 1–28.

Brandt, B. L., Wyle, F. A. & Artenstein, M. S. (1972). Radioactive antigen-binding assay for *Neisseria meningitidis* polysaccharide antibody. *Journal of Immunology*, **108**, 913–20.

Bray, J. (1945). Isolation of antigenically homogeneous strain of *Bact. coli* Neapolitanum from summer diarrhoea of infants. *Journal of Pathology and Bacteriology*, **57**, 239–47.

Brenner, D. J. (1984). Family I. Enterobacteriaceae. In *Bergey's Manual of Systematic Bacteriology*, vol. 1, eds. N. R. Krieg & J. G. Holt, pp. 408–20. Baltimore: Williams & Wilkins.

Brenner, D. J., Davis, B. R., Steigerwalt, A. G., Riddle, C., McWorter, A., Allen, S. D., Farmer, J. J., III, Saito, Y. & Fanning, G. R. (1982a). Atypical biogroups of *Escherichia coli* found in clinical specimens and description of *Escherichia hermanii* sp. nov. *Journal of Clinical Microbiology*, **15**, 703–13.

Brenner, D. J., McWorter, A., Leete Knutson, J. K. & Steigerwalt, A. G. (1982b). *Escherichia vulneris*: a new species of Enterobacteriaceae associated with human wounds. *Journal of Clinical Microbiology*, **15**, 1133–40.

Buddingh, G. J. & Polk, A. D. (1939). Experimental meningococcus infection of the chick embryo. *Journal of Experimental Medicine*, 70, 485–97.

Burdon, D. W. (1970). Quantitative studies of urinary immunoglobulins in hospital patients, including patients with urinary tract infection. *Clinical and Experimental Immunology*, **6**, 189–96.

Burdon, D. W. (1973a). The bactericidal action of immunoglobulin A. *Journal of Medical Microbiology*, **6**, 131–19.

Burdon, D. W. (1973b). Immunoglobulins in the urinary tract. Discussion on a possible role in urinary tract infection. In *Urinary Tract Infection*, eds. W. Brumfitt & A. W. Asscher, pp. 148–58. London: Oxford University Press.

Burdon, D. W. (1976). Immunological reactions to urinary infection: the nature and function of secretory immunoglobulins. In *The Scientific Foundations of Urology*, eds. D. L. Williams & G. D. Chisolm, pp. 192–6. London: Heinemann.

Burgess, M. N., Bywater, R. J., Cowley, C. M., Mullan, N. A. & Newsome, P. M. (1978). Biological evaluation of a methanol-soluble, heat-stable *Escherichia coli* enterotoxin in infant mice, pigs, rabbits and calves. *Infection and Immunity*, **21**, 526–31.

Burgess, N. R. H., McDermott, S. N. & Whiting, J. (1973). Aerobic bacteria occurring in the hind-gut of the cockroach, *Blatta orientalis*. *Journal of Hygiene, Cambridge*, **71**, 1–7.

Burgio, G. R., Lanzavecchia, A., Plebani. A., Jayakar, S. & Ugazio, A. G. (1980). Ontogeny of secretory immunity: levels of secretory IgA and natural antibodies in saliva. *Pediatric Research*, **14**, 1111–14.

Burroughs, A. K., Butler, P., Sternberg, M. J. E. & Baum, H. (1992). Molecular mimicry in liver disease. *Nature*, **358**, 377–8.

Burroughs, A. K., Rosenstein, I. J., Epstein, O., Hamilton-Miller, J. M., Brumfitt, W. & Sherlock, S. (1984). Bacteriuria and primary biliary cirrhosis. *Gut*, **25**, 133–7.

Butler, P., Valle, F., Hamilton-Miller, J. M. T., Brumfitt, W., Baum, H. & Burroughs, A. K. (1993). M2 mitochondrial antibodies and urinary rough mutant bacteria in patients with primary biliary cirrhosis and in patients with recurrent bacteriuria. *Journal of Hepatology*, **17**, 408–14.

Caprioli, A., Falbo, V. & Ruggeri, F. M. (1987). Cytotoxic necrotising factor production by hemolytic strains of *Escherichia coli* causing extra-intestinal infections. *Journal of Clinical Microbiology*, **25**, 146–9.

Carlsson, B., Gothefors, L., Ahlstedt, S., Hanson. L. Å. & Winberg, J. (1976). Studies of *Escherichia coli* O antigen. Specific antibodies in human milk, maternal serum and cord blood. *Acta Paediatrica Scandinavica*, **65**, 216–24.

Carlsson, B., Kaijser, B., Ahlstedt, S., Gothefors, L. & Hanson, L. Å. (1982). Antibodies against *Escherichia coli* capsular (K) antigens in human milk and serum–their relation to the *E. coli* gut flora of the mother and neonate. *Acta Paediatrica Scandinavica*, **71**, 313–18.

Carter, A. O., Borczyk, A. A., Carlson, J. A. K., Harvey, B., Hockin, J. C., Karmali, M. A., Krishnan, C., Korn, D. A. & Lior, H. (1987). An outbreak of *Escherichia coli* O157:H7-associated haemorrhagic colitis in a nursing home. *New England Journal of Medicine*, **317**, 1496–500.

Casali, P. & Schettino, E. W. (1996). Structure and function of natural antibodies. In *Immunology of Silicones*, eds. M. Potter & N. R. Rose, pp. 167–79. Berlin: Springer.

Cherubin, C. E., Marr, J. S., Sierra, M. F. & Becker, S. (1981). *Listeria* and gram-negative bacillary meningitis in New York City 1972–79: frequent causes of menigitis in adults. *American Journal of Medicine*, **71**, 199–209.

Clarke, R. T. J. & Bauchop, T. (1977). *Microbial Ecology of the Gut*. London: Academic Press.

Coid, C. R., Sanderson, H., Slavin, G. & Altman. D. G. (1978). *Escherichia coli* infection in mice and impaired fetal development. *British Journal of Experimental Pathology*, **59**, 292–7.

Cooke, E. M. & Ewins, S. P. (1975). Properties of strains of *Escherichia coli* isolated from a variety of sources. *Journal of Medical Microbiology*, **8**, 107–11.

Cravioto, A., Tello, A., Navarro, A., Ruiz, J., Villafán, H., Uribe, F. & Eslava, C. (1991). Association of *Escherichia coli* HEp-2 adherence patterns with type and duration of diarrhoea. *Lancet*, **337**, 262–4.

De Rycke, J., Gonzalez, E. A., Blanco, J., Oswald, E., Banco, M. & Boivin, R. (1990). Evidence for two types of cytotoxic necrotising factors in human and animal clinical isolates of *Escherichia coli*. *Journal of Clinical Microbiology*, **28**, 694–99.

Dontas, A. S. (1983). The effect of bacteriuria on survival in old age. *Geriatric Medicine Today*, **2**, 74–82.

Dontas, A. S., Kasviki-Charvati, P., Papanayiotou, P. C. & Marketos, S. G. (1981). Bacteriuria and survival in old age. *New England Journal of Medicine*, **304**, 939–43.

Drasar, B. S. & Hill, J. J. (1974). *Human Intestinal Flora*. London: Academic Press.

Dubos, R., Schaedler, R. W. & Costello, R. (1963). Composition, alteration and effects of intestinal flora. *Federation Proceedings, Federation of American Societies for Experimental Biology*, **22**, 1322–9.

Dudgeon, L. S., Wordley, E. & Bawtree, F. (1921). On *Bacillus coli* infections of the urinary tract, especially in relation to haemolytic organisms. *Journal of Hygiene, Cambridge*, **20**, 137–64.

Dudgeon, L. S., Wordley, E. & Bawtree, F. (1923). On *Bacillus coli* infections of the urinary tract, especially in relation to haemolytic organisms. Second communication. *Journal of Hygiene, Cambridge*, **21**, 168–98.

Dupont, H. L. (1982). *Escherichia coli* diarrhea. In *Bacterial Infections of Humans: Epidemiology and Control*, eds. A. S. Evans & H. A. Evans, pp. 219–34. New York: Plenum.

Dupont, H. L., Formal, S. B., Hornick, R. B., Snyder, M. J., Libonati, J. P., Sheehan, D. G., Labrec, E. H. & Kalas, J. P. (1971). Pathogenesis of *Escherichia coli* diarrhea. *New England Journal of Medicine*, **285**, 1–9.

Durack, D. T. & Beeson, P. B. (1977). Protective role of complement in experimental *Escherichia coli* endocarditis. *Infection and Immunity*, **16**, 213–17.

Edwards, P. R. & Ewing, W. H. (1972). *Identification of Enterobacteriaceae*. Minneapolis, Mn: Burgess.

Eisenstein, B. (1981). Phase variation of type I fimbriae in *Escherichia coli* is under transcriptional control. *Science*, **214**, 337–9.

Escherich, T. (1885). Dïe Darmbakterien der Säuglings und Neugeborenen. *Fortschritte der Medizin*, **3**, 515–22.

Evans, D. A., Kass, E. H., Hennekens, C. H., Rosner, B., Miao. L., Kendrick, M.I., Miall, W. E. & Stuart, K. L. (1982). Bacteriuria and subsequent mortality in women. *Lancet*, **1**, 156–8.

Evans, D. G. & Evans, D. J. (1978). New surface-associated heat-labile colonisation factor antigen (CFA/II) produced by enterotoxigenic *Escherichia coli* of serogroups O6 and O8. *Infection and Immunity*, **21**, 638–47.

Evans, D. G., Evans, D. J. Jr. & Dupont, H. L. (1977). Virulence factors of enterotoxigenic *Escherichia coli*. *Journal of Infectious Diseases*, **136**, Supplement, 118–23.

Evans, D. G., Silver, R. P., Evans, D. J., Chase, D. G. & Gorbach, S. L. (1975). Plasmid controlled colonisation factor associated with virulence in *Escherichia coli* enterotoxigenic for humans. *Infection and Immunity*, **12**, 656–66.

Ewing, W. H. & Davies, B. R. (1961). The O-antigen groups of *Escherichia coli* cultures from different sources. Atlanta, GA: Centre for Disease Control.

Farmer, J. J. III, Davis, B. R., Hickman-Brenner, F. W., McWorter, A., Huntley-Carter, G. P., Asbury, M. A., Riddle, C., Wathe-Grady, H. G., Elias, C., Fanning, G. R., Steigerwalt, A. G., O'Hara, C. M., Morris, G. K., Smith, P. B. & Brenner, D. J. (1985a). Biochemical identification of new species and biogroups of Enterobacteriaceae isolated from clinical specimens. *Journal of Clinical Microbiology*, **21**, 46–76.

Farmer, J. J. III, Fanning, G. R., Davis, B. R., O'Hara, C. M., Riddle, C., Hickman-Brenner, F. W., Asbury, M. A., Lowery, V. A. III & Brenner, D. J. (1985b). *Escherichia fergusonii* and *Enterobacter taylorae*: two new species of Enterobacteriaceae isolated from clinical specimens. *Journal of Clinical Microbiology*, **21**, 77–81.

Feng, P. (1995). *Escherichia coli* serotype O157:H7: novel vehicles of infection and emergence of phenotypic variants. *Emerging Infectious Diseases*, **1**, 47–52.

Ferguson, W. W. & June, R. C. (1952). Experiments on feeding adult volunteers with *Escherichia coli* 0111, B4, a coliform organism associated with infant diarrhoea. *American Journal of Hygiene*, **55**, 155–69.

Floreani, A., Basendine, M. F., Mitchison, H., Freeman, R. & James, O. F. (1989). No specific association between primary biliary cirrhosis and bacteriuria? *Journal of Hepatology*, **8**, 201–7.

Fowler, J. E. Jr. & Stamey, T. (1977). Studies of introital colonisation in women with recurrent urinary tract infection. VII. The role of bacterial adherence. *Journal of Urology*, **117**, 472–6.

Freedman, L. R., Phair, J. P., Seki. M., Hamilton. H. B., Nefziger, M. D. & Hirata, M. (1965). The epidemiology of urinary tract infections in Hiroshima. *Yale Journal of Biology and Medicine*, **37**, 262–82.

Fujita, K., Yamamoto, T. & Kitagawa, R. (1991). Binding sites for P and/or type 1-piliated *Escherichia coli* in human ureter. *Journal of Urology*, **146**, 217–22.

Gasser, C., Gautier, E., Steck, A., Siebenmann, R. E. & Oeschlin, R. (1955). Hämolytisch-urämische syndrome: bilaterale nierenrindennekrosen bei acuten erworbenen hämolytischen anämien. *Schweizer Medizinische Wochenschrift*, **85**, 905–9.

Giles, C. & Sangster, G. (1948). An outbreak of infantile gastroenteritis in Aberdeen. The association of a special type of *Bact. coli* with the infection. *Journal of Hygiene, Cambridge*, **46**, 1–9.

Giles, C., Sangster, G. & Smith, J. (1949). Epidemic gastroenteritis of infants in Aberdeen during 1947. *Archives of Disease in Childhood*, **24**, 45–53.

Gindrat, J.-J., Gothefors, L., Hanson, L. Å. & Winberg. J. (1972). Antibodies in human milk against *Escherichia coli* of the serotypes most commonly found in neonatal infections. *Acta Paediatrica Scandinavica*, **61**, 587–90.

Glynn, A. A., Brumfitt, W. & Howard. C. J. (1971). K antigens of *Escherichia coli* and renal involvement in urinary tract infections. *Lancet*, **1**, 514–16.

Gorbach, D. L., Banwell, J. G., Chatterjee, B. D., Jacobs, B. & Sack, R. B. (1971). Acute undifferentiated human diarrhoea in the tropics. I. Alterations in intestinal microflora. *Journal of Clinical Investigation*, **50**, 881–9.

Gorbach, S. L., Kean, B. H., Evans, D. G., Evans, D. J. & Bessudo, D. (1975). Travellers' diarrhoea and toxigenic *Escherichia coli. New England Journal of Medicine*, **292**, 933–5.

Gould, K., Ramirez-Ronda, C. H., Holmes, R. K. & Sanford, J. P. (1975). Adherence of bacteria to heart valves *in vitro. Journal of Clinical Investigation*, **56**, 1364–70.

Grados, O. & Ewing, W. H. (1970). Antigenic relationship between *Escherichia coli* and *Neisseria meningitidis. Journal of Infectious Diseases*, **122**, 100–3.

Gransden, W. R., Eykyn, S. J., Phillips, I. & Rowe, B. (1990). Bacteraemia due to *Escherichia coli*: a study of 861 episodes. *Reviews of Infectious Diseases*, **12**, 1008–18.

Gross, R. J. & Rowe, B. (1985). Serotyping of *Escherichia coli*. In *The Virulence of Escherichia coli*, ed. M. Sussman, pp. 345–63. London: Academic Press.

Gross, R. J., Scotland, S. M. & Rowe, B. (1976). Enterotoxin testing of *Escherichia coli* causing epidemic enteritis in the United Kingdom. *Lancet*, **1**, 629–30.

Grunberg, J., Ofek, I., Perry, R., Wiselka, M., Boulnois, G. & Goldhar, J. (1994). Blood group NN dependent phagocytosis mediated by NFA-3 hemagglutinin of *Escherichia coli. Immunology and Infectious Diseases*, **4**, 28–32.

Gruneberg, R. N. & Bettelheim, K. A. (1969). Geographical variation in serological types of urinary *Escherichia coli. Journal of Medical Microbiology*, **2**, 219–24.

Gruneberg, R. N., Leigh, D. A. & Brumfitt, W. (1968). *Escherichia coli* serotypes in urinary tract infections. Studies in domicilliary antenatal and hospital practice. In *Urinary Tract Infection*, eds. F. O'Grady & W. Brumfitt, pp. 68–79. London: Oxford University Press.

Gruneberg, R. N., Leigh, D. A. & Brumfitt, W. (1969). Relationship of bacteriuria in pregnancy to acute pyelonephritis, prematurity and fetal mortality. *Lancet*, **2**, 1–3.

Guerrant, R. L., Moore, R. A., Kirschenfold, B. A. & Sande, M. A. (1975). Role of toxigenic and invasive bacteria in acute diarrhoea of childhood. *New England Journal of Medicine*, **293**, 567–73.

Guinee. P. A. M. (1963). Preliminary investigations concerning the presence of *E. coli* in man and various species of animals. *Zentralblatt für Bakteriologie, Parasitenkunde, Infektionskrankheiten und Hygiene, Abteilung 1: Originale* **188**, 201–18.

Hagberg, M., Ahlstedt, S. & Hanson, L. Å. (1982). Antibody-dependent cell-mediated cytotoxicity against *Escherichia coli* O antigens. *European Journal of Clinical Microbiology*, **1**, 59–65.

Hanson, L. Å., Ahlstedt, S., Jodal, U., Kaijser, B., Larsson, P., Lidin-Janson, G., Lincoln, K., Lindberg, U., Mattsby, I., Olling, S., Peterson, H. & Sohl, A. (1975). The host-parasite relationship in urinary tract infection. *Kidney International*, **8**, S28–S34.

Hanson, L. Å., Holmgren, J., Jodal, U. & Lomberg, J. (1969). Precipitating antibodies to *Escherichia coli* O antigens: a suggested difference in the antibody response of infants and children with first and recurrent attacks of pyelonephritis. *Acta Paediatrica Scandinavica*, **58**, 506–12.

Hanson, L. Å., Söderström, T., Brinton, C., Carlsson, B., Larson, P., Mellander, L. & Svanborg-Eden, C. (1983). Neonatal colonisation with *Escherichia coli* and the ontogeny of the antibody response. *Progress in Allergy*, **33**, 40–52.

Hanson, L. Å. & Winberg, J. (1966). Demonstration of antibodies of different immunoglobulin types to the O-antigen of the infecting strain in infants and children with pyelonephritis. *Nature*, **212**, 1495–6.

Harber, M. J., Chick, S., Mackenzie, R. & Asscher, A. W. (1982). Lack of adherence to epithelial cells by freshly isolated urinary pathogens. *Lancet*, **1**, 586–8.

Headings, D. L. & Overall, J. C. (1977). Outbreak of meningitis in a newborn intensive care unit caused by a single *Escherichia coli* K1 serotype. *Journal of Pediatrics*, **90**, 99–102.

Hobbs, B. C., Rowe, B., Kendall, M., Turnbull, P. C. B. & Ghosh, A. C. (1976). *Escherichia coli* O27 in adult diarrhoea. *Journal of Hygiene, Cambridge*, **77**, 393–400.

Hobbs, B. C., Rowe, B. & Taylor, J. (1949). School outbreak of gastro-enteritis associated with a pathogenic paracolon bacillus. *Lancet*, **2**, 530–2.

Holmgren, J. & Smith, J. W. (1975). Immunological aspects of urinary tract infection. *Progress in Allergy*, **18**, 289–352.

Hopf, U., Möller, B., Stemerowicz, R., Lobeck, H., Rodloff, A., Freudenberg, M., Galanos, C. & Huhn, D. (1989). Relation between *Escherichia coli* R(rough)-forms in gut, Lipid A in liver, and primary biliary cirrhosis. *Lancet*, **2**, 1419–22.

Horton, R. (1993). Voluntary suspension of Centoxin. *Lancet*, **341**, 298.

Ikari, N. S. (1964). Bactericidal antibody to *Escherichia coli* in germ-free mice. *Nature*, **202**, 879–81.

Ingham, H. R., Sisson, P. R., Tharagonnet, D., Selkon, J. B. & Codd, A. A. (1977). Inhibition of phagocytosis *in vitro* by obligate anaerobes. *Lancet*, **2**, 1252–4.

Ip, S. M., Crichton, P. B., Old, D. C. & Duguid, J. P. (1981). Mannose-resistant and eluting haemaglutinins and fimbriae in *Escherichia coli*. *Journal of Medical Microbiology*, **14**, 223–6.

Jacobsen, S. H., Katouli, M., Tullus, K. & Brauner, A. (1990). Phenotypic differences and characteristics of pyelo-nephritogenic strains of *Escherichia coli* isolated from children and adults. *Journal of Infection*, **21**, 279–86.

Johnson, W. M. & Lior, H. (1988). Production of Shiga toxin and cytolethal distending toxin (CLDT) produced by serogroups of *Shigella* spp. *FEMS Microbiology Letters*, **48**, 235–8.

Kaijser. B. (1973). Immunological studies on some *Escherichia coli* strains with special reference to K antigen and its relation to urinary tract infection. *Journal of Infectious Diseases*, **127**, 670–7.

Kaijser, B. & Ahlstedt, S. (1977). Protective capacity of antibodies against Escherichia coli O and K antigens. *Infection and Immunity*, **17**, 286–9.

Kaijser, B., Hanson, L. Å., Jodal, U., Lidin-Janson, G. & Robbins, J. B. (1977). Frequency of *Escherichia coli* K antigens in urinary tract infections in children. *Lancet*, **1**, 663–4.

Kaijser, B., Jodal, U. & Hanson, L. Å. (1973). Studies on the antibody response and tolerance to *E. coli* K antigens in immunised rabbits and children with urinary tract infection. *International Archives of Allergy*, **44**, 260–73.

Kaijser, B., Larsson, P., Nimmich, W. & Söderström, T. (1983). Antibodies to *Escherichia coli* K and O antigens in protection against acute pyelonephritis. *Progress in Allergy*, **33**, 275–88.

Kaijser, B., Larsson, P. & Olling, S. (1978). Protection against ascending *Escherichia coli* pyelonephritis in rats and significance of local immunity. *Infection and Immunity*, **20**, 78–81.

Kallenius, G. & Winberg, J. (1978). Bacterial adherence to periurethral epithelial cells in girls prone to urinary tract infection. *Lancet*, **2**, 540–3.

Kalmanson, G. M., Harwick, H. J., Turck, M. & Guze, L. B. (1975). Urinary tract infection; localisation and virulence of *Escherichia coli*. *Lancet*, **1**, 134–6.

Karmali, M. A., Steele, B. T., Petrie, H. & Lim, C. (1983). Sporadic cases of haemolytic-uraemic associated with faecal cytotoxin and cytotoxin-producing *Escherichia coli* in stools. *Lancet*, **1**, 619–20.

Kasper, D. L., Winkelhake, J. L., Zollinger, W. D., Brandt, B. C. & Artenstein, M. S. (1973). Immunochemical similarity between polysaccharide antigens of *Escherichia coli* 07:KI(L):NM and group B *Neisseria meningitidis*. *Journal of Immunology*, **110**, 262–8.

Kass, E. H. (1956). Asymptomatic infections of the urinary tract. *Transactions of the Association of American Physicians*, **69**, 56–63.

Kass, E. H. (1960). Bacteriuria and pyelonephritis in pregnancy. *Archives of Internal Medicine*, **105**, 194–8.

Kass, E. H., Miall, W. E., Stuart, K. L. & Rosner, B. (1978). Epidemiologic aspects of infections of the urinary tract. In *Infections of the Urinary Tract*, eds. E. H. Kass & W. Brumfitt, pp. 1–7. Chicago: University of Chicago Press.

Kass, E. H., Savage, W. & Santamarina, B. A. G. (1965). The significance of bacteriuria in preventive medicine. In *Progress in Pyelonephritis*, ed. E. H. Kass, pp. 3–10. Philadelphia, PA: Davis.

Kauffmann, F. (1944). Zur serologie der Coli-Gruppe. *Acta Pathologica et Microbiologica Scandinavica*, **21**, 20–45.

Kauffmann, F. (1954). *Enterobacteriaceae*, 2nd edn. Copenhagen: Munksgaard.

Kauffmann, F. (1966). *The Bacteriology of Enterobacteriaceae*. Copenhagen: Munksgaard.

Keighley, M. R. B. & Burdon, D. W. (1979). *Antimicrobial Prophylaxis in Surgery*. Tunbridge Wells: Pitman Medical.

Kelly, M. J. (1978). The quantitative and histological demonstration of pathogenic synergy between *Escherichia coli* and *Bacteroides fragilis* in guinea-pig wounds. *Journal of Medical Microbiology*, **11**, 513–23.

Kiselius, P. V., Schwan, W. R., Amundsen, S. K., Duncan, J. L. & Schaffer, A. J. (1989). *In vivo* expression and variation of *Escherichia coli* type 1 and P pili in the urine of adults with acute urinary tract infections. *Infection and Immunity*, **57**, 1656–62.

Klipstein, F. A., Rowe, B., Engert, R. F., Short, H. B. & Gross, R. J. (1978). Enterotoxigenicity of enteropathogenic serotypes of *Escherichia coli* isolated from infants with epidemic diarrhoea. *Infection and Immunity*, **21**, 171–8.

Knutton, S., Lloyd, D. R. & McNeish, A. S. (1987). Identification of a new fimbrial structure in enterotoxigenic *Escherichia coli* (ETEC) serotype O148:H28 which adheres to human intestinal mucosa: a potentially new human ETEC colonization factor. *Infection and Immunity*, **55**, 86–92.

Knutton, S., Shaw, R. K., Bhan, M. K., Smith, H. R., McConnell, M. M., Cheasty, T., Williams, P. H. & Baldwin, T. J. (1992). Ability of entero-aggregative *Escherichia coli* strains to adhere *in vitro* to human intestinal mucosa. *Infection and Immunity*, **60**, 2083–91.

Konowalchuk, J., Speirs, J. I. & Stavric, S. (1977). Vero response to a cytotoxin of *Escherichia coli*. *Infection and Immunity*, **18**, 775–9.

Korhonen, T. K. & Rhen, M. (1982). Bacterial fimbriae as vaccines. *Annals of Clinical Research*, **14**, 272–7.

Korhonen, T. K., Valtonen, M. V., Pakinnen, J., Väisänen-Rhen, V., Finne, J., Ørskov, F., Svenson, S. B. & Mäkelä, P. H. (1985). Serotypes, hemolysin production and receptor recognition of *Escherichia coli* strains associated with neonatal sepsis and meningitis. *Infection and Immunity*, **48**, 486–91.

Kunin, C. M. (1966). Asymptomatic bacteriuria. *Annual Review of Medicine*, **17**, 383–406.

Kunin, C. M. (1979). *Detection, Prevention and Management of Urinary Tract Infection*, 3rd edn. Philadelphia, PA: Lea & Febiger.

Kunin, C. M., Deutscher, R. & Paquin, A. (1964). Urinary tract infection in schoolchildren: an epidemiological, clinical and laboratory study. *Medicine (Baltimore)*, **43**, 91–130.

Levin, J., Alving, C. R., Munford, R. S. & Stütz, P. L. (1993). *Bacterial Endotoxins: Recognition and Effector Mechanisms*. Amsterdam: Elsevier.

Levine, M. M., Bergquist, E. J., Nalin, D. R., Waterman, D. H., Hornick, R. B., Young, C. R., Sotman, S. & Rowe, B. (1978). *Escherichia coli* strains that cause diarrhoea but do not produce heat-labile or heat-stable enterotoxins and are not invasive. *Lancet*, **1**, 1119–22.

Levine, M. M., Caplan, E. S., Waterman, D., Cash, R. A., Hornick, R. B. & Snyder, M. J. (1977). Diarrhoea caused by *Escherichia coli* that produce only heat-stable enterotoxin. *Infection and Immunity*, **17**, 78–82.

Levine, M. M., Dupont, H. L., Formal, S. B., Hornick, R. B., Takeuchi, A., Gangarosa, E. J., Snyder, M. J. & Libonati, J. P. (1973). Pathogenesis of *Shigella dysenteriae* I (Shiga) dysentery. *Journal of Infectious Diseases*, **127**, 261–70.

Levine, M. M., Ferreccio, C., Prado, V., Cayazzo, M., Abrego, P., Martinez, J., Maggi, L., Baldini, M. M., Martin, W., Maneval, D., Kay, B., Guers, L., Lior, H., Wasserman, S. S. & Nataro, J. P. (1993). Epidemiologic studies of *Escherichia coli* diarrheal infections in a low socioeconomic level periurban community in Santiago, Chile. *American Journal of Epidemiology*, **138**, 849–68.

Lindberg, U., Hanson, L. Å., Jodal, U., Lidin-Janson, G., Lincoln, K. & Olling, S. (1975). Asymptomatic bacteriuria in schoolgirls. II. Differences in *Escherichia coli* causing asymptomatic and symptomatic bacteriuria. *Acta Paediatrica Scandinavica*, **64**, 432–6.

Liu, T. Y., Gotschlich, E. C., Dunne, F. T. & Jonssen, E. K. (1971). Studies on the meningococcal polysaccharides. II. Composition and chemical properties of the group B and group C polysaccharide. *Journal of Biological Chemistry*, **216**, 4703–12.

Lock, R., Dahlgren, C., Lindén, M., Stendahl, O., Svensbergh, A. & Öhman, L. (1990). Neutrophil killing of two type 1 fimbria-bearing *Escherichia coli* strains: Dependence on respiratory burst activation. *Infection and Immunity*, **58**, 37–42.

Lodinova, R., Jonja, V. & Wagner, V. (1973). Serum immunoglobulins and coproantibody formation in infants after artificial intestinal colonisation with *Escherichia coli* 083 and oral lysozyme administration. *Pediatric Research*, **7**, 659–69.

Lopez-Alvarez, J., Gyles, C. L., Shipley, P. & Falkow, S. (1980). Genetic and molecular characteristics of Vir plasmids of bovine septicemic *E. coli*. *Journal of Bacteriology*, **141**, 758–69.

Mabeck, C. E., Ørskov, F. & Ørskov, I. (1971). *Escherichia coli* serotypes and renal involvement in urinary tract infections in children. *Lancet*, **1**, 1312–14.

Macone, A. B., Pier, G. B., Pennington, J. E., Matthews, W. J. & Goldman, D. A. (1981). Mucoid *Escherichia coli* in cystic fibrosis. *New England Journal of Medicine*, **304**, 1445–9.

Marier, R., Wells, J. G., Swanson, R. C., Callahan, W. & Mehlman, I. J. (1973). An outbreak of enteropathogenic *Escherichia coli* foodborne disease traced to imported cheese. *Lancet*, **2**, 1376–8.

Maslow, J. N., Mulligan, M. E., Adams, K. S., Justis, J. C. & Arbeit, R. D. (1993). Bacterial adhesins and host factors: role in the development and outcome of *Escherichia coli* bacteremia. *Clinical Infectious Diseases*, **17**, 89–97.

McAllister, T. A., Alexander, J. G., Dulake, C., Percival, A., Boyce, J. M. H. & Wormald, P. J. (1971). The sensitivity of urinary pathogens–a survey. *Postgraduate Medical Journal*, **47**, 7–18.

McCabe, W. R. (1981). Gram-negative bacteremia. In *Medical Microbiology and Infectious Diseases*, ed. A. I. Braude, pp. 1387–94. Philadelphia, PA: Saunders.

McCabe, W. R., Carlings, P. C., Bruins, S. & Greely, A. (1975). The relation of K antigen to the virulence of *Escherichia coli*. *Journal of Infectious Diseases*, **131**, 6–10.

McCracken, G. H. (1984). Management of neonatal meningitis 1984. *Journal of Antimicrobial Chemotherapy*, **14** Supplement B, 23–31.

McCracken, G. H. Jr., Sarff, L. D., Glode, M. P., Mize, S. G., Schiffer, M. S., Robbins, J. B., Gotschlich, E. C., Ørskov, I. & Ørskov, F. (1974). Relation between *Escherichia coli* K1 capsular polysaccharide antigen and clinical outcome in neonatal meningitis. *Lancet*, **2**, 246–50.

Mehlman, I. J., Eide, E. L., Sanders, A. C., Fishbein, M. & Alusso, C. C. G. (1977). Methodology for recognition of invasive potential of *Escherichia coli*. *Journal of the Association of Official Analytical Chemists*, **60**, 546–62.

Merson, M. H., Morris, G. K., Sack, D. A., Wells, T. G., Feeley, J. C., Sack, R. B., Creech, W. B., Kapikian, A. Z. & Gangarosa, E. J. (1976). Travellers' diarrhoea in Mexico. *New England Journal of Medicine*, **294**, 1299–305.

Minshew, B. H., Jorgensen, J., Counts, G. W. & Falkow, S. (1978a). Association of hemolysin production, hemagglutination of human erythrocytes and virulence for chicken embryos of extraintestinal *Escherichia coli* isolates. *Infection and Immunity*, **20**, 50–4.

Minshew, B. H., Jorgensen, J., Swanstrum, M., Grootes-Reuvecamp, G. A. & Falkow, S. (1978b). Some characteristics of *Escherichia coli* strains isolated from extraintestinal infections in humans. *Journal of Infectious Diseases*, **137**, 648–54.

Morrison, D. C. & Ryan, J. L. (1992). *Bacterial Endotoxic Polysaccharides*. Boca Raton: CRC Press.

Morrison, D. C. & Ryan, J. L. (1996). *Novel Therapeutic Strategies in the Treatment of Sepsis*. New York: Marcel Dekker.

Morschhäuser, J., Vetter, V., Emödy, L. & Hacker, J. (1994). Adhesin regulatory genes within large, unstable DNA regions of pathogenic *Escherichia coli*: cross-talk between different adhesin clusters. *Molecular Pathogenesis*, **11**, 555–66.

Nalin, D. R., McLaughlin, J. C., Rahaman, M., Yunus, M. & Curlin, G. (1975). Enterotoxigenic *Escherichia coli* and idiopathic diarrhoea in Bangladesh. *Lancet*, **2**, 1116–19.

Nataro, J. P., Kaper, J. B., Robins-Browne, B., Prado, V., Vial, P. A. & Levine, M. M. (1987). Patterns of adherence of diarrhoeagenic *Escherichia coli*. *Pediatric Infectious Diseases*, **6**, 829–31.

Nataro, J. P., Yikang, D., Cookson, S., Cravioto, A., Savarino, J., Guers, L. D., Levine, M. M. & Tacket, C. O. (1995). Hetetrogeneity of entero-aggregative *Escherichia coli* virulence demonstrated in volunteers. *Journal of Infectious Diseases*, **171**, 465–8.

Needell, M. H., Neter, E., Staubitz, E. & Bingham, W. A. (1955). The antibody (haemagglutination) response of patients with infection of the urinary tract. *Journal of Urology*, **74**, 674–82.

Negeleka, M., Martineau-Doize, B. & Fairbrother, J. M. (1994). Septicemia-inducing *Escherichia coli* O115:K"V165"F165, resist killing by porcine polymorphonuclear leukocytes *in vitro*: role of F165$_1$ fimbriae and K"V165" O-antigen capsule. *Infection and Immunity*, **62**, 398–404.

Newcastle Asymptomatic Bacteriuria Research Group (1975). Asymptomatic bacteriuria in schoolchildren in Newcastle upon Tyne. *Archives of Disease in Childhood*, **50**, 90–102.

Nye, F. J. (1979). Travellers' diarrhoea. *Clinics in Gastroenterology*, **8**, 767–81.

O'Brien, A. D. & Holmes, R. K. (1987). Shiga and Shiga-like toxins. *Microbiological Reviews*, **51**, 206–20.

O'Brien, A. D., Lively, T. A., Chen, M. E., Rothman, S. W. & Formal, S. B. (1983). *Escherichia coli* 0157:H7 strains associated with haemorrhagic colitis in the United States produce a *Shigella dysenteriae* I (Shiga) like cytotoxin. *Lancet*, **1**, 702.

Ochman, H., Whittam, T. S., Caugant, D. A. & Selander, R. K. (1983). Enzyme polymorphism and genetic population structure in *Escherichia coli* and *Shigella*. *Journal of General Microbiology*, **129**, 2715–26.

O'Farrell, S. M., Lennox-King, S. M. J., Bettelheim, K. A., Shaw, E. J. & Shooter, R. A. (1976). *Escherichia coli* in a maternity ward. *Infection*, **4**, 146–52.

Ofek, I. & Doyle, R. J. (1994). *Bacterial Adhesion to Cells and Tissues*, pp. 171–94. New York: Chapman & Hall.

Ofek, I., Goldhar, J., Keisari, Y. & Sharon, N. (1995). Nonopsonic phago-cytosis of microoprganisms. *Annual Review of Microbiology*, **49**, 239–76.

Ogawa, H., Nakaumura, A. & Sakazaki, R. (1968). Pathogenic properties of enteropathogenic *Escherichia coli* from diarrheal children and adults. *Japanese Journal of Medical Science and Biology*, **21**, 339–49.

O'Grady, F., Gauci, C. L., Watson, B. W. & Hammond, B. (1968). *In vitro* models simulating conditions of bacterial growth in the urinary tract. In *Urinary Tract Infection*, eds. F. O'Grady & W. Brumfitt, pp. 80–90. London: Oxford University Press.

O'Hanley, P., Lalonde, G. & Ji, G. (1991). α-Hemolysin contributes to the pathogenicity of piliated digalactoside-binding *Escherichia coli* in the kidney: efficacy of an a-hemolysin vaccine in preventing renal injury in the BALB/c mouse model of pyelonephritis. *Infection and Immunity*, **59**, 1153–61.

Olsen, A., Johnson, A. & Normark, S. (1989). Fibronectin binding mediated by a novel class of surface organelles on *Escherichia coli*. *Nature*, **338**, 652–5.

Onderdonk, A. B., Bartlett, J. G., Louie, T., Sullivan-Seigler, N. & Gorbach, S. L. (1976). Microbial synergy in experimental intra-abdominal abscess. *Infection and Immunity*, **13**, 22–6.

Onderdonk, A. B., Louie, T. J., Tally, F. P. & Bartlett, J. G. (1979). Activity of metronidazole against *Escherichia coli* in experimental intra-abdominal sepsis. *Journal of Antimicrobial Chemotherapy*, **5**, 201–10.

Ørskov, F., Ørskov, I., Evans, D. J., Sack, R. B., Sack, D. A. & Wadström, T. (1976). Special *Escherichia coli* serotypes among enterotoxigenic strains from diarrhoea in adults and children. *Medical Microbiology and Immunology*, **162**, 73–80.

Ørskov, F., Ørskov, I., Jann, B., Jann, K., Müller-Seitz, E. & Westphal, O. (1967). Immunochemistry of *Escherichia coli* O antigens. *Acta Pathologica et Microbiologica Scandinavica*, **71**, 339–58.

Ørskov, F., Whittam, T. S., Cravioto, A. & Ørskov, I. (1990). Clonal relationships among classic enteropathogenic *Escherichia coli* (EPEC) belonging to different O groups. *Journal of Infectious Diseases*, **162**, 76–81.

Ørskov, I. & Ørskov, F. (1983). Serology of *Escherichia coli* fimbriae. *Progress in Allergy*, **33**, 80–105.

Ørskov, I., Ørskov, F. & Birch-Andersen, A. (1980). Comparison of *Escherichia coli* fimbrial antigen F7 with type I fimbriae. *Infection and Immunity*, **27**, 657–66.

Ørskov, I., Ørskov, F., Jann, B. & Jann, K. (1977). Serology, chemistry and genetics of O and K antigens of *Escherichia coli*. *Bacteriological Reviews*, **41**, 667–710.

Parkinnen, J., Korhonen, T. K., Pere, A., Hacker, J. & Soinila, S. (1988). Binding sites in the rat brain for *Escherichia coli* S fimbriae associated with neonatal meningitis. *Journal of Clinical Investigation*, **81**, 860–5.

Parry, S. H., Abraham, S. N. & Sussman, M. (1982). The biological and serological properties of adhesion determinants of *Escherichia coli* isolated from urinary tract infections. In *Clinical, Bacteriological and Immunological Aspects of Urinary Tract Infection in Children*, ed. H. Schulte-Wissermann, pp. 113–25. Stuttgart: Thieme.

Parry, S. H., Boonchai, S., Abraham, S. N., Salter, J. M., Rooke, D. M., Simpson, J. M., Bint, A. J. & Sussman, M. (1983). A comparative study of the mannose-resistant and mannose-sensitive haemagglutinins of *Escherichia coli* isolated from urinary tract infections. *Infection*, **11**, 123–8.

Parry, S. H. & Rooke, D. M. (1985). Adhesins and colonisation factors of *Escherichia coli*. In *The Virulence of Escherichia coli*, ed. M. Sussman, pp. 79–155. London: Academic Press.

Percival, A., Brumfitt, W. & De Louvois, J. (1964). Serum antibody levels as an indication of clinically inapparent pyelonephritis. *Lancet*, **2**, 1027–33.

Powell, D. W. (1991). Approach to the patient with diarrhoea. In *Textbook of Gastroenterology*, vol. 1, eds. T. Yamada., D. H. Alpers, C. Owyang & D. W. Powell, pp. 732–78. Philadelphia, PA: Lippincott.

Public Health Laboratory Service (1995). Interim guidelines for the control of infections with Vero cytotoxin producing *Escherichia coli* (VTEC). *Communicable Disease Report Review*, **5**, R77–R81.

Quick, C. A. & Brogan, T. D. (1968). Gram-negative rods and surgical wound infection. *Lancet*, **1**, 1163–7.

Raymond, N. J., Roberson, M. D. & Lang, S. D. R. (1992). Aortic valve endocarditis due to *Escherichia coli*. *Clinical Infectious Disease*, **15**, 749–50.

Riley, L. W., Remis, R. S., Helgerson, S. D., McGee, H. B., Wells, J. G., Davis, B. R., Herbert, R. J., Olcott, E. S., Johnson, L. M., Hargrett, N. T., Blake, P. A. & Cohen, M. L. (1983). Haemorrhagic colitis associated with a rare *Escherichia coli* serotype. *New England Journal of Medicine*, **308**, 681–5.

Ritter, A., Blum, G., Emödy, L., Kerenyi, M., Böck, A., Neuhierl, B., Rabsch, W., Scheutz, F. & Hacker, J. (1995). tRNA genes and pathogenicity islands: influence on virulence and metabolic properties of uropathogenic *Escherichia coli*. *Molecular Pathogenesis*, **17**, 109–21.

Roberts, A. P., Linton, J. D., Waterman, M. M., Gower, P. E. & Koutsaimanis, K. G. (1975). Urinary and faecal *Escherichia coli* O-serotypes in symptomatic urinary tract infection and asymptomatic bacteriuria. *Journal of Medical Microbiology*, **8**, 311–18.

Rolleston, G. L., Making, T. M. J. & Hodson, C. J. (1974). Intrarenal reflux and the scarred kidney. *Archives of Disease in Childhood*, **49**, 531–9.

Rosenberg, M. L., Koplan, J. P., Wachsmuth, J. K., Wells, J. G., Gangarosa, E. J., Guerrant, R. L. & Sack, D. A. (1977). Epidemic diarrhoea at Crater Lake from enterotoxigenic *Escherichia coli*. *Annals of Internal Medicine*, **86**, 711–18.

Rosenstein, I. J., Hazelhurst, G. R., Burroughs, A. K., Epstein, O., Sherlock, S. & Brumfitt, W. (1984). Recurrent bacteriuria and primary biliary cirrhosis: ABO blood group, P1 blood group and secretor status. *Journal of Clinical Pathology*, **37**, 1055–8.

Rowe, B. (1979). The role of *Escherichia coli* in gastroenteritis. *Clinics in Gastroenterology*, **8**, 625–44.

Rowe, B., Taylor, J. & Bettelheim, K. A. (1970) An investigation of travellers' diarrhoea. *Lancet*, **1**, 1–5.

Rowley, D. (1983). Immune responses to enterobacteria presented by various routes. *Progress in Allergy*, **33**, 159–74.

Russell, C. & Mellville, T. H. (1978). Bacteria in the human mouth. *Journal of Applied Bacteriology*, **44**, 163–81.

Sack, D. A., Kaminsky, D. C., Sack, R. B., Wamola. I. A., Ørskov, F., Ørskov, I., Slack, R. C. B., Arthur, R. R. & Kapikian, A. Z. (1977a). Enterotoxigenic *Escherichia coli* diarrhoea in travellers: a prospective study of American Peace Corps volunteers. *Johns Hopkins Medical Journal*, **141**, 63–70.

Sack, D. A., McLaughlin, J. C., Sack, R. B., Ørskov, F. & Ørskov, I. (1977b). Enterotoxigenic *Escherichia coli* isolated from patients at a hospital in Dacca. *Journal of Infectious Diseases*, **135**, 275–80.

Sack, R. B. (1987). Enterohaemorrhagic *Escherichia coli*. *New England Journal of Medicine*, **317**, 1535–7.

Sansonetti, P. J., d'Hautville, H., Formal, S. B. & Toncas, M. (1982). Plasmid-mediated invasiveness of 'Shigella-like' *Escherichia coli*. *Annales de Microbiologie (Paris)*, **132A**, 351–5.

Sarff, L. M., McCracken, G. H. Jr., Schiffer, M. S., Glode, M. P., Robbins, J. B., Ørskov, I. & Ørskov, F. (1975). Epidemiology of *Escherichia coli* Kl in healthy and diseased newborns. *Lancet*, **2**, 1099–104.

Schiffer, M. S., Oliviera, E., Glode, M. P., McCracken, G. H. Jr., Sarff, L. M. & Robbins, J. B. (1976). A review: relation between invasiveness and the Kl capsular polysaccharide of *Escherichia coli*. *Pediatric Research*, **10**, 82–7.

Scotland, S. M., Willshaw, G. A., Smith, H. R., Said, B., Stokes, N. & Rowe, B. (1993). Virulence properties of *Escherichia coli* strains belonging to serogroups O26, O55, O111 and O128 isolated in the United Kingdom in 1991 from patients with diarrhoea. *Epidemiology and Infection*, **111**, 429–38.

Sérény, B. (1955). Experimental *Shigella* keratoconjunctivitis: a preliminary report. *Acta Microbiologica Academiae Scientarum Hungaricae*, **2**, 293–6.

Sharon, N., Eshdat, Y., Silverblatt, F. J. & Ofek, I. (1981). Bacterial adherence to cell surface sugars. In *Adhesion and Microorganism Pathogenicity*, eds. M. O'Connor, J. Whelan & K. Elliott, pp. 119–35. Tunbridge Wells: Pitman Medical.

Shore, E. G., Dean, A. G., Honk, K. J. & Davis, B. R. (1974). Enterotoxin-producing *Escherichia coli* and diarrhoeal disease in adult travellers: a prospective study. *Journal of Infectious Diseases*, **129**, 577–82.

Silva, R. M., Toledo, M. R. F. & Trabulsi, L. R. (1982). Correlation of invasiveness with plasmid in enteroinvasive strains of *Escherichia coli*. *Journal of Infectious Diseases*, **146**, 706.

Siitonen, A. (1992). *Escherichia coli* in faecal flora of healthy adults: serotypes, P and Type 1C fimbriae, non-P mannose-resistant adhesins and hemolytic activity. *Journal of Infectious Diseases*, **116**, 1058–65.

Siitonen, A., Martikainen, R., Ikäheimo, R., Palmgren, J. & Mäkelä, P. H. (1993). Virulence-associated characteristics of *Escherichia coli* in urinary tract infection: a statistical analysis with special attention to type 1C fimbriation. *Microbial Pathogenesis*, **15**, 65–75.

Skinner, F. A. & Carr, J. G. (1974). *The Normal Microbial Flora of Man*. London: Academic Press.

Smith, H. W. (1963). Haemolysins of *Escherichia coli*. *Journal of Pathology and Bacteriology*, **85**, 197–211.

Smith, H. W. (1974). A search for transmissible pathogenic characters in invasive strains of *Escherichia coli*: the discovery of a plasmid-controlled toxin and a plasmid-controlled lethal character closely associated, or identical, with colicin V. *Journal of General Microbiology*, **83**, 95–111.

Smith, H. W. & Gyles, C. L. (1970). The relationship between two apparently different enterotoxins produced by enteropathogenic strains of *Escherichia coli* of porcine origin. *Journal of Medical Microbiology*, **3**, 387–401.

Smith, H. W. & Huggins, M. B. (1976). Further observations on the association of the colicine V plasmid of *Escherichia coli* with pathogenicity and with survival in the alimentary tract. *Journal of General Microbiology*, **92**, 335–50.

Smyth, C. J., Marron, M. & Smith, S. G. J. (1994). Fimbriae of *Escherichia coli*. In *Escherichia coli in Domestic Animals and Man*, ed. C. L. Gyles, pp. 399–435. Wallingford: CAB International.

Sohl-Akerlund, A., Ahlstedt, S., Hanson, L. Å., Lundberg, U. & Olling, S. (1977). Differences of antigenicity of *Escherichia coli* strains isolated from patients with various forms of urinary tract infections. *International Archives of Allergy and Applied Immunology*, **55**, 458–67.

Springer, G. F. (1970). Importance of blood group substances in interactions between man and microbes. *Annals of the New York Academy of Sciences*, **169**, Article 1, 134–52.

Stamey, T. (1980). *Pathogenesis and Treatment of Urinary Tract Infections*. Baltimore, MD: Williams & Wilkins.

Stemerowicz, R., Hopf, U., Möller, B., Willenbrink, C., Rodloff, A., Reinhardt, R., Freudenberg, M. & Galanos, C. (1988). Are antimitochondrial antibodies in primary biliary cirrhosis induced by R (rough) mutants of Enterobacteriaceae. *Lancet*, **2**, 1166–70.

Sussman, M., Abraham, S. N. & Parry, S. H. (1982a). Bacterial adhesion in the host-parasite relationship of urinary tract infection. In *Clinical, Bacteriological and Immunological Aspects of Urinary Tract Infections in Children*, ed. H. Schulte-Wissermann, pp. 103–12. Stuttgart: Thieme.

Sussman, M., Asscher, A. W., Waters, W. E., Evans, J. A. S., Campbell, H., Evans, K. T. & Williams, J. E. (1969). Asymptomatic significant bacteriuria in the non-pregnant woman. 1. Description of a population. *British Medical Journal*, **1**, 799–803.

Sussman, M. & Gower, P. E. (1996). Urinary tract infection. In *Nephrology*. London: Chapman & Hall, in press.

Sussman, M., Parry, S. H., Rooke, D. M. & Lee, M. J. S. (1982b). Bacterial adherence and the urinary tract. *Lancet*, **1**, 1352.

Svanborg Eden, C. (1978). Attachment of *Escherichia coli* to human urinary tract epithelial cells. *Scandinavian Journal of Infectious Diseases, Supplement* **15**, 1–54.

Svanborg-Eden, C., Bjursten, L. M., Hull, R., Magnusson, K.-E. & Leffler, M. (1984). Influence of adhesins on the interaction of *Escherichia coli* with human phagocytes. *Infection and Immunity*, **44**, 672–80.

Svanborg Eden, C., Carlsson, B., Hanson, L. Å., Jann, K., Korhonen, T. K. & Wadström, T. (1979a). Anti-pili antibodies in breast milk. *Lancet*, **2**, 1235.

Svanborg Eden, C., Eriksson, B., Hanson, L. Å., Jodal, U., Kaijser, B., Lidin-Janson. G., Lindberg, U. & Olling, S. (1978). Adhesion to normal human uroepithelial cells of *Escherichia coli* from children with various forms of urinary tract infection. *Journal of Pediatrics*, **93**, 398–403.

Svanborg Eden, C., Hanson, L. Å., Jodal, U., Lindberg, U. & Sohl-Akerlund, A. (1976). Variable adhesion to normal urinary tract epithelial cells of *Escherichia coli* strains associated with various forms of urinary tract infection. *Lancet*, **2**, 490–2.

Svanborg Eden, C., Lidin-Janson, G. & Lindberg, U. (1979b). Adhesiveness to urinary tract epithelial cells of fecal and urinary *Escherichia coli* isolates from patients with symptomatic urinary tract infections or asymptomatic bacteriuria of varying duration. *Journal of Urology*, **122**, 185–8.

Tacket, C. O., Moseley, G., Kay, B., Losonsky, G. & Levine, M. M. (1990). Challenge studies in volunteers using *Escherichia coli* strains with diffuse adherence to HEp-2 cells. *Journal of Infectious Diseases*, **162**, 550–2.

Tamura, K., Sakazaki, R., Kosako, Y. & Yoshizaki, E. (1986). *Leclercia adecarboxylata* gen. nov. comb. nov. formerly known as *Escherichia adecarboxylata*. *Current Microbiology*, **13**, 179–84.

Taylor, J. (1961). Host-specificity and enteropathogenicity of *Escherichia coli*. *Journal of Applied Bacteriology*, **24**, 316–25.

Taylor, J. Powell, B. W. & Wright, J. (1949). Infantile diarrhoea and vomiting: a clinical and bacteriological investigation. *British Medical Journal*, **2**, 117–25.

Taylor, J., Wilkins, M. P. & Payne, J. M. (1961). Relations of rabbit gut reaction to enteropathogenic *Escherichia coli*. *British Journal of Experimental Pathology*, **42**, 43–52.

Teng, N. N. H., Kaplan, H. S., Hebert, J. M., Moore, C., Douglas, H., Wunderlich, A. & Braude, A. I. (1985). Protection against Gram-negative bacteremia and endotoxemia with human monoclonal IgM antibodies. *Proceedings of the National Academy of Science USA*, **82**, 1790–4.

Thomson, S. (1955). The role of certain varieties of *Bacterium coli* in gastro-enteritis of babies. *Journal of Hygiene, Cambridge*, **53**, 357–67.

Thomson, S., Watkins, A. G. & Gray, O. P. (1956). *Escherichia coli* gastro-enteritis. *Archives of Disease in Childhood*, **31**, 340–5.

Tourville, D., Bienenstock, J. & Tomasi, T. B. (1968). Natural antibodies of human serum, saliva and urine reactive with *Escherichia coli*. *Proceedings of the Society for Experimental Biology and Medicine*, **128**, 722–7.

Tulloch, E. F., Ryan, K. J., Formal, S. B. & Franklin, F. A. (1973). Invasive enteropathic *Escherichia coli* dysentery. An outbreak of 28 adults. *Annals of Internal Medicine*, **79**, 13–17.

Turck, M., Petersdorf, R. G. & Fournier, M. R. (1962). The epidemiology of non-enteric *Escherichia coli* infections: prevalence of serological groups. *Journal of Clinical Investigation*, **41**, 1760–5.

Tzipori, S., Montanaro, J., Robins-Browne, R. M., Vial, P., Gibson, R. & Levine, M. M. (1992). Studies with enteroaggregative *Escherichia coli* in the gnotobiotic piglet gastroenteritis model. *Infection and Immunity*, **60**, 5302–6.

Van Dijk, W. C., Verbrugh, H. A., Peters, R., Van Der Tol, M. E., Peterson, P. K. & Verhoef, J. (1977). *Escherichia coli* K antigen in relation to serum-induced lysis and phagocytosis. *Journal of Medical Microbiology*, **10**, 123–30.

Van Dijk, W. C., Verbrugh, H. A., Van Erne-Van der Tol, M . E., Peters, R. & Verhof, J. (1981). *Escherichia coli* antibodies in opsonisation and protection against infection. *Journal of Medical Microbiology*, **14**, 381–9.

Verweij, W. R. (1993). Mixed intra-abdominal infections and abscess formation in the rat: a study of cellular host response and bacterial interactions. pp. 85–98. Doctoral Thesis. Department of Medical Microbiology and Parasitology, Medical School, Vrije Universiteit, Amsterdam.

Verweij, W. R., Namavar, F., Schouten, W. F. & MacLaren, D. M. (1991). Early events after intra-abdominal infection with *Bacteroides fragilis* and *Escherichia coli*. *Journal of Medical Microbiology*, **35**, 18–22.

Wadström, T., Aust-Keltis, A., Habte, D., Holmgren, J., Meeuwisse, G., Mollby, R. & Soderlind, D. (1976). Enterotoxin-producing bacteria and parasites in stools of Ethiopian children with diarrhoeal disease. *Archives of Disease in Childhood*, **51**, 865–70.

Wilfert, C. M. (1978). *E. coli* meningitis: K1 antigens and virulence. *Annual Review of Medicine*, **29**, 129–36.

Williams, G. L., Davies, D. K. L., Evans, K. T. & Williams, J. E. (1968). Vesicoureteric reflux in patients with bacteriuria of pregnancy. *Lancet*, **2**, 1202–5.

Watanakunakorn, C. & Kim, J. (1992). Mitral valve endocarditis caused by a serum resistant strain of *Escherichia coli*. *Clinical Infectious Disease*, **14**, 501–5.

Wolberg, G. & DeWitt, D. (1969). Mouse virulence of K(L) antigen-containing strains of *Escherichia coli*. *Journal of Bacteriology*, **100**, 730–7.

Wright, R. (1982). The liver. In *Clinical Aspects of Immunology*, eds. P. J. Lachmann & D. K. Peters. pp. 878–902. Oxford: Blackwell.

Ziegler, E. J., Fisher, C. J., Sprung, C. L., Straube, R. C., Sadoff, J. C., Foulke, G. E., Wortel, C. H., Fink, M. P., Dellinger, R. P., Teng, N. N. H., Allen, I. E., Berger, H. J., Knatterud, G. L., LoBuglio, A. F., Smith, C. R. & the HA-1A Sepsis Study Group (1991). Treatment of Gram-negative bacteremia and septic shock with HA-1A human monoclonal antibody against endotoxin. *New England Journal of Medicine*, **324**, 429–36.

2

Escherichia coli infections in farm animals

C. WRAY and M. J. WOODWARD

It has long been known that *Escherichia coli*, though a normal inhabitant of the intestinal tract, can be associated with a variety of pathological conditions in farm animals, including poultry. This review brings up to date the account, by Morris & Sojka (1985), of the more important aspects of *E. coli* infections.

In veterinary practice *E. coli* infections occur most frequently in young animals and are usually referred to as colibacillosis. Two main forms, enteric colibacillosis and systemic colibacillosis, are recognised. Another manifestation of *E. coli* infection is coliform mastitis in adult cattle, and there are a number of other sporadic diseases, such as urinary tract infection, which are associated with the organism.

The factors that contribute to the virulence of *E. coli* are becoming better understood. Irrespective of serotype or host, enteric colibacillosis involves the following series of sequential steps, oral infection, colonisation of the intestine after site-specific adhesion to the intestinal mucosa, release of toxins and the pathological consequences of toxin action, which may involve intestinal cells or cells in other organs. Systemic colibacillosis is due to invasive *E. coli* strains that can survive and multiply at extra-intestinal sites. With the advent of sophisticated molecular and cell biological tools, the mechanisms of adherence and the biochemical effects of the various toxins are being clarified. These mechanisms will be considered here mainly as they concern animals, before their relationship to disease conditions in farm animals is described.

The toxins of *Escherichia coli*

Heat-labile enterotoxins

These enterotoxins are inactivated by heat at 60°C and resemble cholera toxin pharmacologically and immunologically (see Chapter 9). A wide range of serogroups of enterotoxigenic *E. coli* (ETEC) of porcine origin produce heat-labile enterotoxin LT1. Most possess the antigenic fimbrial adhesin F4(K88), but LT1 has also been detected in isolates from other farm animals. LT1 produced by *E. coli* from pigs (LTp) has common and unique antigenic determinants when compared with the LT1 produced by *E. coli* of human origin (LTh) (Honda *et al.*, 1981; Geary *et al.*, 1982). LT1 activates adenylate cyclase and so increases the concentration of adenosine 3', 5'-cyclic monophosphate (cAMP) in intestinal epithelial cells, which results in a net secretion of fluid into the intestinal lumen without causing histological damage.

Another heat-labile enterotoxin, LT2, has been detected in *E. coli* isolated from cattle in Thailand. Though it shares many biological properties with LT1, it is not neutralised by antisera against cholera toxin or LT1. The toxin causes rounding of Y1 adrenal cells and Chinese hamster ovary (CHO) cells and activates adenylate cyclase in eukaryotic cells (Green *et al.*, 1983) but, unlike LT1, which is encoded by a plasmid, LT2 appears to be chromosomally determined (Pickett *et al.*, 1986). So far, LT2 has been detected only in *E. coli* from South-East Asia where it is produced by 74 per cent of LT-positive strains of *E. coli* of animal and human origin (Seriwatana *et al.*, 1988).

The molecular weight of LT1 is approximately 88 kDa and it consists of one A polypeptide subunit linked to five B polypeptide subunits that bind to the GM_1 ganglioside receptor of the mucosal cell membrane. LT2 consists of polypeptide subunits of a similar size and mobility to LT1 subunits (Holmes *et al.*, 1986).

Heat-stable enterotoxins

The heat-stable enterotoxins (ST) are proteins of low molecular weight that are resistant to heating at 100°C for 30 minutes and can be divided into two types. The first, STa, is methanol soluble and active in the gastro-intestinal tract of calves, sheep and neonatal mice; it is usually produced by *E. coli* that express the fimbrial adhesins F5(K99), F41 and F6(987P). The second, STb, is insoluble in methanol, induces intestinal secretion in newborn and weaner pigs but has no apparent toxicity in mice. In *E. coli* that produce F4(K88), STb and LT1 production are usually associated, but other toxin combinations have been described (Harnett & Gyles, 1985). STa stimulates guanylate cyclase, which increases the intracellular guanosine 3′, 5′-cyclic monophosphate (cGMP) concentration and inhibits intestinal absorption by a mechanism of action that is unclear.

STa produced by *E. coli* of human, bovine and porcine origin have been purified and slight molecular heterogeneity has been demonstrated, but they are similar in chemical and biological activities. The receptor for STa responsible for specific binding to enterocytes is thought to be a protein or lipoprotein; villus cells contain almost twice as many receptors as crypt cells.

Cytotoxic necrotising factor

Cytotoxic necrotising factor (CNF) was first described to occur in *E. coli* isolated from extra-intestinal infections in humans (Caprioli *et al.*, 1983). It is heat labile and causes giant-cell formation in Vero, Hela and CHO cells and produces necrosis when injected intradermally into rabbits. *Escherichia coli* that produce CNF have subsequently been isolated from pigs, calves, cats and dogs (Gonzalez & Blanco, 1985; McLaren & Wray, 1986; Prada *et al.*, 1991; Pohl *et al.*, 1992). Though CNF has been detected in a wide range of *E. coli* serogroups, most isolates belong to a small range of O-groups including, O2, O4, O6, O22, O32, O75, O83 and O88 (Holland, 1990).

A second type of CNF, CNF2, has also been identified. It differs in causing necrosis in the mouse footpad, moderate fluid accumulation in rabbit intestinal loops and elongation of HeLa cells (De Rycke *et al.*, 1990). Strains that produce CNF2 have been isolated from calves and lambs with diarrhoea and/or septicaemia. Though the two CNF toxins are distinct, they are partially cross-neutralising. CNF1 is chromosomally encoded (Falbo *et al.*, 1992), while CNF2 is encoded on the transmissible Vir plasmid first detected by Smith (1974). Both types of CNF are monomeric proteins of 110–115 kDa (Caprioli *et al.*, 1984; Oswald & De Rycke, 1990).

Unlike strains that produce CNF2, most CNF1-producing strains also produce a haemolysin (Caprioli *et al.*, 1987; Blanco *et al.*, 1990; De Rycke *et al.*, 1990) that is encoded with the CNF genes on a 37-kb fragment of DNA.

Vero cytotoxin

Vero cytotoxigenic *E. coli* (VTEC) were first described by Konowalchuk *et al.* (1977), who showed that culture filtrates of some *E. coli* strains caused irreversible damage to Vero cells and other cell lines such as HeLa cells. The toxin responsible, Vero cytotoxin (VT), is similar, in biological properties, physical properties and antigenicity, to the Shiga toxin of *Shigella dysenteriae* (O'Brien *et al.*, 1982), consequently VT is also known as Shiga-like toxin (SLT). The type of VT neutralised by anti-Shiga toxin was designated VT1 (SLTI). A second type of the toxin, first demonstrated in a strain of *E. coli* O157, is not neutralised by anti-Shiga toxin sera and was termed VT2 (SLTII) (Scotland *et al.*, 1985).

Both types of VT have been purified and consist of A and B subunits with molecular weights of 35 kDa and 10.7 kDa, respectively (Yatsudo *et al.*, 1987). The A subunit possesses the biological activity of the toxin, while the B subunits are thought to mediate specific binding and receptor-mediated toxin uptake. The receptor for VT1 and VT2 is globotriosyl ceramide (Gb_3), which also occurs in hydatid cyst fluid. In several *E. coli* strains the genes that control VT production are phage associated (Scotland *et al.*, 1983; Smith *et al.*, 1983).

Animal isolates of VTEC belong to a wide range of serogroups (Smith *et al.*, 1988; Holland, 1990). They have been implicated in disease in calves and pigs (Holland, 1990), and in the latter they have been isolated from cases of oedema disease (Dobrescu, 1983; Smith *et al.*, 1983). With the exception of O5, O26, O55, O111 and O157, most animal serogroups of VTEC differ from those of human origin.

Although porcine VTEC hybridise with a VT2 probe, cytotoxin that is neutralised by anti-VT2 antibody is produced only at low concentrations (Smith *et al.*, 1988). Another toxin, VT2e, produced by porcine *E. coli*, differs from VT2 in that it is not active on HeLa cells (Blanco *et al.*, 1983). It is more heat labile, not phage mediated and binds to globotetrasyl ceramide (Gb_4) (Marques *et al.*, 1987). On the basis of amino-acid sequence homology, VT2e resembles Shiga toxin and is composed of one A subunit and five B subunits (Donohue-Rolfe *et al.*, 1984). The molecular weights of the A and B subunits are 33 and 7.5 kDa, respectively (MacLeod & Gyles, 1989, 1990). The A subunit of Shiga toxin specifically removes an adenine from eukaryotic 28S rRNA (Saxena *et al.*, 1989) and inhibits protein synthesis.

Fimbrial antigens and putative colonisation factors of *Escherichia coli*

Escherichia coli produce a variety of fimbriae. These act as antigens and as colonisation factors, and they play an important role in the pathogenesis of colibacillosis. Thus, Smith & Linggood (1971) showed that removal of the plasmid that encodes the F4(K88)-antigen from an enterotoxin-producing strain of *E. coli* renders the strain avirulent for piglets.

Type-1 fimbriae (F1)

Most, if not all, *E. coli*, whether pathogenic or not, produce type-1 fimbriae. They are relatively long, about 7 nm in diameter with a subunit molecular weight of 17 kDa (see Chapter 6). These fimbriae are produced at 18°C and 37°C and mediate adherence to certain surfaces, including human type A and guinea-pig erythrocytes. This adherence is termed mannose-sensitive because it is inhibited by D-mannose and its derivatives. The adherence is also mediated by binding to oligosaccharide chains of laminin, an interaction that is abolished by periodate oxidation and enzymatic digestion of laminin saccharides (Westerlund & Karkonen, 1993). The role of type-1 fimbriae in pathogenesis remains unclear. Though they mediate adherence to a wide range of mammalian tissues, including oropharyngeal and bladder mucosa, a non-fimbriate mutant of *E. coli* has been shown to be more virulent on intraperitoneal inoculation into rats than the fimbriate parent strain (May *et al.*, 1993). Type-1 fimbriae are chromosomally encoded and show phase variation that is due to inversion of a small DNA element. Switching is stimulated by aliphatic amino-acids in culture media and depends on global regulators, such as leucine-responsive regulatory protein (Lrp) (Gally *et al.*, 1993; Blomfield *et al.*, 1993), integration host-factor (IHF) (Dorman & Higgins, 1987) and histone-like protein (H-NS) (Kawula & Orndorff, 1991). Other factors that regulate expression of type-1 fimbriae, such as the F-18 colicin plasmid, modulate colonisation (Burghoff *et al.*, 1993; McCormick *et al.*, 1993).

Mannose-resistant adhesin factors and haemagglutinins

Several specific adhesins, whose attachment to erythrocytes and epithelial cells is not inhibited by D-mannose, are important virulence factors in the pathogenesis of diarrhoeal disease in farm animals (Moon, 1990). Some of these, such as K88(F4) and K99(F5), were identified many years ago, while others (see Table 2.1) have been more recently recognised, but it is not always clear whether some of these are true colonisation factors. The rate of discovery of fimbrial antigens is increasing rapidly and there is a need for a standard nomenclature and a reference centre.

Colonisation factors may be associated with ETEC, VTEC and septicaemia strains of *E. coli*, and the encoding genes may be carried on transmissible plasmids or on the chromosome.

There are well recognised associations between the pathogenic *E. coli* serotype, in terms of fimbrial antigen and toxin type, the host animal and the disease syndrome. Thus, for example, F4-positive strains of *E. coli* from pigs produce STb and LT.

F4 (K88 antigen)

These plasmid-encoded protein antigens are true colonisation factors but were originally classified as a capsular antigens. F4 antigen is the commonest adhesin of *E. coli* isolated from pigs (see Wray *et al.*, 1993a) and isogenic variants that lack F4 lack the virulence of the parent strain (Smith & Linggood, 1971). Three antigenic variants, ab, ac and ad, have been identified and their nucleotide sequences and amino-acid sequences have been determined (Dykes *et al.*, 1985). However, F4+ *E. coli* do not adhere to the brush borders of intestinal epithelium from all piglets and Bijlsma *et al.* (1981) have shown, with the *in vitro* brush border test, that several different piglet phenotypes are distinguishable. These appear to be the product of two alleles at a single locus and are inherited in a simple Mendelian manner, the adhesive allele being dominant over the non-adhesive allele (Sellwood *et al.*, 1975). Haemagglutination of porcine erythrocytes mediated by F4 does not depend on the receptors required for adhesion to intestinal brush borders (Cox & Houvenaghel, 1987).

The brush border polar glycolipids of pigs sensitive and resistant to F4 vary, and it has been suggested that the receptor is either a glycoprotein or a glycolipid (Kearns & Gibbons, 1979). It has been shown that receptors for F4 fimbriae are present in the mucus that overlies the epithelial cells of the piglet small intestine and that the amount of K88ab

Table 2.1. *Recently described putative adhesive fimbrial antigens*

Antigen Designation	O-serogroup	*E. coli* type/ disease syndrome	Reference
F42	8	ETEC	(Yano *et al.*, 1986)
F17	8, 9, 15, 78 101, 86	ETEC/ septicaemia in cattle	(FY – Girardeau *et al.*, 1980) (Att 25 – Pohl *et al.*, 1982)
F107(F18)	139, 138	PWD (porcine VTEC)	(Bertschinger *et al.*, 1990)
F107(F18) variants	141, 157	PWD	(Nagy *et al.*, 1992) (Kennan and Monckton, 1990)
8813(F18)	25, 108, 138, 141 147 and 157	Porcine ETEC	(Salajka *et al.*, 1992)
F165	115, 78, 9, 101, 15 7, 117, 4, 18, 4 149	Septicaemia in pigs Septicaemia in cattle	(Fairbrother *et al.*, 1986)
CS31a	18, 17, 78, 117, 23 134, 9, 157, 87, 161	Septicaemia in cattle	(Girardeau *et al.*, 1988)
M326	65	Porcine VTEC	(Aning *et al.*, 1983)
C1213	20, 153, 78, 9	Diarrhoea in cattle	(Varga, 1991)
F11	1, 2, 78	Septicaemia in poultry	(Van den Bosch *et al.*, 1993)

ETEC, enterotoxigenic *E. coli*; PWD, post-wearing diarrhoea; VTEC, Vero cytotoxigenic *E. coli*.

receptor in the mucus is age dependent. In 35-day-old piglets the mucus contains protein and glycolipid galactosyl ceramide receptors (Blomberg *et al.*, 1993). The dominant antigen of F4 is encoded by *faeG*, while other minor proteins are encoded by *faeI*, *faeH*, *faeF* and *faeC*. However, by epitope exchange experiments, Bakker (1991) demonstrated that the adhesive properties of K88ab and K88ac fimbriae can be attributed to particular amino-acid residues in the FaeG protein and that there is a close correlation between the sero-specific epitopes and receptor-binding sites. Indeed, the significance of adherence by F4, F41 and CS31A fimbriae in the pathogenesis of disease has been demonstrated by the passive protection of infant mice against F41[+] ETEC by intravenous administration of F4-specific monoclonal antibodies to their dams (Duchet-Suchaux *et al.*, 1992).

F5 (K99 antigen)

This plasmid-mediated antigen was first detected in strains of *E. coli* from calves and lambs but was subsequently also detected in porcine strains. The host-specificity of F5+ *E. coli* is age-related and mostly confined to the immediate neonatal period (Moon, 1990). Age-dependent resistance is apparently due to the decreasing availability of epithelial cell receptors to the F5 antigen, and adherence of F5+ strains is greater to epithelial cells of one-day-old animals than to those of older animals (Runnels *et al.*, 1980). The distal portion of the small intestine is preferentially colonised by F5+ *E. coli*, and Francis *et al.* (1989) found that expression of the F5 antigen is encouraged by the higher pH values of the ileal fluid. However, Mainil *et al.* (1987) demonstrated loss of F5 determinants with increasing frequency over time after inoculation during the course of natural infection of pigs with *E. coli* O101:K30:K99:F41, which raises questions about selective pressures in the intestine. Various plasma glycoproteins competitively inhibit adhesion of F5+ *E. coli* to mucosal glycoproteins (Mouricout & Julian, 1987) and it has been shown that the ganglioside *N*-glycolyl-GH3 binds laterally to F5 fimbriae at numerous positions (Willemsen & De Graaf, 1993). It is interesting that mixed glycoprotein glycans inhibit the adhesion of F5+ *E. coli* to erythrocytes *in vitro* and they protect colostrum-deprived calves from lethal ETEC infections (Mouricout *et al.*, 1990).

F41

Although the designation F41 was originally used for anionic K99, F41 is now recognised as physically, antigenically and genetically distinct from K99 (Moon, 1990) and also from K88, even though the chromosomal determinants for F41 have considerable sequence homology with the plasmid-borne determinant for K88 (Moseley *et al.*, 1986). Most F41+ ETEC belong to serogroups O9 and O101, and produce K99 as well as F41. Consequently, the role of F41 is difficult to assess, but a K99- F41+ ETEC has been observed to adhere to calf intestinal cells *in vitro* (Morris *et al.*, 1982a). It is possible that F41 is of only minor importance; it is usually accompanied by K99 and most strains originally classified as carrying only F41 also carry K99 genes (Moseley *et al.*, 1986). In our experience the latter are expressed *in vivo* (C. J. Thorns & C. Wray, unpublished) but variants that have lost the genes for K99 remain virulent for newborn pigs (Mainil *et al.*, 1987).

F6 (987P antigen)

This antigen appears to be closely related to type-1 fimbriae and, like it, is subject to phase variation, which often makes it difficult to identify this antigen by culture. Type-1 fimbriae and F6 fimbriae are morphologically identical and have similar physico-chemical properties but differ in amino-acid composition, peptide subunit size, receptor specificity, antigenicity and the inability of F6+ strains to produce haemagglutination. The genes for F6 are chromosomally determined (Klaasen *et al.*, 1990) but strains in which the genetic determinants are plasmid encoded have been described (Schifferli *et al.*, 1990; Casey *et al.*, 1993). Although F6+ *E. coli* are usually isolated from pigs, such strains have been associated with disease in lambs (Duff *et al.*, 1989) and cattle (Wray *et al.*, 1992). Newborn piglets are particularly susceptible and become resistant to colonisation by F6+ *E. coli* by three weeks of age (Dean *et al.*, 1987).

The receptors for F6 are probably galactose- or fucose-containing glycoproteins (Dean & Isaacson, 1985) that may disappear as the piglet ages. The receptors may be released into the bowel lumen, bind the F6 antigen competitively, so facilitating bacterial clearance (Dean *et al.*, 1987). However, reduced expression of F6 antigen by bacteria in the ileal loops of older pigs, as determined by immunofluorescence, has also been noted.

F17 (Att 25 or F-Y)

This fine fimbrial antigen was first detected on ETEC strains that cause diarrhoea in calves (Girardeau *et al.*, 1980; Pohl *et al.*, 1982). They are 3–4 nm in diameter, consist of 20-kDa subunits and do not produce haemagglutination. The genes for F17 production are chromosomal and have been cloned (Lintermans *et al.*, 1988).

The role of F17 in intestinal colonisation has not been conclusively proved, but strains that produce F17 adhere to intestinal villi *in vitro*. There is no correlation between F17 production and enterotoxin production, and F17 antigen has been detected on non-ETEC and also on attaching and effacing *E. coli* (AEEC)(Hall *et al.*, 1988). However, Pohl *et al.* (1984) found a correlation between F17 production and the development of diarrhoea and septicaemia in newborn calves. Antibodies to F17 add to the protection of calves against challenge strains of *E. coli* with F5+, F41+ or F17+ (Contrepois & Girardeau, 1985).

F18/F107 antigen

A strain of *E. coli* serotype O139:K12:H1, isolated from a case of oedema disease, was shown by electron microscopy to express fimbriae after growth on blood agar (Bertschinger *et al.*, 1990). This strain attached strongly *in vitro* to isolated porcine brush border fragments and the fimbriae were demonstrated, by immunofluorescence, in the intestinal contents of pigs. Another isolate from oedema disease did not, however, express the fimbriae on culture but the F107 antigen was demonstrated *in vivo*. These fimbriae have been isolated and are composed of 15-kDa peptide subunits. The gene that encodes the fimbrial subunit has been cloned and sequenced (Imbrechts *et al.*, 1992a) and the presence of the gene has been demonstrated in 24 of 28 oedema disease reference strains, including serogroups O139, O141 and O149 (Imbrechts *et al.*, 1992b). Experiments with pigs suggest that susceptibility to intestinal colonisation by a F107+ strain of *E. coli* is associated with the inheritance of a dominant gene (Bertschinger *et al.*, 1993).

A novel colonisation factor, designated '8813', was detected by Salajka *et al.* (1992) in ETEC from pigs with post-weaning diarrhoea. Strains that express this factor adhere to porcine brush borders *in vitro* and in experimental infections they colonise the intestine and induce diarrhoea. The antigen was detected in 39 per cent of 212 strains of *E. coli* of serogroups O25, O108, O138, O147, O151 and O157. Antigen '8813' has been designated as F18 by the International *E. coli* Reference Centre.

Nagy *et al.* (1990) described a fimbrial adhesin, 2134P, which they detected in *E. coli* isolated from cases of post-weaning diarrhoea. This antigen may be similar to that detected by Kennan & Monckton (1990) on *E. coli* O141 from pigs.

Wittig *et al.* (1994) were able to achieve expression of antigen F107 by growing organisms under microaerobic conditions. On the basis of cross-absorption tests they suggested that there are two variants of the antigen, F107ab (Bertschinger strain) and F107ac (Salajka strain 8813 and Nagy strain 2134P). These strains are probably more correctly described as F18ab and F18ac, respectively.

CS31A antigen

This capsule-like protein, which consists of 2-nm fimbriae, was first detected on strains of *E. coli* isolated from calves with diarrhoea or septicaemia (Contrepois *et al.*, 1986; Girardeau *et al.*, 1988). CS31A has been detected on 20.5 per cent of bovine and 1.2 per cent of porcine *E. coli* of serogroups O8, O20, O78, O86, O117 and O153 from diarrhoeal disease (Contrepois *et al.*, 1989). In the bovine strains, CS31A was also detected in association with the F165 and F5 antigens. Genes for the expression of CS31A are carried on a 105-mDa plasmid and the antigen shares significant amino-acid sequence homology with F4(K88) and with F41, particularly at the amino-terminus (Korth *et al.*, 1991). The accessory genes for F4(K88), F41 and CS31A synthesis share considerable homology, while the antigen-specific genes do not (Moseley *et al.*, 1986; Anderson & Moseley, 1988). Hybridisation between CS31A$^+$ isolates and F4/F41 accessory gene probes has been demonstrated by Casey *et al.* (1990) and it appears that a common cluster of accessory genes provides a common mechanism for expression of fimbriae in distinct serotypes of *E. coli*.

Immunoelectron microscopy, after incubation with specific antisera, revealed a wide capsule-like zone around the bacteria that consists of an abundance of very fine fibrils. Production of CS31A is weak in liquid media and is repressed by L-alanine. The role of global regulation in expression of K88, F41 and CS31A is unclear but a possible role for Lrp is suggested by the effect of alanine on expression.

F165 antigen

This mannose-resistant fimbrial antigen was identified by Fairbrother *et al.* (1986) on strains of *E. coli* O115 isolated from septicaemic piglets. It was subsequently identified on *E. coli* from calves with septicaemia and/ or diarrhoea (Pohl *et al.*, 1986). In experiments with newborn colostrum-deprived piglets, F165$^+$ *E. coli* induces watery diarrhoea or septicaemia (Fairbrother *et al.*, 1989) and the organisms are associated with the ileal mucosa and the large intestine.

F165 fimbriae are long, rigid and have a diameter of *c.* 5–8 nm. The purified fimbrial complex consists of two separate protein subunits, F165$_1$ and F165$_2$, of approximately 19 and 17.5 kDa respectively (Fairbrother *et al.*, 1988). The genetic determinants of F165 have been cloned (Harel *et al.*, 1992) and are chromosomally encoded (Nagelcka *et al.*, 1993). The F165 phenotype is complex and depends on which of the subunit antigens is expressed. The antigen is mostly found on *E. coli* of serogroups O8, O9, O101, O115 and O141 isolated from septicaemic piglets and calves. While other adhesins, such as F4, F5, F41 or F6, may be present on these strains (Fairbrother *et al.*, 1989) the expression of F165 depends on a *pap-*

like (*prs*) gene cluster (Sourindra *et al.*, 1993). Mutants that lack F165 induce only mild diarrhoea and it has been suggested that the $F165_1$ subunit may play a role in extra-intestinal adherence and survival in the host tissues.

Other less well characterised putative adhesins

Porcine isolates of Escherichia coli

Fimbriae, designated F42, were demonstrated by Yano *et al.* (1986) to occur on ETEC from pigs in Brazil. They were shown to adhere to porcine intestinal cells *in vitro* but there is no conclusive proof for their role in the intestine during ETEC infection, and preliminary characterisation of a 31-kDa antigen has been made (Leite *et al.*, 1988). The ability of some porcine isolates of *E. coli* O65 to adhere to isolated brush border preparations was demonstrated by Aning *et al.* (1983), and these isolates were subsequently shown to be Vero toxigenic.

Bovine isolates of Escherichia coli

A common antigen was demonstrated by Varga (1991) to occur on *E. coli* of serogroups O20, O9, O8, O21, O101, O78 and O153 isolated from cases of diarrhoea. They consist of long thin fimbriae and produce mannose-resistant haemagglutination of bovine erythrocytes.

Other putative virulence factors

Curli

A novel class of *E. coli* surface structures called 'curli', morphologically and biochemically distinct from all other surface appendages, was described by Olsen *et al.* (1989). Curli are fibronectin- and laminin-binding fibres expressed at temperatures below 37°C when cultures are grown on colonisation factor antigen (CFA) medium. Regulation of curli expression is complex. The *E. coli* K-12 cloning host HB101 does not naturally express the antigen and initial cloning experiments identified a putative curli gene, *crl*, that transcriptionally activates a cryptic curlin subunit gene, *csgA* (Arnquist *et al.*, 1992; Olsen *et al.*, 1993). Most, if not all, strains of *E. coli* possess *csgA*. Whether curli are true virulence factors is unclear, but there is a correlation between curli expression and auto-agglutination and binding to soluble fibronectin and laminin. The role of the *crl* transcriptional activation gene in curli regulation in strains other than HB101 is also open to question (Provence & Curtiss, 1992). It is significant that curli share homology with a similar thin aggregative fimbria, SEF17, found in salmonellas (Collinson *et al.*, 1991, 1992). The characteristics of the two fimbriae are similar and, as for *csgA*, most if not all salmonellas possess the thin aggregative fimbrial gene, *agfA*. Because of their common amino-terminal amino-acid sequences (glycine–valine–valine–proline–glutamine), this class of fimbriae has been termed GV-VPQ (Collinson *et al.*, 1992; Doran *et al.*, 1993). The widespread occurrence of these genes raises questions as to the selective advantage they confer and whether homologous fimbriae are encoded by other Enterobacteriaceae.

Type-IV pilins

These have been described on many unrelated bacterial species, share a high degree of homology at the amino-termini of their respective amino-acid sequences and have unusually short signal sequences for secretion through the membrane (Sohel *et al.*, 1993). As was noted above [in 'F17 (Att 25 or F-Y)'], AEEC show localised adherence that is not only associated with a plasmid-encoded adherence factor termed EAF but also fimbriae described as 'bundle-forming pili' (Giron *et al.*, 1991). Interestingly, DNA sequences that share homology with the fimbrial gene *bfp* (Donnenberg *et al.*, 1992) have been found in some strains of diffuse adherent *E. coli* (DAEC), AAEC and enteroinvasive *E. coli* (EIEC) and many serotypes of *Salmonella* (Sohel *et al.*, 1993).

Nfa antigen

This non-fimbrial adhesin was described by Aubel *et al.* (1993) to occur on ETEC strain 8786 that had originally been isolated from a human infection but was probably of animal origin (Blackes *et al.*, 1982). The Nfa antigen shares significant homology with the recently described SEF14 fimbrial antigen of *Salmonella enteritidis* (Collinson *et al.*, 1993; Turcotte & Woodward, 1993). The *nfa* gene is plasmid borne, while the *sefA* gene is chromosomal. The distribution of *sefA* is limited exclusively to some group D salmonellas, while the distribution of *nfa* is less clear.

These examples of putative virulence determinants make it clear that many of the genes are widespread, not necessarily associated with human or animal infection but possibly both, and that the potential promiscuity of the encoding genes is due to plasmid carriage.

Diseases of farm animals due to *Escherichia coli*

Colibacillary diarrhoea

Colibacillary diarrhoea occurs most frequently in calves, lambs and piglets one to three days after birth and is the most common cause of enteric disease in young animals in the United Kingdom. The disease is often acute and is due to ETEC, which cause severe diarrhoea that gives rise to fluid and electrolyte imbalances, dehydration and death. At autopsy no specific lesions can be observed and the intestinal mucosa is undamaged. Large numbers of *E. coli* (more than 10^8 per gram of contents) are present, closely associated with the mucosa of the small and large intestine. These ETEC belong to relatively few serogroups, and in calves and lambs the OK groups are usually the same, while the OK isolated from pigs are seldom isolated from other species (Sojka, 1971).

In England and Wales the most common serogroups of *E. coli* isolated from pigs with diarrhoea are O149, O8, O138, O147 and O157 (Wray *et al.*, 1993a). Antigen F4 was detected in 21 per cent of cultures, while the other adhesins, F5, F6 and F41, were present in only up to three per cent of the isolates in any year. Heat-labile enterotoxin was produced by more than 17 per cent of the isolates, which generally also produced STb, usually in association with F4 antigen (Smith & Gyles, 1970). STa was detected in 5.3 per cent of the porcine isolates. The most common serogroups among the porcine isolates were the same as those reported by Sojka (1971), which suggests that the ETEC population in pigs remained unchanged. The most frequent serogroup, O149, has also commonly been isolated in many other countries (Murray, 1987; Soderlind *et al.*, 1988; Harel *et al.*, 1991; Wittig & Fabricius, 1992). In some of these countries the incidence of F5 and F6 strains is generally higher than in the United Kingdom, and in Germany 20 per cent of the isolates produced F5 (Wittig & Fabricius, 1992). It has been suggested that in Sweden vaccination of sows has reduced the frequency of F4+ strains and allowed F5+ strains to predominate (Soderlind *et al.*, 1982).

Other serogroups, such as O8, O9, O64 and O101, which commonly produce STa and/or F5 or F6 are also a frequent cause of neonatal diarrhoea in piglets (Harnett & Gyles, 1983, 1985; Harel *et al.*, 1991). Woodward *et al.* (1993) examined O9, O20 and O101 strains which, although lacking the common fimbrial adhesins, were thought to be involved in the aetiology of porcine diarrhoea. The isolates were extremely diverse and it was estimated that there were 18, 16 and 12 clones respectively of the three serogroups. It was concluded that pathogenicity may be directly related to the somatic antigen type, rather than to the wide distribution of a small number of virulent clones.

In cattle and sheep the commonest serogroups were O8, O9 and O101 (Wray *et al.*, 1993a), which is similar to the results of other surveys (Linton *et al.*, 1979; Murray, 1987). The F5 adhesin was detected on 9.1 per cent of bovine isolates and on 11.1 per cent of ovine isolates, usually in association with STa production. Harnett & Gyles (1985) found F5 and STa genes on the same plasmid and suggested that further dissemination of the genes may result from antibiotic selection pressure.

Most ETEC from calves are mucoid and possess the A type of K-antigen (Sivasvamy & Gyles, 1976). Isaacson *et al.* (1977) reported that capsules and fimbriae were involved in the colonisation of the porcine intestine by some ETEC strains and suggested that the capsule may protect the organism in the intestine or that it may be involved in adherence to the mucosa. Our experiments have shown that non-capsulated ETEC are relatively avirulent when used to challenge lambs (Sojka *et al.*, 1978).

In spite the development of effective vaccines, neonatal colibacillosis remains an important disease of farm animals and there appears to have been little change in the ETEC serogroups responsible or their virulence determinants.

Colibacillary toxaemia in pigs

Three syndromes in pigs, due to relatively few *E. coli* serogroups, namely O45, O138, O139 and O141, have been described. These are shock in weaner syndrome, haemorrhagic enteritis and oedema disease.

Shock in weaner syndrome

In this syndrome, one or two piglets in a litter die suddenly (Schimmelpfennig, 1970) and oedema is observed in the intestine, lungs and kidneys and central nervous system. Serous exudate is common in the body cavities and in severe cases blood may pass into the intestinal lumen.

Haemorrhagic colitis

This is a form of enteritis in post-weaning piglets, characterised by sudden death and haemorrhagic lesions in the gastro-intestinal mucosa and associated lymph nodes. The pathogenesis of this and shock in weaner syndrome may be related and involve the rapid absorption of endotoxin from the bowel.

Oedema disease

Oedema disease was first described by Shanks (1938) and remains an important post-weaning disease of pigs. The aetiology is complex, because changes in food composition, temperature and loss of passive protection from the sow are all involved in the pathogenesis. Postmortem examination reveals oedema in the sub-cutis, colonic mesentery and gastric sub-mucosa (Sojka, 1965). Oedema disease is usually seen one to two weeks after weaning, when various nutritional and environmental factors may predispose to the disease. The responsible *E. coli* strains usually belong to a small range of serotypes, O138:K81, O139:K82, O141:K85, which are not invasive and are usually confined to the bowel.

Smith & Halls (1968) infected pigs with *E. coli* O141:K85 and suggested that its pathogenicity is related to its ability to adhere to the intestinal epithelium. It is only recently that adhesion factors have been demonstrated in two oedema disease strains of *E. coli* O139:K12:H1 (Bertschinger *et al.*, 1990).

The clinical signs of oedema disease have been experimentally reproduced by injecting pigs intravenously with the supernatant fluid from the intestinal contents of affected animals (Timoney, 1950). The clinical signs usually appear 24–48 hours after administration of the supernatant, which suggests that oedema disease strains produce a toxin in the intestine. The ultrastructural changes in the vasculature of the intestinal mucosa include endothelial swelling or vacuolation and perivascular oedema (Methiyapun *et al.*, 1984); the neurological signs are, therefore, a consequence of oedema in the central nervous system. It has been suggested that the toxic substance responsible for the oedema be called oedema disease principle (EDP) (Nielsen & Clugston, 1971). An experimental model for subclinical oedema disease was developed in weaners by Kausche *et al.* (1992). Three-week-old pigs were inoculated intragastrically with 10^{10} colony-forming units of a VT2e$^+$ strain of *E. coli* and examined post-mortem 14 days later, when vascular lesions were detected in the brain and ileum. The lesions consisted of segmental myocyte necrosis in the tunica media of small arteries and arterioles.

Lysates of oedema disease strains of *E. coli* possess Vero cytotoxicity (Dobrescu, 1983) and there is a correlation between strains isolated from clinical oedema disease and verocytotoxin production (Linggood & Thompson, 1987). The verocytotoxicity of oedema disease strains can be transferred by DNA to *E. coli* K-12, and pigs inoculated with such a strain develop the clinical and pathological lesions of the disease (Smith *et al.*, 1983). The genetic determinants that code for the toxin were identified by Gannon *et al.* (1989), and pigs inoculated with transformants that carry the complete toxin operon developed the disease. The purified toxin reproduced the disease when injected into pigs but without signs of endotoxaemia (Macleod & Gyles, 1991).

Porcine post-weaning diarrhoea

The pathogenesis of *E. coli*-induced porcine post-weaning diarrhoea (PWD) is more complicated than that of neonatal diarrhoea and may be attributed to factors associated with weaning that interact with the organism. Among these are the stress of weaning and decreased gastric bactericidal activity due to a temporary increase in gastric pH. After weaning, pigs are no longer protected by milk factors (Svendsen & Larsen, 1977; Deprez *et al.*, 1986) and *E. coli* may cause diarrhoea. Rotavirus has also been associated with PWD, often in conjunction with haemolytic *E. coli* (Lecce *et al.*, 1982; Nabuurs *et al.*, 1993). PWD has also been attributed partly to the feeding regimen, which may cause hypersensitivity of the intestinal mucosa to dietary antigens (Miller *et al.*, 1984). The one unifying finding, however, is the marked increase in numbers of haemolytic *E. coli* that occurs two to seven days after weaning (Thomlinson, 1969). Nabuurs *et al.* (1993) showed that ETEC numbers increased and were subsequently superseded by the VT-producing serotype O139:K82.

A reproducible model of PWD colibacillosis was developed by Sarmiento *et al.* (1988a) by controlling management and environmental variables to simulate conditions often seen at weaning. Sucking pigs were briefly exposed to a starter diet at one week of age, weaned at three weeks of age, held at ambient temperature and again given the starter diet. One day after weaning each pig was given 10^{10} *E. coli*. Some piglets developed acute fatal diarrhoea, others moderate diarrhoea with weight loss and faecal shedding of the inoculum strain, while others remained clinically normal although shedding the inoculum strain. Later experiments (Sarmiento *et al.*, 1988b, 1990) indicated that weaning or restricted creep feeding were unnecessary for the induction of PWD but that it may increase its severity.

Nagy *et al.* (1990) examined 205 K88+ *E. coli* isolates from cases of PWD. The commonest (61 per cent) K88-positive serogroup was O149 and 61 per cent of these produced LT and STb. Of 70 K88- strains, 17 produced VT and most belonged to serogroups O138, O139, O141 and

O149. A fimbrial adhesin that adheres better to the microvilli of older pigs than to those of newborn pigs has been detected on ETEC strains of serogroups O157 and O141 (Nagy *et al.* 1992). These strains are pathogenic and cause diarrhoea when given to pigs (Casey *et al.*, 1992).

Disease due to enteropathogenic Escherichia coli

Escherichia coli that attach intimately to enterocytes of the intestinal mucosa with loss (effacement) of microvilli are known as attaching and effacing *E. coli* (AEEC) (Moon *et al.*, 1983). The attaching and effacing (AE) lesions are detectable only by transmission electron microscopy, unless specific staining techniques are used. Such lesions are increasingly recognised in a variety of animal species (Holland, 1990). They may be mild and scattered throughout the small and large intestine or more severe and restricted to the large intestine. The caecum and colon are most often involved, but the distal jejunum and ileum may also be affected. Large numbers of bacteria attach to the intestinal epithelium, so that the adherent bacteria appear to be attached to the cells at raised, cuplike projections called pedestals. Pedestal formation appears to involve disorganisation of the cytoskeleton and polymerisation of actin adjacent to sites of bacterial attachment. Within a few days destruction of the microvillus border can be observed. The mechanisms by which AE lesions are produced is not fully understood, because expression of an attachment factor and production of cytotoxin are important but not essential. The AE lesions due enteropathogenic strains are associated with a bacterial chromosomal gene, *eae* (Jerse *et al.*, 1990). A plasmid-encoded adherence factor has been detected in enteropathogenic *E. coli* (EPEC) strains from humans and has been termed EAF. This has been shown to mediate adherence to cells *in vitro* and to the porcine intestine (Baldini *et al.*, 1983). The adhesin is a *c.* 94-kDa outer-membrane protein that is found in many, but not all, EPEC (Chart *et al.*, 1988). A fuller review of the mechanisms of attachment is provided by Tesh & O'Brien (1992) (see also Chapter 14).

Many strains of AEEC from animals produce VT (Konowalchuk *et al.*, 1977) of which two main types have been recognised. These may occur singly or in combination in bovine *E. coli* isolates, and VT2e predominates in porcine isolates. VTEC have been isolated from a wide range of animal species and a number of experimental studies with VTEC have reproduced the characteristic intestinal lesions and blood-stained diarrhoea (Holland, 1990).

In a survey of *E. coli* submitted for serological identification, 4.7 per cent of porcine isolates, 2.8 per cent of bovine isolates and 6.1 per cent of ovine isolates produced VT (Wray *et al.*, 1993a). One VT-negative strain of *E. coli* has been isolated from a calf with AE lesions in the small and large intestine (Pearson *et al.*, 1989). In a longitudinal study of VT-producing *E. coli* in two cohorts of 10 and 16 calves, Tokhi *et al.* (1993) found that 53 per cent of faecal isolates were positive for VTEC. At any one time 20–80 per cent of animals excreted VTEC of a number of serogroups, and their presence was associated with diarrhoea. Mainil *et al.* (1993) showed that 24 per cent of *E. coli* from calves with diarrhoea hybridised with the *eae* probe. Of these, 56 per cent hybridised with the VT1 probe, one strain with the VT2 probe and three strains produced both VT1 and VT2. However, ten *eae* probe-positive isolates were negative with both VT probes. Some of the other isolates hybridised with probes from enteroadherent *E. coli*. AE lesions were produced in the intestines of gnotobiotic pigs after infection with an *eae*-positive, VT-negative strain of *E. coli* O45 isolated from a case of post-weaning diarrhoea (Zhu *et al.*, 1994).

Zoonotic aspects of VTEC infection

In humans, VTEC, frequently of serogroup O157, are associated with haemorrhagic colitis (HC) and haemolytic-uraemic syndrome (HUS) (see Chapters 10 and 15). Such strains have also been isolated from the faeces of cattle by several investigators (see Karmali, 1989), and the frequent association between VTEC infection in humans and the consumption of beef and dairy products suggests that cattle are a reservoir of VTEC. After an epidemiological investigation of two sporadic cases of HUS associated with milk, Wells *et al.* (1991) identified VTEC, which included *E. coli* O157, in 8.4 per cent (13/154) of healthy dairy cattle. *E. coli* O157 have also been isolated from cattle in the United Kingdom (Chapman *et al.*, 1989) and in Germany (Montenegro *et al.*, 1990). In Scotland, Synge & Hopkins (1992) isolated the organism from scouring calves. In the faeces of cattle *E. coli* O157 are usually present in small numbers and the extent of the bovine reservoir is unknown. However, with more sensitive immunomagnetic separation techniques Wright *et al.* (1994) found that infection was widespread in a herd associated with milk-borne infection.

Infection with cytotoxic-necrotising-factor-producing Escherichia coli

Escherichia coli that produce CNF were first detected by Caprioli *et al.* (1983) in young children with diarrhoea. They have subsequently been detected in calves, pigs, cats and dogs (Gonzalez and Blanco, 1985; McLaren and Wray, 1986; De Rycke *et al.*, 1987; Prada *et al.*, 1991; Pohl *et al.*, 1992). Though CNF+ *E. coli* are usually isolated from cases of enteric disease, they have also been isolated from extra-intestinal and urinary tract infections. CNF+ *E. coli* usually belong to serogroups O2, O4, O6, O22, O32, O75, O78 and O88 (Holland *et al.*, 1990).

Wray *et al.* (1993a) detected CNF+ *E. coli* in 6.8 per cent of porcine isolates, 8.3 per cent of bovine isolates and 9.1 per cent of ovine isolates. In Spain, Blanco *et al.* (1993) detected CNF2+ *E. coli* in 20 per cent of isolates from ill calves and in 34 per cent of isolates from healthy controls; CNF1+ strains were detected in one healthy and two ill calves. Although CNF+ *E. coli* were isolated from healthy calves, animal experiments have demonstrated their pathogenicity. The effect of the intravenous injection into young lambs of a partially purified extract of CNF from a bovine isolate of *E. coli* has been investigated by De Rycke & Plassiart (1990). All the lambs developed severe clinical neurological signs and mucoid diarrhoea six hours after inoculation. Oedema and haemorrhages were found in the central nervous system and foci of coagulative necrosis in the myocardium. Of a litter of six piglets infected orally with a CNF+ strain of *E. coli* O88, two died and three developed blood stained diarrhoea (Wray *et al.*, 1993b). The pathological changes consisted of an early enteritis that progressed to enterocolitis and there was septicaemic spread to the lungs. The histopathological changes were characteristic of toxaemic effects in brain, heart, liver and kidney, and characterised by congestion, oedema and exudation. Infection with a CNF+ *E. coli* of serogroup O32 produced a similar but milder enterocolitis.

CNF-producing *E. coli* have been isolated from a wide range of clinical conditions in humans and animals, including diarrhoea, extra-intestinal and urinary infections. Though animal experiments have indicated their toxicity, further studies are desirable because of their association with a number of different disease syndromes.

Systemic colibacillosis

Systemic colibacillosis occurs frequently in calves, lambs and poultry. Septicaemia strains of *E. coli* pass through the alimentary or respiratory mucosa and enter the bloodstream, where they may cause either a generalised infection (colisepticaemia) or a localised infection such as meningitis and/or arthritis in calves and lambs, or air sacculitis and pericarditis in poultry. Systemic colibacillosis is less frequently encountered in piglets.

Systemic colibacillosis in calves and lambs

This occurs commonly in colostrum-deprived animals but may also occur in some colostrum-fed animals that have failed to absorb immunoglobulins. If colostrum is to be effective it must be ingested within a few hours of birth, because little or no immunoglobulin absorption takes place after 24–36 hours. Systemic colibacillosis occurs in one-day-old to 14-week-old lambs, but it is most common at two to three weeks of age. The severity of the disease in calves and lambs can be related to the degree of deficiency of serum λ-globulins, particularly IgM (Penhale *et al.*, 1970).

Generalised infection follows an acute, usually fatal, course. Diarrhoea may occur but is not a constant feature, and many of the signs and symptoms observed in infected animals may be due to endotoxin. In some animals the course of the disease is more chronic and *E. coli* localises in the joints and meninges. More recently, a new diarrhoea syndrome with ataxia in young calves has been described by Espinasse *et al.* (1991). The *E. coli*, which can usually be isolated in pure culture from generalised infections, belong to a small number of serogroups, of which O78:K80 is the most common.

Systemic colibacillosis in poultry

Colibacillosis is primarily a disease of two- to three-week-old birds and often appears to be secondary to respiratory infections, such as with Infectious Bronchitis virus and *Mycoplasma gallisepticum*. The strains of *E. coli* belong to relatively few serological groups, the most common are O78:K80, O1:K1 and O2:K1.

Virulence determinants in septicaemia strains of Escherichia coli

Septicaemia strains have special properties that enable them to resist the host defence mechanisms. Many strains carry plasmids with genes for colicin V (ColV), and have a greater ability to survive in blood and peritoneal fluid. The determinants for serum resistance and ColV production are closely linked (Binns *et al.*, 1979). Similarly, plasmid genes associated with ColV encode a specific high-affinity iron-uptake mechanism that consists of aerobactin, a hydroxamate siderophore, and an inducible outer-membrane protein, which acts as a receptor for the ferric–aerobactin complex. In this way, the organism is able to multiply under iron-restricted conditions (see Chapter 12).

The ability of *E. coli* to grow under iron-limited conditions is highly correlated with its lethality for one-day-old chicks (Dho and Lafont, 1984). It has been shown with gene probes that the aerobactin gene system is present and expressed in virulent isolates but is absent from most avirulent avian *E. coli* isolates (Lafont *et al.*, 1987). Similarly, Ou Said *et al.* (1988) showed that most bacteraemia strains from calves produce aerobactin and are serum resistant. Aerobactin is released *in vivo* by *E. coli* in gnotobiotic lambs and assists in the spread of the organism from the mesenteric lymph nodes to other organs, where it can multiply and survive (Der Vartanian *et al.*, 1992).

Another independent plasmid, Vir, has been detected in an ovine strain of *E. coli* (Smith, 1974). Such strains produce a protein toxin that is lethal for mice, chickens and calves and, more recently, Oswald *et al.* (1989) have shown that CNF2 cytotoxicity is encoded by the Vir plasmid. They were, however, unable to ascribe a role to CNF2 in the aetiology of septicaemia (Oswald *et al.*, 1991). The Vir phenotype is also characterised by the production of a surface antigen (Smith, 1974) and Morris *et al.* (1982b) showed that Vir$^+$ strains of *E. coli* can attach *in vitro* to a number of cell preparations. Since Vir plasmids hybridise with F17A probes, it has been suggested that the Vir surface antigen may be a variant of the F17 adhesin, the molecular mass of their pilins is similar and both adhere to similar intestinal receptors (Oswald *et al.*, 1991).

Other surface antigens that are putative adhesins include CS31a (Contrepois *et al.*, 1986) and F165 (Fairbrother *et al.*, 1986), which were first identified in *E. coli* from calves and piglets respectively. Later, Contrepois *et al.*, (1989) showed that these antigens may occur on *E. coli* isolated from both species.

Fimbriae have been identified on *E. coli* from poultry (Nagaraja *et al.*, 1983), and it has been suggested that their virulence for turkeys is associated with better persistence in the respiratory tract (Arp *et al.*, 1980). Similarly, Dho & Lafont (1984) showed that 64 per cent of the *E. coli* strains that are lethal for one-day-old chickens adhere to isolated epithelial cells. Various types of fimbriae are expressed by *E. coli* strains of avian origin. Thus, type-1A-like fimbriae have been demonstrated to be present on O78 strains (Dho-Moulin *et al.*, 1990) and several type-1-like fimbriae have been described to be present on O1 strains (Suwanichkul and Panigrahy 1987). The heterogeneous nature of these fimbriae, with major subunits of different molecular weights, including serological variants, is similar to that of P-fimbriae (De Ree *et al.*, 1985). Recently, Van den Bosch *et al.* (1993) identified F11 fimbriae on avian strains of *E. coli* that belong to the class of P-fimbriae, but they were unable to link expression of F11 with adherence to chicken cells. The most commonly encountered serotypes associated with avian colibacillosis were O1:K1, O2:K1, O35 and O78:K80 and 96 per cent expressed F11.

Mastitis

Escherichia coli are an important cause of bovine mastitis. It was the most common cause in 45,000 incidents of mastitis in 378 herds in the United Kingdom (Wilesmith *et al.*, 1986). The subject has been extensively reviewed by Jones (1990) and only the most salient features will be presented here.

Many cases of *E. coli* mastitis are mild, with a transient increase in numbers of *E. coli* followed by rapid elimination of the organism, before clinical signs are apparent. The symptoms include clots, milk discoloration and swelling of the udder with little loss of milk production. At the other extreme, severe mastitis may occur shortly after parturition and result in death of the animal.

It has not been possible to distinguish *E. coli* strains that cause mastitis from strains in normal faeces. Amongst 279 *E. coli* isolates from cattle with mastitis, 67 different O-serogroups were demonstrated (Linton *et al.*, 1979) and a search for common virulence factors has been unrewarding (Wray *et al.*, 1983; Sanchez-Carlo *et al.*, 1984; Jones, 1990). It has been suggested that serum resistance is a possible factor (Carroll *et al.*, 1973) that correlates with the presence of a capsule (Ward & Sebunya, 1981). Endotoxin is regarded as playing a major role in the inflammatory response and the profound toxaemia that characterise the acute form of the disease (Frost & Brooker, 1983). A second toxin, which is cytotoxic, has been associated with necrosis of the superficial layer of the teat and lactiferous sinuses (Frost *et al.*, 1982). CNF-producing *E. coli* have been isolated from cases of bovine mastitis (Pohl *et al.*, 1993).

Adhesion of fimbriate *E. coli* to udder epithelium is not a feature of the isolates (Jones, 1990). However, *E. coli* isolated from bovine mastitis binds to fibronectin, mediated by the novel coiled surface structures called curli that were described above in the section entitled, 'other putative virulence factors' (Olsen *et al.*, 1989). Experimental mastitis can be produced by inoculating the mammary gland of lactating cows with as few as 50 viable *E. coli* cells and endotoxin infusion produces similar signs to those of the natural disease (Frost *et al.*, 1982).

A close relationship has been demonstrated between coliform contamination of bedding and the occurrence of coliform mastitis. This supports the current view that the *E. coli* that cause mastitis are environmental contaminants.

References

Aning, K. G., Thomlinson, J. R., Wray, C., Sojka, W. J. & Coulter, J. (1983). Adhesion factor distinct from K88, K99, 987P, CFAI and CFAII in porcine *Escherichia coli*. *Veterinary Record*, **112**, 251.

Anderson, D. G. & Moseley, S. L. (1988). *Escherichia coli* F41 adhesin: genetic organisation, nucleotide sequence, and homology with the K88 determinant. *Journal of Bacteriology*, **170**, 4890–6.

Arnquist, A., Olsen, A., Pfeifer, J., Russell, D. G. & Normark, S. (1992). The Crl protein activates cryptic genes for curli formation and fibronectin binding in *Escherichia coli* HB101. *Molecular Microbiology*, **6**, 2443–52.

Arp, L. H., Graham, C. L. G. & Cheville, N. F. (1979). Comparison of clearance rates of virulent and avirulent *Escherichia coli* in turkeys after aerosol exposure. *Avian Diseases*, **23**, 386–91.

Aubel, D., Darfeuille-Michand, A. & Joly, B. (1993). New adhesive factor (antigen 8786) on a human enterotoxigenic *Escherichia coli* O117:H4 strain isolated in Africa. *Infection and Immunity*, **59**, 1290–9.

Bakker, D. (1991). Studies on the K88 fimbriae of enteropathogenic *Escherichia coli*. PhD Thesis. Vrije Universiteit, Utrecht, The Netherlands.

Baldini, M. M., Kaper, J. B., Levine, M. M., Candy, D. C. A. & Moon, M. W. (1983). Plasmid-mediated adhesion in enteropathogenic *Escherichia coli* to HEp2 cells is not dependent on the presence of fimbriae. *Journal of Pediatric Gastroenterology and Nutrition*, **2**, 534–8.

Bertschinger, H. U., Bachmann, M., Mettler, C., Pospischil, A., Schraner, E. M., Stamm, M., Sydler, T. & Wild, P. (1990). Adhesive fimbriae produced in vivo by *Escherichia coli* O139:K12(B):H1 associated with enterotoxaemia in pigs. *Veterinary Microbiology*, **25**, 267–81.

Bertschinger, H. U., Stamm, M. & Vogeli, P. (1993). Inheritance of resistance to oedema disease in the pig: experiments with an *Escherichia coli* strain expressing fimbriae 107. *Veterinary Microbiology*, **35**, 79–89.

Bijlsma, S. W., de Nys, A. & Frik, J. F. (1981). Adherence of *Escherichia coli* to porcine intestinal brush borders by means of serological variants of the

K88 antigen. *Antonie van Leeuwenhoek Journal of Microbiology and Serology*, **47**, 467–8.

Binns, M. M., Davies, D. L. & Hardy, K. G. (1979). Cloned fragments of the plasmid Col V 1-K94 specifying virulence and serum resistance. *Nature*, **279**, 778–81.

Blackes, R. E., Brown, K. M., Becker, S., Abdul Alim, A. R. M. & Huq, I. (1982). Longitudinal studies of infectious diseases and physical growth of children in Rural Bangladesh. II. Incidence of diarrhoea and association with known pathogens. *American Journal of Epidemiology*, **115**, 315–24.

Blanco, J., Alonso, M. P., Gonsalez, E. A., Blanco, M. & Garabal, I. (1990). Virulence factors of bacteraemic *Escherichia coli* with particular reference to production of cytotoxic necrotising factor (CNF) by P-fimbriated strains. *Journal of Medical Microbiology*, **31**, 175–83.

Blanco, J., Gonzalez, E. A., Bernardez, I. & Requerio, B. (1983). Differential biological activities of Vero cytotoxins (VT) released by human and porcine *Escherichia coli* strains. *FEMS Microbiology Letters*, **20**, 167–70.

Blanco, M., Blanco, J., Blanco, J. E. & Ramos, J. (1993). Enterotoxigenic, verotoxigenic and necrotoxigenic *Escherichia coli* isolated from cattle in Spain. *American Journal of Veterinary Research*, **54**, 1446–51.

Blomberg, L., Krivan, H. C., Cohen, P. S. & Conway, P. L. (1993). Piglet ileal mucus contains protein and glycolipid (Galactosylceramide) receptors specific for *Escherichia coli* K88 fimbriae. *Infection and Immunity*, **61**, 2526–31.

Blomfield, I. C., Calie, P. J., Eberhardt, K. J., McClain, M. S. & Eisenstein, B. I. (1993). Lrp stimulates phase variation of type 1 fimbriation in *Escherichia coli* K-12. *Journal of Bacteriology*, **175**, 27–36.

Burghoff, R. L., Pattersen, L., Kragfelt, K. A., Newman, J. V., Richardson, M., Bliss, J. L., Laux, D. C. & Cohen, P. S. (1993). Utilisation of the mouse large intestine to select an *Escherichia coli*. *Infection and Immunity*, **61**, 1293–1300.

Caprioli, A., Donelli, G., Falbo, V., Possenti, R., Roda, L. G., Roscetti, G. & Ruggeri, F. M. (1984). A cell-division active protein from *Escherichia coli*. *Biochemistry and Biophysical Research Communications*, **118**, 587–93.

Caprioli, A., Falbo, V., Roda, L. G., Ruggeri, F. M. & Zona, C. (1983). Partial purification and characterisation of an *Escherichia coli* toxic factor that induces morphological cell alterations. *Infection and Immunity*, **39**, 1300–1306.

Caprioli, A., Falbo, V., Ruggeri, F. M., Baldassari, L., Biscchia, R., Ippolito, G., Romoli, E. & Donnelli, G. (1987). Cytotoxic necrotising factor production by hemolytic strains of *Escherichia coli* causing extra-intestinal infections. *Journal of Clinical Microbiology*, **25**, 146–9.

Carroll, E. J., Jain, N. C., Schalm, O. W. & Lasmanis, J. (1973). Experimentally induced coliform mastitis: inoculation of udders with serum-sensitive and serum-resistant organisms. *American Journal of Veterinary Research*, **34**, 1143–6.

Casey, T. A., Moseley, S. L. & Moon, H. W. (1990). Characterisation of bovine septicemic, bovine diarrhoeal and human enteroinvasive *Escherichia coli* that hybridise with K88 and F41 accessory gene probes but do not express these antigens. *Microbial Pathogenesis*, **8**, 383–92.

Casey, T. A., Nagy, B. & Moon, H. W. (1992). Pathogenicity of porcine enterotoxigenic *Escherichia coli* that do not express K88, K99, F41 or 987P adhesins. *American Journal of Veterinary Research*, **53**, 1488–92.

Casey, T. A., Schneider, R. A. & Dean-Nystrom, E. A. (1993). Identification of plasmid and chromosomal copies of 987P pilus genes in enterotoxigenic *Escherichia coli* 987. *Infection and Immunity*, **61**, 2249–52.

Chapman, P. A., Wright, D. J. & Norman, P. (1989). Verotoxin-producing *Escherichia coli* infection in Sheffield: cattle as a possible source. *Epidemiology and Infection*, **102**, 439–45.

Chart, H., Scotland, S. M., Willshaw, G. A. & Rowe, B. (1988). Hep2 adhesion by strains of *Escherichia coli* belonging to enteropathogenic serogroups. *Journal of General Microbiology*, **134**, 1315–21.

Collinson, S. K., Doig, P. C., Doran, J. L., Clouthier, S., Trust, T. J. & Kay, W. W. (1993). Thin aggregative fimbriae mediate binding of *Salmonella enteritidis* to fibronectin. *Journal of Bacteriology*, **175**, 12–18.

Collinson, S. K., Emody, L., Muller, K.-M., Trust, T. J. & Kay, W. W. (1991). Purification and characterisation of thin, aggregative fimbriae from *Salmonella enteritidis*. *Journal of Bacteriology*, **173**, 4773–81.

Collinson, S. K., Emody, L., Trust, T. J. & Kay, W. W. (1992). Thin aggregative fimbriae from diarrheagenic *Escherichia coli*. *Journal of Bacteriology*, **174**, 4490–5.

Contrepois, M., Dubourguier, H. C., Parodi, A. L., Girardeau, J.-P. & Ollier, J. L. (1986). Septicaemic *Escherichia coli* and experimental infections of calves. *Veterinary Microbiology*, **12**, 109–18.

Contrepois, M., Fairbrother, J. M., Kaura, Y. K. & Girardeau, J.-P. (1989). Prevalence of CS31A and F165 surface antigens in *Escherichia coli* isolates from animals in France, Canada and India. *FEMS Microbiology Letters*, **59**, 310–24.

Contrepois, M. & Girardeau, J.-P. (1985). Additive protective effects of colostral antipili antibodies in calves experimentally infected with enterotoxigenic *Escherichia coli*. *Infection and Immunity*, **50**, 947–9.

Cox, E. & Houvenaghel, A. (1987). *In vitro* adhesion of K88ab-, K88ac- and K88ad-positive *Escherichia coli* and intestinal villi, to buccal cells and to erythrocytes of weaned piglets. *Veterinary Microbiology*, **15**, 201–7.

Dean, E. A. & Isaacson, R. E. (1985). Purification and characterisation of a receptor for the 987P pilus of *Escherichia coli*. *Infection and Immunity*, **47**, 98–105.

Dean, E. A., Whipp, S. C. & Moon, H. W. (1987). The role of epithelial receptors for 987P pili in age-specific intestinal colonisation by enterotoxigenic *Escherichia coli*. In: *Advances in research on cholera and related diarrhoeas*, eds. R.B. Sack & Y. Zinnaka, Proceedings of the US-Japan Conference on Cholera. Tokyo: KTH Scientific.

Deprez, P., Van den Hende, C., Muylle, E. & Oyaert, W. (1986). The influence of the administration of sow's milk on the post-weaning excretion of the hemolytic *E. coli* in the pig. *Veterinary Research Communications*, **10**, 469–78.

De Ree, J. M., Schwillens, P. & Van den Bosch, J. F. (1985). Monoclonal antibodies that recognise the P-fimbriae $F7_1$, $F7_2$, F9 and F11 from uropathogenic *Escherichia coli*, *Infection and Immunity*, **50**, 900–4.

De Ree, J. M. & Van den Bosch, J. F. (1989). Fimbrial serotypes of *Escherichia coli* strains isolated from extra-intestinal infections. *Journal of Medical Microbiology*, **29**, 95–9.

De Rycke, J., Gonzalez, E. A., Blanco, J., Oswald, E., Blanco, M. & Boivin, R. (1990). Evidence for two types of cytotoxic necrotising factor in human and animal clinical isolates of *Escherichia coli*. *Journal of Clinical Microbiology*, **28**, 694–9.

De Rycke, J., Guillot, J. F. & Boivin, R. (1987). Cytotoxins in non-enterotoxigenic strains of *Escherichia coli* isolated from faeces of diarrhoeic calves. *Veterinary Microbiology*, **15**, 137–57.

De Rycke, J. & Plassiart, G. (1990). Toxic effects for lambs of cytotoxic necrotising factor from *Escherichia coli*. *Research in Veterinary Science*, **49**, 349–54.

Der Vartanian, M., Jaffeux, B., Contrepois, M., Chavarot, M., Girardeau, J.-P., Bertin, Y. & Martin, C. (1992). Role of aerobactin in systemic spread of an opportunistic strain of *Escherichia coli* from the intestinal tract of Gnotobiotic lambs. *Infection and Immunity*, **60**, 2800–7.

Dho, M. & Lafont, J. P. (1984). Adhesive properties and iron uptake ability in *Escherichia coli* lethal and nonlethal for chicks. *Avian Diseases*, **28**, 1016–25.

Dho-Moulin, M., Van den Bosch, J. F., Girardeau, J. P., Bree, A., Barat, T. & Lafont, J. P. (1990). Surface antigens from *Escherichia coli* O2 and O78 strains of avian origin. *Infection and Immunity*, **58**, 740–5.

Dobrescu, L. (1983). New biological effect of edema disease principle (*Escherichia coli* neurotoxin) and its use as an *in vitro* assay for this toxin. *American Journal of Veterinary Research*, **44**, 31–4.

Donnenberg, M. S., Giron, J. A., Nataro, J. P. & Kaper, J. B. (1992). A plasmid-encoded type IV fimbrial gene of enteropathogenic *Escherichia coli* associated with localised adherence. *Molecular Microbiology*, **6**, 3427–37.

Donohue-Rolphe, A., Keusch, G. T., Edson, C., Thorley-Lawson, D. & Jacewicz, M. (1984). Pathogenesis of *Shigella* diarrhoea. IX. Simplified high yield purification of *Shigella* toxin and characterisation of subunit composition and function by the use of monoclonal and polyclonal antibodies. *Journal of Experimental Medicine*, **160**, 1767–81.

Doran, J. L., Collinson, S. K., Burian, J., Sarlos, G., Todd, E. C. D., Munro, C. K., Kay, C. M., Banser, P. A., Peterkin, P. I. & Kay, W. W. (1993). DNA-based diagnostic tests for *Salmonella* species targeting *agfA*, the structural gene for thin aggregative fimbriae. *Journal of Clinical Microbiology*, **31**, 2263–73.

Dorman, C. J. & Higgins, C. F. (1987). Fimbrial phase variation in *Escherichia coli*: dependance upon integration host factor and homologies with other site-specific recombinases. *Journal of Bacteriology*, **169**, 3840–3.

Duchet-Suchaux, M., Menanteau, P. & Zijderveld, F. G. (1992). Passive protection against enterotoxigenic *Escherichia coli* strains by intravenous inoculation of dams with monoclonal antibodies against F41. *Infection and Immunity*, **60**, 2828–34.

Duff, J. P. & Hunt, B. W. (1989). Lambs die from porcine *E. coli*. *Veterinary Record*, **125**, 404.

Dykes, C. W., Halliday, I. J., Read, M. J., Hobden, A. N. & Harford, S. (1985). Nucleotide sequences of fair variants of the K88 gene of porcine *Escherichia coli*. *Infection and Immunity*, **50**, 279–83.

Espinasse, J., Navetat, H., Contrepois, M., Baroux, D. & Schelcher, F. (1991). A new diarrhoeic syndrome with ataxia in young Charolais calves: clinical and microbiological findings. *Veterinary Record*, **128**, 422–5.

Falbo, V., Famiglietti, M. & Caprioli, A. (1992). Gene block encoding production of Cytotoxic Necrotising Factor 1 and hemolysin in *Escherichia coli* isolates from extraintestinal infections. *Infection and Immunity*, **60**, 2182–7.

Fairbrother, J. M., Broes, A., Jacques, M. & Lariviere, S. (1989). Pathogenicity of *Escherichia coli* O115:K'V165' strains isolated from pigs with diarrhoea. *American Journal of Veterinary Research*, **50**, 1029–36.

Fairbrother, J. M., Lallier, R., Leblanc, L., Jacques, M. & Lariviere, S. (1988). Production and purification of *Escherichia coli* fimbrial antigen F165. *FEMS Microbiology Letters*, **56**, 247–52.

Fairbrother, J. M., Lariviere, S. & Lallier, R. (1986). New fimbrial antigen F165 on *Escherichia coli* serogroup O115 strains isolated from piglets with diarrhoea. *Infection and Immunity*, **51**, 10–15.

Francis, D. H., Allen, S. D. & White, R. G. (1989). Influence of bovine intestinal fluid on the expression of K99 pili by *Escherichia coli*. *American Journal of Veterinary Research*, **50**, 822–6.

Frost, A. J. & Brooker, B. E. (1983). The effect of *Escherichia coli* endotoxin and culture filtrate on the dry bovine mammary gland. *Journal of Comparative Pathology*, **93**, 211–18.

Frost, A. J., Hill, A. W. & Brooker, B. E. (1982). Pathogenesis of experimental bovine mastitis following a small inoculum of *Escherichia coli*. *Research in Veterinary Science*, **33**, 105–12.

Gally, D. L., Bogan, J. A., Eisenstein, B. I. & Blomfield, I. C. (1993). Environmental regulation of the fim switch controlling type 1 phase variation in *Escherichia coli* K-12: effects of temperature and media. *Journal of Bacteriology*, **175**, 6186–93.

Gannon, V. P. J., Gyles, C. L. & Wilcock, B. P. (1989). Effects of *Escherichia coli* Shiga-like toxins (verotoxins) in pigs. *Canadian Journal of Veterinary Research*, **53**, 306–12.

Geary, S. J., Marchlewicz, B. A. & Finkelstein, R. A. (1982). Comparison of heat labile enterotoxin from porcine and human strains of *E. coli*. *Infection and Immunity*, **36**, 215–20.

Girardeau, J.-P., Dubourguier, H. C. & Contrepois, M. (1980). Attachement des *E. coli* enteropathogènes à la muqueuse intestinale. *Bulletin des Groupements Techniques Vétérinaires*, **4B**, 190, 49.

Girardeau, J.-P., der Vartanian M., Ollier, J. L. & Contrepois, M. (1988). CS31A, a new K88-related fimbrial antigen on bovine enterotoxigenic and septicaemic *Escherichia coli* strains. *Infection and Immunity*, **56**, 2180–8.

Giron, J. A., Ho, A. S. & Schoonik, G. K. (1991). An inducible bundle-forming pilus of enteropathogenic *Escherichia coli*. *Science*, **254**, 710–13.

Gonzalez, E. A. & Blanco, J. (1985). Production of cytotoxin VT in enteropathogenic and non-enteropathogenic *Escherichia coli* strains of porcine origin. *FEMS Microbiology Letters*, **26**, 127–30.

Green, B. A., Neill, R. J., Ruyechan, W. T. & Holmes, R. K. (1983). Evidence that a new enterotoxin of *E. coli* which activates adenyl cyclase in eukaryotic target cells is not plasmid mediated. *Infection and Immunity*, **41**, 383–90.

Hall, G. A., Chanter, N. & Bland, A. P. (1988). Comparison in gnotobiotic pigs of lesions caused by verotoxigenic and non-verotoxigenic *Escherichia coli*. *Veterinary Pathology*, **25**, 205–10.

Harel, J., Forget, C., Saint-Amand, J., Daigle, F., Dubreuil, D., Jacques, M. & Fairbrother, J. M. (1992). Molecular cloning of a determinant coding for fimbrial antigen F1651, a Prs-like fimbrial antigen from porcine septicaemic *Escherichia coli*. *Journal of General Microbiology*, **138**, 1495–502.

Harel, J., Lapointe, H., Fallora, A., Lartie, L. A., Bigras-Poulin, M., Lariviere, S. & Fairbrother, J. M. (1991). Detection of genes for fimbrial antigens and enterotoxins associated with *Escherichia coli* serogroups isolated from pigs with diarrhoea. *Journal of Clinical Microbiology*, **29**, 745–52.

Harnett, N. M. & Gyles, C. L. (1983). Enterotoxigenicity of bovine and porcine *Escherichia coli* of O groups 8, 9, 20, 64, 101 and X46. *American Journal of Veterinary Research*, **43**, 41–9.

Harnett, N. M. & Gyles, C. L. (1985). Enterotoxin plasmids in Bovine and Porcine enterotoxigenic *Escherichia coli* O groups 9, 20, 64 and O101. *Canadian Journal of Comparative Medicine*, **49**, 79–87.

Holland, R. E. (1990). Some infectious causes of diarrhoea in young farm animals. *Clinical Microbiology Reviews*, **3**, 345–75.

Holmes, R. K., Twiddy, E. M. & Pickett, C. L. (1986). Purification and characterisation of type II heat-labile enterotoxin of *E. coli*. *Infection and Immunity*, **53**, 464–73.

Honda, T., Tsuji, T., Takeda, Y. & Miwantani, T. (1981). Immunological non-identity of heat labile enterotoxins from human and porcine enteropathogenic *E. coli*. *Infection and Immunity*, **34**, 337–40.

Imbrechts, H., De Greve, H. & Lintermans, P. (1992a). The pathogenesis of oedema disease in pigs: a review. *Veterinary Microbiology*, **31**, 221–33.

Imbrechts, H., De Greve, H., Schliker, C., Bouchet, H., Pohl, P., Charlier, G., Bertschinger, H., Wild, P., Van Dekerckhove, J., Van Damme, J., Van Montagu, M. & Lintermans, P. (1992b). Characterisation of F107 fimbriae of *Escherichia coli* 107/86, which causes Edema Disease in pigs and nucleotide sequence of the F107 major fimbrial subunit gene *fedA*. *Infection and Immunity*, **60**, 1963–71.

Issacson, R. E., Nagy, B. & Moon, H. W. (1977). Colonisation of porcine small intestine by *Escherichia coli*: colonisation and adhesion factors of pig enteropathogens that lacks K88. *Journal of Infectious Diseases*, **135**, 531–9.

Jerse, A. E., Yu, J., Tall, B. D. & Kaper, J. B. (1990). A genetic loci of enteropathogenic *E. coli* necessary for the production of attaching and effacing lesions in tissue culture cells. *Proceedings of the National Academy of Science, USA*, **87**, 7839–43.

Jones, T. O. (1990). *Escherichia coli* mastitis in dairy cattle–a review of the literature. *Veterinary Bulletin*, **60**, 205–31.

Karmali, M. A. (1989). Infection by verocytotoxin-producing *Escherichia coli*. *Clinical Microbiological Reviews*, **2**, 15–38.

Kausche, F. M., Dean, E. A., Arp, L. H., Samuel, J. E. & Moon, H. W. (1992). An experimental model for subclinical edema disease (*Escherichia coli* enterotoxemia) manifest as vascular necrosis in pigs. *American Journal of Veterinary Research*, **53**, 281–7.

Kawula, T. H. & Orndorff, P. E. (1991). Rapid site-specific DNA inversion in *Escherichia coli* mutants lacking the histone-like protein. *Journal of Bacteriology*, **173**, 4116–23.

Kearns, M. J. & Gibbons, R. A. (1979). The possible nature of the pig intestinal receptor for the K88 antigen of *Escherichia coli*. *FEMS Microbiology Letters*, **6**, 165–8.

Kennan, R. M. & Monckton, R. P. (1990). Adhesive fimbriae associated with porcine enterotoxigenic *Escherichia coli* of the O141 serotype. *Journal of Clinical Microbiology*, **28**, 2006–11.

Klaasen, P., Woodward, M. J., Zijderveld, F. & de Graaf, F. K. (1990). The 987P gene cluster in enterotoxigenic *E. coli* contains an Stpa transposon that activates 987P expression. *Infection and Immunity*, **58**, 801–7.

Konowalchuk, J., Speirs, J. I. & Stavrik, S. (1977). Vero response to a cytotoxin of *Escherichia coli*. *Infection and Immunity*, **18**, 775–9.

Korth, M. J., Schneider, R. A. & Moseley, S. L. (1991). An F41-K88-related genetic determinant of bovine septicaemic *Escherichia coli* mediates expression of CS31A fimbriae and adherence to epithelial cells. *Infection and Immunity*, **59**, 2333–40.

Lafont, J. P., Dho, M., D'Hauteville, H. M., Bree, A. & Sansonetti, P. J. (1987). Presence and expression of aerobactin genes in virulent avian strains of *Escherichia coli*. *Infection and Immunity*, **55**, 193–7.

Lecce, J. G., Balsbaugh, R. K., Clare, D. A. & King, M. W. (1982). Rotavirus and hemolytic enteropathogenic *Escherichia coli* in weanling diarrhoea of pigs. *Journal of Clinical Microbiology*, **16**, 715–23.

Leite, D. S., Yano, T. & Pestana De Castro, A. F. (1988). Production, purification and partial characterisation of a new adhesive factor (F42) produced by enterotoxigenic *Escherichia coli* isolated from pigs. *Annals de l'Institut Pasteur, Microbiology*, **139**, 295–306.

Lingood, M. A. & Thompson, J. M. (1987). Verotoxin production among porcine strains of *Escherichia coli* and its association with oedema disease. *Journal of Medical Microbiology*, **25**, 359–62.

Lintermans, P. F., Pohl, P., Bertels, A., Charlier, G., Van Dekerckhove, J., Van Damme, J., Schoup, J., Sscliker, C., Korhonen, T., De Greve, H. & Van Montagu, M. (1988). Characterisation and purification of the F17 adhesin on the surface of bovine enteropathogenic and septicemic *Escherichia coli*. *American Journal of Veterinary Research*, **49**, 1794–9.

Linton, A. H., Howe, K., Sojka, W. J. & Wray, C. (1979). A note on the range of *Escherichia coli* O-serotypes causing clinical bovine mastitis and their antibiotic resistance spectra. *Journal of Applied Bacteriology*, **46**, 585–90.

Macleod, D. L. & Gyles, C. L. (1989). Effects of culture condtions on yield of Shiga-like toxin IIv from *Escherichia coli*. *Canadian Journal of Microbiology*, **35**, 623–9.

Macleod, D. L. & Gyles, C. L. (1990). Purification and characterisation of an *Escherichia coli* Shiga-like toxin-II variant. *Infection and Immunity*, **58**, 1232–9.

Macleod, D. L., Gyles, C. L. & Wilcock, B. P. (1991). Reproduction of edema disease of swine with purified Shiga-like toxin-II variant. *Veterinary Pathology*, **28**, 66–73.

Mainil, J. G., Jacquemin, E. R., Kaeckenbeeck, A. E. & Pohl, P. (1993). Association between the effacing (eae) gene and the Shiga-like toxin-encoding genes in *cherichia coli* isolates from cattle. *American Journal of Veterinary Research*, **54**, 1064–8.

Mainil, J. G., Sadowski, P. L., Tarsio, M. & Moon, H. W. (1987). *In vivo* emergence of enterotoxigenic *Escherichia coli* variants lacking genes for K99 fimbriae and heat-stable enterotoxin. *Infection and Immunity*, **55**, 3111–16.

Marques, L. R. M., Peiris, J. S. M., Cryz, S. J. & O'Brien, A. D. (1987). *Escherichia coli* strains isolated from pigs with edema disease produce a variant of Shiga-like toxin II. *FEMS Microbiology Letters*, **44**, 33–8.

May, A., Block, C. A., Sawyer, R. G., Spengler, M. D. & Pruett, T. L. (1993). Enhanced virulence of *Escherichia coli* bearing a site-targetted mutation on the major structural subunit of type 1 fimbriae. *Infection and Immunity*, **61**, 1667–73.

McCormick, B. A., Klemm, P., Krogfelt, K. A., Burghoff, R. L., Pallesen, L. Laux, D. C. & Cohen, P. S. (1993). *Escherichia coli* F-18 place locked 'on' for expression of type 1 fimbriae is a poor coloniser of the streptomycin-treated mouse large intestine. *Microbial Pathogenesis*, **14**, 33–43.

McLaren, I. & Wray, C. (1986). Another animal *E. coli* cytopathic factor. *Veterinary Record*, **119**, 576–7.

Methiyapun, S., Panlenz, J. F. L. & Bertschinger, H. U. (1984). Ultrastructure of the intestinal mucosa in pigs experimentally inoculated with an edema disease producing strain of *Escherichia coli* (O139:K12:H1). *Veterinary Pathology*, **21**, 516–20.

Miller, B. G., Newby, T. J., Stokes, C. R. & Bourne, F. J. (1984). Influence of diet on post-weaning malabsorption and diarrhoea in the pig. *Research in Veterinary Science*, **36**, 187–93.

Montenegro, M. A., Bulte, M., Trumpf, T., Aleksic, S., Reuter, G., Bulling, B. & Helmuth, R. (1990). Detection and characterisation of faecal verotoxin-producing *Escherichia coli* from healthy cattle. *Journal of Clinical Microbiology*, **28**, 1417–21.

Moon, H. W. (1990). Colonisation factor antigens of enterotoxigenic *Escherichia coli* in animals. *Current Topics in Microbiology and Immunology*, **151**, 147–65.

Moon, H. W., Whipp, S. C., Argenzio, R. A., Levine, M. M. & Giannarella, R. A. (1983). Attaching and effacing activities of rabbit and human enteropathogenic *Escherichia coli* in pig and rabbit intestine. *Infection and Immunity*, **41**, 1340–51.

Morris, J. A. & Sojka, W. J. (1985). *Escherichia coli* as a pathogen in animals. In *The Virulence of Escherichia coli*, ed. M. Sussman, pp. 47–77. London: Academic Press.

Morris, J. A., Thorns, C. J., Scott, A. C. & Sojka, W. J. (1982b). Properties associated with the Vir plasmid: a transmissible pathogenic characteristic associated with strains of invasive *Escherichia coli*. *Journal of General Microbiology*, **128**, 2097–103.

Morris, J. A., Thorns, C. J., Scott, A. C., Sojka, W. J. & Wells, G. A. (1982a). Adhesion *in vivo* associated with an adhesive antigen (F41) produced by a K99 mutant of the reference strain *Escherichia coli* B41. *Infection and Immunity*, **36**, 1146–53.

Moseley, S. L., Dougan, G., Schneider, R. A. & Moon, H. W. (1986). Cloning of chromosomal DNA encoding the F41 adhesin of enterotoxigenic *Escherichia coli* and genetic homology between adhesins F41 and K88. *Journal of Bacteriology*, **167**, 799–804.

Mouricout, M. & Julian, R. (1987). Pilus mediated binding of bovine enterotoxigenic *Escherichia coli* to calf small intestinal mucins. *Infection and Immunity*, **55**, 1216–23.

Mouricout, M., Petit, J. M., Carias, J. R. & Julian, R. (1990). Glycoprotein glycans that inhibit adhesion of *Escherichia coli* mediated by K99 fimbriae: treatment of experimental colibacillosis. *Infection and Immunity*, **58**, 98–106.

Murray, C. J. (1987). *Salmonella* and *Escherichia coli* from veterinary and human sources in Australia during 1985 and 1986. *Australian Veterinary Journal*, **64**, 256–7.

Nabuurs, M. J. A., Van Zijderveld, F. G. & De Leeuw, P. W. (1993). Clinical and microbiological field studies in The Netherlands of diarrhoea in pigs at weaning. *Research in Veterinary Science*, **55**, 70–7.

Nagaraja, K. V., Enery, D. A., Newman, J. A. & Pomeroy, B. S. (1983). Identification and isolation of somatic pili from pathogenic *Escherichia coli* of turkeys. *American Journal of Veterinary Research*, **44**, 284–7.

Nagelcka, M., Jacques, M., Martineau-Doize, B., Daigle, F., Harel, J. & Fairbrother, J. M. (1993). Pathogenicity of an *Escherichia coli* O115:K'V165' mutant negative for F165, fimbriae in septicemia of gnotobiotic pigs. *Infection and Immunity*, **61**, 836–43.

Nagy, B., Casey, T. A. & Moon, H. W. (1990). Phenotype and genotype of *Escherichia coli* isolated from pigs with post-weaning diarrhoea in Hungary. *Journal of Clinical Microbiology*, **28**, 651–3.

Nagy, B., Casey, T. A., Whipp, S. C. & Moon, H. W. (1992). Susceptibility of porcine intestine to Pilus-mediated adhesion by some isolates of piliated enterotoxigenic *Escherichia coli* increases with age. *Infection and Immunity*, **60**, 1285–94.

Nielsen, N. O. & Clugston, R. E. (1971). Comparison of *E. coli* endotoxin shock and acute oedema disease in young pigs. *Annals of the New York Academy of Science*, **176**, 176–89.

O'Brien, A. D., La Veck, G. D., Thompson, M. R. & Formal, S. B. (1982). Production of *Shigella dysenteriae* type 1-like cytotoxin by *Escherichia coli*. *Journal of Infectious Diseases*, **146**, 763–9.

Olsen, A., Arnquist, A., Hammer, M., Sukupolvi, S. & Normark, S. (1993). The RpoS sigma factor relieves H-NS-mediated transcriptional repression of csgA, the subunit gene of fibronectin-binding curli in *Escherichia coli*. *Molecular Microbiology*, 7, 523–36.

Olsen, A., Jonsson, A. & Normark, S. (1989). Fibronectin binding mediated by a novel class of surface organelles on *Escherichia coli*. *Nature*, **338**, 652–5.

Oswald, E. & De Rycke, J. (1990). A single protein of 110 kDa is associated with the multinucleating and necrotising activity coded by the Vir plasmid of *Escherichia coli*. *FEMS Microbiology Letters*, **68**, 279–84.

Oswald, E., De Rycke, J., Guillot, J. F. & Bolvin, R. (1989). Cytotoxic effect of multinucleation in HeLa cell cultures associated with the presence of Vir plasmid in *Escherichia coli*. *FEMS Microbiology Letters*, **58**, 95–100.

Oswald, E., De Rycke, J., Lintermans, P., Van Muylem, K., Mainil, J., Daube, G. & Pohl, P. (1991). Virulence factors associated with cytotoxic necrotising factor two (CNF2) in bovine diarrheic and septicemic strains of *Escherichia coli*. *Journal of Clinical Microbiology*, **29**, 2522–7.

Ou Said, A. M., Contrepois, M. G., Der Vartanian, M. & Girardeau, J. P. (1988). Virulence factors and markers in *Escherichia coli* from calves with bacteremia. *American Journal of Veterinary Research*, **49**, 1657–60.

Pearson, G. R., Watson, C. A., Hall, G. A. & Wray, C. (1989). Natural infection with an attaching and effacing *Escherichia coli* in the small and large intestines of a calf with diarrhoea. *Veterinary Record*, **124**, 297–9.

Penhale, W. J., McEwan, A. D., Selman, I. & Fisher, E. W. (1970). Quantitative studies on bovine immunoglobulins. II. Plasma immunoglobulin levels in market calves and their relationship to neonatal infection. *British Veterinary Journal*, **126**, 30–7.

Pickett, C. L., Twiddy, E. M., Belisle, B. W. & Holmes, R. K. (1986). Cloning of genes that encode a new heat-labile enterotoxin of *Escherichia coli*. *Journal of Bacteriology*, **165**, 348–52.

Pohl, P., Lintermans, P., Moury, J., Van Muylem, K. & Marin, M. (1986). Facteurs de virulence chez les *Escherichia coli* septicemiques et saprophytes du veau. *Annales de Médicine Vétérinaire*, **130**, 515–20.

Pohl, P., Lintermans, P. & Van Muylem, K. (1984). Fréquence des adhésines K99 et Att 25 chez les *E. coli* du veau. *Annales de Médicine Vétérinaire*, **128**, 555–8.

Pohl, P., Lintermans, P., Van Muylem, K. & Schotte, M. (1982). Colibacilles entérotoxigenes du veau possédent un antigène d'attachment différent de l'antigène K99. *Annales de Médicine Vétérinaire*, **126**, 569–71.

Pohl, P., Mainil, J., Devriese, L., Haesebrouck, F., Broes, A., Lintermans, P. & Oswald, E. (1992). *Escherichia coli* productrices de la toxine cytotoxique nécrosant de type 1 (CNF1) isolées à partir de processus pathologiques chez des chats et des chiens. *Annales de Médicine Vétérinaire*, **137**, 21–5.

Pohl, P., Oswald, E., Van Muylem, K., Jacquemin, E., Lintermans, P. & Mainil, J. (1993). *Escherichia coli* producing CNF1 and CNF2 cytotoxins in animals with different disorders. *Veterinary Research*, **24** (4)

Prada, J., Baljer, G., De Rycke, J., Steinrück, H., Zimmermann, S., Stephan, R. & Beutin, L. (1991). Characteristics of α-haemolytic strains of *Escherichia coli* isolated from dogs with gastro-enteritis. *Veterinary Microbiology*, **29**, 59–73.

Provence, D. L. & Curtiss, R. (1992). Role of *crl* in avian pathogneic *Escherichia coli*: a knockout mutation of *crl* does not affect hemagglutination activity, fibronectin binding or curli production. *Infection and Immunity*, **60**, 4460–7.

Runnels, P. L., Moon, H. W. & Schneider, R. A. (1980). Development of resistance with host age to adhesion of K99+ *Escherichia coli* to isolated intestinal epithelial cells. *Infection and Immunity*, **28**, 298–300.

Salajka, E., Salajkova, Z., Alexa, P. & Hornich, M. (1992). Colonisation factor different from K88, K99, F41 and 987P in enterotoxigenic *Escherichia coli* strains isolated from post-weaning diarrhoea in pigs. *Veterinary Microbiology*, **32**, 163–75.

Sanchez-Carlo, V., McDonald, J. S. & Packer, R. A. (1984). Virulence factors of *Escherichia coli* isolated from cows with acute mastitis. *American Journal of Veterinary Research*, **45**, 1775–7.

Sarmiento, J. I., Casey, T. A. & Moon, H. W. (1988a). Postweaning diarrhea in swine: experimental model of enterotoxigenic *Escherichia coli* infection. *American Journal of Veterinary Research*, **49**, 1154–9.

Sarmiento, J. I., Dean, E. A. & Moon, H. W. (1988b). Effects of weaning on diarrhea caused by enterotoxigenic *Escherichia coli* in three-week-old pigs. *American Journal of Veterinary Research*, **49**, 2030–3.

Sarmiento, J. I., Runnels, P. L. & Moon, H. W. (1990). Effects of preweaning exposure to a starter diet on enterotoxigenic *Escherichia coli*-induced postweaning diarrhea in swine. *American Journal of Veterinary Research*, **51**, 1180–3.

Saxena, S. K., O'Brien, A. D. & Ackerman, E. J. (1989). Shiga toxin, Shiga-like toxin II variant and ricin are all single-site RNA N-glycosidases of 28 S RNA when microinjected into *Xenopus* oocytes. *Journal of Biological Chemistry*, **264**, 596–601.

Schifferli, D. M., Beachey, E. H. & Taylor, R. K. (1990). The 987P fimbrial gene cluster of enterotoxigenic *Escherichia coli* is plasmid encoded. *Infection and Immunity*, **58**, 149–56.

Schimmelpfennig, H.-H. (1970). Untersuchungen zur Aetiologie der Oedemkrankheit des Schweines. *Fortschritte der Veterinarmedizin*, **13**, 1–80.

Scotland, S. M., Smith, H. R. & Rowe, B. (1985). Two distinct toxins active on Vero cells from *Escherichia coli* O157. *Lancet*, **2**, 885–6.

Scotland, S. M., Smith, H. R., Willshaw, G. A. & Rowe, B. (1983). Vero cytotoxin production in a strain of *Escherichia coli* is determined by genes carried on a bacteriophage. *Lancet*, **2**, 216.

Sellwood, R., Gibbons, R. A., Jones, G. W. & Rutter, M. J. (1975). Adhesion of enteropathogenic *Escherichia coli* to pig intestines brush borders: the existence of two pig phenotypes. *Journal of Medical Microbiology*, **8**, 405–11.

Seriwatana, J., Echeverria, P., Taylor, D. N., Rasrinant, L., Brown, E. J., Peiris, J. S. M. & Clayton, C. L. (1988). Type II heat-labile enterotoxin-producing *E. coli* isolated from animals and humans. *Infection and Immunity*, **56**, 1158–61.

Shanks, P. L. (1938). An unusual condition affecting the digestive organs of the pig. *Veterinary Record*, **50**, 356–8.

Sivasvamy, G. & Gyles, C. L. (1976). The prevalence of enterotoxigenic *Escherichia coli* in faeces of calves with diarrhoea. *Canadian Journal of Comparative Medicine*, **40**, 241–6.

Smith, H. R., Scotland, S. M., Willshaw, G. A., Wray, C., McLaren, I. M., Cheasty, T. & Rowe, B. (1988). Vero cytotoxin production and presence of VT genes in *Escherichia coli* strains of animal origin. *Journal of General Microbiology*, **134**, 829–34.

Smith, H. W. (1974). A search for transmissible pathogenic characters in invasive strains of *Escherichia coli*: the discovery of a plasmid-controlled toxin and a plasmid controlled lethal character closely associated or identical with Colicine V. *Journal of General Microbiology*, **83**, 95–111.

Smith, H. W., Green, P. & Parsell, Z. (1983). Vero cell toxins in *Escherichia coli* and related bacteria: transfer by phage and conjugation and toxic action in laboratory animals, chickens and pigs. *Journal of General Microbiology*, **129**, 3121–37.

Smith, H. W. & Gyles, C. L. (1970). The relationship between two apparently different enterotoxins produced by enteropathogenic strains of *Escherichia coli* of porcine origin. *Journal of Medical Microbiology*, **3**, 387–401.

Smith, H. W. & Halls, S. (1968). The production of oedema disease and diarrhoea in weaned pigs by the oral administration of *Escherichia coli*: factors that influence the course of experimental disease. *Journal of Medical Microbiology*, **1**, 45–59.

Smith, H. W. & Linggood, M. L. (1971). Observation on the pathogenic properties of the K88, Hly and Ent plasmids of enteropathogenic *Escherichia coli* with particular reference to porcine diarrhoea. *Journal of Medical Microbiology*, **11**, 471–92.

Soderlind, O., Olsson, E., Smyth, C. J. & Mollby, R. (1982). Effects of parenteral vaccination of dams on intestinal *Escherichia coli* in piglets with diarrhoea. *Infection and Immunity*, **36**, 900–6.

Soderlind, O., Thafvelin, B. & Mollby, R. (1988). Virulence factors in *Escherichia coli* strains isolated from Swedish pigs with diarrhoea. *Journal of Clinical Microbiology*, **26**, 879–84.

Sohel, I., Puente, J. L., Murray, W. J., Vupio-Varkila, J. & Schoolnik, G. A. (1993). Cloning and characterisation of bundle-forming pilin gene of enteropathogenic *Escherichia coli* and its distribution in Salmonella serotypes. *Molecular Microbiology*, 7, 563–75.

Sojka, W. J. (1965). *Escherichia coli in domestic animals and poultry*, pp. 104–124. Farnham Royal, Bucks, England: Commonwealth Agricultural Bureaux.

Sojka, W. J. (1971). Enteric disease in newborn piglets, calves and lambs due to *Escherichia coli* infection. *Veterinary Bulletin*, 41, 509–22.

Sojka, W. J., Wray, C. & Morris, J. A. (1978). Passive protection in lambs against experimental colibacillosis by colostral transfer of antibodies from K99 vaccinated ewes. *Journal of Medical Microbiology*, 11, 493–9.

Sourindra, N. M., Harel, J. & Fairbrother, J. M. (1993). Structure and copy number analyses of pap, sfa and afa related gene clusters in F165 positive bovine and porcine *Escherichia coli* isolates. *Infection and Immunity*, 61, 2453–61.

Suwanichkul, A. & Panigrahy, B. (1987). Diversity of pilus subunits of *Escherichia coli* isolated from avian species. *Avian Diseases*, 32, 822–5.

Svendsen, J. & Larsen, J. L. (1977). Studies of the pathogenesis of enteric *Escherichia coli* infections in weaned pigs. The significance of the milk of the dam. *Nordisk Veterinaer Medicine*, 29, 533–8.

Synge, B. A. & Hopkins, G. F. (1992). Verotoxigenic *Escherichia coli* O157 in Scottish cattle. *Veterinary Record*, 130, 583.

Tesh, V. L. & O'Brien, A. D. (1992). Adherence and colonisation mechanisms of enteropathogenic and enterohemorrhagic *Escherichia coli*. *Microbial Pathogenesis*, 12, 245–54.

Thomlinson, J. R. (1969). Post-weaning enteritis and dysentery. *Veterinary Record*, 85, 298–300.

Timoney, F. (1950). Oedema disease of swine. *Veterinary Record*, 62, 748–56.

Tokhi, A. M., Peiris, J. S. M., Scotland, S. M., Willshaw, G. A., Smith, H. R. & Cheasty, T. (1993). A longitudinal study of Vero cytotoxin producing *Escherichia coli* in cattle calves in Sri Lanka. *Epidemiology and Infection*,. 110, 197–208.

Turcotte, C. & Woodward, M. J. (1993). Cloning, DNA nucleotide sequence and distribution of the gene encoding the SEF14 fimbrial antigen of *Salmonella enteritidis*. *Journal of General Microbiology*, 139, 1477–85.

Van den Bosch, J. F., Hendriks, J. H. I. M., Gladigau, I., Willems, H. M. C., Storm, P. K. & de Graaf, F. K. (1993). Identification of F11 fimbriae in chicken *Escherichia coli* strains. *Infection and Immunity*, 61, 800–6.

Varga, J. (1991). Characterisation of a new fimbrial antigen present in *Escherichia coli* strains isolated from calves. *Journal of Veterinary Medicine*, B38, 689–700.

Ward, G. E. & Sebunya, T. K. (1981). Somatic and capsular factors of coliforms which affect resistance to bovine serum bactericidal activity. *American Journal of Veterinary Research*, 42, 1937–40.

Wells, J. G., Shipman, L. D., Greene, K. D., Sowers, E. G., Green, J. H., Cameron, D. N., Downes, F. P., Martin, M. L., Griffin, P. M., Ostroff, S. M., Potter, M. E., Tauxe, R. V. & Wachsmuth, I. K. (1991). Isolation of *Escherichia coli* O157:H7 and other Shiga-like toxin producing *E. coli* from dairy cattle. *Journal of Clinical Microbiology*, 29, 985–9.

Westerlund, B. & Karkonen, T. K. (1993). Bacterial proteins binding to the mammalian extracellular matrix. *Molecular Microbiology*, 9, 687–94.

Wilesmith, J. W., Francis, P. G. & Wilson, C. D. (1986). Incidence of clinical mastitis in a cohort of British dairy herds. *Veterinary Record*, **118**, 199–204.

Willemsen, P. T. J. & de Graaf, F. K. (1993). Multivalent binding of K99 fimbriae to the N-glycolyl-GM3 ganglioside receptor. *Infection and Immunity*, **61**, 4518–22.

Wittig, W. & Fabricius, C. (1992). *Escherichia coli* types isolated from porcine *E. coli* infections in Saxony from 1963 to 1990. *Zentralblatt für Bakteriologie A*, **277**, 389–402.

Wittig, W., Prager, R., Stamm, M., Strekel, W. & Tschäpe, H. (1994). Expression and plasmid transfer of genes coding for the fimbrial antigen F107 in porcine *Escherichia coli* strains. *Zentralblatt für Bakteriologie A*, **281**, 130–9.

Woodward, J. M., Connaughton, I. D., Fahy, V. A., Lymberg, A. J. & Hampson, D. J. (1993). Clonal analysis of *Escherichia coli* of serogroups O9, O20 and O101 isolated from Australian pigs with neonatal diarrhoea. *Journal of Clinical Microbiology*, **31**, 1185–8.

Wray, C., Callow, R. J. & Sojka, W. J. (1983). An examination of *Escherichia coli* strains isolated from cases of bovine mastitis for possible virulence determinants. *Veterinary Microbiology*, **8**, 141–5.

Wray, C., McLaren, I. M. & Carroll, P. J. (1993a). *Escherichia coli* isolated from farm animals in England and Wales between 1986 and 1991. *Veterinary Record*, **133**, 439–42.

Wray, C., Piercy, D. W. T., Carroll, P. J. & Cooley, W. A. (1993b). Experimental infection of neonatal pigs with CNF toxin-producing strains of *Escherichia coli*. *Research in Veterinary Science*, **54**, 290–8.

Wray, C., Piercy, D. W. T., Carroll, P. J., Johnson, C. T. & Higgins, R. J. (1992). Bovine haemorrhagic colitis associated with CNF+ and F6+ (987p) *E. coli*. *Veterinary Record*, **131**, 220.

Wright, D. J., Chapman, P. A. & Siddow, C. A. (1994). Immunomagnetic separation as a sensitive method for isolating *Escherichia coli* O157 from food samples. *Epidemiology and Infection*, **113**, 31–9.

Yano, T., Leite, D. D. S., De Carmargo, I. J. B. & De Castro, A. F. P. (1986). A probable new adhesive factor (F42) produced by enterotoxigenic *Escherichia coli* isolated from pigs. *Microbiology and Immunology*, **30**, 495–508.

Yatsudo, T., Nakabayashi, N., Hirayama, T. & Takeda, Y. (1987). Purification and some properties of a Vero toxin from *Escherichia coli* O157:H7 that is immunologically unrelated to Shiga toxin. *Microbial Pathogenesis*, **3**, 21–30.

Zhu, C., Harel, J., Jacques, M., Desautels, C., Donnenberg, M. S., Beaudry, M. & Fairbrother, J. M. (1994). Virulence properties and attaching-effacing activity of *Escherichia coli* O45 from swine postweaning diarrhea. *Infection and Immunity*, **62**, 4153–9.

3

Escherichia coli in the normal flora of humans and animals

K. A. BETTELHEIM

Inter faeces urinumque homo est natus.
Man is born between the faeces and the urine.
(Latin Proverb)

The dual nature of *Escherichia coli* as pathogen and commensal has long intrigued microbiologists. When Escherich first studied the faecal flora of neonates, he did so to gain a better understanding of the pathogenesis of enteric infections (Escherich, 1885, 1988; Bettelheim, 1986). As a result he discovered what he called *Bacterium coli commune,* which now bears his name as *Escherichia coli* and this species is now known to be closely related to the enteric pathogens *Shigella* and *Salmonella.* The need to differentiate between 'commensal' *E. coli* and bowel pathogens at first led to the development of the biochemical tests that became the basis of modern bacterial taxonomy, notably the taxonomy of the Enterobacteriaceae in general and *E. coli* in particular. The Enterobacteriaceae have been redefined by Farmer *et al.* (1985). The major contribution of Kauffmann (1947) was to establish the serology of *E. coli,* which permitted a greater understanding of the ecology of these organisms. Other methods of typing have also successfully been applied to *E. coli,* including biotyping, the use of antibiotic resistance patterns (resistotyping) (Crichton & Old, 1992) and isoenzyme patterns (Goullet & Picard, 1986). The clonal nature of *E. coli* has been specifically addressed in a number of ways (Achtman, 1985; Whittam, 1989). Though there is a very extensive body of literature on the presence of *E. coli* and other Enterobacteriaceae in human faeces, it should be recognised that they are only a very small part of the faecal flora. According to Mitsuoka & Hayakawa (1972) the total bacterial count of faeces is about 10^{10} per gram, while the count of enterobacteria is 10^8 to 10^9 per gram. The faeces of neonates by comparison contain higher counts of Enterobacteriaceae.

Acquisition of *Escherichia coli* by the newborn

Acquisition of commensal Escherichia coli *from the mother*

Early studies were directed towards understanding the acquisition of enteropathogenic *E. coli* (EPEC) by the newborn. These generally showed that EPEC were derived at birth from the genital tract of the mother (Ocklitz & Schmidt, 1957). Since commensal *E. coli* may not necessarily have the same ability to colonise as EPEC, colonisation by the former was studied by Bettelheim *et al.* (1974a,b), who found that babies tended to acquire the faecal flora of their mother, generally by the oral route. The faecal flora of babies tended not to be as diverse as that of their mothers and genetic variation was observed in the strains during transmission (O'Farrell & Bettelheim, 1976; Shinebaum *et al.*, 1977). In normally delivered babies, predominantly looked after by their own mothers, it appears that the major source of commensal strains of *E. coli* is the faecal flora of the mother (Bettelheim *et al.*, 1983b). This is, however, not always the case and no clear reason could be found why some babies failed to acquire their mother's faecal *E. coli*. The only factor that might have played a part was the length of labour. The longer the period of labour, the more likely babies were to be colonised by their mother's faecal *E. coli*. *Escherichia coli* derived from those who handled the babies, other than the mothers, served to cloud the issue.

Other sources of commensal Escherichia coli *in babies*

Four babies born by Caesarean section were studied by Bettelheim *et al.* (1974c), who found that, though they had no contact with their maternal faecal flora, they were colonised by *E. coli* at the same time and to the same extent as normally delivered babies, but not by strains derived from their mothers. Occasionally, strains appeared to be transmitted between mothers and their babies, the strains undergoing phenotypic variation in the process.

Other observations of babies born by Caesarean section suggested that the routes by which they had acquired *E. coli* were: from nurses' hands directly or by way of feeding bottles, from maternal faeces during extended labour before Caesarean section, from the maternal faeces by way of the mother's hand, possibly after contamination of the breast, from gastric lavage tubes via the nurse's hands or during oxygen administration (Bettelheim & Lennox-King, 1976; O'Farrell *et al.*, 1976;

Lennox-King *et al.*, 1976a,b). In this study nurses attended to most of the needs of the infants, so enhancing the possibility of cross-infection and maintaining a relatively high level of *E. coli* in the environment. Similar conclusions were reached by Graham & Taylor (1976).

Since the first strains that colonise neonates may persist for up to 18 months, Kühn *et al.* (1986) suggested that colonisation should not be left to chance. Murono *et al.* (1993) also concluded that the spread of *E. coli* to neonates in hospitals is much more significant than acquisition from the mother. The separation of infants after birth for eight to 72 hours and their subsequent care by nursery staff enhanced horizontal transmission. Direct transmission from mothers to their babies was related to greater contact between them.

Colonisation by feeding

The O-serogroup composition of commensal *E. coli* in beast-fed babies is less complex than in bottle-fed babies, while in general the O-serogroup distribution was similar (Ørskov and Sørenson, 1975). Faecal strains of *E. coli* from breast-fed infants are more sensitive to human serum and are more often autoagglutinating (Gothefors *et al.*, 1975). Since human milk inhibits *E. coli*, though variably from strain to strain (Dolby & Honor, 1975), mutant strains of reduced virulence may be favoured.

Borderon *et al.*(1978) infected neonates in an intensive therapy unit with 10^8 to 10^9 azide-resistant *E. coli* and demonstrated variability in the interaction between *E. coli* and neonates. In all but one baby, the strain became the whole or part of the faecal Enterobacteriaceae flora for a number of days. Similarly, Lodinova *et al.* (1979) artificially colonised neonates with a strain of *E. coli* O83 in order to prevent colonisation with EPEC, but it is possible that EPEC have characteristics that allow them successfully to compete with other *E. coli* strains.

The spread of *E. coli* in child day-care centres has been investigated in relation to the type of diaper (napkin) worn by the children (Van *et al.*, 1991). When clothing was worn over the diaper, faecal coliform contamination of the environment was significantly reduced and use of paper diapers further significantly reduced this contamination. A high contamination rate with faecal *E. coli* was observed for most of the animate and inanimate items in the environment. In the case of small sterile toy balls, which had been introduced into the day-care centres, contamination reached 46 per cent. Eleven environmental trimethoprim-resistant *E. coli* that were isolated had plasmid profiles unique to the centre from which they were isolated. This showed that children can be foci for the spread of *E. coli* and that faecal–oral transmission is most probable.

Distribution of *Escherichia coli* in the gastro-intestinal tract

Babies

Enterobacteriaceae were isolated from the duodenal aspirates of children aged between three and 36 months from shanty town homes, with poor sanitation, in Peru (Penny *et al.*, 1992), but there was no relationship between species of Enterobacteriaceae isolated and the source of the specimen. In the majority of aspirates only one species could be identified; where more than one species was present one usually predominated, but organisms of other groups were often present. About one-quarter of the aspirates yielded only one serotype, while a mixture of serotypes was found in the others.

The distribution of *E. coli* along the length of the intestinal tract of babies was investigated by Bettelheim *et al.* (1992). Specimens were obtained from three sites along the intestine of seven babies, six of whom had died at between the ages of 1.5 and 5.5 months, and the other at 12 months. For six of the babies the cause of death was sudden infant death syndrome (SIDS), the other baby also died suddenly but from another cause. In only one of the babies was a single O-serogroup found (O2). In the others between two and four serogroups were present. Generally, strains present in the proximal bowel could also be isolated from the rectum, which suggests that faeces provide a reasonable indication of the distribution of *E. coli* along the length of the bowel.

Adults

A wide variety of *E. coli* types may be present in adult faeces, but usually only a few of these can, at any one time, be isolated from the faeces of healthy individuals. As new types are ingested, they either pass through or colonise by displacing previous types. While certain majority types predominate, there may also be a resident minority of the *E. coli* flora, which is much more difficult to detect. Bettelheim *et al.* (1972) obtained ten evenly spaced samples along the length of nine fully formed stool specimens obtained from five female and four male subjects aged between 19 and 36 years. At least ten *E. coli*-like colonies were selected from each, to ensure the greatest diversity of colonial types. These nine

Table 3.1. *Typical O-serogroup distributions of* Escherichia coli *in faeces*

Specimen	Serogroup	Sample									
		1	2	3	4	5	6	7	8	9	10
Aᵃ	O60	40	10	9	10	39	10	10	10	9	39
	O21										1
	Rough									1	
	NT			1		1					
Bᵃ	O81	8	6	7	30	3	5	6	5	2	15
	O4		1								
	O1		1								6
	O7			1					1	1	6
	O11										3
	O20								1		
	O27								2		1
	O35										2
	O126								1		
	Rough			3		7	2	2		4	6
	NT							1			
D	Rough	7	39	8	8	6	2	2	26	5	2
E	O64			1	2	5	2	3	14	3	3
	O43/41										1
	Rough	10	28	8	6		1		3	2	
Iᵇ	O3			1		1					2
	O7	10	9	9	49	9	9	10	46	9	96
	O11				1				1		
	O55		1						3	1	2

ᵃ Strains of the same O-serogroup but differing in antibiotic sensitivity were isolated.
ᵇ *E. coli* O69 was isolated on antibiotic susceptibility media.
After Bettelheim *et al.* (1972).

stools yielded 1580 strains with a mean of 3.8 O-serogroups, but the distribution of strains differed (Table 3.1). It was clear that each site from all specimens yielded the predominant O-serogroup of the specimen, but with conventional sampling some minor groups will have been missed.

Studies by Gorbach *et al.* (1967) and Drasar *et al.* (1969) had shown that a Gram-positive microflora predominates in the human ileum, while Gram-negative bacteria tend to be found only in its distal region. Gorbach and Tabaqchali (1969) found that in patients with small-intestinal bacterial overgrowth (stagnant loop syndrome) the bacteria present were qualitatively similar to those present in the faeces. The serotypes of *E. coli* present along the entire length of the gastro-intestinal tract in patients with stagnant loop syndrome were studied by Tabaqchali *et al.* (1977), who found that a number of closely related strains were present simultaneously along the length of the bowel. This confirmed many earlier observations that *E. coli* in the bowel is the subject of considerable genetic interchange. Thus, in one patient there were strains of *E. coli* ORough:H32 of four different biotypes and one strain of O-untypable:H32. This patient also yielded two pairs of strains, each of the same biotype but of different serotype, i.e. ORough:H19 and O104:H19 in one case and O129:H30 and O129:H- in the other. After treatment for six weeks with tetracycline, these types were replaced by a completely different group of strains. Food appeared not to affect the variety of serotypes and biotypes but the numbers increased in the post-prandial samples. A possible onward movement of serotypes along the gastro-intestinal tract was not found.

There is also an indirect way in which conclusions may be drawn about the role of *E. coli* in the human adult bowel. Serotypes present may induce detectable serum antibodies. While patients with inflammatory bowel disease are more likely to develop circulating antibacterial antibodies, healthy individuals may also develop such antibodies, particularly to their dominant types. Tabaqchali *et al.* (1978) examined the sera, from patients with and without inflammatory bowel disease and from healthy individuals, for the presence of agglutinating antibodies against all the then recognised *E. coli* O-serogroups. The highest antibody titres were found in patients with Crohn's disease, a chronic inflammatory disease of the gastro-intestinal tract, and to a lesser extent in those with ulcerative colitis, but the controls also had significant antibody levels. The O-serogroups to which the control sera most commonly contained antibodies included O2, O8, O14, O60, O70 O136 and O144. The highest titre, of mainly IgM, was against O60 (1:400). This demonstrates that the lipopolysaccharide O-antigen of the *E. coli* intestinal flora of healthy adults can gain access to the bloodstream, but probably only in small amounts.

Factors that affect the human intestinal Escherichia coli *flora*

To gain a better understanding of the possible acquisition of *E. coli* by healthy adults, nine individuals were observed for two to five months (Shooter *et al.*, 1977) and their faecal *E. coli* serotyped. The subjects were eight women aged between 42 and 56 years, and the 61-year-old husband of one of them. They usually ate at home, four went on holiday during the period and one also ate at a canteen. Some of the subjects yielded only very few *E. coli* serotypes. One yielded only *E. coli* O2:H6 throughout a three-month study period. Three others yielded only three, four and seven different serotypes each. Seven of the 12 specimens from one of the subjects contained only *E. coli* O22, O106 and ORough, which shared the same flagellar antigen H1. The other subjects carried a greater variety of serotypes, but one persisted over a period of months. The subject who ate in canteens had the greatest variety of serotypes, the husband and wife carried the same serotype (O1:H7), while the wife's variety of serotypes was lower (i.e. seven) than that of the husband (i.e. 21).

The effect of diet on the human *E. coli* flora was examined (Bettelheim *et al.*, 1977b) in six nurses in a London hospital. They were the subject of a specific protocol over eight weeks. During the first and last two weeks the nurses consumed a normal diet, including some meals in the hospital canteen, while during the middle four weeks they ate a diet exclusively of tinned food and ultraheat-treated milk with vitamin supplements. All cutlery was autoclaved and only disposable plates and cups were used. Their tooth brushes were soaked in hydrogen peroxide and sterile water was used for tooth cleaning. Specimens from all faeces passed were cultured for *E. coli* and ten colonies representative of as many different colonial variants as possible were examined.

The mean number of serotypes per specimen for each nurse before, during and after the sterile diet was calculated and a clear trend was apparent. Before the sterile diet the mean number of serotypes for the six nurses was 1.31 (range 0.82 to 1.71), which fell to 0.51 (range 0.22 to 0.91) during the sterile diet period, and rose to 1.84 (range 1.00 to 3.00) on return to the normal diet. During the sterile diet phase, new serotypes were observed that may previously have been present and missed (Bettelheim *et al.*, 1972), but non-compliance with the strict dietary requirements could not be excluded. Occasionally the new serotypes shared antigens with types already present.

The role of food was also the main reason for the changes in *E. coli* flora noted in a group of students who had travelled from many parts of the world to Dublin, Ireland (Majed *et al.*, 1978). Faeces specimens were collected before the departure of the students and then weekly for four months in Dublin. Little overlap in serotypes from one specimen to the next was observed, but a certain trend was noted. This suggested a persistent flora, representatives of which could not always be isolated from a given specimen, but which could be found weeks later on a number of occasions. Transient serotypes were isolated on single occasions or

Table 3.2. *Distribution of* E. coli *OH serotypes in the faeces of a student travelling from Norway to Dublin*

Place and date				
Norway 22.7.71	Norway	Dublin 10.9.71	Dublin 15.9.71	Dublin 20.9.71
E. coli serotypes				
O19:H7	O19:H7	O115:H10	O1:H7	O1:H7
O19:Hnt	O19:H10	O152:H8	O1:H33	O1:H⁻
O145:H33	O115:H10	ORough:H10		Ont:H4
		ORough:Hnt		Ont:H7
		ORough:H⁻		

Source: Majed *et al.* (1978).

several times and serological variation among the serotypes was also noted (Table 3.2).

Similar continuous changes in *E. coli* serotypes have also been observed in Peace Corps volunteers who were stationed in Morocco (Ørskov *et al.*, 1984). The flora changed after the volunteers arrived and continued to change, regardless of the development of diarrhoea, which was usually associated with acquisition of an enterotoxigenic *E. coli* (ETEC) serotype. In a survey of *E. coli* from the faeces of healthy adults in Finland (Siitonen, 1992), strains with O- and K-antigens associated with extra-intestinal infections were prevalent, while strains with other known virulence-associated characteristics were comparatively rarely found.

These studies show that at any time there may be a diversity of *E. coli* in the adult bowel and that new types of *E. coli*, which may persist for long periods, may be acquired mainly from the diet. These new types may displace a major type or they may only be transient colonisers. Phenotypic variation also occurs within the bowel.

Microbial factors that affect the human intestinal Escherichia coli

Soon after the discovery of colicines it was thought that these may play a role in the intestinal microbial ecology, giving colicinogenic strains a selective advantage. In humans given mixtures of pairs of *E. coli* strains, the ColV plasmid promoted intestinal survival, while the ColE plasmid did not (Smith and Huggins, 1976). A spontaneous chromosomal mutant of a faecal isolate resistant to sodium nalidixate survived in the intestinal tract for six to ten days after oral administration (Smith and Huggins, 1978). The survival of a number of plasmid-bearing derivatives of this strain was determined, but they did not persist for very long and considerable experimental variation was noted. It is nevertheless significant that some of the plasmid-bearing strains were recoverable a number of days after inoculation.

In order to colonise, *E. coli* must, at least to some extent, adhere to the intestinal epithelial cells. The observation that adherence of *E. coli* to mucosal cells is mediated by mannose receptors (Ofek *et al.*, 1977) is, therefore, significant, since mannose is common in the surface of mucosal cells.

Certain strains of *E. coli* carry S-fimbriae that adhere to the sialic-acid-containing surface glycoproteins of mucosal cells. Schroten *et al.*, (1992) examined the binding of S-fimbriate *E. coli* to buccal epithelial cells of humans of different ages and found that the mean number of organisms bound per cell rose slightly with age, though not sufficiently to explain the age-linked differences in susceptibility to *E. coli* meningitis and sepsis. Such adherence may reflect the ability of the S-fimbriate organism to displace resident strains.

Acquisition of pathogenic *Escherichia coli*

Intestinal pathogenic Escherichia coli

Enteropathogenic *E. coli* (EPEC) have caused many outbreaks of infantile gastro-enteritis (Robins-Browne, 1987) but seem largely to have disappeared from the developed world, though they are still of major importance in the developing world.

EPEC appear to have a capacity to infect the newborn (Bettelheim *et al.*, 1983a). In a maternity ward, where the earlier studies of neonatal colonisation had been carried out, an outbreak of gastro-enteritis due to EPEC (O125:H21) occurred in spite of careful precautions, including cancellation of new admissions and barrier nursing. This EPEC strain spread to 16 babies, while other serotypes spread at most to each of three babies. A two-year-old child in a separate ward block was infected 25 days after the index case; the only connection was the medical staff. The ease of spread of EPEC may be linked to their ability to establish colonisation from a very low infective dose. To demonstrate its pathogenic potential, 10^8 organisms of an EPEC strain were deliberately fed to a baby, which, as a result, became colonised (Neter *et al.* 1955), but a much lower dose is sufficient to set up a human infection under natural conditions. Similarly, Rowe *et al.* (1970) studied British troops in Aden and showed that an *E. coli* strain (O148:H21), later shown to be enterotoxigenic (ETEC), can spread rapidly and cause travellers' diarrhoea. The presence on ETEC of specific fimbrial colonisation factor antigens (CFA) (Evans *et al.*, 1975) is important, but is probably only a part of the effective means by which they colonise.

A good example of the ability of pathogenic *E. coli* to spread and colonise is the astonishing rise of *E. coli* O157:H7. This was first described as a 'rare' *E. coli* serotype (Riley *et al.*, 1983) that caused an outbreak of haemorrhagic colitis (enterohaemorrhagic *E. coli*; EHEC). It was not found amongst the *E. coli* strains from a variety of sources (Bettelheim, 1978). Since then this serotype has been responsible for many outbreaks of food-poisoning in North America, Europe and other parts of the world, including the largest ever outbreak, reported in the United States of America in 1992–1993 (Preliminary report, 1993). Only a low dose of EHEC may be necessary to cause human infection (Griffin and Tauxe, 1991) and in the 1992–1993 outbreak the hamburger patties later recalled contained fewer than 100 organisms each before cooking, so that the number of *E. coli* O157:H7 ingested by each affected person was probably even lower. Pai *et al.* (1988) demonstrated that asymptomatic human carriage can occur. *Escherichia coli* O157 that produce Shiga-like toxin (SLT) have been isolated from asymptomatic cattle associated with outbreaks and those in surveys (Ørskov *et al.*, 1987; Wells *et al.*, 1991; Wieler *et al.*, 1992; Beutin *et al.*, 1993;). These organisms seem particularly suited to living and surviving in the rumen of cattle, particularly if these are underfed (Rasmussen *et al.*, 1993). The very low infectious dose that can cause disease is clear from an outbreak associated with apple cider (Zhao *et al.*, 1993).

Knowledge of the factors that contribute to this low infective dose of EHEC would be valuable for an understanding of the pathogenicity of *E. coli* and probably also of enteropathogenic Enterobacteriaceae such as *Salmonella* and *Shigella*.

Uropathogenic Escherichia coli

Urinary tract infection is more common in women than in men and the ascending route of infection is the most important by which faecal *E. coli* reach the urinary tract. There is a close correlation between introital

Table 3.3. *Distribution of* E. coli
*O-serogroups that cause urinary
tract infection*

O-serogroup	No. of isolates
1	137
2	79
4	209
6	208
7	89
9	18
11	19
18	51
39	5
75	134
Others	822
Total	1771

Source: Gruneberg & Bettelheim
(1969).

colonisation and the carriage of the organisms in the anterior urethra
(O'Grady *et al.*, 1970) and, in women who develop urinary tract infection
after genitourinary surgery, the causative *E. coli* is predominant in the
faecal flora before surgery (Bettelheim *et al.*, 1971). Similarly, a faecal
origin is suggested by the urinary tract infection in a woman working in a
microbiology research laboratory, who probably ingested the particular
strain (Parry *et al.*, 1981). In recurrent urinary tract infection similar types
reappeared after they had apparently been cleared from the urinary tract,
suggesting that these strains are part of the normal faecal flora (Brauner *et
al.*, 1992).

Ten O-serogroups, with geographical differences in distribution, account for between 43 and 81 per cent of the smooth *E. coli* isolated from
the urine (Table 3.3), and their prevalence in urinary tract infection
correlates with those present in normal faeces (Grueneberg *et al.*, 1968;
Grueneberg & Bettelheim, 1969; Roberts *et al.*, 1975).

In a two-year study of urinary tract infection, Spencer *et al.* (1968)
showed that small clusters of infection were due to certain *E. coli*
serogroups. While these strains may have been 'more transmissible' or
'more able to cause urinary tract infection', their source was probably
from the faecal flora and simultaneous colonisation from a common
source, such as food, was thought likely. Haemolytic strains of *E. coli*

present in the faeces (Hacker *et al.*, 1983) may be a pool of potential urinary pathogens.

The possibility that faecal colonisation precedes colonisation of the urinary tract and the development of pyelonephritis and septicaemia, particularly by children, has been extensively studied in Sweden (Tullus *et al.*, 1986, 1987; Tullus, 1988). Faecal colonisation by P-fimbriate strains of *E. coli* correlated with the incidence of urinary infection with the same type. Though there was no correlation between P-fimbriation and ability to colonise the bowel of neonates, the presence of these *E. coli* in the intestine was associated with urinary tract infection.

Escherichia coli in animals

Pigs

The bacterial flora of piglets has been reviewed by Smith (1971). During their first day of life the stomach pH is high and the alimentary tract becomes flooded with large numbers of *E. coli* and other bacteria. As the pH falls the bacterial numbers decrease, except in the case of lactobacilli.

Jones and Rutter (1974) described an antigen (K88) that aided the adherence of virulent *E. coli* in the pig intestine. The possible role of this antigen in colonisation by non-virulent strains had not been assessed. The significance of fimbriae for the colonisation by *E. coli* of the porcine intestinal tract was demonstrated in a series of specific colonisation experiments (Nagy *et al.*, 1977). These showed that fimbriae facilitate intestinal adhesion and colonisation by K88-negative strains. Sellwood (1979) found that the receptor for the K88 antigen is genetically determined in the pig population and the different variants of the K88 antigen have significantly different receptor-binding properties (Payne, 1994).

The faecal colonisation by *E. coli* of two pigs throughout their 210-day life was studied by Linton *et al.* (1978). In the absence of selection pressure by antibiotics, some serogroups persisted for long periods, while others appeared and disappeared. Antibiotics caused the selection of certain resistant serogroups, but only some of these persisted. Hinton *et al.* (1985a) demonstrated a highly complex *E. coli* flora with many serogroups present in weaned and unweaned pigs. The presence of an ETEC serotype dominated the flora, which became much more restricted. There are marked similarities between the normal *E. coli* flora of humans and pigs.

Cattle

The alimentary tract of newborn calves is flooded with large numbers of bacteria, but to a lesser extent than in piglets (Smith, 1971). This may be because calves are less contaminated with faecal matter than are piglets. In addition, bovine colostrum is bactericidal for *E. coli* (Reiter and Brock, 1975) and acts as a defence mechanism against colonisation.

Howe and Linton (1976) sampled 400 healthy calves in Southern Britain ranging from birth to eight weeks of age over a period of ten months. Of the 93 O-serogroups found, O8, O9 and O17 predominated. A similar complexity of types was noted when these studies were extended (Howe *et al.*, 1976a) and the serotypes found on the carcass surfaces were similar to those found in the rectum (Howe *et al.*1976b). Antigen K99 appears to play a similar role in the calf to that played by the K88 antigen in piglets (Burrows *et al.*, 1976).

Calves, like humans, acquire their *E. coli* from their mothers (Smith and Crabbe, 1956; Hinton *et al.*, 1985b). With increasing age the diversity of the *E. coli* of farm animals decreases (Hinton, 1985).

Cats and dogs

Enteropathogenic *E. coli* serogroups O26, O55 and O111 are present in 12 per cent of dogs and eight per cent of cats (Mian, 1959). Similarly, Mackel *et al.* (1960) found serogroups O55, O114, O126 and O128 in kittens. A study of the carriage of antibiotic-resistant *E. coli* by healthy cats and dogs revealed that 60 per cent of dogs and 26 per cent of cats carried such strains, many of which were multiresistant and the resistance of 60 per cent of these strains was transferable (Moss and Frost, 1984).

Rats and mice

Coliforms are present in very small numbers in the stomach of mice less than 12 days old (Mushin and Dubos, 1965). The numbers then rose and fell again by the age of 21 months. The numbers in the duodenum were very small, while they were large in the colon. Similarly, the numbers rose until the eighteenth day and then fell again. *Escherichia coli* could be isolated from the faeces at all times.

Germ-free mice fed with individual strains of *E. coli* K-12 that differ in genetic composition become colonised but, when they are fed with more than one strain at a time, the strains are in competition and a colonising order of the different phenotypes can be demonstrated (Onderdonk *et al.*, 1981). In the course of a study of antagonism between isogenic strains of *E. coli* in the intestines of gnotobiotic mice, it was shown that strains can become host 'adapted' and the dominant population. Culture, *in vitro*, of such strains in broth led to loss of the 'adaptation' (Duval-Iflah *et al.*, 1981). Berg and Owens (1979) suggested that strict anaerobes form a layer in the mucin on the mucosal epithelia that physically inhibits introduced strains of *E. coli* from approaching and penetrating it.

Domestic poultry

As part of the investigations of reservoirs of antibiotic-resistant *E. coli*, Howe *et al.* (1976c) found that some serogroups, such as O9, O83 and O96, persisted throughout the life of chickens, while serogroup O15, O18 and O131 strains appeared early but later disappeared. Serogroups O3, O8, O65, O70, O78 and O114 appeared late but persisted until slaughter. These serogroups, which were isolated from at least five per cent of the droppings of individual birds, probably have a particular ability to colonise the chicken intestinal tract.

Birds

Dott *et al.* (1981) studied recreational lakes and bathing areas for the *E. coli* flora of sea-bird droppings, mainly gulls. On the basis of biotyping they suggested that these birds carry kinds of *E. coli* different from humans.

The effect of antibiotics on intestinal *Escherichia coli*

The development and transfer of resistance

Escherichia coli plays a particularly important role in the development of the antibiotic resistance of enteric pathogens. The discovery of antibiotic-resistance transfer (R) factors, by Watanabe (1963), explained how such resistance spreads between certain Gram-negative organisms, though both plasmid- and chromosomally mediated antibiotic resistance are regularly observed.

Organisms that produce extended-spectrum β-lactamase, which is plasmid mediated, are resistant to most penicillins, cephalosporins and aztreonam (Philippon *et al.*, 1989; Weber *et al.*, 1990) and to currently available β-lactamase-inhibiting β-lactam drug combinations. Many *E. coli* chromosomally mediated β-lactamases have also been distinguished (Matthew and Harris, 1986). *Escherichia coli* can increase the level of β-lactamase production by increasing the number of β-lactamase gene copies, by altering the promoter or attenuator regions that affect gene transcription, or by changing the complex regulatory apparatus of inducible β-lactamase expression (Lindberg and Normark, 1986; Sanders, 1992).

The development of a structurally altered DNA gyrase (Wolfson *et al.*, 1989) permits *E. coli* to resist the quinolone drugs. It may also decrease their outer membrane permeability by reducing the number of porins (Bedard *et al.*, 1989). *Escherichia coli* can readily become resistant to ziduvidine (AZT), a thymine analogue active against the human immunodeficiency virus, by the loss of thymidine kinase, which converts AZT to its active triphosphate form (Lewin *et al.*, 1990).

Reves *et al.* (1990) showed that the faecal *E. coli* of children in a day-care centre frequently acquire trimethoprim resistance as compared with children not attending such centres. These resistant strains of *E. coli* were unique to each centre and likely to be transmitted from the children into the community. The prevalence of such spread was highest to mothers and siblings, least to fathers and it was not linked to household antibiotic use (Fornasini *et al.*, 1992).

The behaviour of resistant Escherichia coli *in the human bowel*

When cultures in gelatin capsules containing 10^{10} to 10^{11} viable R-factor-carrying *E. coli* are ingested by healthy adults, the R-factor-bearing strains rapidly disappear. This may be due to the ecological disadvantage of such bacteria in an environment that lacks the selective pressure to maintain the R-factors (Anderson, 1974).

In the natural situation in humans there is no significant difference in residence times between resistant and sensitive strains of *E. coli* and a low level of plasmid-carrying strains is maintained (Hartley and Richmond, 1975). Under these conditions, R-factors are less widespread in O-serogroups known to persist well in the human intestinal tract, such as O1, O2, O4, O5 and O75, than other serogroups. Strains of *E. coli* that carry R-plasmids are regularly found in the faeces of patients in hospitals, and the plasmids as well as the *E. coli* that carry them can be transmitted (Avril and Gerbaud, 1976).

For plasmids to be maintained in *E. coli* in the natural environment they must confer a selective advantage on the host organism (Gordon, 1992). Cooksey *et al.* (1990) noted a great diversity of plasmids that conferr β-lactam resistance in hospital isolates of *E. coli*, and this suggests that such strains are widely distributed in the community. In the developed world, significant carriage of resistant *E. coli*, probably derived from the food chain, has been found in the healthy population (Bonten *et al.*, 1992).

Escherichia coli in the food chain

Escherichia coli *in abattoirs*

Animal carcasses are generally contaminated with their intestinal *E. coli* even under good slaughter-house conditions (Shooter *et al.*, 1970). There is considerable contamination of carcasses by the animals' own intestinal *E. coli* and there is extensive interchange of *E. coli* between carcasses. On a sheep-slaughtering line in an abattoir of high hygienic standard, Bettelheim (1981) noted that the rectal *E. coli* of animals tended to be washed away during the very heavy hosing down that follows removal of the intestines, but recontamination by environmental *E. coli* occurred, presumably derived from other animals. Extensive spread of both *E. coli* and antibiotic-resistance markers was observed.

During a survey of a poultry packing station by Shooter *et al.* (1970, 1974), *E. coli* was isolated from the chickens and their giblets throughout the processing stages, and from the various waters used in the feather-softening processes and cooling tanks. An extensive study of the contamination of pig carcasses in two abattoirs by Linton *et al.* (1976) showed the presence of certain *E. coli* O-serogroups throughout, while others made only a transient appearance. A high level of antibiotic resistance was found in the strains and strains survived the chilling process. The persistently high infection rate with Gram-negative enteric pathogens, including *E. coli* O157, suggests that this contamination in abattoirs still continues.

Escherichia coli *in food*

A high correlation between the faecal *E. coli* serotypes of hospital patients and those that contaminate their food was demonstrated by Cooke *et al.* (1970). In a survey of over 4000 samples of retail processed foods in the United Kingdom (Pinegar and Cooke, 1985), an overall

E. coli contamination rate of 12 per cent was noted, and over a quarter of the cakes and confectionery were contaminated as compared with only nine per cent of meat and meat-based products, but the meat product isolates were more likely to be antibiotic resistant. A contamination level of 10^3 *E. coli* per gram was found in 27 per cent of foods.

In the developing world food is often associated with the transmission of pathogenic *E. coli* and Kaul *et al.* (1990) found ETEC on raw meat, as well as on the hands of operatives and their equipment. Similarly dairy products yield both pathogenic and antibiotic-resistant *E. coli* (Abbar & Kaddar, 1991).

In a series of feeding experiments by Cooke *et al.* (1972), 25 human volunteers ingested between 10^5 and 10^8 organisms of specific *E. coli* serotypes, approximating the numbers found in hospital food. In 24 of 25 such feeding experiments the ingested serotype could subsequently be recovered from the faeces of the volunteer and in four it persisted for more than a month. This shows that ingested *E. coli* will bring about colonisation.

Conclusions

At present more is probably known about *E. coli* than about any other organism in the biosphere, including humans, and the genome of *E. coli* is one of the most extensively mapped of any organism. Humans have a continuing intimate relationship with *E. coli* and it is more intriguing than almost any other, considering that each week more than 100 papers on this organism are published. In spite of this, however, there continue to be many gaps in our knowledge of its interactions with humans. Though the relationship with these organisms is generally smooth, those who have spent many hours intrigued by them are aware that this love as with 'the love of woman! It is a lovely and a fearful thing.' (Byron).

References

Abbar, F. & Kaddar, H. Kh. (1991). Bacteriological studies on Iraqi milk products. *Journal of Applied Bacteriology*, **71**, 497–500.
Achtman, M. (1985). Clonal groups and virulence factors among *Escherichia coli*K1 strains. In *Enterobacterial Surface Antigens: Methods for Molecular Characterization*. eds T. K. Korhonen, E. A. Dawes, & P. H. Mäkelä, pp. 65–74. Amsterdam: Elsevier.
Anderson, J. D. (1974). The effect of R-factor carriage on the survival of *Escherichia coli* in the human intestine. *Journal of Medical Microbiology*, **7**, 85–90.

Avril, J.-L. & Gerbaud, G. R. (1976). Indépendence des plasmides hébergés par *Escherichia coli* de malades hospitalisés sans antibiothérapie. *Annales du Microbiologie (Paris)*, **127B**, 167–75.

Bachmann, B. J. (1990). Linkage map of *Escherichia coli* K-12, edition 8. *Microbiological Reviews*, **54**, 130–97.

Bedard, J., Chanberland, S., Wong, S., Schollaardt, T. & Bryan, L. E. (1989). Contribution of permeability and susceptibility to inhibition of DNA synthesis in determining susceptibilities of *Escherichia coli*, *Pseudomonas aeruginosa*, and *Alcaligenes faecalis* to ciprofloxacin. *Antimicrobial Agents and Chemotherapy*, **33**, 1457–64.

Berg, R. D. & Owens, W. E. (1979). Inhibition of translocation of viable *Escherichia coli* from the gastrointestinal tract of mice by bacterial antagonism. *Infection and Immunity*, **25**, 820–27.

Bettelheim, K. A. (1978). The sources of 'OH' serotypes of *Escherichia coli*. *Journal of Hygiene, Cambridge*, **80**, 83–113.

Bettelheim, K. A. (1981). The isolation of *Escherichia coli* from a sheep slaughtering line in an abattoir. *Comparative Immunology, Microbiology and Infectious Diseases*, **4**, 93–100.

Bettelheim, K. A. (1986). Commemoration of the publication 100 years ago of the papers by Dr. Th. Escherich in which are described for the first time the organisms that bear his name. *Zentralblatt für Bakteriologie und Hygiene A*, **261**, 255–65.

Bettelheim, K. A., Breadon, A., Faiers, M. C., O'Farrell S. M. & Shooter, R. A. (1974a). The origin of 'O' serotypes of *Escherichia coli* in babies after normal delivery. *Journal of Hygiene, Cambridge*, **73**, 67–70.

Bettelheim, K. A., Bushrod, F. M., Chandler, M. E., Cooke, E. M., O'Farrell, S. & Shooter, R. A. (1977a). *Escherichia coli* serotype distribution in man and animals. *Journal of Hygiene, Cambridge*, **73**, 467–71.

Bettelheim, K. A., Cooke, E. M., O'Farrell, S. & Shooter, R. A. (1977b). The effect of diet on intestinal *Escherichia coli*. *Journal of Hygiene, Cambridge*, **79**, 43–5.

Bettelheim, K. A., Drabu, Y., O'Farrell, S., Shaw, E. J., Tabaqchali, S. & Shooter, R. A. (1983a). Relationship of an epidemic strain of *Escherichia coli* O125.H21 to other serotypes of *E. coli* during an outbreak situation in a neonatal ward. *Zentralblatt für Bakteriologie und Hygiene A*, **253**, 509–14.

Bettelheim, K. A., Dulake, C. & Taylor, J. (1971). Postoperative urinary tract infections caused by *Escherichia coli*. *Journal of Clinical Pathology*, **24**, 442–3.

Bettelheim, K. A., Faiers, M. & Shooter, R. A. (1972). Serotypes of *Escherichia coli* in normal stools. *The Lancet*, **2**, 1224–6.

Bettelheim, K. A., Goldwater, P. N., Evangelidis, H., Pearce, J. L. & Smith, D. L. (1992). Distribution of toxigenic *Escherichia coli* serotypes in the intestines of infants. *Comparative Immunology, Microbiology and Infectious Diseases*, **15**, 65–70.

Bettelheim, K. A. & Lennox-King, S. M. J. (1976). The acquisition of *Escherichia coli* by newborn babies. *Infection*, **4**, 174–9.

Bettelheim, K. A., Peddie, B. A. & Chereshsky, A. (1983b). The ecology of *Escherichia coli* in a maternity ward in Christchurch, New Zealand. *Zentralblatt für Bakteriologie und Hygiene B*, **178**, 389–93.

Bettelheim, K. A., Teoh-Chan, C. H., Chandler, M. E., O'Farrell, S. M.,

Rahamin, L., Shaw, E. J. & Shooter, R. A. (1974b). Further studies of *Escherichia coli* in babies after normal delivery. *Journal of Hygiene, Cambridge*, **73**, 277–85.

Bettelheim, K. A., Teoh-Chan, C. H., Chandler, M. E., O'Farrell, S. M., Rahamin, L., Shaw, E. J. & Shooter, R. A. (1974c). Spread of *Escherichia coli* colonizing new-born babies and their mothers. *Journal of Hygiene, Cambridge*, **73**, 383–7.

Beutin, L., Geier, D., Steinrück, H., Zimmermann, S. & Scheutz, F. (1993). Prevalence and some properties of Verotoxin (Shiga-like toxin)-producing *Escherichia coli* in seven different species of healthy domestic animals. *Journal of Clinical Microbiology*, **31**, 2483–8.

Bonten, M., Stobberingh, E., Philips, J. & Houben, A. (1992). Antibiotic resistance of *Escherichia coli* in fecal samples of healthy people in two different areas in an industrialized country. *Infection*, **20**, 258–62.

Borderon, J. C., Laugier, J. & Gold, F. (1978). Essai d'établissement d'une souche de *Escherichia coli* sensible aux antibiotiques dans l'intestin du nouveau-né. *Annales de Microbiologies (Paris)*, **129B**, 581–96.

Brauner, A., Jacobson, S. H. & Kühn, I. (1992). Urinary *Escherichia coli* causing recurrent infections–a prospective follow-up of biochemical phenotypes. *Clinical Nephrology*, **38**, 318–23.

Burrows, M. R., Sellwood, R. & Gibbons, R. A. (1976). Haemagglutinating and adhesive properties associated with the K99 antigen of bovine strains of *Escherichia coli*. *Journal of General Microbiology*, **96**, 269–75.

Chatkaemorakot, A., Echeverria, P., Taylor, D. N., Bettelheim, K. A., Blacklow, N. R., Sethabutr, O., Seriwatana, J. & Kaper, J. (1987). HeLa cell-adherent *Escherichia coli* in children with diarrhoea in Thailand. *Journal of Infectious Diseases*, **156**, 669–72.

Cooke, E. M., Hettiaratchy, I. G. T. & Buck, A. C. (1972). Fate of ingested *Escherichia coli* in normal persons. *Journal of Medical Microbiology*, **5**, 361–9.

Cooke, E. M., Shooter, R. A., Kumar, P. J., Rousseau, S. A. & Foulkes, A. (1970). Hospital food as a possible source of *E. coli* in patients. *Lancet*, **1**, 436–7.

Cooksey, R., Swenson, J., Clark, N., Gay, E. & Thornsberry, C. (1990). Patterns and mechanisms of β-lactam resistance among isolates of *Escherichia coli* from hospitals in the United States. *Antimicrobial Agents and Chemotherapy*, **34**, 739–45.

Crichton, P. B. & Old, D. C. (1992). Numerical index of the discriminatory ability of biotyping and resistotyping for strains of *Escherichia coli*. *Epidemiology and Infection*, **108**, 279–86.

Dolby, J. M. & Honor, P. (1975). Bacteriostasis of *Esch. coli* by milk. *Archives of Diseases of Childhood*, **10**, 823.

Dott, W., Wolff, H. J. & Botzenhart, K. (1981). Zur hygienschen Beschaffenheit von Freibadegewässern. 2. Mitteilung: Vergleich der Biotypen von *Escherichia coli* aus Seewasser und Vogelfaeces. *Zentralblatt für Bakteriologie und Hygiene B*, **173**, 233–41.

Drasar, B. S., Shiner, M., & McLeod, G. M. (1969). Studies on the intestinal flora. I. The bacterial flora of the gastrointestinal tract in healthy and achlorhydric persons. *Gastroenterology*, **56**, 71–9.

Duval-Iflah, Y., Raibaud, P. & Rousseau, M. (1981). Antagonisms among isogenic strains of *Escherichia coli* in the digestive tracts of gnotobiotic mice. *Infection and Immunity*, **34**, 957–69.

Escherich, Th. (1885). Die Darmbakterien des Neugeboren und Sauglings. *Fortschritte der Medizin*, **3**, 515–22, 547–54.

Escherich, Th. (1988). The intestinal bacteria of the neonate and breast-fed infant (Translated by K. A. Bettelheim). *Review of Infectious Diseases*, **10**, 1220–5.

Evans, D. G., Silver, R. P., Evans, D. J. Jr., Chase, D. G. & Gorbach, S. L. (1975). Plasmid-controlled colonization factor associated with virulence in *Escherichia coli* enterotoxigenic for humans. *Infection and Immunity*, **12**, 565–7.

Farmer, J. J. III, Davis, B. R., Hickman-Brenner, F. W., McWorter, A., Huntley-Carter, G. P., Asbury, M. A., Riddle, C., Wathe-Grady, H. G., Elias, C., Fanning, G. R., Steigerwalt, A. G., O'Hara, C. M., Morris, G. K., Smith, P. B. & Brenner, D. J. (1985). Biochemical identification of new species and biogroups of Enterobacteriaceae isolated from clinical specimens. *Journal of Clinical Microbiology*, **21**, 46–76.

Fornasini, M., Reves, R. R., Murray, B. E., Morrow, A. L. & Pickering, L. K. (1992). Trimethoprim-resistant *Escherichia coli* in households of children attending day care centers. *Journal of Infectious Diseases*, **166**, 326–30.

Gorbach, S. L., Plaut, A. G., Nahas, L. & Weinstein, L. (1967). Studies of intestinal microflora. II. Microorganisms of the small intestine and their relations to oral and fecal flora. *Gastroenterology*, **53**, 856–67.

Gorbach, S. L. & Tabaqchali, S. (1969). Bacteria bile and the small bowel. *Gut*, **10**, 963–72.

Gordon, D. M. (1992). Rate of plasmid transfer among *Escherichia coli* strains isolated from natural populations. *Journal of General Microbiology*, **138**, 17–21.

Gothefors, L., Olling, S. & Winberg, J. (1975). Breast feeding and biological properties of faecal *E. coli* strains. *Acta Paediatrica Scandinavica*, **64**, 807–12.

Goullet, P. & Picard, B. (1986). Comparative esterase electrophoretic polymorphism of *Escherichia coli* isolates obtained from animal and human sources. *Journal of General Microbiology*, **132**, 1843–51.

Graham, J. M. & Taylor, J. (1976). Serogroups of *Escherichia coli* isolated from infants nursed in a premature baby unit. *Journal of Applied Bacteriology*, **41**, xxi.

Griffin, P. M. & Tauxe, R. V. (1991). The epidemiology of infections caused by *Escherichia coli* O157:H7, other enterohaemorrhagic *E. coli*, and the associated haemolytic uraemic syndrome. *Epidemiological Reviews*, **13**, 60–98.

Grueneberg, R. N. & Bettelheim, K. A. (1969). Geographical variation in serological types of urinary *Escherichia coli*. *Journal of Medical Microbiology*, **2**, 219–24.

Grueneberg, R. N., Leigh, D. A. & Brumfitt, W. (1968). *Escherichia coli* serotypes in urinary tract infections. Studies in domiciliary antenatal and hospital practice. In *Urinary Tract Infection*, eds. F. O'Grady & W. Brumfitt, pp. 68–79. London: Oxford University Press.

Hacker, J., Schröter, G., Schrettenbrunner, A., Hughes, C. & Goebel, W. (1983). Hemolytic *Escherichia coli* strains in the human fecal flora as potential urinary pathogens. *Zentralblatt für Bakteriologie und Hygiene A*, **254**, 370–8.

Hartley, C. L. & Richmond, M. H. (1975). Antibiotic resistance and survival of *E. coli* in the alimentary tract. *British Medical Journal*, **4**, 71–4.

Hinton, M. (1985). The sub-specific differentiation of *Escherichia coli* with particular reference to ecological studies in young animals including man. *Journal of Hygiene, Cambridge*, **95**, 595–609.

Hinton, M., Hampson, D. J., Hampson, E. & Linton, A. H. (1985a). A comparison of the ecology of *Escherichia coli* in the intestine of healthy unweaned pigs and pigs after weaning. *Journal of Applied Bacteriology*, **58**, 471–8.

Hinton, M., Linton, A. H. & Hedges, A. J. (1985b). The ecology of *Escherichia coli* in calves reared as dairy-cow replacements. *Journal of Applied Bacteriology*, **58**, 131–8.

Howe, K. & Linton, A. H. (1976). The distribution of O-antigen types of *Escherichia coli* in normal calves, compared with man, and their R plasmid carriage. *Journal of Applied Bacteriology*, **40**, 317–30.

Howe, K., Linton, A. H. & Osborne, A. D. (1976a). A longitudinal study of *Escherichia coli* in cows and calves with special reference to the distribution of O-antigen types and antibiotic resistance. *Journal of Applied Bacteriology*, **40**, 331–40.

Howe, K., Linton, A. H. & Osborne, A. D. (1976b). An investigation of calf carcass contamination by *Escherichia coli* from the gut contents at slaughter. *Journal of Applied Bacteriology*, **41**, 37–45.

Howe, K., Linton, A. H. & Osborne, A. D. (1976c). The effect of tetracycline on the coliform gut flora of broiler chickens with special reference to antibiotic resistance and O-serotypes of *Escherichia coli*. *Journal of Applied Bacteriology*, **41**, 453–64.

Jones, G. W. & Rutter, J. M. (1974). The association of K88 antigen with haemagglutinating activity in porcine strains of *Escherichia coli*. *Journal of General Microbiology*, **84**, 135–44.

Kauffmann, F. (1947). The serology of the coli group. *Journal of Immunology*, **57**, 71–100.

Kaul, M., Pabley, S. & Chibber, S. (1990). Virulence of *Escherichia coli* isolated from raw meat, food handlers and equipment of meat shops. *World Journal of Microbiology and Biotechnology*, **6**, 7–9.

Kühn, I., Tullus, K. & Möllby, R. (1986). Colonization and persistance of *Escherichia coli* phenotypes in the intestines of children aged 0 to 18 months. *Infection*, **14**, 9–12.

Lennox-King, S. M. J., O'Farrell, S. M., Bettelheim, K. A. & Shooter, R. A. (1976a). Colonization of caesarian section babies by *Escherichia coli*. *Infection*, **4**, 134–8.

Lennox-King, S. M. J., O'Farrell, S. M., Bettelheim, K. A. & Shooter, R. A. (1976b). *Escherichia coli* isolated from babies delivered by caesarian section and their environment. *Infection*, **4**, 139–45.

Lewin, C. S., Allen, R. & Amyes, A. G. B. (1990). Zidovudine-resistance in *Salmonella typhimurium* and *Escherichia coli*. *Antimicrobial Agents and Chemotherapy*, **25**, 706–8.

Lindberg, F. & Normark, S. (1986). Contribution of chromosomal β-lactamases to β-lactam resistance in enterobacteria. *Review of Infectious Diseases*, **8**, Supplement 3, S292–S304.

Linton, A. H., Handley, B. & Osborne, A. D. (1978). Fluctuations in *Escherichia coli* O-serotypes in pigs throughout life in the presence and absence of antibiotic treatment. *Journal of Applied Bacteriology*, **44**, 285–98.

Linton, A. H., Handley, B., Osborne, A. D., Shaw, B. G., Roberts, T. A. & Hudson, W. R. (1976). Contamination of pig carcasses at two abattoirs by

Escherichia coli with special reference to O-serotypes and antibiotic resistance. *Journal of Applied Bacteriology*, **42**, 89–110.

Lodinova, R., Jouja, V., Vinsova, N. & Vocel, J. (1979). Prevention and treatment of gastrointestinal infections by oral colonization with a non-enteropathogenic *E. coli* strain O83 in infants. *Folia Microbiologica, Praha*, **24**, 84–6.

Mackel D. C., Weaver, R. E., Langley, L. F. & De Capito, T. M. (1960). Observations on occurrence in cats of *Escherichia coli* pathogenic for man. *American Journal of Hygiene*, **71**, 176–8.

Majed, N. I., Bettelheim, K. A., Shooter, R. A. & Moorhouse, E. (1978). The effect of travel on faecal *Escherichia coli* serotypes. *Journal of Hygiene, Cambridge*, **81**, 481–7.

Matthew, M. & Harris, A. M. (1986). Identification of β-lactamase by analytical isolelectric focussing: correlation with bacterial taxonomy. *Journal of General Microbiology*, **94**, 55–67.

Mian, K. A. (1959). Isolation of enteropathogenic *Escherichia coli* from household pets: relation to infantile diarrhea. *Journal of the American Medical Association*, **171**, 1957–61.

Mitsuoka, T. & Hayakawa, K. (1972). Die Faecalflora bei Menschen. I. Mitteilung: Die Zusammensetzung der Faecalflora der verschiedenen Altersgruppen. *Zentralblatt für Bakteriologie und Hygiene A*, **223**, 333–42.

Moss, S. & Frost, A. J. (1984). The resistance to chemotherapeutic agents of *Escherichia coli* from domestic dogs and cats. *Australian Veterinary Journal*, **61**, 82–4.

Murono, K., Fujita, K., Yoshikawa, M., Saijo, M., Inyaku, F., Kakehashi, H. & Tsukamoto, T. (1993). Acquisition of nonmaternal Enterobacteriaceae by infants delivered in hospitals. *Journal of Pediatrics*, **122**, 120–5.

Mushin, R. & Dubos, R. (1965). Colonization of the mouse intestine with *Escherichia coli*. *Journal of Experimental Medicine*, **122**, 745–57.

Nagy, B., Moon, H. W. & Isaacson, R. E. (1977). Colonization of porcine intestine by enterotoxigenic *Escherichia coli*: selection of piliated forms *in vivo*, adhesion of piliated forms to epithelial cells *in vitro*, and incidence of a pilus antigen among porcine enteropathogenic *Escherichia coli* . *Infection and Immunity*, **16**, 344–52

Neter, E., Westphal, O., Lüderitz, O., Gino, R. M. & Gorzynski, E. A. (1955). Demonstration of antibodies to enteropathogenic *Escherichia coli* in sera of children of various ages. *Pediatrics*, **16**, 801–8.

Ocklitz, H. W. & Schmidt, R. F. (1957). Enteropathogenic *Escherichia coli* serotypes: infection of the new-born through mother. *British Medical Journal*, **2**, 1036–8.

O'Farrell, S. M. & Bettelheim, K. A. (1976). Antigenic degradation in *Escherichia coli*. *Zentralblatt für Bakteriologie und Hygiene A*, **235**, 399–403.

O'Farrell, S. M., Lennox-King, S. M. J., Bettelheim, K. A. Shaw, E. J. & Shooter, R. A. (1976). *Escherichia coli* in a maternity ward. *Infection*, **4**, 146–52.

Ofek, I., Mirelman, D & Sharon, N. (1977). Adherence of *Escherichia coli* to human mucosal cells mediated by mannose receptors. *Nature, London*, **265**, 623–5.

O'Grady, F. W., Richards, B., McSherry, M. A., O'Farrell, S. M. & Cattell, W. R. (1970). Introital enterobacteria, urinary infection and the urethral syndrome. *Lancet*, **2**, 1208–10.

Onderdonk, A., Marshall, B., Cisneros, R. & Levy, S. B. (1981). Competition between congenic *Escherichia coli* K-12 strains *in vivo*. *Infection and Immunity*, **32**, 74–9.

O'Neill, P. M., Talboys, C. A., Roberts, A. P. & AzAdian, B. S. (1990). The rise and fall of *Escherichia coli* O15 in a London Teaching Hospital. *Journal of Medical Microbiology*, **33**, 23–7.

Ørskov, F., Ørskov, I. & Villar, J. A. (1987). Cattle as a reservoir of verotoxin-producing *Escherichia coli*. O157.H7. *Lancet*, **2**, 276.

Ørskov, F., Sack, R. B., Ørskov, I. & Froelich, J. L. (1984). Changing fecal *Escherichia coli* flora during travel. *European Journal of Clinical Microbiology*, **3**, 306–9.

Ørskov, F. & Sørenson, K. B. (1975). *Escherichia coli* serogroups in breast-fed and bottle-fed infants. *Acta Pathologica et Microbiologica Scandinavia*, **B83**, 25–30.

Pai, C. H., Ahmed, N. & Lior, H., Johnson, W. M., Sims, H. V. & Woods, D. E. (1988). Epidemiology of sporadic diarrhoea due to verocytotoxin-producing *E. coli*: a two year prospective study. *Journal of Infectious Diseases*, **157**, 1054–7.

Parry, S. H., Abraham, S. N., Feavers, I. M., Lee, M., Jones, M. R., Bint, A. J. & Sussman, M. (1981). Urinary tract infection due laboratory-aquired *Escherichia coli*: relation to virulence. *British Medical Journal*, **282**, 949–50.

Payne, D. (1994). A study of K88-mediated haemagglutination by entero-toxigenic *Escherichia coli* (ETEC). *Microbiologica*, **17**, 99–110.

Penny, M. E., Scotland, S. M., Smith, H. R., McConnell, M. M., Knutton, S. K. & Sack, R. B. (1992). Virulence properties of Enterobacteriaceae isolated from the small intestine of children with diarrea. *Pediatric Infectious Diseases*, **11**, 623–30.

Philippon, A., Labia, R. & Jacoby, G. (1989). Extended spectrum β-lactamases. *Antimicrobial Agents and Chemotherapy*, **34**, 1131–6.

Pinegar, J. A. & Cooke, E. M. (1985). *Escherichia coli* in retail processed food. *Journal of Hygiene, Cambridge*, **95**, 39–46.

Preliminary Report (1993). Foodborne Outbreak of *Escherichia coli* O157:H7 infections from hamburgers – Western United States, 1992–1993. *Morbidity and Mortality Weekly Report*, **42**, 85–6.

Rasmussen, M. A., Cray, W. C. Jr., Casey, T. A. & Whipp, S. C. (1993). Rumen contents as a reservoir of enterohaemorrhagic *Escherichia coli*. *FEMS Microbiology Letters*, **114**, 79–84.

Reiter, B. & Brock, J. H. (1975). Inhibition of *Escherichia coli* by bovine colostrum and post-colostral milk. *Immunology*, **28**, 7182.

Reves, R. R., Fong, M., Pickering, L. K., Bartlett, A. III, Alvarez, M. & Murray, B. E. (1990). Risk factors for fecal colonization with trimethoprim- and multi-resistant *Escherichia coli* among children in day care centers in Houston. *Antimicrobial Agents and Chemotherapy*, **34**, 429–34.

Riley, L. W., Remis, R. S., Helgerson, S. D., McGee, H. B., Wells, G. J., Davis, B. R., Hebert, R. J., Olcott, E. S., Johnson, L. M., Hargrett, N. T., Blake P. A. & Cohen, M. L. (1983). Hemorrhagic colitis associated with a rare *Escherichia coli* serotype. *New England Journal of Medicine*, **308**, 681–5.

Roberts, A. P., Linton, J. D., Waterman, M. M., Gower, P. E. & Koutsaimanis, K. G. (1975). Urinary and faecal *Escherichia coli*

O-serotypes in symptomatic urinary tract infection and asymptomatic bacteriuria. *Journal of Medical Microbiology*, **8**, 311–18.

Robins-Browne, R. M. (1987). Traditional enteropathogenic *Escherichia coli*. *Review of Infectious Diseases*, **9**, 28–53.

Rowe, B., Taylor, J. & Bettelheim, K. A. (1970). An investigation of travellers' diarrhea. *The Lancet*, **1**, 1–5.

Sanders, C. C. (1992). b-Lactamases of gram-negative bacteria: new challenges for new drugs. *Clinical Infectious Diseases*, **14**, 1089–99.

Schroten, H., Steinig, M., Plogman, R., Hanisch, F. G., Hacker, J., Herzig, P. & Wahn, V. (1992). S-Fimbriae mediated adhesion of *Escherichia coli* to human buccal epithelial cells is age independent. *Infection*, **20**, 273–5.

Sellwood, R. (1979). *Escherichia coli* diarrhoea in pigs with and without the K88 receptor. *Veterinary Record*, **105**, 228–30.

Shinebaum, R., Shaw, E. J., Bettelheim, K. A. & Dickerson, A. G. (1977). Transfer of invertase production from a wild strain of *Escherichia coli*. *Zentralblatt für Bakteriologie und Hygiene A*, **237**, 189–95.

Shooter, R. A., Bettelheim, K. A., Lennox-King, S. M. J. & O'Farrell, S. (1977). *Escherichia coli* serotypes in the faeces of healthy adults over a period of several months. *Journal of Hygiene, Cambridge*, **78**, 95–8.

Shooter, R. A., Cooke, E. M., O'Farrell, S., Bettelheim, K. A., Chandler, M. E. & Bushrod, F. M. (1974). The isolation of *Escherichia coli* from a poultry packing station and an abattoir. *Journal of Hygiene, Cambridge*, **73**, 245–7.

Shooter, R. A., Cooke, E. M., Rousseau, S. A. & Breaden, A. L. (1970). Animal sources of common serotypes of *Escherichia coli* in the food of hospital patients. Possible significance in urinary tract infection. *Lancet*, **2**, 226–8.

Siitonen, A. (1992). *Escherichia coli* in fecal flora of healthy adults: serotypes, P and type 1C fimbriae, non-P mannose-resistant adhesins, and haemolytic activity. *Journal of Infectious Diseases*, **166**, 1058–65.

Smith, H. W. (1971). The bacteriology of the alimentary tract of domestic animals suffering from *Escherichia coli* infection. *Annals of the New York Academy of Sciences*, **176**, 110–25.

Smith, H. W. & Crabb, W. E. (1956). The typing of *Escherichia coli* by bacteriophage: its application in the study of the *E. coli* populations of the intestinal tract of healthy calves and calves suffering from white scours. *Journal of General Microbiology*, **15**, 556–74.

Smith, H. W. & Huggins, M. B. (1976). Further observations on the association of the colicine V plasmid of *Escherichia coli* with pathogenicity and with survival in the alimentary tract. *Journal of General Microbiology*, **92**, 335–50.

Smith, H. W. & Huggins, M. B. (1978). The effect of plasmid-determined and other characteristics on the survival of *Escherichia coli* in the alimentary tract of two human beings. *Journal of General Microbiology*, **109**, 375–9.

Smith, H. W. & Jones, J. E. T. (1963). Observations on the alimentary tract and its bacterial flora in healthy and diseased pigs. *Journal of Pathology and Bacteriology*, **86**, 387–412.

Spencer, A. G., Mulcahy, D., Shooter, R. A., O'Grady, F. W., Bettelheim, K. A. & Taylor, J. (1968). *Escherichia coli* serotypes in urinary-tract infection in a medical ward. *Lancet*, **2**, 839–42.

Tabaqchali, S., Howard, A., Teoh-Chan, C. H., Bettelheim, K. A. & Gorbach, S. L. (1977). *Escherichia coli* serotypes throughout the gastrointestinal tract of patients with intestinal disorders. *Gut*, **18**, 351–5.

Tabaqchali, S., O'Donoghue, D. P. & Bettelheim, K. A. (1978). *Escherichia coli* antibodies in patients with inflammatory bowel disease. *Gut*, **19**, 108–13.

Tullus, K. (1988). Fecal colonization with P-fimbriated *Escherichia coli* as a predictor of acute pyelonephritis in infancy–a prospective study. *Infection*, **16**, 267–8.

Tullus, K., Kühn, I., Källenius, G., Wrangsell, G., Ørskov, F., Ørskov, I. & Svenson, S. (1986). Fecal colonization with pyelonephritic *Escherichia coli* in neonates as a risk factor for pyelonephritis. *European Journal of Clinical Microbiology*, **5**, 643–8.

Tullus, K., Kühn, I., Kalin, M., Mollby, R., Olin, A, Svenson, S. & Kallenius, G. (1987). Epidemiological aspects of faecal colonization with P-fimbriated *Escherichia coli* in neonates. *Infection*, **15**, 25–31.

Update (1993). Multistate outbreak of *Escherichia coli* O157:H7 infections from hamburgers–Western United States, 1992–1993. *Morbidity and Mortality Weekly Report*, **42**, 258–63.

Van, R., Wun, C.-C., Morrow, A. L. & Pickering, L. K. (1991). The effect of diaper type and overclothing on faecal contamination in day-care centres. *Journal of the American Medical Association*, **265**, 1840–4.

Watanabe, T. (1963). Infective heredity of multiple drug resistance in bacteria. *Bacteriological Reviews*, **27**, 87–115.

Weber, D. A., Sanders, C. C., Bakken, J. S. & Quinn, J. P. (1990). A novel chromosomal TEM derivative and alterations in outer membrane proteins together mediate selective ceftazidime resistance in *Escherichia coli*. *Journal of Infectious Diseases*, **162**, 460–5.

Wells, J. G., Shipman, L. D., Greene, K. D., Sowers, E. G., Green, J. H., Cameron, D. N., Downes, F. P., Morton, M. I., Griffin, P. M., Ostroff, S. M., Potter, M. E., Tauxe, R. V. & Wachsmuth, I. K. (1991). Isolation of *Escherichia coli* serotype O157:H7 and other shiga-like-toxin producing *E. coli* from dairy cattle. *Journal of Clinical Microbiology*, **29**, 985–9.

Whittam, T. S. (1989). Clonal dynamics of *Escherichia coli* in its natural habitat. *Antonie van Leeuwenhoek Journal of Microbiology*, **55**, 23–32.

Wieler, L. H., Bauerfeind, R. & Baljer, G. (1992). Characterization of Shiga-like toxin producing *Escherichia coli* (SLTEC) from calves with and without diarroea. *Zentralblatt für Bakteriologie, International Journal of Medical Microbiology, Virology, Parasitology and Infectious Diseases*, **276**, 243–53.

Wolfson, J. S., Hooper, D. C. & Swartz, M. N. (1989). Mechanisms of action of and resistance to quinolone antimicrobial agents. In *Quinolone antimicrobial agents*, eds. J. S. Wolfson & D. C. Hooper, pp. 5–34. Washington, D.C.: American Society for Microbiology.

Zhao, T., Doyle, M. P. & Besser, R. E. (1993). Fate of enterohemorrhagic *Escherichia coli* O157:H7 in apple cider with and without preservatives. *Applied Environmental Microbiology*, **56**, 2526–30.

Part two
Virulence factors

4

Capsules of *Escherichia coli*

K. JANN and B. JANN

Gram-negative bacteria such as *Escherichia coli* characteristically have an outer membrane external to their murein layer. Lipopolysaccharide, a typical component of this outer membrane, is the O-antigen of wild-type bacteria. Though antibodies directed against the O-antigen usually agglutinate these bacteria, serological studies of *E. coli* (Kauffmann, 1954; Ørskov *et al.*, 1977) have shown that agglutination of many strains by homologous O-antisera occurs only after heating. This inhibitory effect is due to the presence of antigens distinct from O-antigens that are present as an extracellular envelope, or capsule, which covers the O-antigenic lipopolysaccharide. These are termed capsular or K-antigens ('Kapselantigene') and can be demonstrated by light microscopy. With proper contrast and stabilisation, they can also be studied by electron microscopy (Bayer & Thurow, 1977; Bayer *et al.*, 1985; Bayer, 1990: Kröncke *et al.*, 1990; Bronner *et al.*, 1993).

Capsules protect pathogenic bacteria against non-specific host defences, notably the action of complement and phagocytes. Thus, encapsulated bacteria are often virulent, and their capsules are virulence factors. K-specific antibodies, formed at a late stage of infection, overcome the protective action of the capsules, but some capsules are not recognised as foreign by the host. As a result, antibodies are not produced and the host is vulnerable to the pathogen.

Knowledge about *E. coli* capsules and K-antigens has increased greatly in recent years. In the light of the biomedical significance of capsules, a synopsis of structural, biochemical and genetic information of *E. coli* capsules is desirable and the molecular aspects of capsular (K) antigens and their biological significance will be considered.

General chemical characteristics of capsular antigens

Capsular antigens are acid polysaccharides with a regular structure, made up of repeating oligosaccharide units. Some strains express capsules at all growth temperatures (group I), while others do so only above about 25°C (group II) (Ørskov *et al.*, 1984). These organisms and their capsules have been further analysed and several distinct features characteristic of the two groups of organisms have been established (Jann & Jann, 1990, 1992). The classification of the *E. coli* capsular polysaccharides is shown in Table 4.1.

Strains with group I capsules, which are expressed at all temperatures, belong to serogroups O8, O9 and O20. Their capsules are determined by chromosomal genes close to the *his* locus and, in some strains, also close to *trp* (Schmidt *et al.*, 1977; Laakso *et al.*, 1988). The capsular acid polysaccharides of group I usually have large repeating units, tetra- to hexasaccharides, and the most common acid components are hexuronic acid and pyruvate. The group can be subdivided on the basis of the sugar composition of their capsular polysaccharides, some of which do not contain amino sugars (group Ia), while others contain one or two amino sugars per repeating unit (group Ib). The polysaccharides of group Ia resemble the capsular polysaccharides of *Klebsiella*.

Strains with group II capsules, which are only expressed at about 25°C and above, occur in many O-groups and co-expression with lipopolysac-charide is not regulated. Group II capsules of *E. coli* are chromosomally determined by the *kps* gene cluster, which is close to *serA*. These polysaccharides have smaller, usually di- or trisaccharide, repeating units than group I capsules. Their acidic components are more diverse than those of group I, with hexuronic acids, *N*-acetylneuraminic acid, 3-deoxy-*manno*-D-octulosonic acid (KDO), mannosaminuronic acid or phosphate as possible representatives. Some group II capsular poly-saccharides are similar in structure and general characteristics to those of *Neisseria meningitidis* and *Haemophilus influenzae* (Jann & Jann, 1990, 1992). It has recently been observed that *E. coli* strains with group II polysaccharides have greatly elevated CMP (cytidine 5'-monophosphate-KDO synthetase (CKS) activity, but only after growth at capsule-permissive temperatures.

Some *E. coli* strains have capsular polysaccharides, chemically similar to those of group II capsules, that are determined by a chromosomal site proximal to *serA*, which is not temperature regulated and the CKS activity of these strains is not elevated. These capsules (K3, K10, K11, K54, K96, K98), although closely related to group II capsules, appear to

Table 4.1. *Classification of the capsular polysaccharides of* Escherichia coli

	Capsular polysaccharide group	
	I	II
Acidic component	Glucuronic acid	Glucuronic acid
	Galacturonic acid	NeuNAc
	Pyruvate	KDO
		ManNAcA
		Phosphate
Expressed below 20°C	Yes	No
Co-expression with O-antigens	O8, O9, O20	Many O-antigens
Lipid at the reducing end	Core-lipid A	Phosphatidic acid
Chromosomal determination (close to)	*rfb* (*his*), *rfc* (*trp*)	*kpsA* (*ser*)
CMP–KDO synthetase activity raised	No	Yes
Intergeneric relationship with	*Klebsiella* (Ia)	*H. influenzae*, *N. meningitidis*

CMP, cytidine 5'-monophosphate; KDO, 3-deoxy-*manno*-D-octulosonic acid; NeuNAc, *N*-acetylneuraminic acid; ManNAcA, mannosaminuronic acid.

belong to a subclass of group II. It is suggested that they be termed group III capsules, although they may turn out to be a heterogeneous group.

During structural analysis it became evident that capsular polysaccharides are terminated by a lipid substituent at their reducing end. Polysaccharides of group Ib have core-lipid A at their reducing end and so are really lipopolysaccharide (Jann & Jann, 1990; Jann *et al.*, 1992), and there are indications that group Ia capsular polysaccharides also terminate in core-lipid A (Homonylo *et al.*, 1988; Whitfield *et al.*, 1989). Polysaccharides of group II have a phosphatidic acid substituent (Gotschlich *et al.*, 1981; Schmidt & Jann, 1982). This is shown in Figure 4.1 for the K12 polysaccharide. The fatty acid spectrum of this lipid has the expected composition for the membrane phospholipids of *E. coli*. It is of interest that the related capsular polysaccharides of *N. meningitidis* and *H. influenzae* type b (Hib) also have phosphatidic acid at their reducing end (Gotschlich *et al.*, 1981; Kuo *et al.*, 1985). In the group II polysaccharides so far analysed, the lipid substituent was present in only 40–60 per cent of the preparations. This may have been due to the pronounced lability of the glycosyl-phosphodiester linkage. It is assumed that the lipid end may function as a membrane anchor for the capsular polysaccharides and to assist in the formation of a cell-associated capsule.

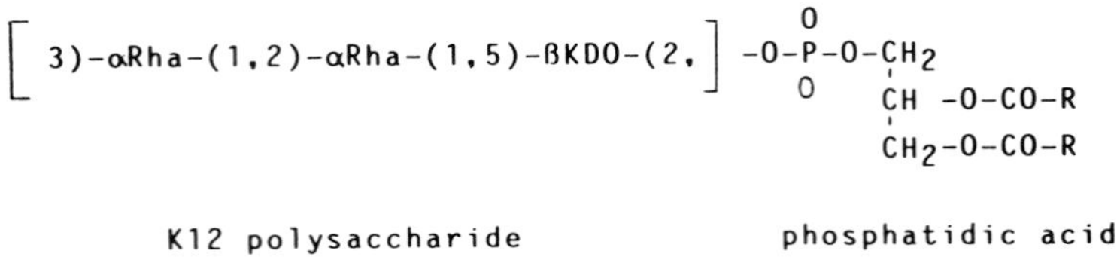

$$\left[\text{ 3})-\alpha Rha-(1,2)-\alpha Rha-(1,5)-\beta KDO-(2,} \right] \quad \begin{array}{c} O \\ -O-P-O-CH_2 \\ O \quad CH-O-CO-R \\ CH_2-O-CO-R \end{array}$$

K12 polysaccharide   phosphatidic acid

Fig. 4.1. Structure of K12 capsular polysaccharide (K12 antigen) with terminally substituted phosphatidic acid. KDO, 3-Deoxy-*manno*-D-octulosonic acid.

Structures

More than 70 distinct *E. coli* capsular polysaccharide antigens are recognised and the structures of most have been elucidated. Since it is beyond the scope of this chapter to discuss them all, they are listed in Table 4.2 with their group assignment, composition and the relevant references.

A number of K-specific capsular polysaccharides have the same structure as the O-specific polysaccharides of certain lipopolysaccharides (O-antigens). Thus, the polysaccharides of K9 and O104, K85 and O141 and K87 and O32 are identical (Jann *et al.*, 1971; Kogan *et al.*, 1992).

Group II polysaccharides of particular interest

Certain polysaccharides of group II are of special interest with respect to their biochemistry, genetics and their significance in infections.

Polysaccharides that contain 3-deoxy-manno-D-octulosonic acid

3-Deoxy-*manno*-D-octulosonic acid has been thought of as a characteristic constituent of lipopolysaccharide and as providing the linkage between lipid A and the carbohydrate moiety of lipopolysaccharide (Jann & Westphal, 1975). It is, however, also a major constituent of a number of capsular polysaccharides. While lipopolysaccharide contains only some two to five per cent KDO, this sugar constitutes 40–60 per cent of the capsular polysaccharide mass. KDO has been reviewed by Unger (1981).

KDO occurs in many types of linkages, in pyranose and furanose ring forms, mostly as the β-anomer but also as the α-anomer. The various substitution patterns of KDO in capsular polysaccharides and in lipopolysaccharide are illustrated in Figure 4.2. The capsular polysaccharide of *N. meningitidis* 29-e contains seven-linked KDO (Bhattacharjee *et al.*, 1978).

Table 4.2. *Composition of* Escherichia coli *capsular polysaccharides*

Antigen	Composition		Structure elucidated by
	Acidic component	Other components	
Group Ia			
K26	GlcA-Prv	Gal, L-Rha	Beynon & Dutton (1988)
K27	GlcA	Gal, Glc, L-Fuc	Jann et al. (1968, 1995)
K28	GlcA	Gal, Glc, L-Fuc	Altman & Dutton (1985)
K29	GlcA-Prv	Gal, Glc, Man	Choy et al. (1975)
K30	GlcA	Gal, Man	Chakraborty et al. (1980)
K31	GlcA	Gal, Glc, L-Rha	Dutton et al. (1990)
K32	GlcA	Gal, Glc, L-Rha	Anison et al. (1987)
K33	GlcA-Prv	Gal, Glc, L-Fuc	H. Parolis, personal communication
K34	GlcA	Gal, Glc	Dutton & Kuma-Mintha (1987)
K35	GlcA	Gal, Glc, Man	Hackland & Parolis (1992)
K36	GalA	Gal, Man	Parolis et al. (1988)
K37	Prv	Gal, Glc	Anderson et al. (1987)
K39	GlcA	Gal, Glc, Man	Parolis et al. (1989)
K42	GalA	Gal, Fuc	Niemann et al. (1978)
K55	GlcA-Prv	Man	Anderson & Parolis (1988)
K102	GlcA	Gal, Glc	de Bruin et al. (1992b)
K103	Prv	Gal, Rha	M. R. Grue, H. Parolis & L. A. S. Parolis, *in press*
Group Ib			
K8	GlcA	**GlcNAc, GalNAc,** Gal	Parolis & Parolis (1988)
K9	NeuNAc	**GalNAc,** Gal	Dutton et al. (1987)
K38	GalA	**GlcNAc, GalNAc,** Gal, Rib	Hackland et al. (1991)
K40	GlcA-Ser	**GlcNAc**	Dengler et al. (1986)
K44	GlcA	**GlcNAc, GalNAc,** Rha	Dutton et al. (1988)
K45	GalA	**GlcNAc, FucNAc**	Grue et al. (1993b)
K46	GroP	**GlcNAc,** Gal, Glc, Rha	Dutton et al. (1992)
K47	Prv	**GlcNAc,** Gal, Man	de Bruin et al. (1992a)

Table 4.2. (cont.)

Antigen	Composition		Structure elucidated by
	Acidic component	Other components	
K48	GlcA	GlcNAc, **DAS**[a]	D. V. Whittaker, H. Parolis and L. A. S. Parolis, in press
K49	GlcA-Thr	**GlcNAc**, Gal, Glc	Beynon (1988)
K50	Prv	**GlcNAc**, **ManNAc**, Man, Rha	M. R. Grue, H. Parolis & L. A. S. Parolis, in press
K57	GalA	**GlcNAc**, Gal, Rib	Parolis et al. (1990a)
K83	GalA	**GlcNAc**, Gal, Man, Rha	D. V. Whittaker, H. Parolis & L. A. S. Parolis, in press
K85	GlcA	**GlcNAc**, Man, Rha	Jann et al. (1966)
K87	GlcA	**GlcNAc**, **FucNAc**, Gal, Glc	Tarcsay et al. (1971) Parolis et al. (1990b)
K101	GlcA	**GlcNAc**, **GalNAc**, Gal	Grue et al. (1993a)
Group II			
K1	NeuNAc		Ørskov et al. (1979)
K2a	GroP	Gal	Jann et al. (1980)
K2ab	GroP	Gal	Jann & Schmidt (1980)
K4	GlcA	GalNAc	Rodriguez et al. (1988a)
K5	GlcA	GlcNAc	Vann et al. (1981)
K6	KDO	Rib	Jennings et al. (1982)
K7 (K56)	ManNAcA	Glc	Tsui et al. (1982)
K12	KDO	Rha	Schmidt & Jann (1983)
K13	KDO	Rib	Vann & Jann (1979)
K14	KDO	GalNAc	Jann et al. (1983)
K15	KDO	GlcNAc	Jann & Jann (1990)
K16	KDO	Rib	Lenter et al. (1990a)
K18	Rit*P*	Rib	Rodriguez et al. (1988b)
K19	KDO	Rib	Jann et al. (1988)
K20	KDO	Rib	Vann et al. (1983)

K22	Rit$P$	Rib	Rodriguez et al. (1988b)
K23	KDO	Rib	Vann et al. (1983)
K24	KDO, Gro$P$		Lenter et al. (1990b)
K51	GlcNAcP		Jann et al. (1985)
K52	Gal$P$	Fru	Hofmann et al. (1985a)
K53	GlcA	Gal	Bax et al. (1988)
K74	KDO	Rib	Ahrens et al. (1988)
K92	NeuNAc		Lifely et al. (1985)
K93	GlcA	Gal	Bax et al. (1988)
K95	KDO	Rib	Dengler et al. (1985)
K97	KDO	Rib	Jann unpublished
K100	Rit$P$	Rib	Rodriguez et al. (1988b)

Group III[b]

K3	KDH	Rha	Dengler et al. (1988)
K10	Qui4NMal	Rha	Sieberth et al. (1993)
K11	Glc$P$	Glc, Fru	Rodriguez et al. (1989)
K54	GlcA-Thr	Rha	Hofmann et al. (1985b)
K96	GlcA	Rha	Jann et al. (1993)
K98	GlcA	Rha	Hahne et al. (1991)

[a] DAS is 2,3-diacetamido-2,3,6-trideoxy-β-L-mannopyranose.

[b] This is a provisional designation for a heterogeneous group of K-antigens. Its members differ genetically and biochemically from those in Groups I and II. See text for details.

The amino sugars of group Ib capsular polysaccharides are shown in bold to emphasise their difference from group Ia capsular polysaccharides, which do not contain amino sugars.

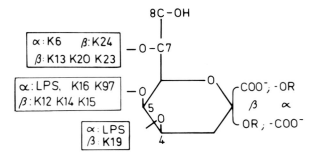

Not yet found : 8 - KDOp

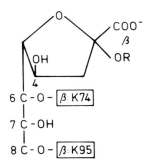

Not yet found : 4- KDOf , 7- KDOf

Fig. 4.2. 3-Deoxy-*mano*-D-octulosonic acid (KDO) linkages that occur in group II capsular polysaccharides and in the lipopolysaccharides (LPS) of *Escherichia coli*.

Antigen K24 has the unusual combination of KDO with glycerol phosphate and, therefore, also belongs to the group of phosphate-containing polymers (see below).

A KDO-related 4-deoxy-2-hexulosonic acid (4KDH in Table 4.2) is present in antigen K3 of *E. coli*. This is a substituent of a polysaccharide backbone that consists of -2)-α-L-rhamnosyl-(1,3)-α-L-rhamnosyl-(1,3)-α-L-rhamnosyl repeating units.

Phosphate-containing polymers

These capsular antigens are not strictly polysaccharides, but are comparable to the complex teichoic acids of certain Gram-positive bacteria (Wicken & Knox, 1980). They may contain glycerol phosphate (K2a,

Table 4.3. *Structures of the capsular antigens of* Escherichia coli *K18, K22, K100 and* Haemophilus influenzae *type b (Hib)*

Type	Structure	Reference
K22	2)-β-Rib-(1→2)-Rit-(5-*P*-	Rodriguez *et al.* (1988b)
K18[a]	2)-β-Rib-(1→2)-Rit-(5-*P*-3-OAc	Rodriguez *et al.* (1988b)
K100	3)-β-Rib-(1→2)-Rit-(5-*P*-	Rodriguez *et al.* (1988b)
Hib	3-)β-Rib-(1→1)-Rit-(5-*P*-	Branefors-Hellander *et al.* (1976)

[a] On average, every second repeating unit is acetylated. For interpretation, see text.

K2ab), ribitol phosphate (K18, K22, K100) or they may form a sugar phosphate polymer, which may or may not be substituted by other sugars.

Antigens K18, K22 and K100 are ribosyl-ribitol phosphates, structurally closely related to the capsular polysaccharide of Hib (Branefors-Helander *et al.*, 1976). Since Hib causes severe and often lethal infections in small children, and the Hib capsular antigen is an important virulence determinant (Moxon & Vaughn, 1981), attempts at cross-protection have been made with the related and serologically cross-reacting *E. coli* K100 polysaccharide (Schneerson & Robbins, 1975). These attempts were discontinued when it became evident that *E. coli* K100 may itself be virulent for children.

The primary structures of *E. coli* K18, K22, K100 and Hib antigens are shown in Table 4.3. Antigen K18 differs from K22 in being about 40 per cent O-acetylated at C-3 of the 2-linked ribose. NMR spectroscopy and computer-aided molecular modelling (M. L. Rodriguez, A. Neszmelyi & Jann, unpublished) indicates that antigens K18, K22 and K100 and Hib capsular antigen form helices that differ in the pitch and tilt of their turns. This results in different exposures of their epitopes on the helical surface and correlates with their recognition by antibodies, and this explains the observed cross-reactivities (Schneerson & Robbins, 1975). The extent to which these polymer chains are helical is unknown.

Polysaccharides that contain glucuronic acid

Two of the four glucuronic-acid-containing group II polysaccharides listed in Table 4.2 are of particular interest.

4)-β-GlcA-1→3)-β-GalNAc-(1

3

↑

2-β-Fru

(A) (Rodriguez *et al.*, 1988a)

4)-β-GlcA-(1→4)-GlcNac-(1

(B) Vann *et al.*, 1981)

Polysaccharide K4 (A) is a fructosylated chondroitin, the fructose of which splits off under very mild acid conditions. X-ray diffraction measurements suggest that the polysaccharide may have a spatial structure that resembles chondroitin sulphate. Both polymers consist of helices with the substituent on the inside, fructose in the case of the K4 and sulphate in the case of chondroitin sulphate, with the chondroitin backbone pointing outwards (A. T. Atkins, personal communication).

Polysaccharide K5 (B) has the same primary structure as *N*-acetyl heparosan, the first polymeric intermediate in the biosynthesis of heparin (Navia *et al.*, 1983). NMR analysis and structure calculations (D. R. Ferro and A. Torii, personal communication) show that the polysaccharide chain, or parts of it, form a multiple helix.

Polysaccharides that contain N-*acetylneuraminic acid*

Two capsular polysaccharides of group II are known to contain *N*-acetylneuraminic acid (NeuNAc). The repeating unit of polysaccharide K1 is -8)-α-NeuNAc-(2, (Ørskov *et al.*, 1979), which has the same structure as the capsular polysaccharide of *N. meningitidis* type b. Another member of this group of polysialic acids is the capsular polysaccharide of *N. meningitidis* type c that has the repeating unit, -9)-α-NeuNAc-(2→9)-α-NeuNAc-(2 (Lifely *et al.*, 1985). The K92 polysaccharide of *E. coli* combines the polysaccharides substructures of *E. coli* K1 and the *N.-meningitidis* type c in an alternating sequence.

The effect of structural modification on the serological specificity

O-acetylation

Certain sugars of the repeating units of many capsular polysaccharides are O-acetylated and the acetyl substituent is usually an immuno-dominant part of the serological epitope. Though not every repeating unit in the polysaccharide is substituted, O-acetylation is not random; the same hydroxyl group of the same sugar residue is always acetylated. Two related types of epitopes are, therefore, always present in such polysaccharide preparations. One of these is defined by the non-acetylated sugar and the other by its acetylated form. Sometimes an acetyl group is the only difference between otherwise identical structures of distinct polysaccharide antigens. For example, antigen K2ab (formerly antigen K62), the acetylated form of antigen K2a (Larsen *et al.*, 1980), antigen K1, which occurs in an acetylated and non-acetylated form (Ørskov *et al.*, 1979; Jann *et al.*, 1980; Jann & Schmidt, 1980), antigens K53 and K93, in which the same polysaccharide backbone is substituted with one (K53) or two (K93) acetyl groups in each repeating unit (Bax *et al.*, 1988), and antigen K18, which is the acetylated form of K22 antigen (Rodriguez *et al.*, 1988b).

The significance of partial O-acetylation has been studied by immuno-electron microscopy by comparing the reaction with absorbed antisera of the non-acetylated antigen K22 and antigen K18 acetylated to about 40 per cent (M. L. Rodriguez, K. D. Kröncke & K. Jann, unpublished). All the K22 bacteria reacted with an anti-K22 serum and had a capsule but they did not react with an absorbed anti-K18 serum specific for 3-*O*-acetylribose and no capsule was detected. In contrast, only about 40 per cent of the K18 bacteria reacted with the absorbed acetylribose-specific antiserum and some 60 per cent reacted with the K22 serum. This shows that *E. coli* K18 is a mixture of organisms that differ in their ability to acetylate their capsular antigen. The same was found with the partially acetylated *E. coli* K1 capsular polysaccharide (Ørskov *et al.*, 1979). It is assumed that partial O-acetylation is due to a specific transacetylase, active or present in only a part of the bacterial population. The enzyme activity is probably controlled by a genetic element that switches enzyme activity on or off at a constant rate. This phenomenon, first analysed with *Salmonella* lipopolysaccharide, was termed O-antigen form variation (Mäkelä & Stocker, 1969).

Other substitutions

Several capsular polysaccharides are substituted with pyruvate, mainly at α-Gal or α-Man residues, in a ketosidic linkage (Table 4.2). This introduces a charge, sometimes as in K26, K29 and K33, in addition to another charged constituent such as a hexuronic acid.

The charge on polysaccharides K40 and K49 is due to amide substitution of the carboxyl group of a hexuronic acid by an amino-acid (Table 4.2). This is also encountered in the polysaccharides of other genera and removal of the substituent with alkali does not alter the charge density of the polysaccharide. The negative charge of polysaccharide K10 is due to amidation of the amino group of the 4,6-dideoxy-4-aminoglucose residue with one of the carboxyl groups of malonic acid (Sieberth *et al.*, 1993).

Genetics of capsular polysaccharides

Genetics of group I capsular polysaccharides

The expression of polysaccharide K27 (group Ia) is determined by a *his*-linked gene cluster that encodes, amongst others, the transferases for the synthesis of the repeating unit and, by way of a *trp*-linked gene, it determines a polymerase that joins the repeating units (Schmidt *et al.*, 1977). The *his*-linked genes and the *trp*-linked gene, respectively, correspond to the *rfb* genes and the *rfc* gene of lipopolysaccharide (Mäkelä & Stocker, 1969). It has also been shown that antigen K30, also of group Ia, is directed only from the *his*-linked genes (Whitfield *et al.*, 1989). This is reminiscent of the genetic determination of *Salmonella* lipopolysaccharide, where the polymerase gene may be either within or outside the *his*-linked *rfb* gene cluster.

Expression of group Ia capsular polysaccharide is subject to the rcs (regulation of capsule synthesis) system (McCallum & Whitfield, 1991; Keenleyside *et al.*, 1992, 1993), which has been described for the mucus antigen of rough *E. coli* K-12 strains (Gottesman & Stout, 1991). This is essentially a two-component regulatory system fine-tuned by the lon-protease of *E. coli*.

The organisation of group I capsule genes and their functions in capsule expression is still unclear.

Genetics of group II capsular polysaccharides

In comparison with group I capsules, much more is known about the genetics of group IIa capsules. The *kps* genes responsible for the synthesis (polymerisation) and surface expression of these polysaccharides have been extensively studied with *E. coli* K1 and K5 strains (see Boulnois & Roberts, 1990; Silver *et al.*, 1993). The genes have been mapped to 64 minutes, near *serA* on the *E. coli* chromosome (Ørskov & Nymann, 1974; Vimr, 1990), and they are organised into three gene regions. A central region, region 2, determines the polymerisation of the respective K polysaccharides but differs in strains with different capsule types, and its size depends on the structure and size of the polysaccharide repeating unit (Boulnois *et al.*, 1992). Region 2 is flanked by regions 1 and 3, which contain genes that direct the translocation of the polysaccharide across the inner (cytoplasmic) membrane and its transport through periplasm and outer membrane on to the cell surface. Transport regions 1 and 3 can be exchanged, functionally intact, between *E. coli* strains with different capsular polysaccharides (Boulnois *et al.*, 1987; Roberts *et al.*, 1988). Region 1 of *E. coli* K5 has been sequenced and a number of open reading frames (ORF) defined and characterised (Pazzani *et al.*, 1993). Region 3 contains two genes that were identified independently for *E. coli* K5 (Smith *et al.*, 1990) and *E. coli* K1 (Vimr *et al.*, 1989; Pavelka *et al.*, 1991). The region 2 genes of the K5 capsule gene cluster have been sequenced (Petit *et al.*, 1995) and, because they are K5 specific, have been termed *kfi* (kapsel antigen five). The region 2 genes of *E. coli* K1 are known as *neu* genes (activation and transfer of *N*-acetylneuraminic acid) (Vimr *et al.*, 1989; Silver *et al.*, 1993). The capsule genes, *kps* and *kfi*, of *E. coli* K5, their ORF and putative functions are summarised in Figure 4.3.

Expression of group II capsular polysaccharides is not regulated by the rcs system, but is under the control of the *rfaH* gene (Stevens *et al.*, 1994). Since RfaH also affects synthesis of the lipopolysaccharide core (Pradel & Schnaitman, 1991), it has been ascertained, with appropriate recombinant strains of K5, that this is not an indirect effect on capsule expression. In the non-coding region upstream of several gene clusters that direct the production of various polysaccharides in enteric bacteria, including group II capsule genes, a 39-bp DNA sequence (JUMPstart sequence) has been identified (Hobbs & Reeves, 1994). Since the JUMPstart sequence is homologous to sequences found in RfaH-regulated genes, a common mode of regulation of these polysaccharides by RfaH seems possible.

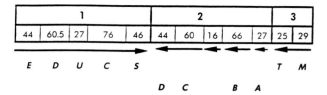

Region	Kps	Kfi	Location	Putative function
1	E		Inner membrane	Transport protein
1	D		Periplasm	Transport protein
1	U		Cytoplasm	CKS (KDO for export)
1	C		Cytoplasm	Synthesis of phosphatidyl-KDO
1	S		Inner membrane (?)	and its ligation with the PS
2		D	Cytoplasm	UDPGlc-DH
2		C	Inner membrane	GlcA- and GlcNAc-TF°
2		B	?	?
2		A	?	?
3	T		Cytoplasm	Translocation energiser
3	M		Inner membrane	Translocator (channel)

Fig. 4.3. The organisation of the genes that determine the expression of *Escherichia coli* group II capsular K5 polysaccharide. Gene regions 1 and 3 contain *kps* genes, determining expression, and region 2 contains the *kfi* (K five antigen) genes determining synthesis of the K5 polysaccharide. The arrows indicate the direction of transcription. The putative sizes of the gene products, as calculated from the DNA sequences of the genes, are indicated in kilodaltons (boxed). The figure also shows the authors' interpretation of the functions of the products (KpsEDUCS and KfiCD) of the genes (*kpsEDUC* and *kfiCD*).[a] TF, transferase.

Not much is known about the genetics of group III capsular polysaccharides. As in the case of *E. coli* K10 and K54, these capsule genes consist of three regions. Region 2 is type-specific. Region 1 contains transport genes, some of which, such as *kpsE* and *kpsD*, can substitute for the corresponding genes in region 1 of capsule group II. Region 3 appears to be unrelated genetically to that of capsule group II (Pearce & Roberts, 1995). Hybridisation studies indicated that group III is genetically heterogeneous. Its classification as group III is therefore provisional and at present the group is best characterised as, 'neither group I nor group II'.

Biosynthesis of capsular polysaccharides

The expression of bacterial capsules is a complex process that involves various cellular compartments. Activation and interconversion of sugar constituents take place in the cytoplasm, while polymerisation (biosynthesis) of the polysaccharide by transfer of the sugar units from their activated (nucleotide) forms is achieved by specific sugar transferases associated with the cytoplasmic membrane. Polymerisation may follow either of two mechanisms, (i) assembly of lipid-linked oligosaccharide repeating units or (ii) chain elongation by addition of sugars, directly from their activated forms.

Biosynthesis of group I capsular polysaccharides

Little is known about the biosynthesis of group I capsular polysac-charides. The studies by Troy *et al.* (1971, 1972, 1992) on the biosynthesis of a *Klebsiella* capsular polysaccharide remain some of the best sources of information. The capsular polysaccharide is synthesised by polymerisa-tion of oligosaccharide repeating units linked to undecaprenol pyrophosphate, and there is evidence that this mechanism also operates in the biosynthesis of *E. coli* K27 and K30 polysaccharides (K. Jann & B. Jann, unpublished; C. Whitfield, unpublished).

Biosynthesis of group II capsular polysaccharides

Systematic studies of the polymerisation of group II capsular poly-saccharides, *in vivo* and *in vitro*, have been carried out with polysialic acid antigen K1 and K5, which consists of glucuronic acid and *N*-acetyl-glucosamine. Only the essential features will be considered here.

Biosynthesis of the K1 polysaccharide

Studies of the polymerisation of the K1 polysaccharide *in vitro*, based on the isolation of sialyl-monophosphoundecaprenol, suggest that un-decaprenol phosphate is a co-factor in the polymerisation (Troy & McClosky, 1979; Troy, 1992; Whitfield *et al.*, 1984). Biosynthesis of the structurally identical capsular polysialic acid of *N. meningitidis* B is similar (Masson & Holbein, 1985). Polysialic acid and its fragments can be used as exogenous acceptors in the elongation of K1 polysaccharide *in vitro* (Whitfield & Troy, 1984) but the nature of the primary endogenous acceptor and the initiating reaction by which transfer of the first sugar constituent takes place remain unknown. Since K1 antigen, as isolated from the capsule, has *N*-acetylneuraminic acid (sometimes known as sialic acid) at its reducing end (Gotschlich *et al.*, 1981), it is possible that the first sugar transferred is *N*-acetylneuraminic acid. The sialyl linkage is, however, very labile and the results could have been due to breakage of the polysaccharide during the determination. If that is so, the true terminal reducing sugar may have escaped detection (see below).

Biosynthesis of K5 polysaccharide

Polymerisation of K5 antigen takes place on the cytoplasmic face of the inner membrane, chain elongation is at the non-reducing end of the chain and no lipid co-factor is necessary. Chain elongation proceeds stepwise by direct sequential transfer of *N*-acetylglucosamine and glucuronic acid from their uridine 5'-diphosphate (UDP) forms, without intermediary formation of undecaprenol diphosphate mono- or oligosaccharides (Finke *et al.*, 1991; Bronner *et al.*, 1993a,b). The capacity of the sugar transferases to use K5 polysaccharide or oligosaccharides with glucuronic acid or *N*-acetylglucosamine at the reducing end as exogenous acceptors *in vitro* has been tested with membranes from recombinant *E. coli* K5. These exogenous acceptors became elongated, and the extent of sugar transfer depended on the ability of the exogenous acceptors to associate with the membrane (Sieberth *et al.*, submitted for publication).

Since polysaccharide K5, as isolated from the capsule, contains KDO and phosphatidic acid, as phosphatidyl-KDO, at its reducing end (Schmidt & Jann, 1982), the cytoplasmic membrane-associated polymerisation product was also expected to have KDO at the reducing end. This was not the case, however, and the nature of the reducing sugar, and thus that of the initiation reaction remain unknown. As with K1 antigen, information is limited to chain elongation (polymerisation).

Two genes from region 2 of the K5 capsule gene cluster (see Figure 4.3) have been cloned and their products analysed. The KfiD protein was found to be a UDP-glucose dehydrogenase (UDP-GlcDH) that provides UDP-gluconic acid (UDP-GlcA), one of the substrates for the biosynthesis of the K5 polysaccharide (Sieberth *et al.*, 1995). The KfiC protein appeared to be a tranferase for both glucuronic acid, from UDP-GlcA, and *N*-acetylglucosamine, from UDP-GlcNAc (Petit *et al.*, 1995; V. Sieberth & Jann, unpublished). Similar results had been reported for the biosynthesis of the capsular hyaluronate of group A streptococci, where the genes for UDP-GlcDH (*hasB*) and hyaluronate synthetase (*hasA*) are within the same capsule gene locus (Dougherty & van de Rijn, 1993, 1994).

It is noteworthy that the mechanism for the polymerisation of polysaccharide K5, i.e. chain growth at the non-reducing end without participation of undecaprenol phosphate as co-factor, is the same as that for the biosynthesis of *N*-acetylheparosan, the first polymeric intermediate of heparin (Lindahl, 1972; Lidholt *et al.*, 1994). Furthermore, there are strong indications that, also in heparin synthesis, both sugar constituents, GlcA and GlcNAc, are transferred by a single enzyme (Lidholt *et al.*, 1992; Lind *et al.*, 1993). On the basis of these findings it is possible to conclude that the genes for K5 biosynthesis in *E. coli* and mammalian cells may be related. Capture of the genes by an invasive strain of *E. coli* may be an explanation for these facts, particularly because the region 2 genes have a GC content that is not characteristic of *E. coli* (Petit *et al.*, 1995; I. S. Roberts, personal communication). Gene capture may also be the cause of the presence of region 2 genes (*neu* genes) in *E. coli* K1.

Expression of capsular polysaccharides on the bacterial surface

Bacterial polysaccharides are expressed on the bacterial surface in three stages, translocation across the inner membrane, transport through the periplasm and passage of the outer membrane.

Polysaccharide translocation across the cytoplasmic membrane appears to depend on whether the mechanism of polymerisation is by polysaccharide assembly from lipid-linked oligosaccharides or by continuous elongation of the polysaccharide without the formation of lipid-linked intermediates. Lipid-linked oligosaccharides, formed at the inner side of the cytoplasmic membrane, probably cross the membrane by a flip-flop mechanism (McGrath & Osborn, 1991) and are then assembled at the outer face of the membrane, without the need for polysaccharide translocation. Polysaccharides completely polymerised at the cytoplasmic side of the membrane have to be translocated with the help of special (translocator) protein(s).

Transport of the polysaccharides through the periplasm requires the participation of transport (shuttle) proteins. Channel-forming proteins in the outer membrane are thought to make possible their surface expression. The appearance of lipopolysaccharides (Mühlradt *et al.*, 1973) and capsular polysaccharides (see below) occurs at surface sites where the inner and outer membrane are in close apposition. Such sites, described by Bayer (1975), were shown to play a role in the transport of macromolecules across the cell wall.

While there is little information about the surface expression of group I capsular polysaccharides (but see Bayer & Thurow, 1977), the export of group II capsular polysaccharides is the subject of intensive study and a picture of the export process is emerging.

Surface expression of group II capsular polysaccharides

Expression of group II capsular polysaccharides on the bacterial surface has been studied mainly with the K1 and K5 polysaccharide representatives of group IIa. Since their expression is temperature regulated, it is possible to follow *de novo* capsule formation by shifting the growth conditions from a restrictive to a permissive temperature. Sudden appearance of K1, K5 and K12 capsules can be observed 25–30 minutes after such a temperature shift (Whitfield *et al.*, 1984; Kröncke *et al.*, 1990a,b). Newly formed capsular polysaccharide appears on the cell surface at discrete sites, indicating the presence of special exit ports. Immunoelectron microscopy with the immunogold method showed that these sites were associated with membrane adhesion sites, which have also been implicated in the surface transport of other bacterial polysaccharides (Bayer, 1990). The translocation of these group II polysaccharides is sensitive to membrane de-energisation (Whitfield *et al.*, 1984; Kröhncke *et al.*, 1990b).

Comparative studies show that expression of group II capsules coincides with an increased activity of the cytoplasmic enzyme CMP–KDO synthetase (CKS), which is responsible for the formation of activated KDO. In *E. coli* with group II capsules this increase was observed only at capsule-permissive temperatures (Finke *et al.*, 1989, 1990). At first, a possible explanation appeared to be involvement of CMP–KDO in the initiation of polysaccharide biosynthesis. However, experiments with recombinant *E. coli* have shown that KDO is implicated in the transport of polysaccharide K5 across the cytoplasmic membrane (Bronner *et al.*, 1993a). The gene responsible for CKS in capsule expression, *kpsU*, was located in region 1 that harbours the transport genes. The over-expressed product, KpsU (K-CKS), differs in amino-acid sequence (70 per cent similarity; 44 per cent identity) and in its kinetics data from the enzyme involved in lipopolysaccharide biosynthesis (L-CKS) (Rosenow *et al.*, 1994); thus, K-CKS and L-CKS are isoenzymes. The three-dimensional structure of K-CKS has been determined (Jelakovic *et al.*, 1996).

Cytoplasmic polysaccharide K5 preparations from translocation-deficient strains did not have KDO at the reducing end, while periplasmic polysaccharide K5 from a transport mutant was substituted with KDO and phosphatidic acid (Bronner *et al.*, 1993). Thus, membrane translocation of polysaccharide K5 and its substitution with phosphatidyl-KDO appear to be concerted reactions, but the mechanism of translocation is unknown. It is possible that the products of region 3 genes (*kpsM*, *kpsT*) act as translocator and energiser in a system also postulated for export of the capsular polysaccharide of Hib (Kroll *et al.*, 1990) and *N. meningitidis* (Frosch *et al.*, 1991). The KpsM and KpsT proteins are thought to form the ABC-2 translocator (Reizer *et al.*, 1992; Saier, 1994), a specialised subclass of ABC transporters (Higgins *et al.*, 1990).

Gene region 1 of *E. coli* K5 (Figure 4.3) has been completely sequenced and the individual transport genes have been subcloned (Pazzani *et al.*, 1993). The transport protein products of these genes (Rosenow *et al.*, 1995; P. Hänfling & K. Jann, unpublished) indicate that KpsE and KpsD proteins are associated with the inner membrane, and are, to a large extent, exposed to the periplasmic space. It is not yet possible to give the functions of the KpsC and KpsS proteins with certainty. Both are, however, engaged in membrane translocation of the K5 polysaccharide and/or phosphatidyl-KDO substitution.

It was shown with recombinant *E. coli* K5 that the products of region 2 are not by themselves able to synthesise polysaccharide (Bronner *et al.*, 1993a,b), although this region was originally defined as a polymerisation region (Roberts *et al.*, 1988; Boulnois & Jann, 1989). For efficient polysaccharide synthesis, gene products from region 1 (*kpsS* and *kpsC*) and from region 3 (*kpsT*) are necessary. The products of these genes outside region 2 are probably important to hold together the transferase and the growing polysaccharide and/or to keep the transferase in an active state by protein–protein interaction. It is, therefore, evident that expression of *E. coli* capsules is a complex process in the course of which co-ordinate interaction of many proteins is necessary (Bliss & Silver, 1996).

The significance of capsules in infection

The role of capsules in non-specific host defence

The interaction of bacterial surfaces with the complement system is an important mechanism by which invasive bacteria evade non-specific host defences. This interaction results in an impairment of bacteriolysis and/or phagocytosis, processes that are effected by the terminal membrane attack complex (MAC) and complement component C3b, respectively. Normally, the complement system is activated either by interaction with antibodies with bacterial surface components (classical pathway) or by triggering of the properdin (alternative) pathway (Loos, 1985; Cross, 1990).

The mechanism by which bacterial capsules interfere with complement activity are not entirely clear, but several observations are helpful for an understanding of the complicated interplay between the bacteria and host defence. The classical and alternative complement pathways are subject to regulation and control. As far as is known, it is largely interference with regulatory proteins by capsular polysaccharides that inhibits complement action. Complement component C3 is the first and pivotal factor that the classical and alternative pathways have in common, before the terminal MAC components are sequentially activated. Conversion of C3 to the active form, C3b, is brought about by the classical convertase C2bC4b, which is under the control of the C4-binding protein C4bp (Nussenzweig & Melton, 1981). Some capsular polysaccharides appear to bind C4bp and so interrupt the complement cascade (Cross, 1990). Activation of C3 to C3b is controlled by factors B and H that regulate the affinity of C3b for bacterial cell surfaces.

Certain capsules decrease the affinity of C3b for factor B, while others increase its affinity for factor H (Loos, 1985; Cross, 1990). In both cases surface deposition of complement, opsonic C3b or the lytic MAC is decreased and encapsulated bacteria escape phagocytosis and the bactericidal activity of complement. Capsules that consist of or contain *N*-actylneuraminic acid, such as polysaccharides K1 and K92 of *E. coli*, the capsules of *N. meningitidis* types B and C, and group B *Streptococcus* polysaccharides, appear to exert their anti-complementary action in this way (Stevens *et al.*, 1978; Wessels *et al.*, 1989; Cross, 1990).

Another explanation for the protective action that capsules have for bacteria may simply be that encapsulated bacteria bind complement too far from the bacterial surface to be harmful (Rowley, 1954; Cross, 1990). Such an interpretation has also been given for the resistance of *E. coli* O111 to complement, in which long-chain lipopolysaccharide plays a role (Joiner, 1985).

A general view of the role of *E. coli* capsules as virulence determinants is not possible. For instance, while the K1 capsule interacts with complement as described above, the K5 capsule does not appear to endow serum resistance to *E. coli*. Thus, the serum resistance of mutants of *E. coli* O18:K5 that are K5-negative is the same as that of their encapsulated parent strain (Cross, 1990). It may be that complement sensitivity depends not only on the chemical nature of the capsular polysaccharide (K-antigen), but also on the cell wall lipopolysaccharide (O-antigen). It may be, therefore, that the combination of K-antigens with O-antigens determines the outcome of the bacterium–host interaction in immunity to infection. The fact that only a limited number of O–K combinations is encountered in invasive strains of *E. coli* tends to support this notion.

Table 4.4. *Immune response to capsular polysaccharides of* Escherichia coli *K1 and K92, and* Neisseria meningitidis *groups B and C*

Capsular antigen	Structure	Immuno-genicity	Determinant
E. coli K1	8)-α-NeuNac-(2,	No	–
N. meningitidis B			
N. meningitidis C	9)-α-NeuNAc-(2,	Yes	9)-α-NeuNAc-(2,
E. coli K92	8)-α-NeuNAc-(2→9)-α-NeuNAc-(2,	Yes	9)-α-NeuNAc

Immunogenicity and molecular mimicry

Although *E. coli* capsules generally induce the formation of anti-capsular antibodies that are active in infection immunity, their immunogenicity often depends on the age of the host. Thus, many encapsulated *E. coli* and related *Neisseria* and *Haemophilus* serotypes are not immunogenic in the newborn or in young children (Jennings, 1990). This is documented in the age-related susceptibility to infection with encapsulated invasive bacteria, and in the poor immune response of infants to many poly-saccharide vaccines.

In adults, too, some *E. coli* capsules are non-immunogenic or only poorly immunogenic. This is due to the identity of such capsules with certain substances found in the host. As a result, the host does not recognise the bacterial structures as foreign and so is unable to raise anti-capsular antibodies. This phenomenon of molecular mimicry enables the bacteria to escape the host immune recognition and endows them with virulence. Capsular polysaccharide K1, a poly (α-2,8)-sialic acid, has the same structure as the carbohydrate terminus of the neural cell adhesion molecule n-CAM (Finne, 1982). The immune response to K1 and related *E. coli* and *Neisseria* polysaccharides is compared in Table 4.4. The lack of an α-2,8 specificity is obvious. The structural identity is corroborated by the action of the endosialidase from coliphage K1 on n-CAM, which indicates that an important mammalian glycoprotein can be manipulated with a prokaryotic enzyme (Troy, 1992). Similarly, *E. coli* K5 capsular polysaccharide is identical to *N*-acetyl heparosan, the first polymeric intermediate in the biosynthesis of heparin (Navia *et al.*, 1983). A coliphage K5-borne lyase cleaves not only polysaccharide K5 (Gupta *et al.*, 1983; Hänfling *et al.*, 1996), but also *N*-acetyl heparosan in a β-elimination reaction. Again, a prokaryotic probe can be used to manipulate an important mammalian substance. Capsular polysaccharide K4 appears as a fructosylated chondroitin and its relatively poor immunogenicity may be due to the lability of the fructosyl linkage. Thus, growth of bacteria in body compartments of low pH or their processing in phagolysosomes may convert them from a K4 capsular form, in which they induce and react with anti-K4 antibodies, to a chondroitin-type capsule, in which they no longer do so. These findings emphasise that capsules counteract the host defence not only by interaction with complement components but also by evasion of immune recognition as the result of molecular mimicry.

References

Ahrens, R., Brade, H., Jann, B. & Jann, K. (1988). Structure of the K74 antigen from *Escherichia coli* O44:K74:H18, capsular polysaccharide containing furanosidic β KDO residues. *Carbohydrate Research*, **179**, 223–31.

Altman, E. & Dutton, G. G. S. (1985). Chemical and structural analysis of the capsular polysaccharide from *Escherichia coli* O9:K28(A):H⁻ (K28 antigen). *Carbohydrate Research*, **138**, 293–303.

Anderson, A. N. & Parolis, H. (1988). Investigation of the structure of the capsular polysaccharide of *Escherichia coli* K55 using *Klebsiella* bacteriophage phi 5. *Carbohydrate Research*, **188**, 157–68.

Anderson, A. N., Parolis, H. & Parolis, L. A. S. (1987). Structural investigation of the capsular polysaccharide from *Escherichia coli* O9:K37(A84a). *Carbohydrate Research*, **163**, 81–90.

Anison, G., Dutton, G. G. S. & Altman, G. (1987). Structure of the capsular polysaccharide of *Escherichia coli* O9:K32(A):H19. *Carbohydrate Research*, **168**, 89–102.

Bax, A., Summers, M. F., Egan, W., Guirgis, N., Schneerson, R., Robbins, J. B., Ørskov, F. & Ørskov, I. (1988). Structural studies of the *Escherichia coli* K93 and K53 capsular polysaccharides. *Carbohydrate Research*, **173**, 53–64.

Bayer, M. E. (1990). Visualization of the bacterial polysaccharide capsule. *Current Topics in Microbiology and Immunology*, **150**, 129–57.

Bayer, M. E., Carlemalm, E. & Kellenberger, E. (1985). Capsule of *Escherichia coli* K29: ultrastructural preservation and immunoelectron microscopy. *Journal of Bacteriology*, **162**, 985–91.

Bayer, M. E. & Thurow, H. (1977). Polysaccharide capsule of *E.coli*: microscope study of its size, structure and sites of synthesis. *Journal of Bacteriology*, **130**, 911–36.

Beynon, L. M. (1988). PhD thesis. University of British Columbia, Vancouver.

Beynon, L. M. & Dutton, G. G. S. (1988). Structural studies of *E. coli* K26 capsular polysaccharide using g.l.c.-c.i.-m.s. *Carbohydrate Research*, **179**, 419–23.

Bhattacharjee, A. K., Jennings, H. J. & Kenny, C. P. (1978). Structural elucidation of the 3-deoxy-D-mannosoctulosonic acid containing meningococcal 29-e capsular polysaccharide antigen using carbon-13 NMR. *Biochemistry*, **17**, 645–51.

Bliss, J. M. & Silver, R. P. (1996). Coating the surface: a model for expression of capsular polysialic acid in *Escherichia* coli K1. *Molecular Microbiology*, **21**, 221–31.

Boulnois, G. J., Drake, R., Pearce, R. & Roberts, I. (1992). Genome diversity at the serA-linked capsule locus in *Escherichia coli*. *FEMS Microbiology Letters*, **100**, 121–4.

Boulnois, G. J. & Jann, K. (1989). Bacterial polysaccharide capsule synthesis, export and evolution of structural diversity. *Molecular Microbiology*, **3**, 1819–23.

Boulnois, G. J. & Roberts, I. S. (1990). Genetics of capsular polysaccharide production in bacteria. *Current Topics in Microbiology and Immunology*, **150**, 1–18.

Boulnois, G. J., Roberts, I. S., Hodge, R., Hardy, K., Jann, K. & Timmis, K. N. (1987). Analysis of the K1 capsule biosynthesis genes of *Escherichia coli*: definition of three functional regions for capsule production. *Molecular and General Genetics*, **208**, 242–6.

Branefors-Helander, P., Erbing, C., Kenne, L. & Lindberg, B. (1976). Structural studies of the capsular antigens from *H. influenzae* type b. *Acta Chemica Scandinavica*, **30**, 276–7.

Bronner, D., Sieberth, V., Pazzani, C., Roberts, I. S., Boulnois, G. J., Jann, B. & Jann, K. (1993a). Expression of the capsular K5 polysaccharide of *Escherichia coli*: biochemical and electron microscopic analyses of mutants with defects in region 1 of the K5 gene cluster. *Journal of Bacteriology*, **175**, 5984–92.

Bronner, D., Sieberth, V., Pazzani, C., Smith, A., Boulnois, G., Roberts, I., Jann, B. & Jann, K. (1993b). Synthesis of the K5 (Group II) capsular polysaccharide in transport deficient recombinant *Escherichia coli*. *FEMS Microbiology Letters*, **113**, 279–84.

de Bruin, A. H., Parolis, H. & Parolis, L. A. S. (1992a). Structural elucidation of the capsular polysaccharide of *E. coli* serotype K47. *Carbohydrate Research*, **233**, 195–204.

de Bruin, A. H., Parolis, H. & Parolis, L. A. S. (1992b). The capsular antigen of *Escherichia coli* serotype O8:K102:H⁻. *Carbohydrate Research*, **235**, 199–209.

Chakraborty, A. K., Friebolin, N. & Stirm, S. (1980). Primary structure of the *E. coli* serotype K30 capsular polysaccharide. *Journal of Bacteriology*, **141**, 971–2.

Choy, Y. M., Fehmel, F., Frank, N. & Stirm, S. (1975). *Escherichia coli* capsule bacteriophages. VI. Primary structure of the bacteriophage 29 receptor, the *E. coli* serotype 29 capsular polysaccharide. *Journal of Virology*, **16**, 581–90.

Cross, A. S. (1990). The biologic significance of bacterial encapsulation. *Current Topics in Microbiology and Immunology*, **150**, 87–97.

Dengler, T., Himmelspach, K., Jann, B. & Jann, K. (1988). Structure of the K3 antigen of *Escherichia coli* O4:K3:H44, a polysaccharide containing a 4-deoxy-2-hexulosonic acid. *Carbohydrate Research*, **178**, 191–201.

Dengler, T., Jann, B. & Jann, K. (1985). Structure of the K95 antigen from *Escherichia coli* O75:K95:H5, a capsular polysaccharide containing furanosidic KDO residues. *Carbohydrate Research*, **142**, 269–76.

Dengler, T., Jann, B. & Jann, K. (1986). Structure of the serine containing capsular polysaccharide K40 antigen from *E. coli* O8:K40:H9. *Carbohydrate Research*, **150**, 233–40.

Dougherty, B. A. & van de Rijn, I. (1993). Molecular characterization of *hasB*from an operon required for hyaluronic acid synthesis in group A streptococci. Demonstration of UDP-glucose dehydrogenase activity. *Journal of Biological Chemistry*, **268**, 7118–24.

Dougherty, B. A. & van de Rijn, I. (1994). Molecular characterization of *hasA* from an operon required for hyaluronic acid synthesis in group A streptococci. *Journal of Biological Chemistry*, **269**, 169–75.

Dutton, G. G. S., Karunaratne, D. N. & Lim, A. V. S. (1988). *Escherichia coli* serotype K44: an acidic capsular polysaccharide containing two 2-acetamido-2-deoxyhexoses. *Carbohydrate Research*, **183**, 111–22.

Dutton, G. G. S. & Kuma-Mintah, A. (1987). Structure of *Escherichia coli* capsular antigen K34, *Carbohydrate Research*, **169**, 213–20.

Dutton, G. G. S., Kuma-Mintah, A., Ng, S. K., Parolis, H., Dell, A. & Reason, A. (1992). Determination of the structure of the capsular antigen of *Escherichia coli* O8:K46:H30, using FABMS and 2D-NMR spectroscopy. *Carbohydrate Research*, **231**, 39–50.

Dutton, G. G. S., Kuma-Mintah, A. & Parolis, H. (1990). The structure of *Escherichia coli* K31 antigen. *Carbohydrate Research*, **197**, 171–80.

Dutton, G. G. S., Parolis, H. & Parolis, L. A. S. (1987). The structure of the neuraminic acid containing capsular polysaccharide of *E. coli* serotype K9. *Carbohydrate Research*, **170**, 193–206.

Finke, A., Bronner, D., Nikolaev, A. V., Jann, B. & Jann, K. (1991). Biosynthesis of the *Escherichia coli* K5 polysaccharide, a representative of group II polysaccharides: polymerization *in vitro* and characterization of the product. *Journal of Bacteriology*, **173**, 4088–94.

Finke, A., Jann, B. & Jann, K. (1990). CMP-KDO synthetase activity in *Escherichia coli* expressing capsular polysaccharides. *FEMS Microbiology Letters*, **69**, 129–34.

Finke, A., Roberts, I., Pazzani, C., Boulnois, G. & Jann, K. (1989). Activity of CMP-KDO synthetase in *E. coli* expressing the capsular K5 polysaccharide–implication for biosynthesis of the K5 polysaccharide. *Journal of Bacteriology*, **171**, 374–9.

Finne, J. (1982). Occurrence of unique polysialosyl carbohydrate units in glycoproteins of developing brain. *Journal of Biological Chemistry*, **257**, 11966–70.

Frosch, M., Edwards, U., Bousset, K., Krauße, B. & Weisgerber, C. (1991). Evidence for a common molecular origin of the capsule gene loci in Gram-negative bacteria expressing group II capsular polysaccharides. *Molecular Microbiology*, **5**, 1251–63.

Gotschlich, E. C., Frazer, B. A., Nishimura, O., Robbins, J. B. & Liu, T. Y. (1981). Lipid on capsular polysaccharides of Gram-negative bacteria. *Journal of Biological Chemistry*, **256**, 8915–21.

Gottesman, S. & Stout, V. (1991). Regulation of capsular polysaccharide synthesis in *Escherichia coli* K-12. *Molecular Microbiology*, **5**, 1599–606.

Grue, M. R., Parolis, H. & Parolis, L. A. S. (1993a). Structural elucidation of the capsular polysaccharide of *Escherichia coli* serotype K101 by high resolution NMR spectroscopy. *Carbohydrate Research*, **246**, 283–90.

Grue, M. R., Parolis, H. & Parolis, L. A. S. (1993b). *Escherichia coli* serotype K45 capsular antigen: a glycan containing 3-acetamido-3,6-dideoxygalactopyranose. *Carbohydrate Research*, **248**, 191–8.

Gupta, D. S., Jann, B. & Jann, K. (1983). Enzymatic degradation of capsular K5 antigen of *E. coli* by coliphage K5. *FEMS Microbiology Letters*, **16**, 13–17.

Hackland, P. L. & Parolis, H. (1992). The structure of the capsular polysaccharide of *Escherichia coli* O9:K35:H⁻. *Carbohydrate Research*, **235**, 211–20.

Hackland, P. L., Parolis, H. & Parolis, L. A. S. (1991). *Escherichia coli* O9:K38 capsular antigen: another ribofuranose containing glycan. *Carbohydrate Research*, **219**, 193–201.

Hahne, M., Jann, B. & Jann, K. (1991). Structure of the capsular polysaccharide (K98 antigen) of *E. coli* O7:K98:H6. *Carbohydrate Research*, **222**, 245–53.

Hänfling, P., Shashkov, A. S., Jann, B. & Jann, K. (1996). Analysis of the enzymatic cleavage (β elimination) of the capsular K5 polysaccharide of *Escherichia coli* by K5-specific coliphage: a reexamination. *Journal of Bacteriology*, **178**, 4747–50.

Higgins, C. F., Hyde, S. C., Mimmack, M. M., Gileadi, U., Gil, D. R. & Gallagher, M. P. G. (1990). Binding protein-dependent transport systems. *Journal of Bioenergetics and Biomembranes*, **22**, 571–92.

Hobbs, M. & Reeves, P. (1994). The JUMPstart sequence: a 39 bp element common to several polysaccharide gene clusters. *Molecular Microbiology*, **12**, 855–6.

Hofmann, P., Jann, B. & Jann, K. (1985a). Structure of the fructose containing K52 capsular polysacccharide of uropathogenic *E. coli* O4:K52:H⁻. *European Journal of Biochemistry*, **147**, 601–9.

Hofmann, P., Jann, B. & Jann, K. (1985b). Structure of the amino acid containing capsular polysaccharide (K54 antigen) from *E. coli* O6; K54:H10. *Carbohydrate Research*, **139**, 261–71.

Homonylo, M. K., Wilmont, S. J., Lam, J. S., MacDonald, L. A. & Whitfield, C. (1988). Monoclonal antibodies against the capsular K antigen of *Escherichia coli* (O9:K30(A):H12): characterisation and use in analysis of K antigen organisation on the cell surface. *Canadian Journal of Microbiology*, **34**, 1159–65.

Jann, B., Ahrens, R., Dengler, T. & Jann, K. (1988). Structure of the capsular polysaccharide (K19 antigen) from uropathogenic *E. coli* O25:K19:H12. *Carbohydrate Research*, **177**, 273–7.

Jann, B., Dengler, T. & Jann, K. (1985). The capsular (K51) antigen of *Escherichia coli* O1:K51:H⁻, an O-acetylated poly-*N*-acetylglucosamine phosphate. *FEMS Microbiology Letters*, **29**, 257–61.

Jann, B., Hofmann, P. & Jann, K. (1983). Structure of the 3-deoxy-D-manno-octulosonic acid (KDO) containing capsular polysaccharide (K14 antigen) from *Escherichia coli* O6:K14:H31. *Carbohydrate Research*, **120**, 131–42.

Jann, B. & Jann, K. (1990). Structure and biosynthesis of the capsular antigens of *Escherichia coli*. *Current Topics in Microbiology and Immunology*, **150**, 19–43.

Jann, B., Jann, K., Schmidt, G., Ørskov, F. & Ørskov, I. (1971). Comparative immunochemical studies of the surface antigens of *Escherichia coli* strains O8:K87(B?):H19 and (O32):K87(B?):H45. *European Journal of Biochemistry*, **23**, 515–22.

Jann, B., Kochanowski, H. & Jann, K. (1993). Structure of the capsular K96 polysaccharide (K96 antigen) from *Escherichia coli* O77:K96:H and comparison with the capsular K54 polysaccharide (K54 antigen) from *Escherichia coli*. *Carbohydrate Research*, **253**, 323–7.

Jann, B., Shashkov, A. S., Kochanowski, H. & Jann, K. (1995). NMR reinvestigation of the capsular K27 polysaccharide (K27 antigen) from *Escherichia coli* O8:K27:H-*Carbohydrate Research*, **277**, 353–8.

Jann, K., Dengler, T. & Jann, B. (1992). Core-lipid A on the K40 polysaccharide of *Escherichia coli* O8:K40:H9, a representative of group I capsular polysaccharides. *Zentralblatt für Bakteriologie und Hygiene A*, **276**, 196–204.

Jann, K. & Jann, B. (1992). Capsules of *Escherichia coli*, expression and biological significance. *Canadian Journal of Microbiology*, **38**, 705–10.

Jann, K., Jann, B., Ørskov, F. & Ørskov, I. (1966). Immunchemische Untersuchungen an K Antigenen von *Escherichia coli*. III Isolierung und Untersuchung der chemischen Struktur des sauren Polysaccharids aus *E. coli* O141:K85(B):H4 (K85 Antigen). *Biochemische Zeitschrift*, **346**, 368–85.

Jann, K., Jann, B., Schmidt, M. A. & Vann, W. F. (1980). Structure of the *E. coli* K2 capsular antigen, a teichoic acid-like polymer. *Journal of Bacteriolology*, **143**, 1108–15.

Jann, K., Jann, B., Schneider, K. F., Ørskov, F. & Ørskov, I. (1968). Immunochemistry of K antigens of *Escherichia coli*. 5. The K antigen of *E. coli* O8:K27(A):H⁻. *European Journal of Biochemistry*, **5**, 456–65.

Jann, K. & Schmidt, M. A. (1980). Comparative chemical analysis of two variants of the *Escherichia coli*K2 antigens. *FEMS Microbiology Letters*, **7**, 79–81.

Jann, K. & Westphal, O. (1975). Microbial polysaccharides. In *The Antigens*, vol. 3, ed. M. Sela, pp. 1–123, New York: Academic Press.

Jelakovic, S., Jann, K. & Schulz, G. E. (1996). The three-dimensional structure of capsule-specific CMP: 2-keto-3-deoxy-*manno* -octonic acid synthetase from *Escherichia coli*. *FEBS Letters*, **391**, 157–61.

Jennings, H. J. (1990). Capsular polysaccharides as vaccine candidates. *Current Topics in Microbiology and Immunology*, **150**, 97–129.

Jennings, H. J., Rosell, K. G. & Johnson, K. G. (1982). Structure of 3-deoxy-D-manno-octulosonic acid containing polysaccharide (K6 antigen) from *Escherichia coli* LP1092. *Carbohydrate Research*, **105**, 45–56.

Joiner, K. (1985). Studies on the mechanism of bacterial resistance to complement mediated killing and on the mechanism of action of bacteriocidal antibody. *Current in Topics Microbiology and Immunology*, **121**, 99–133.

Kauffmann, F. (1954). In *Enterobacteriaceae*, 2nd edn., pp. 19–48. Copenhagen: Munksgaard.

Keenleyside, W. J., Bronner, D., Jann, K., Jann, B. & Whitfield, C. (1993). Coexpression of colanic acid and serotype specific capsular polysaccharides in *Escherichia coli* strains with group II K antigens. *Journal of Bacteriology*, **175**, 6725–30.

Keenleyside, W., Jayaratne, P., MacLachlan, P. R. & Whitfield, C. (1992). The rcsA gene of *Escherichia coli* O9:K30:H12 is involved in the expression of the serotype-specific group I K (capsular antigen). *Journal of Bacteriology*, **174**, 8–16.

Kogan, G., Jann, B. & Jann, K. (1992). Structure of the *Escherichia coli* O104 polysaccharide and its identity with the capsular K9 polysaccharide. *FEMS Microbiology Letters*, **91**, 135–40.

Krönke, K. D., Boulnois, G., Roberts, I., Bitter-Suermann, D., Golecki, J. R., Jann, B. & Jann, K. (1990a). Expression of the *Escherichia coli* K5 capsular antigen: immunoelectron microscopic and biochemical studies with recombinant *E. coli. Journal of Bacteriology*, **172**, 1085–91.

Krönke, K. D., Golecki, J. R. & Jann, K. (1990b). Further electron microscopic studies on the expression of *Escherichia coli* group II capsules. *Journal of Bacteriology*, **172**, 3469–72.

Kroll, J. S., Loynds, B., Brophy, L. N. & Moxon, E. R. (1990). The bex locus in encapsulated *Haemophilus influenzae*: a chromosomal region involved in capsule polysaccharide export. *Molecular Microbiology*, **4**, 1853–62.

Kuo, J. S. C., Doelling, V. W., Graveline, J. F. & McCoy, D. W. (1985). Evidence for covalent attachment of phospholipid to the capsular polysaccharide of *Haemophilus influenzae* type b. *Journal of Bacteriology*, **163**, 769–73.

Laakso, D. H., Homonylo, M. K., Wilmot, S. J. & Whitfield, C. (1988). Transfer and expression of the genetic determinants for O and K antigen synthesis in *Escherichia coli* O9:K30(A) and *Klebsiella* sp O1:K20, in *E. coli* K-12. *Canadian Journal of Microbiology*, **34**, 987–92.

Larsen, J. C., Ørskov, F., Ørskov, I., Schmidt, M. A., Jann, B. & Jann, K. (1980). Crossed immunoelectrophoresis and chemical structural analysis used for characterization of two varieties of *Escherichia coli* K2 polysaccharide antigens. *Medical Microbiology Immunology*, **168**, 191–200.

Lenter, M. C., Jann, B. & Jann, K. (1990a). Structure of the K16 antigen of *Escherichia coli*O7:K16:H⁻, a KDO containing capsular polysaccharide. *Carbohydrate Research*, **197**, 197–204.

Lenter, M. C., Jann, B. & Jann, K. (1990b). Structure of the K24 antigen of *E. coli* O83:K24:H, a polymer that consists of α-KDO and glycerol phosphate. *Carbohydrate Research*, **208**, 139–44.

Lidholt, K., Fjelstad, M., Jann, K. & Lindahl, U. (1994). Substrate specificities of glycosyl transferases involved in formation of heparin precursor and *E. coli* K5 capsular polysaccharides. *Carbohydrate Research*, **255**, 87–101.

Lidholt, K., Weinke, J. L., Kiser, C. S., Lugemwa, F. N., Bame, K. J., Cheifetz, S., Massague, J., Lindahl, U. & Esko, J. D. (1992). A single mutation affects both *N*-acetylglucosaminyl transferase and glucuronlytransferase activities in a chinese hamster ovary cell mutant defective in heparan sulfate biosynthesis. *Proceedings of the National Academy of Science, USA*, **89**, 2267–71.

Lifely, M. R., Lindon, J. C., Williams, J. M. & Moreno, C. (1985). Structural and conformational features of the *Escherichia coli* K92 capsular polysaccharide. *Carbohydrate Research*, **143**, 191–205.

Lind, T., Lindahl, U. & Lidholt, K. (1993). Biosynthesis of heparin/heparan sulfate. Identification of a 70 kDa protein catalyzing both the D-glucuronosyl- and the *N*-acetyl-D-glucosaminyl transferase reactions. *Journal of Biological Chemistry*, **268**, 20705–8.

Lindahl, U. (1972). Enzymes involved in the formation of the carbohydrate structure of heparin. *Methods in Enzymology*, **28**, 676–84.

Loos, M. (1985). The complement system: activation and control. *Current Topics in Microbiology and Immunology*, **121**, 7–18.

Mäkelä, P. H. & Stocker, B. A. D. (1969). Genetics of polysaccharide biosynthesis. *Annual Reviews of Genetics*, **3**, 291–322.

Masson, L. & Holbein, B. E. (1985). Role of lipid intermediate(s) in the synthesis of serogroup b *Neisseria meningitidis* capsular polysaccharide. *Journal of Bacteriology*, **161**, 861–7.

McCallum, K. L. & Whitfield, C. (1991). The rcsA gene of *Klebsiella pneumoniae* O1:K20 is involved in expression of the serotype-specific K (capsular) antigen. *Infection and Immunity*, **59**, 494–502.

McGrath, B. C. & Osborn, M. J. (1991). Localization of the terminal steps of O-antigen synthesis in *Salmonella typhimurium*. *Journal of Bacteriology*, **173**, 649–54.

Moxon, E. R. & Vaughn, K. A. (1981). The type b capsular polysaccharide as a virulence determinant of *H. influenzae*: studies using clinical isolates and laboratory transformants. *Journal of Infectious Diseases*, **143**, 517–24.

Mühlradt, P. F., Menzel, J., Golecki, J. R. & Speth, V. (1973). Outer membrane of *Salmonella*. Sites of export of newly synthesized lipopolysaccharide on the bacterial surface. *European Journal of Biochemistry*, **35**, 471–481.

Navia, J. L., Riesenfeld, J., Vann, W. F., Lindahl, U. & Roden, L. (1983). Assay of N-acetylheparosan deacetylase with a capsular polysaccharide from *Escherichia coli* K5 as substrate. *Analytical Biochemistry*, **135**, 134–40.

Niemann, H., Chakraborty, A. K., Friebolin, H. & Stirm, S. (1978). Primary structure of the *Escherichia coli* serotype K42 capsular polysaccharide and its serological identity with the *Klebsiella* K63 polysaccharide. *Journal of Bacteriology*, **133**, 390–1.

Nussenzweig, V. & Melton, R. (1981). Human C4 binding protein (C4bp). *Methods in Enzymology*, **80**, 124–33.

Ørskov, F., Ørskov, I., Sutton, A., Schneerson, R., Lind, W., Egan, W., Hoff, G. E. & Robbins, J. R. (1979). Form variation in *Escherichia coli* K1: determined by *O*-acetylation of the capsular polysaccharide. *Journal of Experimental Medicine*, **149**, 669–85.

Ørskov, F., Sharma, V. & Ørskov, I. (1984). Influence of growth temperature on the development of *Escherichia coli* polysaccharide K antigens. *Journal of General Microbiology*, **130**, 2681–4.

Ørskov, I. & Nyman, K. (1974). Genetic mapping of the antigenic determinants of two polysaccharide antigens, K10 and K54 in *Escherichia coli*. *Journal of Bacteriology*, **120**, 43–51.

Ørskov, I., Ørskov, F., Jann, B. & Jann, K. (1977). Serology, chemistry and genetics of O and K antigens of *Escherichia coli*. *Bacteriological Reviews*, **41**, 667–710.

Parolis, H., Parolis, L. A. S. & Stanley, S. M. R. (1988). The use of bacteriophage-mediated depolymerization in the structural investigation of the capsular polysaccharide from *Escherichia coli* serotype K36. *Carbohydrate Research*, **175**, 77–83.

Parolis, H., Parolis, L. A. S., Stanley, S. M. R. & Dutton, G. G. S. (1990a). A structural investigation of the capsular polysaccharide of *Escherichia coli* O9:K57:H32. *Carbohydrate Research*, **200**, 449–56.

Parolis, H., Parolis, L. A. S., Stanley, S. M. R. & Dutton, G. G. S. (1990b). The stucture of the capsular antigen from *Escherichia coli* O8:K87:H19. *Carbohydrate Research*, **205**, 361–70.

Parolis, H., Parolis, L. A. S. & Venter, R. D. (1989). *Escherichia coli* serotype-39 capsular polysaccharide: primary structure and depolymerization by a bacteriophage-associated glycanase. *Carbohydrate Research*, **185**, 225–32.

Parolis, L. A. S. & Parolis, H. (1988). Structure of the capsular antigen of *Escherichia coli* O8:K8:H4. *Carbohydrate Research*, **193**, 157–63.

Pavelka, M. S., Wright, L. F. & Silver, R. P. (1991). Identification of two genes, kpsM and kpsT, in the region 3 of the polysialic acid gene cluster of *Escherichia coli* K1. *Journal of Bacteriology*, **173**, 4603–10.

Pazzani, C., Rosenow, C., Boulnois, G. J., Bronner, D., Jann, K. & Roberts, I. S. (1993) Molecular analysis of region 1 of the *Escherichia coli* K5 antigen gene cluster: a region encoding proteins involved in cell surface expression of capsular polysaccharides. *Journal of Bacteriology*, **175**, 5978–83.

Pearce, R. & Roberts, I. S. (1995). Cloning and analysis of gene clustetrs for production of the *Escherichia coli* K10 and K54 antigens: identification of a new group of serA-linked capsule gene clusters. *Journal of Bacteriology*, **177**, 3992–7.

Petit, C., Rigg, G. P., Pazzani, C., Smith, A., Sieberth, V., Stevens, M., Boulnois, G., Jann, K. & Roberts, I. S. (1995). Analysis of region 2 of the *Escherichia coli* K5 gene cluster: a region encoding proteins for the bio-synthesis of the K5 polysaccharide. *Molecular Microbiology*, **17**, 611–20.

Pradel, E. & Schnaitman, C. (1991). Effect of *rfaH* (*sfrB*) and temperature on expression of *rfa* genes of *Escherichia coli* K-12. *Journal of Bacteriology*, **173**, 6428–31.

Reizer, J., Reizer, A. & Saier, M. H. Jr. (1992). A new subfamily of bacterial ABC-type transport systems catalyzing export of drugs and carbohydrates. *Protein Science*, **1**, 1326–32.

Roberts, I. S., Mountford, R., Hodge, R., Jann, K. B. & Boulnois, G. J. (1988) Common organization of gene clusters for production of different capsular polysaccharides (K antigens) in *E. coli. Journal of Bacteriology*, **170**, 1305–10.

Rodriguez, M. L., Jann, B. & Jann, K. (1988a). Structure and serological characteristic of the capsular K4 antigen of *Escherichia coli* O5:K4:H4, a fructose containing polysaccharide with a chondroitin backbone. *European Journal of Biochemistry*, **177**, 117–24.

Rodriguez, M. L., Jann, B. & Jann, K. (1988b). Comparative structural elucidation of the K18, K22 and K100 antigens of *E. coli* as related ribosylribitol phosphates. *Carbohydrate Research*, **173**, 243–53.

Rodriguez, M. L., Jann, B. & Jann, K. (1990). Structure and properties of the capsular K11 antigen of *Escherichia coli* O13:K11:H11, a fructose containing polysaccharide with a diglucosylphosphate backbone. *Carbohydrate Research*, **196**, 101–9.

Rosenow, C., Roberts, I. S. & Jann, K. (1994). Isolation from recombinant *Escherichia coli* and characterization of CMP-KDO synthetase, involved in the expression of the capsular K5 polysaccharide (K-CKS). *FEMS Microbiology Letters*, **125**, 159–64.

Rosenow, C., Esumeh, F., Roberts, I. S. & Jann, K. (1995). Characterization and localization of the KpsE protein of *Escherichia coli,* which is involved in polysaccharide export. *Journal of Bacteriology*, **177**, 1137–43.

Rowley, D. (1954). The virulence of *Bacterium coli* for mice. *British Journal of Experimental Pathology*, **35**, 528–38.

Saier, M. H. Jr. (1994). Computer-aided analysis of transport protein sequences gleaning evidence concerning function, structure, biogenesis, and evolution. *Microbiological Reviews*, **58**, 71–93.

Schmidt, G., Jann, B., Jann, K., Ørskov, I. & Ørskov, F. (1977). Genetic determinants of the synthesis of the polysaccharide capsular antigen K27(A) of *Escherichia coli. Journal of Geneneral Microbiology*, **100**, 355–61.

Schmidt, M. A. & Jann, K. (1982). Phospholipid substitution of capsular (K) polysaccharide antigens from *Escherichia coli*causing extraintestinal infection. *FEMS Microbiology Letters*, **14**, 74–9.

Schmidt, M. A. & Jann, K. (1983). Structure of the 2-keto-3-deoxy-D-mannooctonic acid containing capsular polysaccharide (K12 antigen) of the urinary tract infective *E. coli* O4:K12:H⁻. *European Journal of Biochemistry*, **131**, 509–17.

Schneerson, R. & Robbins, J. B. (1975). Induction of serum *Haemophilus influenzae* type b capsular antibodies in adult volunteers fed cross reacting *Escherichia coli* O75:K100:H5. *New England Journal of Medicine*, **292**, 1093–6.

Sieberth, V., Jann, B. & Jann, K. (1993). Structure of the K10 capsular antigen from *Escherichia coli* O11:K10:H10, a polysaccharide containing 4,6-dideoxy- 4-malonylamino-D-glucose. *Carbohydrate Research*, **246**, 219–28.

Sieberth, V., Rigg, G. P., Roberts, I. & Jann, K. (1995). Expression and characterization of UDPGlc dehydrogenase (KfiD), which is encoded in the type specific region of the *E.coli* K5 capsule genes. *Journal of Bacteriology*, **177**, 4562–5.

Silver, R. P., Annunziato, P., Pavelka, M. S., Pidgeon, R. P., Wright, L. F. & Wunder, D. E. (1993). Genetic and molecular analyses of the polysialic acid gene cluster of *Escherichia coli*. In *Polysialic Acid*, eds. J. Roth, U. Rutishauser & F. A. Troy, pp. 59–71. Basle: Birkhäuser Verlag.

Smith, A., Boulnois, G. J. & Roberts, I. S. (1990). Molecular analysis of the *Escherichia coli* K5 kps locus: identification and characterization of an inner membrane capsular polysaccharide transport system. *Molecular Microbiology*, **4**, 1863–9.

Stevens, M. P., Hänfling, P., Jann, B., Jann, K. & Roberts, I. S. (1994). Regulation of *Escherichia coli* K5 capsular polysaccharide expression: evidence for involvement of RfaH in the expression of group II capsules. *FEMS Microbiology Letters*, **124**, 93–8.

Stevens, P., Huang, S. N. H., Welch, W. D. & Young, L. S. (1978). Restricted complement activation by *Escherichia coli* with the K1 capsular serotype: a possible role in pathogenicity. *Journal of Immunology*, **121**, 2174–80.

Tarcsay, L., Jann, B. & Jann, K. (1971). Immunochemistry of the K antigens of *Escherichia coli*. The K87 antigen from *E. coli* O8:K87(B):H19. *European Journal of Biochemistry*, **23**, 505–14.

Troy, F. A. (1992). Polysialic acid from bacteria to brain. *Glycobiology*, **2**, 5–23.

Troy, F. A., Frerman, F. E. & Heath, E. C. (1971). The biosynthesis of capsular polysaccharide in *Aerobacter aerogenes. Journal of Biological Chemistry*, **246**, 118–33.

Troy, F. A., Frerman, F. E. & Heath, E. C. (1972). Synthesis of capsular polysaccharides of bacteria. *Methods in Enzymology*, **28**, 602–24.

Troy, F. A. & McCloskey, M. A. (1979). Role of a membranous sialyl transferase complex in the synthesis of surface polymers containing polysialic acid in *Escherichia coli*. Temperature-induced alterations in the assembly process. *Journal of Biological Chemistry*, **254**, 7377–87.

Tsui, F. P., Boykins, R. A. & Egan, W. (1982). Structural and immunological studies of the *Escherichia coli* K7(K56) capsular polysaccharide. *Carbohydrate Research*, **102**, 263–71.

Unger, F. M. (1981). The chemistry and biological significance of 3-deoxy-D-manno-2-octulosonic acid (KDO). *Advances in Carbohydrate Chemistry*, **38**, 323–88.

Vann, W. F. & Jann, K. (1979). Structure and serological specificity of the K13 antigenic polysaccharide (K13 antigen) of urinary tract infective *E. coli. Infection and Immunity*, **25**, 85–92.

Vann, W. F., Schmidt, M. A., Jann, B. & Jann, K. (1981). The structure of the capsular polysaccharide (K5 antigen) of urinary tract infective *Escherichia coli* O10:K5:H4. A polymer similar to desulfoheparin. *European Journal of Biochemistry*, **116**, 359–64.

Vann, W. F., Soderstrom, T., Egan, W., Tsui, F. P., Schneerson, R., Ørskov, I. & Ørskov, F. (1983). Serological, chemical and structural analyses of the *Escherichia coli* cross reactive capsular polysacchardes K13, K20 and K23. *Infection and Immunity*, **39**, 623–9.

Vimr, E. (1990). Map position and genomic organization of the kps cluster for polysialic acid synthesis in *Escherichia coli* K1. *Journal of Bacteriology*, **173**, 1335–8.

Vimr, E. R., Aaronson, W. & Silver, R. P. (1989). Genetic analysis of chromosomal mutations in the polysialic acid gene cluster of *Escherichia coli* K1. *Journal of Bacteriology*, **171**, 1106–17.

Wessels, M. R., Craig, E. R., Vicente-Javier, B. and Kasper, D. L. (1989). Definition of a bacterial virulence factor: sialylation of the group B streptococcal capsule. *Proceedings of the National Academy of Sciences USA*, **86**, 8983–7.

Whitfield, C., Adams, D. & Troy, F. A. (1984). Biosynthesis and assembly of the polysialic acid capsule in *Escherichia coli* K1. Role of low density vesicle fraction in activation of the endogenous synthesis of sialyl polymers. *Journal of Biological Chemistry*, **259**, 12776–80.

Whitfield, C., Schoenhals, G. & Graham, L. (1989). Mutants of *E. coli* O9:K30 with altered synthesis and expression of the capsular K30 antigen. *Journal of General Microbiology*, **135**, 2589–99.

Whitfield, C. & Troy, F. A. (1984). Biosynthesis and assembly of the polysialic acid capsule in *Escherichia coli* K1. *Journal of Biological Chemistry*, **259**, 12769–75.

Whitfield, C., Vimr, E. R., Costerton, W. & Troy, F. A. (1984). Protein synthesis is required for *in vivo* activation of polysialic acid synthesis in *E. coli* K1. *Journal of Bacteriology*, **159**, 321–8.

Wicken, A. J. & Knox, K. W. (1980). Bacterial cell surface amphiphiles. *Biochemica et Biophysica Acta*, **604**, 1–26.

5

Escherichia coli lipopolysaccharide in pathogenesis and virulence

S. HULL

Lipopolysaccharide (LPS) is a complex glycolipid that constitutes the major non-protein component of the outer membrane of Gram-negative bacilli, including *Escherichia coli* and other members of the family Enterobacteriaceae. It is also present in many other important genera of human and animal pathogens, such as *Vibrio*, *Pseudomonas* and *Brucella* (Rietschel *et al.*, 1992). A truncated form of LPS, known as lipo-oligosaccharide (LOS), is found in the outer membranes of bacteria of the genera *Neisseria* and *Haemophilus* (Rietschel *et al.*, 1990). LPS has been the subject of intense investigation, because of its great importance as an inducer of septic shock and an extensive literature has been devoted to the subject.

Lipopolysaccharide structure and its importance in the outer membrane

During the last four decades it has been revealed that LPS has a complex chemical structure, which for convenience is usually divided into three parts: (i) lipid A, (ii) the core oligosaccharide, and (iii) the O-polysaccharide (PS) or O-antigen (Raetz, 1991; Rietschel *et al.*, 1990) (Figure 5.1). Complete LPS is termed smooth, or S-form LPS, while LPS that lacks the O-antigen is referred to as rough, because loss of the O-antigen confers a rough, dry appearance on bacterial colonies. Lipopolysaccharide that contains only the inner core, or a part of it, and lipid A is termed 'deep rough'.

Unlike other virulence factors that enhance the capacity of *E. coli* to cause disease, only a minimal part of LPS is absolutely necessary for cell viability. It has proved impossible to isolate mutants that lack lipid A and 3-deoxy-*manno*-D-octulosonic acid (KDO), the inner core sugar

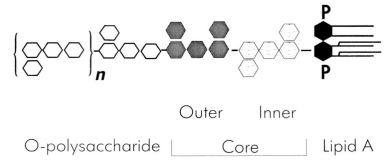

Fig. 5.1. Schematic representation of the structure of lipopolysaccharide (LPS).

proximal to lipid A (Raetz, 1991), probably because of the vital role this molecule plays in the outer membrane. Lipid A is embedded in the outer leaflet of the outer membrane, where it replaces phospholipids (Figure 5.2) and there may be as many as one million molecules of lipid A in each outer membrane (Raetz, 1993). Divalent cations cross-link adjacent LPS molecules into a strong network (Hancock, 1991). Furthermore, lipid A and the inner core are required for the correct assembly and insertion of the major outer-membrane protein, OmpA, and the porin proteins, OmpF, OmpC, and PhoE, into the outer membrane (Sen & Nikaido, 1991; Nikaido, 1992). Deep rough mutants fail to export normal amounts of porins into the outer membrane, and LPS from such mutants fails to trimerise OmpF *in vitro* (Sen & Nikaido, 1991). In addition, *de novo* synthesis of LPS appears to be necessary for the assembly of porins into the outer membrane. Nikaido (1992) suggested that the association between nascent LPS and porin proteins in the outer membrane causes an alteration in the conformation of the proteins, changing them from a stable water-soluble form in the periplasm to a pore-forming structure in the outer membrane. Unfortunately, the mechanisms by which LPS is transported from its site of synthesis, the cytoplasmic membrane, across the periplasm and how it is inserted into the outer membrane are not understood (Raetz, 1990), and many questions remain about the assembly of the outer membrane.

Apart from its importance as a molecular keystone in the outer membrane, LPS is responsible for many of the surface characteristics of *E. coli* and other Gram-negative bacteria, particularly their resistance to detergents, dyes, lysozyme and hydrophobic antibiotics (Hancock, 1991). The capacity of LPS to prevent many compounds from crossing the

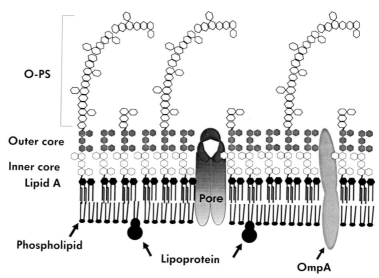

Fig. 5.2. Major features of the outer membrane of *Escherichia coli*, with particular emphasis on lipopolysaccharide. OmpA, outer-membrane protein A; O-PS, O-polysaccharide.

outer membrane and gaining access to the periplasm or peptidoglycan is due to the chemistry of LPS and its three-dimensional structure. Lipopolysaccharide is amphiphilic; lipid A is hydrophobic and lies embedded in the outer membrane, while the O-polysaccharide, which projects from the outer membrane, forms a hydrophilic layer into which hydrophobic compounds penetrate poorly (Rietschel *et al.*, 1990; Hancock, 1991).

Evidence has accumulated that the O-polysaccharide chains do not, as was once thought, merely extend from the surface, but they are flexible and can bend over the surface of the outer membrane and cover incomplete molecules of LPS composed only of lipid A-core and lipid A-core to which only short O-polysaccharide chains are attached (Figure 5.2) (Peterson & McGroarty, 1986; Seydel & Brandenburg, 1992; Seydell *et al.*, 1993). Curiously, even in wild-type bacteria growing under optimal conditions, only some of the LPS molecules are substituted with complete long O-polysaccharide chains. It has been suggested that this endows the surface of the bacterium with a felt-like nap (Peterson & McGroarty, 1986; Seydel & Brandenburg, 1992). This architecture may have a selective advantage for the bacterium, by excluding many compounds, while allowing access to the outer membrane for small hydrophilic molecules, such as amino-acids and sugars. Comprehensive reviews of the three-dimensional structure of LPS have been provided by Seydel & Brandenburg (1992) and Seydel *et al.* (1993).

Lipopolysaccharide genetics and synthesis

Lipopolysaccharide is not a direct gene product but, unlike other protein virulence factors, it is the product of a series of enzymes that must act in the proper sequence. Thus, the genetics and synthesis of LPS are as complex as those of its molecular structure. A broad picture of these mechanisms has emerged, but many details remain unknown. In the last decade considerable progress has been made in cloning the genes for LPS, and this should make available for study the genes and enzymes responsible for LPS synthesis. The genetics and synthesis of LPS have been reviewed by Schnaitman & Klena (1993) and Rick (1987) respectively.

The role of lipid A and inner core regions of lipopolysaccharide in pathogenesis

The role of the lipid A-core portion of LPS in virulence and pathogenicity differs considerably from that of the O-polysaccharide moiety, and each of these parts of the LPS molecule will be discussed in turn.

The endotoxic principle

The signs seen in patients suffering from Gram-negative septicaemia can be reproduced in animals by the injection of killed suspensions of *E. coli* or *Salmonella* bacteria; culture supernatants are less effective in reproducing the symptoms of shock (Raetz, 1991). This observation gave rise to the term 'endotoxin', because it was recognised that a portion of the bacterium itself, rather than a secreted exotoxin, was responsible for the pathological process. Endotoxic (septic) shock is a serious medical condition in which the failure to deliver oxygen eventually leads to multiple organ failure and death ensues rapidly (Shenep, 1992; see Chapter 17). Mortality rates from Gram-negative sepsis and septic shock as high as 60 per cent have been reported, and these figures have changed little since the pre-antibiotic era (Gransden *et al.*, 1990; Ziegler *et al.*, 1991; Martin & Silverman, 1992).

Attempts to identify the principle responsible for the fever and shock in patients infected with Gram-negative bacteria eventually led to the demonstration that the lipid A–KDO portion of LPS is necessary and sufficient to reproduce, in animal models and in cultured mammalian cells, the physiological manifestations and biochemical processes associated with septic shock (Young *et al.*, 1991). Lipid A is the most highly conserved part of LPS and the difference, for example, between *E. coli* LPS and that from *Salmonella* lies in the addition of one extra fatty acid chain in the latter (Rietschel *et al.*, 1990). The exact chemical structure of lipid A from *E. coli* has been published many times (Rietschel *et al.*, 1990; Raetz, 1991; Rietschel *et al.*, 1992). The similarities between the lipid A from various Gram-negative bacteria account for the observation that infections with a variety of these organisms produce very similar symptoms. By way of contrast, the actions of exotoxins are quite specific. The effects of endotoxin administration are numerous and include fever, myocardial depression, coagulopathy, hypotension, acute respiratory distress and multiple organ failure (Cybulski *et al.*, 1988; Shenep, 1992). It is known that the capacity of LPS to produce such a variety of responses is due to the release of cytokines and other metabolites, which are in turn responsible for activation of the acute phase response, in which a number of haematological, metabolic and immunological processes become activated (Glauser *et al.*, 1991). Great progress has been made in the last decade in the understanding of how endotoxin reacts with various components of the immune system.

Stimulation of mammalian cells and factors by endotoxin

Endotoxin binds to a number of surface receptors of macrophages, monocytes and neutrophils, and also with plasma and intercellular proteins (Morrison, 1990; Lei & Chen, 1993). Binding of LPS to macrophages is enhanced if the LPS has first formed a complex with a large protein called the LPS-binding protein (LBP) (Schumann *et al.*, 1990; Tobias *et al.*, 1993). These LPS–LBP complexes then bind to macrophage CD14 molecules (Wright *et al.*, 1990), which stimulates the macrophages to produce the powerful cytokines, tumour necrosis factor (TNF) and interleukin-1 (IL-1). The exact mechanism by which cytokine production by macrophages is induced is unknown, but it is likely to involve protein phosphorylation (Nakano & Shinomiya, 1990; Sibley,

1993). Tumour necrosis factor and IL-1 are key mediators that trigger the pathophysiological events that result in shock (Glauser *et al.*, 1991).

Lipopolysaccharide-binding protein shares homology with another protein, called bactericidal permeability-increasing protein (BPI), which is associated with neutrophil azurophilic granules (Scott *et al.*, 1993). This protein is identical to the protein formerly referred to as cationic anti-microbial protein 57 (CAP57). Bactericidal permeability-increasing protein also binds LPS but, rather than stimulate immune cells, BPI inhibits the activation of neutrophils and its physiological role may be to clear LPS from the circulation (Maarra *et al.*, 1990; Scott *et al.*, 1993). Though it has been reported that BPI is a microbicide, the presence of serum is necessary for this function, and it may in fact merely act to promote the normal complement-mediated lysis of Gram-negative bacteria (Weiss *et al.*, 1993). As a microbicide, BPI is less effective than conventional antibiotics (Scott *et al.*, 1993).

The expression of CD14 on neutrophils is enhanced by TNF, and LPS–LBP complexes bind to CD14 molecules on neutrophils (Wright *et al.*, 1991). This results in an increase, on the surface of neutrophils, in the adhesive capacity of Complement Receptor 3 (CR3), a member of the CD11/CD18 (β_2 integrin) family of integrins (Witthaut *et al.*, 1993). As a result, neutrophils adhere to the walls of small blood vessels and respond with an oxidative burst. This releases toxic products that cause injury to the endothelium, increase its permeability, with resulting haemorrhagic necrosis, a process in which platelets also participate (Piguet, 1993; Winn *et al.*, 1993). Severe sepsis is also often accompanied by neutrophil infiltration in the lungs, where damage to blood vessels allows fluid to enter the alveolar spaces, with a resulting reduction in alveolar gas exchange. The net result is termed adult respiratory distress syndrome, which exacerbates the hypoxaemia caused by circulatory failure, and leads to multiple organ failure. If three or more organs fail, death is almost certain (Martin & Silverman, 1992).

Factor XII, also known as Hageman factor, is among the soluble proteins that bind LPS (Morrison, 1990). Activated Factor XII activates tissue factor, which, in turn, activates the extrinsic coagulation pathway resulting in fibrin deposition in small blood vessels (disseminated intra-vascular coagulation; DIC) (Parrillo *et al.*, 1990), and this contributes to the development of circulatory failure. As in other pathological processes that lead to septic shock, endotoxin-stimulated coagulation is complex and has been reviewed by Van Deventer *et al.*, (1993). Thus, paradox-ically, stimulation by endotoxin can result in both haemorrhage and uncontrolled coagulation. Local damage to blood vessels, caused by activated neutrophils and coagulation, is part of the host defence process designed to contain and destroy invading micro-organisms but, at the extreme, the process can be life-threatening. The importance of this response is aptly illustrated by the susceptibility to Gram-negative infection of C3H/HeJ mice, which are relatively resistant to the lethal effects of administered endotoxin and fail to recruit neutrophils to the site of infection (O'Brien *et al.*, 1979; Svanborg-Eden & Hagberg, 1985). They are, however, extremely susceptible to infection by Gram-negative bacteria (Svanborg-Eden *et al.*, 1988).

Antibodies against endotoxin in the treatment of sepsis

Survival rates from endotoxic shock have improved little since the introduction of antibiotics and there has been a search for other methods of treatment. A number of monoclonal antibodies directed against lipid A or core oligosaccharide has been shown to protect against the lethal effects of endotoxin in animal models, but their adaptation to clinical use has not been as successful (Di Padova *et al.*, 1993; Fang, *et al.*, 1993; Mascelli, *et al.*, 1993). Since lipid A and the inner core are conserved in many Gram-negative bacteria, antibodies to these parts of LPS should be more broadly cross-protective than antibodies directed against the more variable outer core and the O-antigen portions of LPS. Appelmelk & Cohen (1992) have reviewed the studies of anti-core and anti-lipid A monoclonal antibodies and concluded that such antibodies have little effect on the clearing of bacteria from the circulation, because on living bacteria they are directed at structures that are normally hidden by O-polysaccharide and capsules. The protective effects of such monoclonal antibodies may be to neutralise free endotoxin liberated from dead or dying bacteria, before it can bind to LBP and other factors, and stimulate immune cells. If this is correct, lower levels of TNF and IL-1 would be found in animals treated with monoclonal antibodies. No such difference was, however, observed in mice that survived administration of monoclonal antibody against core oligosaccharide as compared with dead untreated control mice (Silva *et al.*, 1990). The precise mechanism by which such monoclonal antibodies afford protection, therefore, remains unclear. In spite of the results observed in experimental animals, the results of clinical trials in humans have been disappointing. Although the survival rates of patients with Gram-negative sepsis who had been given a monoclonal antibody against lipid A are better than those of control patients, the mortality rates for patients already in shock are not signifi-cantly improved (Wolff, 1991).

At least two serious problems have been encountered with the admin-istration of anti-lipid A or anti-core monoclonal antibodies to patients in clinical settings. The first is identification of patients infected with Gram-negative bacteria who would be likely to benefit from such treatment. Since sepsis can very rapidly proceed to shock, the results of blood cultures may not be available before antibody administration. Secondly, in order to be effective, anti-lipid A monoclonal antibody should be administered before cytokine production has been stimulated. In animal experimental models, monoclonal antibodies are often administered before or immediately after endotoxin or bacterial challenge (Appelmelk & Cohen, 1992). This is clearly not possible in the clinical setting. Shinjii *et al.* (1993) have shown that the initial events that lead to increased transcription of mRNA for TNF take place in the first 20 minutes after LPS stimulation. Monoclonal antibodies to lipid A may offer some protection to patients infected with Gram-negative bacteria who are not yet in shock, because further stimulation of the processes leading to shock are inhibited, but these antibodies can do little to reverse the damage in patients who are already in shock.

The virulence of O-polysaccharide and outer core

Serological and chemical variation

While the structure of the lipid A-inner core region of LPS is extremely constant, the outer core and O-polysaccharide chains vary considerably, even within the same species. Indeed, the combination of O-, H- (flagel-lar) and K- (capsular) antigens defines the serotype of *E. coli*. This organism has at least five outer cores (Table 5.1) and 170 different O-antigens can be differentiated by their reaction with polyclonal rabbit antisera (Ørskov *et al.*, 1977, 1984). Precise chemical analysis of the O-polysaccharide from *E. coli* of the same O-serogroup shows hetero-geneity. For example, three different chemotypes have been classified as O1 (Gupta, 1992; Jann *et al.*, 1992) and the 170 different O-antigens may be an underestimate of the true variation. The O-polysaccharides have been further divided into three types based on their structure and migration in an electrical current (Ørskov *et al.*, 1977; Jann & Jann, 1984). These are the neutral homopolymeric, neutral heteropolymeric

Table 5.1. *Structures of the inner core and five outer cores of* Escherichia coli

Core type	Structure	Reference
Inner core of *E. coli* K12:		Blache *et al.*, 1981; Rick, 1987

$$
\begin{array}{cc}
P & P \\
\downarrow & \downarrow \\
4 & 4
\end{array}
$$

HepII (1→3) HepI (1→5) KDO (2→6) Lipid A

$$
\begin{array}{c}
4/5 \\
\uparrow \\
2
\end{array}
$$

KDO 7→ ? PEA

$$
\begin{array}{c}
4 \\
\uparrow \\
2
\end{array}
$$

KDO

Outer cores (hexose region) of five *E. coli* strains:		
R1:	Gal (1→2) Glc (1→3) Glc (1→3) Hep	Rietschel *et al.*, 1990

$$
\begin{array}{cc}
2 & 3 \\
\uparrow & \uparrow \\
1 & 1 \\
\text{Gal} & \text{Glc}
\end{array}
$$

| R2: | Glc (1→2) Glc (1→3) Glc (1→3) Hep | Rietschel *et al.*, 1990 |

$$
\begin{array}{cc}
2 & 6 \\
\uparrow & \uparrow \\
1 & 1 \\
\text{GlcNAc} & \text{Gal}
\end{array}
$$

| R3: | Glc (1→2) Gal (1→3) Glc (1→3) Hep | Rietschel *et al.*, 1990 |

$$
\begin{array}{cc}
2 & 3 \\
\uparrow & \uparrow \\
1 & 1 \\
\text{Glc} & \text{GlcNAc}
\end{array}
$$

| R4: | Gal (1→2) Glc (1→3) Glc (1→3) Hep | Rietschel *et al.*, 1990 |

$$
\begin{array}{cc}
2 & 4 \\
\uparrow & \uparrow \\
1 & 1 \\
\text{Gal} & \text{Gal}
\end{array}
$$

| K12: | Glc (1→2) Glc (1→3) Glc (1→3) Hep | Rietschel *et al.*, 1990 |

$$
\begin{array}{cc}
6 & 6 \\
\uparrow & \uparrow \\
1 & 1 \\
\text{GlcNAc} & \text{Gal}
\end{array}
$$

Abbreviations: Gal, galactose; Glc, glucose; GlcNAc, *N*-acetylglucosamine; Hep, heptose; KDO, 3-deoxy-D-*manno*-octulosonic acid; *P*, phosphate, pyrophosphate or phosphorylethanolamine; and PEA, phosphorylethanolamine. The question mark in the inner core structure indicates that the exact linkage for the PEA has not been established (Rick, 1987). The heptose shown in the outer core structures correspond to HepII of the inner core.

Table 5.2. *Structures of the repeating subunits of selected O-antigens*

O-antigen	Structure	Reference
Neutral homopolysaccharides:		
O8	3)-α-D-Man-(1→2)-α-D-Man-(1→2)-α-D-Man-(1→	Jann & Jann, 1984
O9	3)-α-D-Man-(1→3)-α-D-Man-(1→2)-α-D-Man-(1→2)-α-D-Man-(1→2)-α-D-Man-(1→	
Neutral heteropolysaccharides:		

O1A	3)-α-L-Rhap-(1→3)-α-L-Rhap-(1→3)-β-L-Rhap-(1→4)-β-D-GlcpNAc-(1→
	                              2
	                              ↑
	                              1
	                     β-D-ManpNAc
		Jann et al., 1992

O6	4)-α-D-GalpNAc-(1→3)-β-D-Manp-(1→4)-β-D-Manp-(1→3)-α-D-GlcpNAc-(1→
	                                    2
	                                    ↑
	                                    1
	                              β-D-Glcp
		Jansson et al., 1984

Acidic heteropolysaccharide:		

124	3)-β-D-GalNAc-(1→3)-β-D-Gal-(1→6)-α-D-Gal-(1→
	                                 4
	                                 ↑
	                                 1
	                          α-D-Glc-(1←6)-β-GlcLA
		Jann & Jann, 1984

Abbreviations: Gal, galactose; GalNAc, *N*-acetylgalactosamine; Glc, glucose; GlcLA, glucolactilic acid; GlcNAc, *N*-acetylglucosamine; Man, mannose; ManNAc, mannosamine; Rha, rhamnose.

and acidic heteropolymeric polysaccharides (see Table 5.2 for an example of each).

There is a curious relationship between the pathogenicity of various *E. coli* strains and their O-serogroups. In spite of the large number of O-antigens, a few appear to predominate among isolates recovered from disease, as compared with those isolated from the faeces of normal individuals (Roberts *et al.*, 1975). Thus, a very limited number of O-serotypes is associated with *E. coli* that cause diarrhoea and these do not in general overlap with those frequently associated with urinary tract infection and sepsis (Ørskov & Ørskov, 1977; Ørskov *et al.*, 1982). The O-antigens associated with urinary tract infection, especially upper urinary tract infection (pyelonephritis), and septicaemia overlap because the urinary tract is the most common source of *E. coli* in septicaemia (Johnson, 1991). It has been noted that the O-antigens of enteroinvasive *E. coli*, which cause a dysentery-like disease, are chemically similar to those of *Shigella*, the classical agents of bacillary dysentery (Jann & Jann, 1984).

The various O-antigens associated with particular diseases are listed in Table 5.3. These associations have given rise to the clonal theory of the pathogenicity of *E. coli*. This postulates that pathogenic strains of *E. coli* are the descendants of a few ancestral lines that somehow acquired pathogenic traits (Ørskov & Ørskov, 1977; Ørskov *et al.*, 1982; Achtman & Pluschke, 1986). The ability of these strains of *E. coli* to cause certain diseases is not necessarily due to their particular O-antigens, but rather the genes they carry for other traits that enhance their pathogenicity, such as enterotoxins and colonisation factors. Whether the specific O-antigens of these strains have a role in the disease process has not been determined.

As more genes are cloned that encode the enzymes necessary to produce LPS, it may become possible to 'engineer' novel O-polysaccharides and determine whether the chemical structure, and not merely its presence, affects virulence. A tantalising experiment, which suggested that this may be the case, was carried out by Gemski *et al.* (1972), who, by conjugation, replaced the normal O-antigen of *Shigella flexneri* with two different *E. coli* O-polysaccharides. The *Sh. flexneri* hybrid with the O8 polysaccharide of *E. coli* was not virulent in animal models, while the strain with the O25 polysaccharide was as virulent as the *Sh. flexneri* parent strain. The reason for this difference was not determined and it is not known whether it relates to differences in complement deposition on the bacterial surface.

Table 5.3. *O-antigens associated with disease*

Disease[a]	O-antigens	Reference
Diarrhoea:		
EPEC	O55, O86, O111, O119, O126, O17, O128AB, O142	Levine (1987)
ETEC	O6, O8, O15, O25, O27, O63, O78, O80, O85, O115, O128AC, O139, O148, O159, O167	Levine (1987)
EIEC	O28AC, O29, O124, O136, O143, O144, O152, O164, O167	Levine (1987)
EHEC	O26, O111, O157	Levine (1987)
Urinary tract infection (symptomatic)	O1, O2, O4, O6, O7, O8, O16, O18, O25, O50, O75	Johnson (1991)
Septicaemia	O2, O4, O6, O7, O16, O18	McCabe *et al.* (1978)

[a] EPEC, Enteropathogenic *E. coli*; ETEC, enterotoxigenic *E. coli*; EIEC, enteroinvasive *E. coli*; EHEC, enterohaemorrhagic *E. coli*.

Role of O-polysaccharide in resistance to the bactericidal effect of complement

There is little doubt that O-polysaccharide protects the bacterium from the bactericidal effects of human complement. The complement cascade is one of the pathways that is triggered during the acute phase of the response to infection (Glauser *et al.*, 1991).

Complement consists of at least 20 plasma proteins that act in an exquisitely regulated cascade, which has opsonic, chemotactic and lytic properties. Phagocytic cells have complement receptors and will ingest micro-organisms coated with complement (Vukajilovich, 1992). However, activated complement alone is lytic for Gram-negative bacteria (Joiner, 1988).

Briefly, the complement cascade can be activated in two ways, the classical pathway and the alternative pathway, which can both generate the membrane attack complex (MAC), which forms transmembrane pores in the outer membrane. Classical pathway activation depends on the formation of antigen–antibody complexes. The plasma of normal individuals contains 'natural' antibodies against conserved portions of LPS, probably as a result of continuous contact with Gram-negative bacteria (Taylor, 1985). However, the outer core and long O-polysaccharide chains mask the lipid A of intact bacteria and may hinder the efficient activation of the classical pathway. Endotoxin binds to the first component of complement (C1) and mediates the induction of the complement cascade (Loos *et al.*, 1978). Paradoxically, the O-polysaccharide end of the LPS molecule protects the bacterium from the consequences of the activity of the lipid A moiety at the other end.

The alternative pathway, on the other hand, is independent of specific antibodies, but depends on the presence of a complete, or almost complete, core. In the process of activation of the alternative pathway, molecules of C3b bind to the surface of the bacterium. This involves the formation of ester bonds between C3b and the hydroxyl groups of sugars (Joiner, 1988). Binding of C3b is required for the activation of C5 and its conversion to C5b, which binds to an appropriate surface and triggers the sequential activation and binding of C6 to C9. One molecule each of C5b to C8 bind, followed by the insertion of a number of molecules of C9, which form a ring-like structure, the MAC, in the membrane. The diameter of the ring depends on the number of C9 molecules bound and this may reach as many as 16 (Taylor, 1985). When six to eight molecules of C9 have bound, the ring is complete and a pore is formed (Schröder *et al.*, 1990). This provides lysozyme with access to the peptidoglycan and lysis occurs (Vukajilovich, 1992).

Resistance to complement-mediated lysis

Smooth strains of *E. coli*, particularly those isolated from cases of septicaemia and upper urinary tract infection, are frequently resistant to complement-mediated lysis (Taylor, 1985). This phenomenon is commonly called serum resistance, but complement resistance would be more precise. At one time it was thought that the long O-polysaccharide chains physically prevent the C5b–9 components from binding to bacteria but this is not the case, because smooth, complement-resistant strains also bind and activate complement (Joiner, 1988). The mechanism of resistance of *Salmonella* and *E. coli* O111 has been elucidated, and it has been shown that C3b binds to LPS, but preferentially to the longest O-polysaccharide chains (Goldman *et al.*, 1984; Joiner *et al.*, 1986). As a result, formation of the C5b–9 complex is triggered, but well away from the cell surface and so unable to form the transmembrane pore (Joiner, 1988).

It is strange that not all O-antigens appear able to confer complement resistance; even among strains with the same O-antigen, sensitivity or resistance is not universal (Johnson, 1991). This may be due to the degree of polymerisation of the O-subunits and to the number of cores that are substituted with O-polysaccharide. Bacteria with a high density of O-polysaccharide chains of at least 14 subunits in length are the most resistant to complement (Porat *et al.*, 1987, 1992; Joiner, 1988). Furthermore, the chemistry of the O-antigen is an important factor in complement resistance in *Salmonella* (Liang-Takasaki *et al.*, 1982). The replacement of abequose (3, 6-dideoxy-D-galactose) as a branching sugar in the O-antigen of *S. typhimurium* by tyvelose (3, 6-dideoxy-D-mannose) from *S. enteriditis* resulted in a *Salmonella* hybrid that was less virulent in a mouse model (Mäkelä *et al.*, 1988). This substitution also enhanced the binding of C3b to the surface of the bacteria (Grossman *et al.*, 1986); abequose and tyvelose differ only in the position of a hydroxyl group. Another hybrid that received the O-antigen of *S. montevideo* was even less virulent in the mouse model. The latter O-antigen contains four molecules of mannose in each repeating subunit rather than only one mannose in *S. enteriditis* and *S. typhimurium*. Grossman *et al.* (1986) found that *S. montevideo* binds nearly three times as much C3b as compared with *S. typhimurium*. The *E. coli* O8 antigen, transferred to *Shigella flexneri* in the experiment by Gemski *et al.* (1972) discussed above, is a homopolymer of mannose (see Table 5.2), while that of O25 does not contain mannose (Ørskov *et al.*, 1977).

The resistance of these parent and hybrid strains of *Salmonella* to ingestion by macrophages is parallel to that of resistance to complement (Liang-Takasaki *et al.*, 1982), but when the complement in the serum used in the reaction was inactivated, the differences between the strains were no longer observed. This suggests that recognition of the bacteria by macrophages depends on complement receptors and on the amount of complement bound to the bacteria (Jimenez-Lucho *et al.*, 1990). Thus, the virulence of *Salmonella* is inversely proportional to complement binding.

Comparable experiments with isogenic strains of *E. coli* in appropriate animal models have not yet been done. Iwahi *et al.* (1982) assessed the capacity of 33 wild-type strains of *E. coli* to colonise the bladders and kidneys of mice. Although their study was primarily directed towards determining the role of type-1 fimbriae in colonisation, they also determined the serogroup of the strains and concluded that in this model the O-antigen played no role in virulence. Unfortunately, most of their strains did not carry the O-antigens commonly associated with urinary tract infection. Nevertheless, nine of 15 strains in the avirulent group were rough or non-typable, as compared with only two of eight strains in the most virulent group. Later, Iwahi & Imada (1988) used several strains from this collection and observed a direct correlation between resistance to killing by murine neutrophils and the capacity to colonise the bladder. Treatment of the bacteria with EDTA, at a concentration that did not affect cell viability, decreased both resistance to phagocytosis and bladder colonisation. Treatment with EDTA removes divalent cations that bridge adjacent molecules of LPS and releases LPS from the outer membrane (Leive, 1965; Hancock & Karunatne, 1990). However, treatment with EDTA or loss of LPS may have other, as yet undetermined, effects that would also be relevant to this model system. Therefore, it cannot be absolutely concluded that LPS is responsible for the phagocytosis resistance observed by Iwahi & Imada (1988).

Similar experiments have been carried out by Svanborg-Eden *et al.* (1987) with the refinement that isogenic mutants and recombinants lacking one or more of various putative virulence factors were used. One pair was an O75:K5:H⁻ uropathogenic parent and its O⁻ derivative, into which the *rfb* locus of a rough *E. coli* K-12 had been transferred by conjugation. The O⁻ recombinant was more sensitive to the bactericidal activity of normal human serum, and to ingestion and killing by human neutrophils than its parent. Furthermore, the O⁻ recombinant was cleared from the bladders of immunologically normal mice, but not from the bladders of the LPS non-responder C3H/HeJ mice.

The protective effect of antibodies to O-polysaccharide

Resistance to complement-mediated lysis can be overcome by the addition to the reaction of antibodies specific for the O-antigen of the bacterium (Joiner, 1988) and it has been suggested that the antibodies cause the O-polysaccharide chains to clump. This may have the dual effect of preventing the C3b molecules from binding to the long O-polysaccharide chains and also of providing greater access for C5b–9 to the outer membrane. The capacity of antibodies against the O-antigen to promote the complement-induced lysis of *E. coli*, the so-called bactericidal antibodies, should theoretically be useful for the treatment of *E. coli* sepsis. Unlike antibodies against lipid A and the inner core, which have little effect on intact bacteria, antibodies against the O-polysaccharide actually promote the clearance of the bacteria from the bloodstream (Pollack, 1992).

The effectiveness of antibodies against O-antigens in several different animal models has been tested and has generally been observed to reduce mortality and pathology. For example, Schiff *et al.* (1993) immunised rabbits with a preparation of O18 polysaccharide conjugated to toxin A, and the resulting polyclonal sera significantly protected neonatal rats against death after challenge with an *E. coli* O18:K1 strain. Administration of a monoclonal antibody to O111 polysaccharide increased the survival of mice after challenge with purified LPS, and TNF levels were lower in mice given the monoclonal anti-O111, as compared with those given anti-core or anti-lipid A monoclonal antibody (Baumgartner *et al.* 1990). Similarly, a monoclonal antibody to O111 polysaccharide also increased the survival rates of dogs in a canine sepsis model. Again, dogs that received an anti-core monoclonal antibody were not significantly protected (Pollack, 1992).

The same problems as were noted above in connection with the use of anti-lipid A monoclonal antibodies are encountered when anti-O antibodies are administered to patients infected with *E. coli*; identification of patients who would benefit and the timing of administration. Immunisation of patients with O-polysaccharide or O-polysaccharide-conjugate vaccines might circumvent these problems. Kaisjer & Ahlstedt (1977) immunised mice with whole bacteria of serotypes O6:K13 or O2:K2. The mice produced antibodies to the O- and K-polysaccharides but mice were protected only from challenge with the homologous bacteria. Rhesus monkeys successfully immunised with an O8 polysaccharide–bovine serum albumin conjugate vaccine, and subsequently challenged with a homologous *E. coli* in a model of ascending urinary tract infection, became infected but were protected from renal scarring, while control animals became infected and developed scars. Protection in the immunised monkeys correlated with absence of neutrophil infiltration into the kidneys (Roberts *et al.*, 1993).

Humans have also been successfully immunised with an O-polysaccharide-specific protein conjugate vaccine (Crysz *et al.*, 1991). Volunteers were immunised parenterally with O18 polysaccharide conjugated with cholera toxin or *Pseudomonas aeruginosa* toxin A. The volunteers responded well and few side effects, all regarded as minor, were observed. The serum of the immunised volunteers promoted the uptake and killing by human neutrophils of a strain of *E. coli* O18:K1, and it protected mice from fatal sepsis by the same strain.

Although immunisation with O-polysaccharide is protective, the number of O-antigens synthesised by *E. coli* would seem to make the task of preparing a broadly cross-protective vaccine a daunting endeavour. Even if the O-antigens in a vaccine were limited to those most commonly associated with certain diseases, the vaccines would still have to be polyvalent. A vaccine prepared with O-antigens commonly associated with urinary tract infection and septicaemia would have to contain some ten different O-polysaccharides, and would offer little protection against haemorrhagic enterocolitis. Even though O-antigens are immunogenic and antibodies to O-antigens provide protection against disease, the development of O-polysaccharide vaccines may still be far off. The study of LPS continues to fascinate and frustrate.

References

Achtman, M. & Pluschke, G. (1986). Clonal analysis of descent and virulence among selected *Escherichia coli*. *Annual Reviews of Microbiology*, **40**, 185–210.

Appelmelk, B. J. & Cohen, J. (1992). The protective role of antibodies to the lipopolysaccharide core region. In *Bacterial Endotoxic Lipopolysaccharides*, vol. II, *Immunopharmacology and Pathophysiology*, eds. J. L. Ryan & D. C. Morrison, pp. 375–410. Boca Raton, FL: CRC Press.

Baumgartner, J. D., Heumann, D., Gerain, J., Weinbreck, P., Grau, G. E. & Glauser, M. P. (1990). Association between protective efficacy of anti-lipopolysaccharide (LPS) antibodies and suppression of LPS-induced tumor necrosis factor α and interleukin 6. Comparison of O side chain-specific antibodies with core LPS antibodies. *Journal of Experimental Medicine*, **171**, 889–96.

Blache, D., Bruneteau, M. & Michel, G. (1981). Structure de la region heptose du lipopolysaccharide de *Escherichia coli* K-12 CR34. *European Journal of Biochemistry*, **113**, 563–8.

Crysz, S. J. Jr., Cross, A. S., Sadoff, J. D., Wegmann, A., Que, J. U. & E. Fürer, E. (1990). Safety and immunogenicity of *Escherichia coli* O18 O-specific polysaccharide (O-PS)-toxin A and O-PS-cholera toxin conjugate vaccines in humans. *Journal of Infectious Diseases*, **163**, 1040–5.

Cybulski, M. I., Chan, M. K. W. & Movat, H. Z. (1988). Biology of disease. Acute inflammation and microthrombosis induced by endotoxin, interleukin-1, and tumor necrosis factor and their implication in Gram-negative infection. *Laboratory Investigation*, **58**, 365–78.

Di Padova, F. E., Helmut Brade, H., Barclay, G. R., Poxton, I. R., Liehl, E., Schuetze, E., Kocher, H. P., Ramsay, G., Schreier, M. H., McClelland, B. L. & Rietschel, E. T. (1993). A broadly cross-protective monoclonal antibody binding to *Escherichia coli* and *Salmonella* lipopolysaccharides. *Infection and Immunity*, **61**, 3863–72.

Fang, I. S., Wisniewski, M. A., Huntenburg, C. C., Knight, L. S., Bubbers, J. E. & Schneidkraut, M. J. (1993). Inhibition of lipopolysaccharide-associated endotoxin activities *in vitro* and *in vivo* by the human anti-Lipid A monoclonal antibody SdJ5–1.17.15. *Infection and Immunity*, **61**, 3873–8.

Gemski, P. Jr., Sheahan, D. G., Washington, O. & Formal, S. B. (1972). Virulence of *Shigella flexneri* hybrids expressing *Escherichia coli* somatic antigens. *Infection and Immunity*, **6**, 104–11.

Glauser, M. P., Zanetti, G., Baumgartner, J. D. & Cohen, J. (1991). Septic shock pathogenesis. *Lancet*, **338**, 732–6.

Goldman, R. C., Joiner, K. & Leive, L. (1984). Serum-resistant mutants of *Escherichia coli* O111 contain increased lipopolysaccharide, lack an O antigen-containing capsule, and cover more of their lipid A core with O antigen. *Journal of Bacteriology*, **159**, 877–82.

Gransden, W. R., Eykyn, S. J., Phillips, I. & Rowe, B. (1990). Bacteremia due to *Escherichia coli*: a study of 861 episodes. *Reviews of Infectious Diseases*, **12**, 1008–18.

Grossman, N., Joiner, K. A., Frank, M. M. & Leive, L. (1986). C3b binding, but not its breakdown, is affected by the structure of the O-antigen polysaccharide in lipopolysaccharide from *Salmonellae*. *Journal of Immunology*, **136**, 2208–15.

Grossman, N., Lindberg, A. A., Svenson, S. B., Joiner, K. A., & Leive, L. (1991). Structural aspects of LPS: role in evasion of host defense mechanism. In *Microbial Surface Components and Toxins in Relation to Pathogenesis*, eds. E. Z. Ron & S. Rottem, pp. 143–9. New York: Plenum Press.

Gupta, D. S., Shaskov, A. S., Jann, B. & Jann, K. (1992). Structures of the O1B and O1C lipopolysaccharide antigens of *Escherichia coli*. *Journal of Bacteriology*, **174**, 7963–70.

Hancock, I. C. (1991). Microbial cell surface architecture. In *Microbial Cell Surface Analysis*, eds. N. Mozes, P. S. Hadley, H. J. Busscher & P. G. Rouxhet, pp. 23–59. New York: VCH Publishers.

Hancock, R. E. W. & Karunaratne, D. N. (1990). LPS integration into outer membrane structures. In *Endotoxin Research Series*, vol I. *Cellular and Molecular Aspects of Endotoxin Reaction*, eds. A. Nowotny, J. N. Spitzer & E. J. Ziegler, pp. 191–5. Amsterdam: Elsevier Science Publishers.

Iwahi, T., Abe, Y. & Tsuchiya, K. (1982). Virulence of *Escherichia coli* in ascending urinary tract infection in mice. *Journal of Medical Microbiology*, **15**, 303–16.

Iwahi, T. & Imada, A. (1988). Interaction of *Escherichia coli* with polymorphonuclear leukocytes in pathogenesis of urinary tract infection in mice. *Infection and Immunity*, **56**, 947–53.

Jann, B., Shaskov, A. S., Gupta, D. S., Panasenko, S. M. & Jann, K. (1992). The O1 antigen of *Escherichia coli*: structural characterization of the O1A1-specific polysaccharide. *Carbohydrate Polymers* **18**, 51–7.

Jann, K. & Jann, B. (1984). Structure and biosynthesis of O-antigens. In *Handbook of Endotoxin*, vol 1, *Chemistry of Endotoxins*, ed. E. T. Rietschel, pp. 138–86. Amsterdam: Elsevier Science Publishers.

Jansson, P.-E., Lindberg, B., Lonngren, J., Ortega, C. & Svenson, S. B. (1984). Structural studies of the *Escherichia coli* O-antigen 6. *Carbohydrate Research*, **131**, 277–83.

Jimenez-Lucho, V. E., Leive, L. L. & Joiner, K. A. (1990). Role of the O-antigen of lipopolysaccharide in protection against complement action.

In *The Bacteria*, vol. XI, *Molelcular Basis of Bacterial Pathogenesis*, eds B. H. Iglewski & V. L. Clark, pp. 339–54. New York: Academic Press.

Johnson, J. R. (1991) Virulence factors in *Escherichia coli* urinary tract infection. *Clinical Microbiology Reviews*, **4**, 80–128.

Joiner, K. A. (1988). Complement evasion by bacteria and parasites. *Annual Review of Microbiology*, **42**, 201–30.

Joiner, K. A., Grossman, N., Schmetz, M. & Leive, L. (1986). C3 binds preferentially to long-chain lipopolysaccharide during alternative pathway activation by *Salmonella montevideo*. *Journal of Immunology*, **136**, 710–15.

Kaijser, B. & Ahlstedt, S. (1977). Protective capacity of antibodies against *Escherichia coli* O and K antigens. *Infection and Immunity*, **17**, 286–9.

Lei, M.-G. & Chen, T.-Y. (1992). Cellular membrane receptors for lipopolysaccharide. In *Bacterial Endotoxic Lipopolysaccharides*, vol I, *Molecular Biochemistry and Cellular Biology*, eds. J. L. Ryan & D. C. Morrison, pp. 254–67. Boca Raton, FL: CRC Press.

Leive, L. (1965). Release of lipopolysaccharide by EDTA treatment of *E. coli*. *Biochemical and Biophysical Research Communications*, **21**, 290–6.

Levine, M. M. (1987). Escherichia coli that cause diarrhea: enterotoxigenic, enteropathogenic, enteroinvasive, enterohemorrhagic and entero-adherent. *Journal of Infectious Diseases*, **155**, 377–89.

Liang-Takasaki, C.-J., Makela, P. H. & Leive, L. (1982). Phagocytosis of bacteria by macrophages: changing the carbohydrate of lipopolysaccharide alters interaction with complement and macrophages. *Journal of Immunology*, **128**, 1229–35.

Loos, M., Wellek, B., Thesen, R. & Opferkuch, W. (1978). Antibody-independent interactin of the first component of complement with Gram-negative bacteria. *Infection and Immunity*, **22**, 5–9.

Mäkelä, P. H., Hovi, M., Saxén, H., Valtonen, M. & Valtonen, V. (1988). Role of O antigen in mouse salmonellosis. In *Surface Structures of Microorganisms and their Interactions with the Mammalian Host*, eds. E. Schrinner, M. H. Richmond, G. Seibert & U. Schwarz, pp. 91–8. New York: VCH Publishers.

Marra, M. N., Wilde, C. G., Griffith, J. E., Snable, J. L. & Scott, R. W. (1990). Bactericidal/permeability-increasing protein has endotoxin neutralizing activity. *Journal of Immunology*, **144**, 662–6.

Martin, M. A. & Silverman, H. J. (1992). Gram-negative sepsis and the adult respiratory distress syndrome. *Clinical Infectious Diseases*, **14**, 1213–28.

Mascelli, M. A., Frederick, B., Ely, T., Neblock, D. S., Shealy, D. J., Pak, K. Y. & Daddona, P. E. (1993). Reactivity of the human antiendotoxin immunoglobulin M monoclonal antibody HA-1A with lipopolysaccharides from rough and smooth Gram-negative organisms. *Infection and Immunity*, **61**, 1756–63.

McCabe, W. R., Kajser, B., Olling, S., Uwaydah, M. & Hanson L. Å. (1978). *Escherichia coli* in bacteremia: K and O antigens and serum sensitivity of strains from adults and neonates. *Journal of Infectious Diseases*, **138**, 33–41.

Morrison, D. C. (1990). Diversity of mammalian macromolecules which bind to bacterial lipopolysaccharides. In *Endotoxin Research Series*, vol. I. *Cellular and Molecular Aspects of Endotoxin Reaction*, eds. A. Nowotny, J. N. Spitzer & E. J. Ziegler, pp. 183–9. Amsterdam: Elsevier Press.

Nakano, M. & Shinomiya, H. (1990). Molecular mechanisms of macrophage activation by LPS. In *Endotoxin Research Series*, vol. I, *Cellular and*

Molecular Aspects of Endotoxin Reaction, ed. A. Nowotny, J. N. Spitzer & E. J. Ziegler, pp. 205–14. Amsterdam: Elsevier Press.

Nikaido, H. (1992). Porins and specific channels of bacterial outer membranes. *Molelcular Microbiology*, **6**, 435–442.

O'Brien, A. D., Rosenstreich, D. L., Scher, I., Campbell, G. H., MacDermott, R. P. & Formal, S. B. (1979). Genetic control of susceptibility to *Salmonella typhimurium* infection in mice: role of the *Lps* gene. *Journal of Immunology*, **124**, 20–4.

Ørskov, I. & Ørskov, F. (1977) Special O:K:H: serotypes among enterotoxigenic *E. coli* strains from diarrhea in adults and children. Occurrence of the CF (colonization factor) antigen and of hemagglutinating abilities. *Medical Microbiology and Immunology*, **163**, 99–110.

Ørskov, I., Ørskov, F., Birch-Andersen, A., Kanamori, M., & Svanborg-Eden, C. (1982) O, K, H and Fimbrial antigens in *Escherichia coli* serotypes associated with pyelonephritis and cystitis. *Scandinavian Journal of Infectious Disease*, *Supplement*, **33**, 18–25.

Ørskov, I., Ørskov, F., Jann, B. & Jann, K. (1977). Serology, chemistry, and genetics of O and K antigens of *Escherichia coli*. *Bacteriological Reviews*, **41**, 667–710.

Ørskov, I., Ørskov, F. & Rowe, B. (1984). Six new *E. coli* O groups: O165, O166, O167, O169 and O170. *Acta Pathologica Microbiologica Sandinavica*, Section B, **92**, 189–93.

Parrillo, J. E., Parker, M. M., Natanson, C., Suffredini, A. E., Danner, R. L., Cunnion, R. E. & Ognibene, F. P. (1990), Septic shock in humans. Advances in understanding of pathogenesis, cardiovascular dysfunction, and therapy. *Annals of Internal Medicine*, **113**, 227–42.

Peterson, A. A. & McGroarty, E. J. (1986). Physical properties of short-chain and long-chain fractions of lipopolysaccharide. In *Immunobiology and Immunopharmacology of Bacterial Endotoxins*, eds. A. Szentivanyi, H. Friedman & A. Nowotny, pp. 83–7. New York: Plenum Press.

Piguet, P. F., Vesin, C., Ryser, J. E., Senaldi, G., Grau, G. E. & Tacchini-Cottier, F. (1993). An effector role for platelets in systemic and local lipopolysaccharide-induced toxicity in mice, mediated a CD11a- and CD54-dependent interaction with endothelium. *Infection and Immunity*, **61**, 4182–7.

Pollack, M. (1992). Specificity and function of lipopolysaccharide antibodies. In *Bacterial Endotoxic Lipopolysaccharides*, vol II, *Immunopharmacology and Pathophysiology*, eds. J. L. Ryan & D. C. Morrison, pp 347–74. Boca Raton, FL: CRC Press.

Porat, R., Johns, M. A. & McCabe, W. R. (1987). Selective pressure and lipopolysaccharide subunits as determinants of resistance of clinical isolates of Gram-negative bacilli to human serum. *Infection and Immunity*, **55**, 320–8.

Porat, R., Mosseri, R., Kaplan, E., Johns, M. A. & Shibolet, S. (1992). Distribution of polysaccharide side chains of lipopolysaccharide determine resistance of *Escherichia coli* to the bactericidal activity of serum. *Journal of Infectious Diseases*, **165**, 953–6.

Raetz, C. R. H. (1991). Biochemistry of endotoxins. *Annual Review of Biochemistry*, **59**, 129–70.

Raetz, C. R. H. (1993). The enzymatic synthesis of lipid A. In *Bacterial Endotoxin: Recognition and Effector Mechanisms*, eds. J. Levin, C. R. Alving, R. S. Munford & P. L. Stütz, pp. 39–48. Amsterdam: Elsevier Science Publishers.

Rick, P. D. (1987). Lipopolysaccharide biosynthesis. In Escherichia coli *and* Salmonella typhimurium: *Cellular Molecular Biology*, vol 1, eds. F. C. Neidhardt, J. L. Ingraham, K. B. Low, B. Magasanik, M. Schaechter & H. E. Umbarger, pp. 648–62. Washington, D.C.: American Society for Microbiology Press.

Rietschel, E. T., Brade, L., Holst, O., Kulshin, V. A., Lindner, B., Moran, A. P., Schade, U. F., Zähringer, U. & Brade, H. (1990). Molecular structure of bacterial endotoxin in relation to bioactivity. In *Endotoxin Research Series*, vol I, *Cellular and Molecular Aspects of Endotoxin Reaction*, eds. A. Nowotny, J. N. Spitzer & E. J. Ziegler, pp. 15–32. Amsterdam: Elsevier Science Publishers.

Rietschel, E. T., Brade, L., Lindner, B. & Zähringer, U. (1992). Biochemistry of lipopolysaccharides. In *Bacterial Endotoxic Lipopolysaccharides, vol. I, Molecular Biochemistry and Cellular Biology*, eds. J. L. Ryan & D. C. Morrison, pp. 3–41. Boca Raton, FL: CRC Press.

Robert, A. P., Linton, J. D., Waterman, A. M., Gower, P. E. & Koutsaimanes, K. G. (1975). Urinary and faecal Escherichia coli O-sergogroups in symptomatic urinary-tract infection and asymptomatic bacteriuria. *Journal of Medical Microbiology*, **8**, 311–18.

Roberts, J. A., Kaack, M. B., Baskin, G. & Svenson, S. B. (1993). Prevention of renal scarring from pyelonephritis in nonhuman primates by vaccination with a synthetic Escherichia coli serotype O8 oligosaccharide-protein conjugate. *Infection and Immunity*, **61**, 5214–18.

Schiff, D. E., Wass, C. A., Cryz, S. J. Jr., Cross, A. S. & Kim, K. S. (1993). Estimation of protective levels of anti-O specific lipopolysaccharide immunoglobulin G antibody against experimental Escherichia coli infection. *Infection and Immunity*, **61**, 975–90.

Schnaitman, C. A. & Klena, J. D. (1993). Genetics of lipopolysaccharide biosynthesis in enteric bacteria. *Microbiological Reviews*, **57**, 655–82.

Schröder, G., Brandenburg, K., Brade, L. & Seydel, U. (1990). Pore formation by complement in the outer membrane of Gram-negative bacteria studied with asymmetric planar lipopolysaccharide/phospholipid bilayers. *Journal of Membrane Biology*, **118**, 161–70.

Schumann, R. R., Leong S. R., Flaggs, G. W., Gray, P. W., Wright, S. D., Mathison, J. C., Tobias, P. S. & Ulevitch, R. J. (1990). Structure and function of lipopolysaccharide binding protein. *Science*, **249**, 1429–31.

Scott, R. W., Wilde, C. G., Lane, J. C., Snable, J. L. & Marra, M. M. (1993). Antimicrobial and antiendotoxin activities of bactericidal/permeability-increasing protein *in vitro* and *in vivo*. In *Bacterial Endotoxin: Recognition and Effector Mechanisms*, eds. J. Levin, C. R. Alving, R. S. Munford & P. L. Stütz, pp. 373–8. Amsterdam: Elsevier Press.

Sen, K. & Nikaido, H. (1991). Lipopolysaccharide structure required for in vitro trimerization of Escherichia coli OmpF porin. *Journal of Bacteriology*, **173**, 926–8.

Seydel, U. & Brandenburg, K. (1992). Supramolecular structure of lipopoly-saccharides and lipid A. In *Bacterial Endotoxic Lipopolysaccharides, vol. I, Molecular Biochemistry and Cellular Biology*, eds. J. L. Ryan & D. C. Morrison, pp. 225–50. Boca Raton, FL: CRC Press.

Seydel, U., Labischinski, H., Kastowsky, M. & Brandenburg, K. (1993). Phase behavior, supramolecular structure, and molecular conformation of lipopolysaccharide. *Immunobiology*, **187**, 191–211.

Shenep, J. L. (1992). Septic shock. In *Infections in Immunocompromised*

Infants and Children, ed. C. R. Patrick, pp 277–87. New York: Churchill Livingstone.

Shiniji, H., Akagawa, K. S. & Yoshida, T. (1993). Cytochalasin D inhibits lipopolysaccharide-induced tumor necrosis factor production in macrophages. *Journal of Leukocyte Biology*, **54**, 336–42.

Sibley, C. H. (1993). Introduction to the 70Z/3 model system. In *Bacterial Endotoxin: Recognition and Effector Mechanisms*, eds. J. Levin, C. R. Alving, R. S. Munford & P. L. Stütz, pp. 211–20. Amsterdam: Elsevier Science Publishers.

Silva, A. T., Appelmelk, B. J., Buurman, W. A., Bayston, K. F. & Cohen, J. (1990). Monoclonal antibody to endotoxin core protects mice from *Escherichia coli* sepsis by a mechanism independent of tumor necrosis factor and interleukin-6. *Journal of Infectious Diseases*, **162**, 454–9.

Svanborg-Eden, C. & Hagberg, L. (1985). Urinary white cell excretion related to LPS responsiveness. In *Genetic Control of Host Resistance to Infection and Malignancy*, ed. E. Skamene, pp. 393–8. New York: Alan R. Liss.

Svanborg-Eden, C., Hagberg, L., Hull, R., Hull, S., Magnusson, K.-E. & Öhman, L. (1987). Bacterial virulence host resistance in the urinary tracts of mice. *Infection and Immunity*, **55**, 1224–32.

Svanborg-Eden, C., Shahin, R. & Briles, D. (1988). Host resistance to mucjosal Gram-negative infection. Susceptibility of lipopolysaccharide nonresponder mice. *Journal of Immunology*, **140**, 3180–5.

Taylor, P. W. (1985). Measurement of the bactericidal activity of serum. In *The Virulence of* Escherichia coli, ed. M. Sussman, pp. 445–56. London: Academic Press.

Tobias, P. S., Mathison, J. C., Lee, J. D., Kravchenko, V., Mintz, D., Pugin, J., Han, J., Gegner, J. & Ulevitch, R. F. (1993). LPS binding protein, LPS and CD14 mediated activation of myeloid cells. In *Bacterial Endotoxin: Recognition and Effector Mechanisms*, eds. J. Levin, C. R. Alving, R. S. Munford & P. L. Stütz, pp 135–7. Amsterdam: Elsevier Press.

van Deventer, S. J. H., ten Cate, H., van der Poll, T., Levi, M. & ten Cate, J. W. (1993). Endotoxin-induced coagulation activation: pathogenic role in Gram-negative sepsis and novel intervention strategies. In *Bacterial Endotoxin: Recognition and Effector Mechanisms*, eds. J. Levin, C. R. Alving, R. S. Munford & P. L. Stütz, pp. 305–12. Amsterdam: Elsevier Press.

Vukajilovich, S. W. (1992). Interactions of LPS with serum complement. In *Bacterial Endotoxic Lipopolysaccharides*, vol. II, *Immunopharmacology and Pathophysiology*, ed. J. L. Ryan & D. C. Morrison, pp. 213–35. Boca Raton, FL: CRC Press.

Weiss, J., Elsbach, P., Gazzano-Santoro, H., Parent, J. B., Grinna, L., Horwitz, A. & Theofan, G. (1993). Bactericidal and endotoxin-neutralizing activities of the bactericidal/permeability-increasing protein and its bioactive N-terminal fragment. In *Bacterial Endotoxin: Recognition and Effector Mechanisms*, eds. J. Levin, C. R. Alving, R. S. Munford & P. L. Stütz, pp. 103–11. Amsterdam: Elsevier Press.

Winn, R. K., Thomas, J. R. & Harlan, J. M. (1993). Phagocyte CD11/CD18 adhesion in septic and endotoxic shock. In *Bacterial Endotoxin: Recognition and Effector Mechanisms*, eds. J. Levin, C. R. Alving, R. S. Munford & P. L. Stütz, pp. 463–72. Amsterdam: Elsevier Press.

Witthaut, R., Farhood, A., Smith, C. W. & Jaeschke, H. (1993). Complement and tumor necrosis factor-α contribute to Mac-1 (CD11b/CD18) up-regulation and systemic neutrophil activation during endotoxemia *in vivo*. *Journal of Leukocyte Biology*, **55**, 105–11.

Wolff, S. M. (1991). Monoclonal antibodies and the treatment of Gram-negative bacteremia and shock. *New England Journal of Medicine*, **324**, 486–8.

Wright, S. D., Ramos, R. A., Hermanowski-Vosatka, A., Rockwell, P. & Detmers, P. A. (1991). Activation of the adhesive capacity of CR3 on neutrophils by endotoxin: dependence on lipopolysaccharide binding protein and CD14. *Journal of Experimental Medicine*, **173**, 1281–6.

Wright, S. D., Ramos, R. A., Tobias, P. S., Ulevitch, R. J. & Mathison, J. C. (1990). CD14, a receptor for complexes of lipopolysaccharide (LPS) and LPS binding protein. *Science*, **249**, 1431–3.

Young, L. S., Proctor, R. A., Beutler, B., McCabe, W. R. & Sheagren, J. N. (1991). University of California/Davis interdepartmental conference on Gram-negative septicemia. *Reviews of Infectious Diseases*, **13**, 666–87.

Ziegler, E. J., Fisher, C. J. Jr., Sprung, C. L., Straube, R., Sadoff, J. C., Foulke, G. E., Wortel, C., Fink, M. P., Dellinger, P., Teng, N. N. H., Allen, I. E., Berger, H. J., Knatterud, G. L., LoBuglio, A. F., Smith, C. R. & the HA-1A Sepsis Study Group. (1991). Treatment of Gram-negative bacteremia and septic shock with HA-1A human monoclonal antibody against endotoxin. A randomized, double-blind, placebo-controlled trial. *New England Journal of Medicine*, **324**, 429–36.

6

Type-1 fimbriae of *Escherichia coli*

S. N. ABRAHAM and S. JAISWAL

The type-1 fimbriae of *Escherichia coli*, otherwise known as common fimbriae, are hair-like structures characterised by their ability to bind to D-mannose-containing residues on various surfaces. They were the first bacterial fimbriae to be described (Duguid *et al.*, 1955; Brinton, 1959; Duguid, 1959) and, since then, have become the most widely studied fimbrial structure. Much of this fascination stems from their ability to promote bacterial binding to a wide variety of cells, which is the direct result of their affinity for D-mannose, one of the most ubiquitous sugars on eukaryotic cell surfaces. The ability of type-1 fimbriae to recognise and bind to various human and animal mucosal and inflammatory cells is essential to initiate and sustain bacterial infections in humans and animals.

Genetic organisation

Several genes that reside in a cluster that maps at 98 minutes in the chromosome are involved in the biosynthesis, expression and function of the heteropolymeric type-1 fimbriae of *E. coli* (Bachman, 1983; Freitag & Eisenstein, 1983). The entire gene cluster, which spans 9.5 kbp, was first cloned by Hull *et al.* (1981) and the functions of the various genes were subsequently determined by the mutational inactivation of each gene in turn and examination of the effect on fimbrial expression or function. A genetic and physical map of the type-1 fimbrial gene cluster and the postulated functions of the various gene products are shown in Figure 6.1.

At least four genes encode the subunits that constitute the fimbrial filament. The *fimA* gene encodes the bulk of the filament, and its inactivation results in the loss of fimbriae as determined by traditional electron microscopy (Orndorff & Falkow, 1984; Klemm *et al.*, 1985). Recent

169

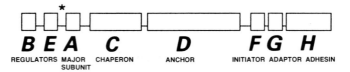

Fig. 6.1. Organisation of genes within the type-1-fimbrial gene cluster. The established and postulated functions of the various gene products are indicated. The asterisk indicates the site of the invertible phase-switch.

studies with high-resolution quick-freeze, deep-etch electron microscopy have, however, revealed that $fimA^-$ mutants express short fibrillar surface structures that comprise the products of at least two genes, $fimH$ and $fimG$, located at the distal end of the fim gene cluster (Jones et al., 1995). The inactivation of $fimH$ results in fimbriae that have lost their capacity to mediate mannose-specific binding and they, therefore, encode the mannose-binding fimbrial 'lectin' (Maurer & Orndorff, 1985; Minion et al., 1986). Though $fimG$ is co-transcribed with $fimH$, and its gene product is closely associated with the FimH protein in the fimbrial structure, its exact function is not clear. It has been suggested that the $fimG$ gene product serves as an adapter that holds FimH in a functionally competent conformation on the fimbriae (Abraham et al., 1987; Klemm & Christiansen, 1987). Evidence that supports this notion comes from the observation that inactivation of $fimG$ reduces the binding of the fimbriae (Klemm & Christiansen, 1987). The $fimF$ gene encodes a protein believed to be another minor subunit of the fimbriae, but evidence for its presence on the fimbrial filament is lacking. It is suggested that FimF plays a role in regulating the length of the fimbriae, because inactivation of $fimF$ results in the formation of extraordinarily long fimbrial filaments (Klemm & Christiansen, 1987; Maurer & Orndorff, 1987; Russell & Orndorff, 1992).

The remaining genes in the cluster encode for proteins involved in the translocation and assembly of fimbrial subunits and the regulation of fimbrial expression. The products of two genes, $fimC$ and $fimD$, play a crucial role in translocation and/or assembly of the fimbriae. Genetic inactivation of either of these genes abolishes fimbrial assembly as determined by electron microscopy (Orndorff & Falkow, 1984; Klemm et al., 1985). The $fimC$ gene encodes a 26-kDa protein located in the bacterial periplasm and its inactivation results in rapid proteolytic degradation of the major and minor fimbrial subunits in the periplasmic space (Jones et al., 1993; Tewari et al., 1993). FimC is a chaperon protein that is believed to attach to newly synthesised subunits as they enter the periplasm from the inner membrane. The functions of FimC are believed to include protection of fimbrial subunits from periplasmic enzymes, maintenance of the nascent proteins in a form competent for assembly and translocation of the subunits to points of assembly at the bacterial outer membrane (Hultgren *et al.*, 1991, 1993). Inactivation of *fimD* also abolishes fimbrial expression (Orndorff & Falkow, 1984; Klemm *et al.*, 1985). The *fimD* gene product is a large 88-kDa outer-membrane protein that forms the base on which the fimbrial filaments are assembled (Klemm & Christiansen, 1990).

Two regulatory genes, *fimB*and *fimE*, situated proximal to *fimA* encode histone-like proteins (Klemm, 1986; Pallesen *et al.*, 1989) that direct the phase-dependent expression of the *fimA* gene, which determines whether or not fimbriae are expressed on the bacterial surface. The mechanisms of phase variation involve the inversion of a 314-base-pair DNA segment that harbours the promoter for the *fimA* gene (Abraham, J. M. *et al.*, 1985; Freitag *et al.*, 1985). Thus, *fimA* is expressed in one orientation (on) but not the other (off). The switching phenomenon is a *RecA*-independent process and requires the function of FimB to direct the switch from on-to-off or from off-to-on (Klemm, 1986; McClain *et al.*, 1991). Unlike FimB, FimE mediates the switch in only one direction, from on-to-off (Blomfield *et al.*, 1991, 1993). In addition to the modulatory effects of FimB and FimE, the phase switch is also affected by at least three global regulators, leucine-responsive regulatory protein (Lrp), integration host-factor (IHF), and the histone-like protein (H-NS) (Dorman & Higgins, 1987; Eisenstein *et al.*, 1987; Blomfield *et al.*, 1991, 1993; Gally *et al.*, 1993).

The structure of type-1 fimbriae

A typically fimbriate strain of *E. coli* expresses some 100–300 peritrichous fimbrial filaments, each about 7 nm wide and 0.2–2 μm long. A single filament consists of a quaternary assembly of several thousand copies of the 17-kDa FimA subunit. X-ray crystallography has revealed that the subunits are arranged in a simple, tight right-handed helix with a central axial hole (Brinton, 1965) and it was predicted that each turn of the helix would consist of 3.14 FimA subunits and that the helical pitch distance would be 2.32 nm. Since these studies were undertaken long before the presence of minor subunits in the fimbriae was known, the predictions do not take account of their presence.

Valuable information about the molecular arrangement of FimA subunits, and the conditions that affect their polymerisation, can be obtained by complete dissociation of the filament into monomeric subunits and determining whether and how reconstitution can take place *in vitro*. The quaternary structure of type-1 fimbriae is extremely stable and, with the exception of guanidine hydrochloride, is resistant to all common dissociating agents (Brinton, 1965). Saturated guanidine hydrochloride completely dissociates type-1 fimbriae and removal of the denaturant results in their reconstitution (Brinton, 1965; Eshdat *et al.*, 1981). Though such reconstituted fimbriae are of the same thickness, they are shorter than native fimbriae (Eshdat *et al.*, 1981; Abraham *et al.*, 1983b). It was possible to monitor the dissociation and reassociation of type-1 fimbriae with a panel of monoclonal antibodies directed against conformation-specific epitopes (Abraham *et al.*, 1983b).

Depolymerisation of fimbrial filaments results in the elimination of several quaternary epitopes and the exposure of several previously buried epitopes on FimA. However, when probed with a panel of monoclonal antibodies, reconstituted fimbriae show the same level of reactivity as the native fimbriae. Furthermore, monoclonal antibodies specific for quaternary structural epitopes display the same periodicity and spiral pattern of binding to reconstituted fimbriae as with native fimbriae, which indicates that the highly ordered subunit packing in the native fimbriae is restored when fimbriae are reconstituted *in vitro* (Abraham *et al.*, 1983b). Though a systematic study was not undertaken, pH, temperature and ionic conditions were found to be critical factors in determining the rate of fimbrial repolymerisation *in vitro* (Eshdat *et al.*, 1981; Abraham *et al.*, 1983b). These reconstitution studies also highlighted the requirement for divalent cations in the polymerisation of type-1 fimbriae; magnesium ions greatly enhance assembly, while EDTA is inhibitory. It is also interesting to note that repolymerisation of fimbrial subunits *in vitro* does not require ATP.

Another approach to the study of the structural arrangement of FimA in the type-1 fimbrial filament was developed by the selective disruption of the hydrophobic and hydrogen bonds that stabilise the helical conformation of the fimbrial polymer. Exposure of type-1 fimbriae to 50 per cent glycerol for four hours at 37°C results in partial and, in some cases, complete disruption of the quaternary fimbrial structure, by selectively unravelling the helices without significant depolymerisation. Electron microscopy study of the linearised fimbrial polymer, rotary shadowed with platinum and carbon, reveals a configuration approximately one-third of the thickness of the native fimbrial filament. Unlike the fully assembled fimbriae, the linearised polymers are highly sensitive to trypsin digestion, which suggests that the quaternary conformation of fimbrial subunits may serve a protective function against proteolytic enzymes (Abraham *et al.*, 1992). This may be relevant to the persistence of *E. coli* in the gastro-intestinal tract, which is replete with digestive enzymes. It should also be noted that the glycerol-induced linearisation of the fimbrial filament lends itself to the mapping of antigenic epitopes that are usually buried in the native structure.

The revelations that the type-1 fimbrial filament is a hetero- and not a homopolymer and that the mannose-binding function does not reside within FimA came 30 years after the seminal studies by Brinton (1965) of the biochemical and physical properties of type-1 fimbriae. Maurer & Orndorff (1985) and Minion *et al.* (1986) showed independently that the inactivation of a gene (*fimH*) at the distal end of the *E. coli fim* locus resulted in fimbriae that had lost their capacity to agglutinate guinea-pig erythrocytes. Careful examination of wild-type and mutant fimbriae failed to reveal any physical or antigenic differences between the two fimbriae indicating that the deleted gene encoded a very minor subunit (Minion *et al.*, 1986). Direct confirmation of the presence of FimH and FimG subunits within the fimbrial structure came from the use of antibody probes directed at synthetic peptides that corresponded to partial peptides of these molecules. Western blot analysis of isolated type-1 fimbriae with antibodies directed against FimH and FimG revealed the presence of proteins of 29 kDa and 14 kDa, respectively (Abraham *et al.*, 1987). These proteins were subsequently purified from isolated type-1 fimbriae (Hansen & Brinton, 1988). Immunoelectron microscopy of fimbriae with antibodies directed against FimH revealed that this subunit was located at the distal tip of the fimbrial filament and intercalated along its length (Abraham *et al.*, 1987, 1988a,b). This spatial arrangement has been confirmed by others (Krogfelt *et al.*, 1990; Chanteloup *et al.*, 1991). It is interesting that certain avian *E. coli* strains have been found to express FimH exclusively at the fimbrial tip (Chanteloup *et al.*, 1991). Attempts to localise FimF and FimG on the fimbrial filament by immunoelectron microscopy have so far been unsuccessful.

A linearised fibrillum-like structure reminiscent of the unique fibrillar structure of P-fimbriae of pyelonephritogenic *E. coli* (Hultgren *et al.*, 1993; see Chapter 8) has been described at the distal tip of the type-1 fimbrial filament of *E. coli*. Unlike the P fibrillar structure, however, the tip configuration of type-1 fimbriae resembled a 'short knob'. Similar structures have also been observed on the type-1 fimbriae of at least three other species of enterobacteria. Immunochemical analysis of these structures indicates that they consist of equal amounts of FimH and FimG (Jones *et al.*, 1995). Further studies are necessary to determine whether these tip structures are present within the fimbrial structure, possibly in a more compressed configuration.

The D-mannose-binding moiety of type-1 fimbriae

Deletion or inactivation of the *fimH* gene in the type-1 fimbrial gene cluster results in loss of fimbrial binding activity (Maurer & Orndorff, 1985; Minion *et al.*, 1986) and antibodies against FimH, but not those against other fimbrial subunits, block fimbrial binding activity (Abraham *et al.*, 1987, 1988a,b). This is compelling evidence to suggest that FimH is the fimbrial moiety that mediates the binding reactions of type-1 fimbriae. Definitive proof of this role can, however, be provided only by the demonstration that FimH, separated from other fimbrial components, mimics the binding activity of intact type-1 fimbriae. The great stability of the type-1 fimbriae and the relatively small amount of FimH present within the filament make it technically difficult to obtain FimH protein from isolated type-1 fimbriae. A novel strategy to obtain FimH has been presented in which *fimH* is cloned and nascent molecules of the incorporated gene product are isolated from the host bacterial periplasm (Tewari *et al.*, 1993). The *fimH* gene was placed behind an inducible promoter in a high-copy plasmid and hyperexpression of FimH was induced by addition of the inducer. The gene product was, however, unstable and partially degraded by the periplasmic proteolytic enzymes.

To stabilise the *fimH* gene product in the periplasm, it was necessary to co-express *fimC*, the chaperon gene of the type-1 fimbrial gene cluster. In this way it was possible to isolate relatively large amounts of the FimH–FimC complex from the host bacterial periplasm. A homogeneous preparation of FimH was obtained by dissociation of the FimH–FimC complex, followed by affinity chromatography of the FimH fraction on a D-mannose affinity column (Tewari *et al.*, 1993). The binding activity of FimH and its specificity for mannose were confirmed by the demonstration that, when immobilised on nitrocellulose strips or inert microspheres, the purified protein mimicked the mannose-inhibitable binding of type-1-fimbriate *E. coli* to inflammatory cells (Tewari *et al.*, 1993; Malaviya *et al.*, 1994a). Moreover, the immobilised FimH protein bound and activated these inflammatory cells to the same extent as type-1-fimbriate *E. coli* (Malaviya *et al.*, 1994b).

Proteins that correspond in size and antigenic properties to *E. coli* FimH have been detected in type-1 fimbriae expressed by other Entero-bacteriaceae (Abraham *et al.*, 1988b; Gerlach & Clegg, 1988). These FimH proteins, like that of *E. coli*, have the same distribution in the filament and appear to be responsible for mannose-inhibitable binding reactions of the fimbriae (Abraham *et al.*, 1988a,b). In spite of the conservation of the structure and function of FimH among the various enterobacteria, there appear to be subtle but distinct differences in the binding specificity of type-1 fimbriae from various species. These are best illustrated by examination of the inhibitory effect of structurally defined mannoglycosides on the binding activity of the various type-1 fimbriae. For example, aromatic α-mannosides and the trisaccharides Man-α3-Man-β4-GlcNAc were weak inhibitors of yeast aggregation by type-1-fimbriate strains of *Salmonella typhimurium* (Firon *et al.*, 1983, 1987). These mannosides were, nevertheless, strong inhibitors of the yeast aggregation by fimbriate strains of *E. coli* and *Klebsiella pneumoniae*. This suggests that there are distinct differences in the type-1 fimbrial mannose-combining sites of *Salmonella* and *E. coli*. On the basis of the potent inhibitory activity of a panel of aromatic mannoglycosides, it was predicted that the shape of the mannose-combining site is in the form of a pocket that corresponds with the size of a trisaccharide and that it is adjacent to a hydrophobic region. By way of contrast, the poor inhibitory activity of the same panel of aromatic compounds on the yeast-aggregating activity of *S. typhimurium* led to the prediction that the putative binding pocket in the type-1 fimbriae of *S. typhimurium* is markedly smaller and devoid of an adjacent hydrophobic region (Firon *et al.*, 1983, 1984, 1987). Since the short oligomannose chains or hybrid units of the glycoproteins on animal cells are preferentially recognised by type-1 fimbriae (Firon *et al.*, 1982, 1985), it is probable that the hetero-geneity in fine-sugar-binding specificity observed amongst the type-1 fimbriae of different Enterobacteriaceae may be responsible for the different haemagglutination patterns of these fimbriae when tested against a panel of animal erythrocytes (Duguid & Old, 1980).

The binding characteristics of the type-1 fimbriae of *E. coli* and *K. pneumoniae* have been compared, to understand better the structural basis of the inter-species differences in sugar binding specificity (Madison *et al.*, 1994). The fimbriae of these species were selected because details of the structural and genetic organisation of their respective gene clusters were known and recombinant clones that express *E. coli* and *K. pneumoniae* type-1 fimbriae and their genetic variants were available (Clegg *et al.*, 1985, 1987; Klemm & Christiansen, 1987; Maurer & Orndorff, 1987; Gerlach & Clegg, 1988; Gerlach *et al.*, 1988). It was possible to discriminate between the sugar binding specificities of *E. coli* and *K. pneumoniae* fimbriae by means of two aromatic mannoglycosides, *p*-nitrophenyl-α-mannoside (*p*-NPαMan) and 4-methylumbelliferyl-α-mannoside (MeUmbαMan) (Madison *et al.*, 1994). The relative inhibitory activity of *p*-NPαMan on *E. coli* and *K. pneumoniae* type-1 fimbriae was 70 and 14 respectively, indicating a fivefold difference in inhibitor affinity for the two fimbriae. An even greater, i.e. 11-fold, difference in affinity between *E. coli* and *K. pneumoniae* fimbriae was observed for MeUmbaMan. Taken together, these findings suggest that *E. coli* and *K. pneumoniae* fimbriae have different sugar-binding specificities.

The molecular mechanisms that underlie these differences have been elucidated by transcomplementation studies. Recombinants were created that express two types of hybrid fimbriae, one consisting of *E. coli* FimH carried on a filament of *K. pneumoniae* FimA subunits and the other of *K. pneumoniae* FimH carried on a filament of *E. coli* FimA subunits. When the binding specificities of these hybrid fimbriae for MeUmbαMan and *p*-NPαMan were determined, the former had a specificity different from that of native *K. pneumoniae* fimbriae but very similar to that of native *E. coli* fimbriae. Conversely, the binding specificity of the latter was different from that of native *E. coli* fimbriae, but similar to that of native *K. pneumoniae* fimbriae. These findings were unexpected, because they suggested that cross-transposition of FimH, the putative binding moiety, between the two fimbriae did not result in a corresponding cross-transposition of sugar-binding specificities. Furthermore, the characteristic binding specificity of each species appeared to be linked with the fimbrial filament. When each of the FimH⁻ fimbrial filaments was tested for its capacity to agglutinate yeast cells, no activity was detected with either fimbrial filament, confirming that the fimbrial filament has no intrinsic binding activity (Madison *et al.*, 1994).

A possible explanation for these findings is that the fimbrial shaft can indirectly affect the adhesin moiety by altering the conformation or presentation of the heterologous FimH molecule. Since the FimA subunits of *K. pneumoniae* and *E. coli* are distinctly different, each transposed FimH must undergo a conformational alteration to fit the quaternary constraints of the heterologous fimbrial filament. Regions of the heterologous FimH that may be altered include the mannose-binding

site. The notion that the fimbrial filament can affect the binding properties of the adhesin moiety by modulating its configuration is intriguing
and suggests that, in spite of the conservation in FimH, type-1 fimbriae of
various enterobacteria display different binding specificities as a result of
the heterogeneity in their FimA subunits. Since subtle structural and
antigenic heterogeneity in FimA subunits are known to exist in type-1
fimbriae, and even among strains of *E. coli*, intraspecies heterogeneity in
sugar-binding specificity may also exist. This could be an effective
mechanism evolved by *E. coli* to bind to alternate receptors in order to
increase its host range.

In addition to regulating the sugar-binding specificities of the FimH
subunit, the fimbrial filament may play a role in determining its binding
affinity for mannoglycosides. Scatchard analysis of data obtained from
the binding of isolated *E. coli* type-1 fimbriae to the mannose-containing
enzyme horseradish peroxidase has revealed that type-1 fimbriae have
two populations of sites with different binding affinities, one with low
affinity (K_a 0.8×10^6 M^{-1} to 3.8×10^6 M^{-1}) and the other high affinity (K_a
0.5×10^8 M^{-1} to 2.0×10^8 M^{-1}). Fragmentation of isolated fimbriae by
repeated freezing and thawing results in a two- to four-fold increase in the
number of high-affinity sites while the number of low-affinity sites
remains unchanged (Ponniah *et al.*, 1991). One conclusion that can be
drawn from these results is that the type-1-fimbrial filament contains
cryptic high-affinity mannose-binding sites that become exposed on
filament fragmentation. The cryptic high-affinity mannose-binding sites
could be FimH molecules intercalated in the fimbrial filament that
become active mannose-binding moieties when, on filament fragmentation, they acquire a distal tip location. Thus, the mannose-binding sites of
internally located FimH molecules are buried within the fimbrial structure and inactive, and only those located at the fimbrial tips bind
mannosylated glycoproteins. It is conceivable that the low-affinity binding sites are high-affinity sites that have been damaged during fimbrial
purification. Alternatively, they may represent longitudinally placed
FimH, partially exposed to display a low level of binding, but further
work is necessary to clarify the structural basis for the two levels of
binding activity displayed by isolated type-1 fimbriae. Taken together,
these studies confirm that FimH is the mannose-binding determinant of
type-1 fimbriae. However, its receptor-binding specificity and affinity are
strictly regulated by the fimbrial filament on which it is borne.

Role in virulence

Epidemiological studies show that a large proportion of clinical isolates of *E. coli* and other species of Enterobacteriaceae express type-1 fimbriae (Clegg & Gerlach, 1987; Eisenstein, 1990; Johnson, 1991). They are also expressed by innocuous gastro-intestinal commensals and bacteria that colonise various environmental sites. It is this ubiquity that makes it difficult to determine their role in virulence. Nevertheless, the remarkable ability of type-1 fimbriae to mediate avid bacterial binding to mucosal surfaces, non-cellular constituents and various host inflammatory cells is a reliable indication of the importance of these structures as determinants of virulence.

Attachment to mucosal surfaces

Most infections caused by *E. coli* are initiated by the colonisation of the host gastro-intestinal, respiratory or urinary tracts (Eisenstein, 1990; Johnson, 1991). *Escherichia coli* is particularly adept at colonising these mucosal surfaces because of its rapid multiplication and ability to attach avidly to cells that line the mucosae. This rapid multiplication rate compensates for loss of bacteria due to constant flushing by mucosal secretions and the exfoliation of epithelial cells laden with adherent bacteria (Freter, 1980; Baddour *et al.*, 1990), and helps to sustain a critical population on the mucosal surface. With a few notable exceptions (McCormick *et al.*, 1989; May *et al.*, 1993), the importance of type-1 fimbriae in facilitating colonisation and infection of mucosal surfaces by *E. coli* and other type-1-fimbriate enterobacteria has been convincingly demonstrated.

When the infectivity of type-1-fimbriate and non-fimbriate phenotypes is compared, the infectivity of the fimbriate organisms is always significantly greater. This has been shown for *E. coli* urinary tract infection (Iwahi *et al.*, 1983; Hultgren, *et al.*, 1985), *K. pneumoniae* urinary tract infection of rats (Fader & Davis, 1982) and *S. typhimurium* gastro-intestinal infection of mice (Duguid *et al.*, 1976). In addition, the specific receptor analogues D-mannose or methyl α-mannoside, but not glucose or methyl α-glucoside, have been shown to inhibit experimental infection and mucosal colonisation by various type-1-fimbriate bacteria (Aronson *et al.*, 1979; Goldhar *et al.*, 1986). Polyclonal and monoclonal antibodies specific for type-1 fimbriae block infection of mouse mucosal surfaces by type-1-fimbriate *E. coli*. D-Mannose-specific monoclonal antibodies directed specifically at the mannosylated receptors on mucosal surfaces also prevent infection by such organisms (Abraham *et al.*, 1985).

Though type-1 fimbriae clearly enable *E. coli* to resist hydrokinetic forces at the mucosal surface, it has been suggested that the close association of bacteria with host cells also preferentially facilitates bacterial growth by enabling the bacteria to take up growth-promoting substances secreted by the host cells. A distinct growth advantage for type-1-fimbriate bacteria in the presence of host cells as compared with non-fimbriate mutants was observed by Zafriri *et al.* (1987). The cytokine interleukin-1 (IL-1), a secreted host cell product, appears significantly to enhance the growth of pathogenic but not non-pathogenic strains of *E. coli* (Porat *et al.*, 1991), but its mode of action remains unknown. The notion that, in mice, type-1 fimbriae confer a growth advantage on bacteria is also supported by observations *in vivo* (Tanaka, 1982; Alkan *et al.*, 1986).

Attachment to non-cellular host constituents

Escherichia coli type-1 fimbriae bind to various non-cellular body constituents, including soluble glycoproteins in body fluids and extracellular matrix proteins. Although most of the binding interactions mediated by type-1 fimbriae appear to be with mannose residues, some may be carbohydrate independent.

Type-1-fimbriate *E. coli* attach to a number of highly mannosylated glycoproteins in body fluids. Such glycoconjugates may attach to and aggregate bacteria, so facilitating their early removal from the host, or they may adsorb to mucosal surfaces and provide an additional matrix for bacterial colonisation. It is, at present, difficult to predict whether these glycoproteins promote or hinder bacterial colonisation but it seems likely that the concentration and physical state of glycoproteins in body fluids are critical determinants of bacterial behaviour. One of the best characterised glycoproteins is Tamm–Horsfall glycoprotein, which is replete with N-linked oligomannose residues and a prominent component of human urine. It binds and aggregates type-1-fimbriate *E. coli* (Ørskov *et al.*, 1980; Chick *et al.*, 1981). It is interesting that type-1-fimbriate *E. coli*, coated with Tamm–Horsfall glycoprotein, are less susceptible to phagocytosis than untreated organisms (Kuriayama & Silverblatt, 1986), which suggests that the bacteria can utilise this glycoprotein to resist host defence factors. Human saliva contains a 60-kDa glycoprotein with a similar capacity to bind to type-1-fimbriate *E. coli* and to block bacterial attachment to buccal epithelial cells (Babu *et al.*, 1986). This glycocon-jugate may play a critical role in modulating the microbial flora of the oral cavity because, in addition to binding to type-1-fimbriate bacteria, the protein part of the molecule binds and aggregates a number of oral pathogens, including *Streptococcus mutans* (Babu *et al.*, 1986). Lysozyme, a constituent of various body secretions, including tears, saliva and nasal secretions, also binds to *E. coli* type-1 fimbriae (Silverblatt & Cohen, 1979).

Type-1 fimbriae of *E. coli* and *Salmonella enterica* bind to immobilised laminin, an extracellular matrix glycoprotein that contains 13–15 per cent by weight of N-linked carbohydrate, which forms a network in basement membranes, and binding was inhibited by D-mannose, suggesting that it was a lectin-like reaction (Kukkonen *et al.*, 1993). The binding of type-1-fimbriate bacteria to laminin is believed to be important in the bacterial colonisation of locally damaged tissue and in bacterial penetration through basement membranes during the metastasis of infections, but direct supportive evidence is not available.

Most Gram-negative bacteria, including *E. coli*, bind poorly to the extracellular matrix protein fibronectin (Abraham *et al.*, 1983a; Hasty *et al.*, 1990). It has, however, been reported that some strains of type-1-fimbriate *E. coli* bind to immobilised, but not to soluble, fibronectin. They adhered primarily to amino-terminal and gelatin-binding domains of the molecule. Treatment of the adherent fibronectin fractions with periodate or endoglycosidase failed to reduce their ability to bind to bacteria (Sokurenko *et al.*, 1992). Moreover, type-1 fimbriae isolated from these strains bound in a mannose-inhibitable manner to a synthetic peptide that was a copy of a portion of the amino-terminal domain of fibronectin. This suggests that, paradoxically, certain *E. coli* type-1 fimbriae can mediate, in a D-mannose-inhibitable manner, protein–protein binding interactions with non-cellular host constituents.

Attachment to inflammatory cells

Once bacteria have penetrated or circumvented the mucosal barrier, they encounter a variety of host inflammatory cells. The several consequences of the subsequent interactions have a significant impact on the ability of the pathogen to survive and on the severity of the resulting disease (Hoepelman & Tuomanen, 1992). The survival of the bacteria depends on their ability to evade, neutralise or resist the bactericidal activities of neutrophils, macrophages and other inflammatory cells. The interaction of bacteria with these inflammatory cells also triggers the unregulated release of pharmacologically active mediators such as cytokines, proteases and toxic oxygen metabolites, many of which are harmful to the host. Indeed, much of the tissue destruction, fever, pain and swelling that accompany bacterial infection has been ascribed to the toxicity of these inflammatory mediators.

Mast cells are preferentially localised to the portals of entry of bacteria, including the skin, respiratory, gastro-intestinal and urinary tracts (Galli, 1993) and are, therefore, likely to be among the first inflammatory cells encountered by invading *E. coli*. Activated mast cells release an array of inflammatory mediators that have numerous biological effects at the site of infection and elsewhere in the body (Gordon *et al.*, 1990; Galli, 1993).

Type-1-fimbriate, but not non-fimbriate *E. coli* or a FimH⁻ isogenic mutant, recognise and adhere avidly to mouse mast cells and bring about their extensive degranulation. The extent of this degranulation is directly related to the number of adherent organisms. A scanning electron micrograph of a bone marrow-derived mouse mast cell with adherent type-1-fimbriate *E. coli* is shown in Figure 6.2. Degranulation of peritoneal mast cells and the release of histamine *in vivo* has been demonstrated by the injection of type-1-fimbriate *E. coli* into the mouse peritoneum (Malaviya *et al.*, 1994b). Although mast cells are not known

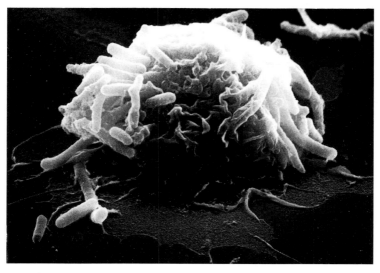

Fig. 6.2. Scanning electron micrograph showing several adherent type-1-fimbriated *Escherichia coli* on teh surface of a mouse mast cell.

to have bactericidal properties, the association of type-1-fimbriate *E. coli* with mouse bone-marrow-derived mast cells triggers phagocytosis and killing by these cells. Examination of thin sections of mast cells after exposure to type-1-fimbriate *E. coli* revealed several bacteria within vacuoles. Mast cells share some bactericidal mechanisms with traditional phagocytes, including acidification of phagocytic vacuoles and the release of superoxide anions (Malaviya *et al.*, 1994a). The secreted chemotactic products of activated mast cells include leukotrienes and tumour necrosis factor-α, which cause a rapid influx of neutrophils to the site of inflammation (Gordon and Galli, 1990).

Neutrophils are the most important host phagocytic cells and one of the first type of cell to migrate to sites of bacterial infection. Type-1 fimbriae promote attachment of *E. coli* to neutrophils resulting in phagocytosis (Goetz & Siverblatt, 1987; Iwahi & Imada, 1988). Though it has been observed that adherent type-1-fimbriate bacteria are ingested and killed by neutrophils and macrophages (Ofek & Sharon, 1990; Gbarah *et al.*, 1993), other observations suggest that such organisms are at least partially resistant to the cidal action of neutrophils (Ohman *et al.*, 1982; Goetz *et al.*, 1987; Lock *et al.*, 1990). Unopsonised *E. coli* bound to neutrophils by type-1 fimbriae are significantly more resistant to killing by neutrophils compared to similar opsonised bacteria (Goetz *et al.*, 1987). It was suggested that the neutrophils released smaller amounts of bactericidal agents in response to unopsonised than opsonised organisms.

The notion that type-1 fimbriae, and particularly FimH, actually impede killing by phagocytic cells was extended by Keith *et al.* (1990), who showed that type-1-fimbriate *E. coli* were some threefold more resistant to killing by mouse macrophages than isogenic FimH⁻ or nonfimbriate bacteria. Whether or not FimH promotes killing by bacteria remains the subject of debate, but it is not in dispute that it causes the release of many pharmacologically active mediators by neutrophils and other activated inflammatory cells. This unregulated release of mediators damages surrounding tissue and is potentially very harmful to the host.

Isolated type-1 fimbriae can also bind avidly to B lymphocytes, trigger T-cell-independent proliferation of these cells and induce the secretion of IgM. This interaction can be attributed to FimH, because mutant FimH deficient fimbriae failed to evoke this response from lymphocytes (Ponniah *et al.*, 1989, 1991, 1992). This 'non-specific' lymphocyte activation may be a mechanism by which bacteria subvert the ability of the host to mount a specific immune response.

Membrane receptors on host cells

Four prospective neutrophil membrane glycoprotein receptors of relative molecular weight (M_r) 70, 80, 100 and 150 have been purified (Rodriguez-Ortega *et al.*, 1987). The two largest of these form a heterodimer, CD11/CD18, that belongs to the integrin receptor superfamily (Gbarah *et al.*, 1992). These integrin molecules bind to type-1 fimbriae by way of oligomannose and hybrid units (Gbarah *et al.*, 1991). The CD11/CD18 heterodimer antigens contain only N-linked oligosaccharides, 38 per cent of which are of the oligomannose type and five per cent are of the hybrid type (Asada *et al.*, 1991).

A well-characterised membrane glycoprotein of granulocytes, macrophages and lung epithelium is non-specific cross-reacting antigen (NCA), a member of the immunoglobulin supergene family. It has been shown that type-1-fimbriate *E. coli* and isolated type-1 fimbriae bind to mannose moieties on some glycoforms of NCA. In addition, on activation with the bacterial peptide formylmethionyl–leucyl–phenylalanine, surface expression of NCA on neutrophils is increased. This is consistent with a role for this molecule in mediating the inflammatory response to bacteria (Sauter *et al.*, 1991). A 65-kDa type-1 fimbrial receptor has been isolated from guinea-pig erythrocytes (Giampapa *et al.*, 1988) but limited structural analysis precludes comparison with other membrane glycoprotein receptors for type-1 fimbriae.

Vaccine prospects

Recognition that adherence is a prerequisite for bacterial infection and the importance of type-1 fimbriae in promoting bacterial adherence have led to the notion that they might be used as vaccines. The underlying rationale is that antibodies evoked against these fimbriae would prevent the attachment of bacteria to the mucosal surface and also serve as opsonins to enhance phagocytosis if tissue invasion takes place (Rene *et al.*, 1982). Thus, rats immunised with type-1 fimbriae are protected against *E. coli*-induced ascending urinary tract infection. In an unimmunised group, ten of 15 animals (67 per cent) acquired infection, while only three of 16 immunised animals (18.8 per cent) became infected. The number of organisms in the kidneys of the immunised animals was significantly lower than in the kidneys of the controls (Silverblatt & Cohen, 1979). Passively administered monoclonal antibody that blocks the binding of *E. coli* type-1 fimbriae to bladder epithelium protects mice against ascending pyelonephritis after intravesical administration of *E. coli* (Abraham, S. N. *et al.*, 1985).

Not all attempts to use type-1 fimbriae as a vaccine have, however, been successful (Levine *et al.*, 1983; O'Hanley *et al.*, 1985). In a trial in humans, administration of isolated type-1 fimbriae from *E. coli* evoked high concentrations of serum anti-fimbrial antibodies but failed to protect against gastro-intestinal colonisation (Levine *et al.*, 1983). This may be due, at least in part, to the high level of antigenic heterogeneity among type-1 fimbriae (Fader *et al.*, 1982; Adegbola & Old, 1987).

Comparison of the amino-acid sequences of FimA of type-1 fimbriae from several species of Enterobacteriaceae has revealed that although the amino-acid sequence homology was up to 79 per cent, there was little or no antigenic cross-reactivity (Buchanan *et al.*, 1985; Abraham & Beachey, 1987). The antigenic heterogeneity may be the result of differences in the tertiary structural conformation of FimA (Fader & Davis, 1982). Multiple variants of the major fimbrial subunit have been described in several other fimbrial types, especially in *N. gonorrhoeae* where extensive serological studies have demonstrated hundreds of fimbrial serotypes (Lim *et al.*, 1979; Brinton *et al.*, 1982). The many antigenic variants of the *E. coli* type-1 fimbriae would clearly be a potential problem in the design of a broad-spectrum vaccine, if FimA were the determinant of adherence. However, the minor fimbrial subunit, FimH, and not the antigenically heterogeneous FimA, is responsible for the D-mannose-binding function (Abraham *et al.*, 1988b; Tewari *et al.*, 1993). Furthermore, antibodies against FimH of *E. coli* type-1 fimbriae react with FimH from type-1 fimbriae of clinical strains of Enterobacteriaceae, including *E. coli*, *K. pneumoniae*, *Citrobacter* spp. and *Serratia* spp. (Abraham *et al.*, 1988b). These antibodies also block adherence *in vitro* of each of these strains to host mucosal cells in adherence assays (Abraham *et al.*, 1988a,b).

The *fimH* genes from *E. coli* and *K. pneumoniae* have recently been cloned and their DNA sequences determined (Klemm & Christiansen, 1987; Gerlach *et al.*, 1988). Comparison of the predicted amino-acid sequences of their gene products, FimA and FimH, showed that, in contrast to FimA, there was up to 85 per cent homology in the primary structure of FimH. Thus, in addition to similar sugar-binding specificities, the adhesive FimH subunits of the various type-1 fimbriae are structurally and antigenically conserved among the different bacterial species. This has encouraged attempts to determine whether antibodies against the *E. coli* FimH molecule can prevent adherence of *E. coli* and *K. pneu-*

moniae to the mucosal surface *in situ* and whether mice immunised actively or passively against FimH are better protected against bacterial infection by type-1-fimbriate organisms compared to controls. The results showed that antibodies against the entire FimH molecule or a synthetic copy, s-T1FimH(1-25)C, of its amino-terminus prevented the attachment of type 1 fimbriate *E. coli* and *K. pneumoniae* to the mouse bladder wall *in situ*. Furthermore, mice passively immunised by intraperitoneal administration of these FimH-specific antibodies were protected against bladder colonisation with type-1-fimbriate strains of *E. coli* and *K. pneumoniae* (Sun *et al.*, 1991; B. Madison & S. N. Abraham, unpublished). Active immunisation of mice with the isolated FimH or the synthetic FimH peptide was also highly effective in reducing *E. coli-* and *K. pneumoniae*-induced bladder colonisation. These observations provide definitive evidence that bacterial colonisation *in vivo* can be inhibited or reduced by antibodies directed specifically against the bacterial fimbrial adhesin protein. Such adhesin- or FimH-specific antibodies appear to be equally effective against infections by different type-1-fimbriate species of Enterobacteriaceae (B. Madison & S. N. Abraham, unpublished). These findings are encouraging and, for the first time, suggest that antibodies against the minor adhesin of type-1 fimbriae may provide broad protection against infections by enterobacteria.

Acknowledgements

We wish to thank Vourdonna Knoeppel for secretarial assistance, and Elizabeth Abraham and Jennifer MacGregor for critical reading of the manuscript. Work by the authors was supported by National Institutes of Health PHS grant AI 13550, a grant from Monsanto-Searle-Washington University Biomedical Research Agreement and an award from Searle (Arthritis and Postaglandin Research Challenge).

References

Abraham, J. M., Freitag, C. S., Clements, J. R. & Eisenstein, B. I. (1985). An invertible element of DNA controls phase variation of type 1 fimbriae of *Escherichia coli. Journal of Bacteriology*, **82**, 5724–7.

Abraham, S. N., Babu, J. P., Giampapa, C. S., Hasty, D. L., Simpson, W. A. & Beachey, E. H. (1985). Protection against *Escherichia coli*-induced urinary tract infections with hybridoma antibodies directed against type 1 fimbriae or complementary D-mannose receptors. *Infection and Immunity*, **48**, 625–8.

Abraham, S. N. & Beachey, E. H. (1987). Assembly of a chemically synthe-sized peptide of *Escherichia coli* type 1 fimbriae into fimbria-like antigenic structures. *Journal of Bacteriology*, **169**, 2460–5.

Abraham, S. N., Beachey, E. H. & Simpson, W. A. (1983a). Adherence of *Streptococcus pyogenes*, *Escherichia coli* and *Pseudomonas aeruginosa* to fibronectin coated and uncoated epithelial cells. *Infection and Immunity*, **41**, 1261–8.

Abraham, S. N., Goguen, J. D. & Beachey, E. H. (1988a). Hyperadhesive mutant of type 1 fimbriated *Escherichia coli* associated with the formation of FimH organelles (fimbriosomes). *Infection and Immunity*, **56**, 1023–9.

Abraham, S. N., Goguen, J. D., Sun, D., Klemm, P. & Beachey, E. H. (1987). Identification of two ancillary subunits of *Escherichia coli* type 1 fimbriae by using antibodies against synthetic oligopeptides of *fim* gene products. *Journal of Bacteriology*, **169**, 5530–5.

Abraham, S. N., Hasty, D. L., Simpson, W. A. & Beachey, E. H. (1983b). Antiadhesive properties of a quaternary structure-specific hybridoma anti-body against type 1 fimbriae of *Escherichia coli*. *Journal of Experimental Medicine*, **158**, 1128–44.

Abraham, S. N., Land, M., Ponniah, S., Endres, R. O., Hasty, D. & Babu, J. P. (1992). Glycerol-induced unravelling of the tight helical conformation of *Escherichia coli* type 1 fimbriae. *Journal of Bacteriology*, **174**, 5145–8.

Abraham, S. N., Sun, D., Dale, J. B. & Beachey, E. H. (1988b). Con-servation of the D-mannose-adhesion protein among type 1 fimbriated members of the family Enterobacteriaceae. *Nature*, **336**, 682–4.

Adegbola, R. A. & Old, D. C. (1987). Antigenic relationships among type-1 fimbriae of Enterobacteriaceae revealed by immunoelectronmicroscopy. *Journal of Medical Microbiology*, **24**, 21–8.

Alkan, M. L., Wong, L. & Silverblatt, F. J. (1986). Change in degree of type 1 piliation of *Escherichia coli* during experimental peritonitis in the mouse. *Infection and Immunity*, **54**, 549–54.

Aronson, M., Medalia, O., Schori, L., Mirelman, D., Sharon, N. & Ofek, I. (1979). Prevention of colonization of the urinary tract of mice with *Escherichia coli* by blocking of bacterial adherence with methyl α-D-mannopyranoside. *Journal of Infectious Diseases*, **139**, 329–32.

Asada, M., Furukawa, K., Kantor, C. & Kobata, A (1991). Structural study of the sugar chains of human leukocyte adhesion molecules CD11/CD18. *Biochemistry*, **30**, 1561–71.

Babu, J. P., Abraham, S. N., Dabbous, M. K. & Beachey, E. H. (1986). Interaction of a 60-kilodalton D-mannose-containing glycoprotein with type 1 fimbriae of *Escherichia coli*. *Infection and Immunity*, **54**, 104–8.

Babu, J. P., Beachey, E. H., Hasty, D. L. & Simpson, W. A. (1986). Isolation and characterization of a 60-kilodalton salivary glycoprotein with specific agglutinating activity against strains of *Streptococcus mutans*. *Infection and Immunity*, **51**, 414–18.

Bachman, B. J. (1983). Linkage map of *Escherichia coli* K-12. edition 7. *Microbiological Reviews*, **47**, 180–230.

Baddour, L. M., Christiansen, G. D., Simpson, W. A. & Beachey, E. H. (1990). Microbial adherence. In *Principles and Practice of Infectious Disease*, vol. 2, eds. G. L. Mandell, R. G. Douglas & J. E. Bennett, pp. 9–25. New York: Churchill Livingstone.

Blomfield, I. C., Calie, P. J., Eberhardt, K. J., McClain, M. S. & Eisenstein, B. I. (1993). Lrp stimulates phase variation of type 1 fimbriation in *Escherichia coli* K-12. *Journal of Bacteriology*, **175**, 27–36.

Blomfield, I. C., McClain, M. S. & Eisenstein, B. I. (1991). Type 1 fimbriae mutants of *Escherichia coli* K12: characterization of recognized afimbriate strains and construction of new *fim* deletion mutants. *Molecular Microbiology*, **5**, 1439–45.

Brinton, C. C. Jr. (1959). Non-flagellar appendices of bacteria. *Nature*, **183**, 782–6.

Brinton, C. C. (1965). The structure, function, synthesis and genetic control of bacterial pili and a molecular model for DNA and RNA transport in gram-negative bacteria. *Annals of the New York Academy of Sciences*, **27**, 1003–54.

Brinton, C. C., Wood, S. W., Brown, A., Labik, A. M. & Bryan, J. R. (1982). The development of neisserial pilus vaccine for gonorrhea and meningococcal meningitis. In *Bacterial Vaccines. Seminars in Infectious Diseases*, vol. 4, eds. L. Wernstein & B. Fields, pp. 140–59. Stuttgart: Thieme.

Buchanan, K., Falkow, S., Hull, R. A. & Hull, S. I. (1985). Frequency among Enterobacteriaceae of the DNA sequences encoding type 1 pili. *Journal of Bacteriology*, **162**, 799–803.

Chanteloup, N. K., Dho-Moulin, M., Esnault, E. & Lafont, J.-P. (1991). Serological conservation and location of the adhesin of avian *Escherichia coli* type 1 fimbriae. *Microbial Pathogenesis*, **10**, 271–80.

Chick, S., Harber, M. J., MacKenzie, R. & Asscher, A. W. (1981). Modified method for studying bacterial adhesion to isolated uroepithelial cells and uromucoid. *Infection and Immunity*, **34**, 256–61.

Clegg, S. & Gerlach, G. F. (1987). Enterobacterial fimbriae. *Journal of Bacteriology*, **169**, 934–8.

Clegg, S., Hull, S., Hull, R. & Pruckler, J. (1985). Construction and comparison of recombinant plasmids encoding type 1 fimbriae of members of the family Enterobacteriaceae. *Infection and Immunity*, **48**, 275–9.

Clegg, S., Purcell, B. K. & Pruckler, J. (1987). Characterization of genes encoding type 1 fimbriae of *Klebsiella pneumoniae, Salmonella typhimurium*, and *Serratia marcescens*. *Infection and Immunity*, **55**, 281–7.

Dorman, C. J. & Higgins, C. F. (1987). Fimbrial phase variation in *Escherichia coli*: dependence on integration host factor and homologies with other site-specific recombinases. *Journal of Bacteriology*, **169**, 3840–3.

Duguid, J. P. (1959). Fimbriae and adhesive properties in *Klebsiella* strains. *Journal of General Microbiology*, **21**, 271–8.

Duguid, J. P., Darekar, M. R. & Wheater, D. W. F. (1976). Fimbriae and infectivity in *Salmonella typhimurium*. *Journal of Medical Microbiology*, **9**, 459–73.

Duguid, J. P. & Old, D. C. (1980). Adhesive properties of Enterobacteriaceae. In *Bacterial Adherence, Receptor, and Recognition*, series B, vol. 6, ed. E. H. Beachey, pp. 185–217. London: Chapman & Hall.

Duguid, J. P., Smith, I. W., Dempster, G. & Edmunds, P. N. (1955). Non-flagellar filamentous appendices fimbriae and hemagglutinating activity in *Bacterium coli*. *Journal of Pathology and Bacteriology*, **70**, 335–41.

Eisenstein, B. I. (1990). Enterobacteriaceae. In *Principles and Practice of*

Infectious Diseases, eds. G. L. Mandell, R. G. Douglas & J. E. Bennett, pp. 1658–1673. New York: Churchill Livingstone

Eisenstein, B. I., Sweet, D. S., Vaughn, V. & Friedman, D. I. (1987). Integration host factor is required for the DNA inversion that controls phase variation in *Escherichia coli*. *Proceedings of the National Academy of Sciences, USA*, **84**, 6506–10.

Eshdat, Y., Silverblatt, F. J. & Sharon, N. (1981). Dissociation and reassembly of *Escherichia coli* type 1 pili. *Journal of Bacteriology*, **148**, 308–14.

Fader, A. & Davis, C. P. (1982). *Klebsiella pneumoniae*-induced experimental pyelitis: the effect of piliation on infectivity. *Journal of Urology*, **128**, 197–201.

Fader, R. C., Duggy, L. D., Davies, C. P. & Kurosky, A. (1982). Purification and chemical characterization of type 1 pili isolated from *Klebsiella pneumoniae*. *Journal of Biological Chemistry*, **257**, 3301–5.

Firon, N., Ashkenazi, S., Mirelman, D., Ofek, I. & Sharon, N. (1987). Aromatic alpha-glycosides of mannose are powerful inhibitors of the adherence of type 1 fimbriated *Escherichia coli* to yeast and intestinal epithelial cells. *Infection and Immunity*, **55**, 472–6.

Firon, N., Duksin, D. & Sharon, N. (1985). Mannose-specific adherence of *Escherichia coli* to BHK cells that differ in their glycosylation patterns. *FEMS Microbiology Letters*, **27**, 161–5.

Firon, N., Ofek, I. & Sharon, N. (1982). Interaction of mannose containing oligosaccharides with the fimbrial lectin of *Escherichia coli*. *Biochemical and Biophysical Research Communications*, **105**, 1426–32.

Firon, N., Ofek, I. & Sharon, N. (1983). Carbohydrate specificity of the surface lectins of *Escherichia coli*, *Klebsiella pneumoniae* and *Salmonella typhimurium*. *Carbohydrate Research*, **120**, 235–49.

Firon, N., Ofek, I. & Sharon, N. (1984). Carbohydrate-binding sites of the mannose-specific lectins of *Enterobacteria*. *Infection and Immunity*, **43**, 1088–90.

Freitag, C. S., Abraham, J. M., Clements, J. R. & Eisenstein, B. I. (1985). Genetic analysis of the phase variation control of expression of type 1 fimbriae in *Escherichia coli*. *Journal of Bacteriology*, **162**, 668–75.

Freitag, C. S. & Eisenstein, B. I. (1983). Genetic mapping and transcriptional orientation of the *fimD* gene. *Journal of Bacteriology*, **156**, 1052–8.

Freter, R. (1980). Prospects for preventing the association of harmful bacteria with host mucosal surface. In *Bacterial Adherence, Receptor and Recognition*, series B, vol. 6, ed. E. H. Beachey, pp. 439–58. London: Chapman & Hall.

Galli, S. J. (1993). New concepts about the mast cells. *New England Journal of Medicine*, **328**, 257–65.

Gally, D. L., Bogan, J. A., Eisenstein, B. I. & Blomfield, I. C. (1993). Environmental regulation of the *fim* switch controlling type 1 fimbrial phase variation in *Escherichia coli* K-12: effects of temperature and media. *Journal of Bacteriology*, **175**, 6186–93.

Gbarah, A., Gahmberg, C. G., Ofek, I., Jacobi, U. & Sharon, N. (1991). Identification of the leukocyte adhesion molecules CD11 and CD18 as receptors for type 1 fimbriated (mannose-specific) *Escherichia coli*. *Infection and Immunity*, **59**, 4524–30.

Gbarah, A., Mirelman, D., Sansonetti, P. J., Verdon, R., Bernhard, W. & Sharon, N. (1993). *Shigella flexneri* transformants expressing type 1 (mannose-specific) fimbriae bind to, activate, and are killed by phagocytic cells. *Infection and Immunity*, **61**, 1687–93.

Gerlach, G. F. & Clegg, S. (1988). Characterization of two genes encoding antigenically distinct type 1 fimbriae of *Klebsiella pneumoniae*. *Gene*, **64**, 2321–40.

Gerlach, G. F., Clegg, S. & Allen, B. (1988). Identification and characterization of the genes encoding the type 3 and type 1 fimbrial adhesins of *Klebsiella pneumoniae*. *Journal of Bacteriology*, **171**, 1262–70.

Giampapa, C. S., Abraham, S. N., Chiang, T. M. & Beachey, E. H. (1988). Isolation and characterization of a receptor for type 1 fimbriae of *Escherichia coli* from guinea pig erythrocytes. *Journal of Biological Chemistry*, **263**, 5362–7.

Goetz, M. B., Kuriyama, S. M. & Siverblatt, F. J. (1987). Phagolysosome formation by polymorphonuclear neutrophilic leukocytes after ingestion of *Escherichia coli* that express type 1 pili. *Journal of Infectious Diseases*, **156**, 229–33.

Goetz, M. B. & Silverblatt, F. J. (1987). Stimulation of human polymorphonuclear leukocyte oxidative metabolism by type 1 pili from *Escherichia coli*. *Infection and Immunity*, **55**, 534–40.

Goldhar, J., Zilberberg, A. & Ofek, I. (1986). Infant mouse model of adherence and colonization of intestinal tissues by enterotoxigenic strains of *Escherichia coli* isolated from humans. *Infection and Immunity*, **52**, 205–8.

Gordon, J. R., Burd, P. R. & Galli, S. J. (1990). Mast cells as a source of multifunctional cytokines. *Immunology Today*, **11**, 458–64.

Hansen, M. S. & Brinton, C. C. (1988). Identification and characterization of *E. coli* type 1 pilus tip adhesion protein. *Nature*, **332**, 265–8.

Hasty, D. L., Beachey, E. H., Courtney, H. S. & Simpson, W. A. (1990). Interactions between fibronectin and bacteria. In *Fibronectin in Health and Disease*, ed. S. Carsons, pp. 89–112. Boca Raton, FL: CRC Press.

Hoepelman, A. I. M. & Tuomanen, E. (1992). Consequences of microbial attachment directing host cell functions with adhesins. *Infection and Immunity*, 60, 1729–33.

Hull, R. A., Gill, R. E., Hsu, P., Minshew, B. H. & Falkow, S. (1981). Construction and expression of recombinant plasmids encoding type 1 or D-mannose-resistant pili from a urinary tract infection *Escherichia coli* isolate. *Infection and Immunity*, **33**, 933–8.

Hultgren, S. J., Abraham, S., Caparon, M., Falk, P., St. Geme J. W. III & Normark, S. (1993). Pilus and nonpilus bacterial adhesins: assembly and function in cell recognition. *Cell*, **73**, 887–901.

Hultgren, S. J., Normark, S. & Abraham, S. N. (1991). Chaperone-assisted assembly and molecular architecture of adhesive pili. *Annual Review of Microbiology*, **45**, 383–415.

Hultgren, S. J., Porter, T. N., Schaeffer, A. J. & Duncan, J. L. (1985). Role of type 1 pili and effects of phase variation on lower urinary tract infections produced by *Escherichia coli*. *Infection and Immunity*, **50**, 370–7.

Iwahi, T., Abe, Y., Nakao, M., Imada, A. & Tsuchiya, K. (1983). Role of type 1 fimbriae in the pathogenesis of ascending urinary tract infection induced by *Escherichia coli* in mice. *Infection and Immunity*, **39**, 1307–15.

Iwahi, T. & Imada, A. (1988). Interaction of *Escherichia coli* with polymorphonuclear leukocytes in pathogenesis of urinary tract infection in mice. *Infection and Immunity*, **56**, 947–53.

Johnson, J. R. (1991). Virulence factors in *Escherichia coli* urinary tract infection. *Clinical Microbiology Reviews*, **4**, 80–128.

Jones, C. H., Pinkner, J. S., Nicholes, A. V., Slonim, L. N., Abraham, S. N. & Hultgren, S. J. (1993). FimC is a periplasmic PapD-like chaperone that directs assembly of type 1 pili in bacteria. *Proceedings of the National Academy of Sciences, USA*, **90**, 8397–401.

Jones, C. H., Pinkner, J. S., Roth R., Heuser, J., Abraham, S. N. & Hultgren, S. J. (1995). FimH adhesin of type 1 pili is presented in a fibrillar tip structure in the Enterobacteriaceae. *Proceedings of the National Academy of Sciences USA*, **92**, 2081–5.

Keith, B. R., Harris, S. L., Russel, P. W. & Orndorff, P. (1990). Effect of type 1 piliation on *in vitro* killing of *Escherichia coli* by mouse peritoneal macrophages. *Infection and Immunity*, **58**, 3448–54.

Klemm, P. (1986). Two regulatory *fim* genes, *fimB* and *fimE*, control the phase variation of type 1 fimbriae in *Escherichia coli*. *EMBO Journal*, **5**, 1389–93.

Klemm, P. & Christiansen, G. (1987). Three *fim* genes required for the regulation of length and mediation of adhesion of *Escherichia coli* type 1 fimbriae. *Molecular and General Genetics*, **208**, 439–445.

Klemm, P. & Christiansen, G. (1990). The *fimD* gene required for cell surface localization of *Escherichia coli* type 1 fimbriae. *Molecular and General Genetics*, **220**, 334–8.

Klemm, P., Jorgensen, B. J., van Die, I., de Ree, H. & Bergmans, H. (1985). The *fim* genes responsible for synthesis of type 1 fimbriae in *Escherichia coli*, cloning and genetic organization. *Molecular and General Genetics*, **199**, 410–14.

Krogfelt, K. A., Bergmans, H. & Klemm, P. (1990). Direct evidence that the FimH protein is the adhesin of *Escherichia coli* type 1 fimbriae. *Infection and Immunity*, **58**, 1995–8.

Kukkonen, M., Raunio, T., Virkola, R., Lahteenmaki, K., Makela, P. H., Klemm, P., Clegg, S. & Korhonen, T. K. (1993). Basement membrane carbohydrate as a target for bacterial adhesion: binding of type 1 fimbriae of *Salmonella enterica* and *Escherichia coli* to laminin. *Molecular Microbiology*, **7**, 229–37.

Kuriyama, S. M. & Silverblatt, F. J. (1986). Effect of Tamm-Horsfall urinary glycoprotein on phagocytosis and killing of type 1-fimbriated *Escherichia coli*. *Infection and Immunity*, **51**, 193–8.

Levine, M. M., Black, R. E., Brinton, C. C., Clements, M. L., Fusco, P., Highes, T. P., O'Donnell, S., Robins-Browne, R., Wood, S. & Young, C. R. (1983). Reactogenicity, immunogenicity and efficacy of *Escherichia coli* type 1 somatic pili parenteral vaccine in man. *Scandinavian Journal of Infectious Diseases, Supplement*, **33**, 83–95.

Lim, S., McMichael, J., Polen, S., Rogers, K., Agnes, C.-C. & To, S. C.-M. (1978). Uses of pili in gonorrhea control: role of bacterial pili in disease, purification and properties of gonococcal pili, and progress in the development of a gonococcal pilus vaccine for gonorrhea. In *Immunobiology of Neisseria gonorrhoeae*, ed. G. F. Brooks, pp. 155–78. Washington DC: American Society for Microbiology.

Lock, R., Dahlgren, C., Linden, M., Stendahl, O., Svensbergh, A. & Ohman, L. (1990). Neutrophil killing of two type 1 fimbria-bearing *Escherichia coli* strains: dependence on respiratory burst activation. *Infection and Immunity*, **58**, 37–42.

Madison, B., Ofek, I., Clegg, S. & Abraham, S. N. (1994). Type 1 fimbrial shafts of *Escherichia coli* and *Klebsiella pneumoniae* influence the sugar binding specificity of their FimH adhesins. *Infection and Immunity*, **62**, 843–8.

Malaviya, R., Ross, E., Jakschick, B. A, & Abraham, S. N. (1994b). Mast cell degranulation induced by type 1 fimbriae of *Escherichia coli* in mice. *Journal of Clinical Investigation* 93, 1645–53.

Malaviya, R., Ross, E., MacGregor, J. I., Ikeda, T., Little, J. R., Jakschick, B. A. & Abraham, S. N. (1994a). Mast cell phagocytosis of FimH-expressing enterobacteria. *Journal of Immunology* 152, 1907–14.

Maurer, L. & Orndorff, P. E. (1985). A new locus *pilE*, required for the binding of type 1 piliated *Escherichia coli* to erythrocytes. *FEMS Microbiology Letters*, **30**, 59–66.

Maurer, L. & Orndorff, P. E. (1987). Identification and characterization of genes determining receptor binding and pilus length of *Escherichia coli* type 1 pili. *Journal of Bacteriology*, **169**, 640–5.

May, A. K., Bloch, C. A., Sawyer, R. G., Spengler, M. D. & Pruett, T. L. (1993). Enhanced virulence of *Escherichia coli* bearing a site-targeted mutation in the major structural subunit of type 1 fimbriae. *Infection and Immunity*, **61**, 1667–73.

McClain, M. S., Blomfield, I. C. & Eisenstein, B. I. (1991). Roles of *fim*B and *fim*E in site-specific DNA inversion associated with phase variation of type 1 fimbriae in *Escherichia coli*. *Journal of Bacteriology*, **173**, 5308–14.

McCormick, B. A., Franklin, D. P., Laux, D. C. & Cohen, P. C. (1989). Type 1 pili are not necessary for colonization of the streptomycin-treated mouse large intestine by type 1-piliated *Escherichia coli* F-18 and *E. coli* K-12. *Infection and Immunity*, **57**, 3022–9.

Minion, F. C., Abraham, S. N., Beachey, E. H. & Goguen, J. D. (1986). The genetic determinant of adhesive function in type 1 fimbriae of *Escherichia coli* is distinct from the gene encoding the fimbrial subunit. *Journal of Bacteriology*, **165**, 1033–6.

Ofek, I. & Sharon, N. (1990). Adhesins as lectins; specificity and role in infections. *Current Topics in Microbiology and Immunology*, **151**, 91–113.

O'Hanley, P., Lark, D., Falkow, S. & Schoolnik, G. (1985). Molecular basis of *Escherichia coli* colonization of the upper urinary tract in BALB/c mice. Gal-gal pili immunization prevents *Escherichia coli* pyelonephritis in the BALB/c mouse model of human pyelonephritis. *Journal of Clinical Investigation*, **75**, 347–60.

Ohman, L., Hed, J. & Stendahl, O. (1982) Interaction between human polymorphonuclear leukocytes and two different strains of type 1 fimbriae-bearing *Escherichia coli*. *Journal of Infectious Diseases*, **146**, 751–7.

Orndorff, P. E. & Falkow, S. (1984). Organization and expression of genes responsible for type 1 piliation in *Escherichia coli*. *Journal of Bacteriology*, **159**, 736–44.

Ørskov, I., Ørskov, F. & Birch-Andersen, A. (1980). Comparison of *Escherichia coli* fimbrial antigen F7 with type 1 fimbriae. *Infection and Immunity*, **27**, 657–66.

Pallesen, L., Madsen, O. & Klemm, P. (1989). Regulation of the phase switch controlling expression of type 1 fimbriae in *Escherichia coli*. *Molecular Microbiology*, **3**, 925–31.

Ponniah, S., Abraham, S. N., Dockter, M., Wall, C. D. & Endres, R. O.

(1989). Mitogenic stimulation of human B lymphocytes by the mannose-specific adhesin on *Escherichia coli* type 1 fimbriae. *Journal of Immunology*, **142**, 992–8.

Ponniah, S., Abraham, S. N. & Endres, R. O. (1992). T-cell-independent stimulation of immunoglobulin secretion in resting human B lymphocytes by the mannose-specific adhesin of *Escherichia coli* type 1 fimbriae. *Infection and Immunity*, **60**, 5197–203.

Ponniah, S., Endres, R. O., Hasty, D. L. & Abraham, S. N. (1991). Fragmentation of *Escherichia coli* type 1 fimbriae exposes cryptic D-mannose-binding sites. *Journal of Bacteriology*, **173**, 4195–202.

Porat, R., Clark, B. D., Wolff, S. M. & Dinarello, C. A. (1991). Enhancement of growth of virulent strains of *Escherichia coli* by interleukin-1. *Science*, **254**, 430–2.

Rene, P., Dinolfo, M. & Silverblatt, F. J. (1982). Serum and urogenital antibody responses to *Escherichia coli* pili in cystitis. *Infection and Immunity*, **38**, 542–7.

Rodriguez-Ortega, M., Ofek, I. & Sharon, N. (1987). Membrane glycoproteins of human polymorphonuclear leukocytes that act as receptors for mannose-specific *Escherichia coli*. *Infection and Immunity*, **55**, 968–73.

Russell, P. W. & Orndorff, P. E. (1992). Lesions in two *Escherichia coli* type 1 pilus genes alter pilus number and length without affecting receptor binding. *Journal of Bacteriology*, **174**, 5923–35.

Sauter, S. L., Rutherford, S. M., Wagener, C. & Hefta, S. A. (1991). Binding of nonspecific cross reacting antigen, a granulocyte membrane glycoprotein, to *Escherichia coli* type 1 fimbriae. *Infection and Immunity*, **59**, 2485–93.

Silverblatt, F. J. & Cohen, L. S. (1979). Antipili antibody affords protection against experimental ascending pyelonephritis. *Journal of Clinical Investigation*, **64**, 333–6.

Sokurenko, E. V., Courtney, H. S., Abraham, S. N., Klemm, P. & Hasty, D. L. (1992). Functional heterogeneity of type 1 fimbriae of *Escherichia coli*. *Infection and Immunity*, **60**, 4709–19.

Sun, D., Madison, B. & Abraham, S. N. (1991). Antiadhesive properties of conformation-specific hybridoma antibodies against FimH proteins of *Escherichia coli* type 1 fimbriae. *Life Science Advances*, **10**, 23–9.

Tanaka, Y. (1982). Multiplication of the fimbriate and nonfimbriate *Salmonella typhimurium* organisms in the intestinal mucosa of mice treated with antibodies. *Japanese Journal of Veterinary Science*, **44**, 523–7.

Tewari, R., MacGregor, J. I., Ikeda, T., Little, J. R., Hultgren, S. J. & Abraham, S. N. (1993). Neutrophil activation by nascent FimH subunits of type 1 fimbriae purified from the periplasm of *Escherichia coli*. *Journal of Biological Chemistry* **268**, 3009–15.

Zafriri, D., Oron, Y., Eisenstein, B. I. & Ofek, I. (1987). Growth advantage and enhanced toxicity of *Escherichia coli* adherent to tissue culture cells due to restricted diffusion of products secreted by the cells. *Journal of Clinical Investigation*, **79**, 1210–16.

7

Fimbriae of enterotoxigenic *Escherichia coli*

F. K. DE GRAAF and W. GAASTRA

Escherichia coli associated with intestinal infections possess a variety of fimbrial adhesins. Apart from type-1 fimbriae, which are present on virtually all strains, other fimbriae appear to be host related. While some fimbrial adhesins are found exclusively on either human, porcine or bovine strains, other fimbriae are less host specific and may, for example, occur on strains of porcine, bovine and ovine origin. At present, no adhesins are known that occur on strains of both human and animal origin. The reasons for this apparent host specificity have not been investigated in detail but the available evidence suggests that it is related

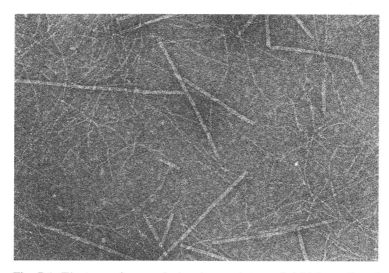

Fig. 7.1. Electron micrograph showing a mixture of rigid (type-1) and flexible (K99) fimbriae.

Table 7.1. *The relationship between fimbrial type, serogroup, toxin production and susceptible host in enterotoxigenic* Escherichia coli

Type	Serogroup	Toxins	Host
K88 (F4)	O8, O45, O138, O141, O147, O149, O157	LT, STa, STb	Pigs
F41	O9, O20, O64, O101	STa	Pigs, calves, lambs
CS31A	O8, O9, O20, O23		Calves
K99 (F5)	O8, O9, O20, O64, O101	STa, STb	Calves, lambs, pigs
987P (F6)	O8, O9, O20, O46, O101, O138, O141, O147, O149	STa, STb	Pigs
CFA/I (F2)	O4, O7, O20, O25, O63, O78, O110, O126, O128, O136, O153, O159	STa, LT	Human
CFA/II (F3)			Human
CS1+CS3	O6, O139	STa, LT	
CS2+CS3	O6	STa, LT	
CS3	O8, O9, O78, O80, O115, O128, O139, O168	STa, LT	
CFA/III+CS6	O25	LT	Human
CFA/IV			Human
CS4+CS6	O25	STa, LT	
CS5+CS6	O6, O29, O92, O114, O115, O167	LT	
CS6	O27, O92, O148, O153	STa, LT	Human
CS7	O15, O114, O128	STa, LT	Human
CS17	O5, O15, O48, O114, O146	LT	Human
PCFO166	O20, O71, O98, O166	STa, LT	Human

CFA, colonisation factor antigen; CS, coli-surface-associated; LT, heat-labile enterotoxin; PCF, putative colonisation factor; ST, heat-stable enterotoxin.

to the presence of specific receptors for the adhesins on the host epithelium.

The electron microscope shows that most fimbriae appear as rigid, hair-like, filamentous structures with a diameter of 5–7 nm. Certain fimbriae, such as K88, K99 and CS3, have a much smaller diameter and, as a result, are very thin and flexible filaments, often referred to as fibrillae (Figure 7.1). Both types of fimbrial structure are composed of protein subunits that are assembled into a helical structure but with different numbers of subunits per helical turn.

Each particular fimbrial type is associated with a limited number of serogroups of enterotoxic *E. coli* (ETEC) (Table 7.1). The enterotoxins produced by ETEC are also listed in Table 7.1 and the genes that encode these toxins are located on plasmids.

The operons that encode fimbriae may be located on plasmids or on the chromosome. Human ETEC often produce serotype-specific combinations of two adhesins encoded on two different plasmids. Plasmids have also been found that encode an adhesin and a toxin, such as the plasmids that carry genes for 987P or K99 fimbriae and the heat-stable enterotoxin STa.

Structural relationships and antigenic properties

The major fimbrial subunits of the various types of fimbriae can be separated into two groups depending on their molecular weights. The subunits of the K88, F41 and CS31A fimbriae of animal strains and of CS13 fimbriae of human strains are composed of large subunits (*c.* 27 kDa), that share limited sequence homology. Genetic studies of the operons that encode these adhesins have shown that, apart from the gene that encodes the major fimbrial subunit, the operons are very similar in structural organisation and nucleotide sequence (Anderson & Moseley, 1988; Girardeau *et al.*, 1991). This close relationship is clear from the fact that when CS13 fimbrial subunits are overproduced under the control of the accessory genes of the K88 and F41 operons, functional CS13 fimbriae are produced. It has been suggested that the K88, F41, CS31A and CS13 adhesins may have originated from a common ancestor that, by horizontal gene transfer, became adapted to different host receptors during evolution and/or escaped from the host immune response.

The second group of fimbrial subunits has a lower molecular weight and shows more similarities in amino-acid sequence than does the K88 family, with the exception of the fimbrial subunits of human ETEC. In the latter group, a common ancestor has been suggested for the operons that encode CFA/I, CS1, CS2, CS4, PCFO166 and CS17 fimbriae.

Three subtypes of K88 fimbriae, K88ab, K88ac and K88ad, can be distinguished serologically (de Graaf & Mooi, 1986). These fimbriae have one or more common epitopes 'a', while 'b', 'c' and 'd' represent subtype-specific epitopes. The K88 antigen has at least 11 epitopes, designated a1 to a7, b1, b2, c and d. The antigenic formulae for the various K88 subtypes are as follows (van Zijderveld *et al.*, 1990):

K88ab, a1a2a3a4a5a6b1b2
K88ac, a1a2a3(a4)a5a6a7c
K88ad, a1a2a3a4a7d

Monoclonal antibodies (MAbs) directed against conformational epitopes recognise K88-positive bacteria *in vivo*. Oral administration of MAbs against K88 protects piglets against infection with K88-positive ETEC. Regions in the K88 primary structure that belong to some of these epitopes have been identified by studies with recombinant K88 subunit genes, in which part of the nucleotide sequence has been replaced by heterologous determinants (Bakker *et al.*, 1990).

At least five epitopes have been found on F41 fimbriae (van Zijderveld *et al.*, 1989). MAbs directed against one of these inhibited the adhesion of F41-fimbriate bacteria *in vitro*. Similar experiments with MAbs directed against K88 showed that MAbs against the subtype-specific epitopes b, c and d inhibit adhesion, but those against the common a epitopes do not.

The smaller K99 fimbrial subunit probably contains only a single dominant epitope. MAbs directed against K99 inhibit adhesion of K99-positive ETEC to piglet enterocytes and have prophylactic and therapeutic uses in the control and treatment of neonatal diarrhoea.

MAbs directed against fimbriae of human ETEC have been used for diagnostic and epidemiological purposes. Epitopes on the CFA/I fimbrial subunit have been mapped with MAbs. Six potential antigenic determinants were predicted on the CFA/I subunit protein (Klemm & Mikkelsen, 1982) and two of these are located within the 46 amino-terminal amino-acid residues. Comparison of four MAbs against CFA/I in enzyme-linked immunosorbant assay (ELISA) and immunoblot assays (Worobec *et al.*, 1983) with six types of fimbriae showed that three of the MAbs are specific for CFA/I. The fourth MAb showed distinct cross-reactivity in the ELISA assay with K99 fimbriae, indicating a common structural element in the two fimbriae. In this connection, it should be noted that K99 and CFA/I fimbriae bind to receptor molecules with terminal sialic acid residues (Faris *et al.*, 1980). In spite of the similarity of the complete amino-acid sequence of CFA/I and CS1 subunits and of the amino-termini of the CFA/I, CS1, CS2, CS4, PCFO166 and CS17 fimbrial subunits, these proteins are antigenically unrelated in immunodiffusion tests and ELISA (McConnell *et al.*, 1989). However, polyclonal rabbit antisera raised against CS4 fimbriae cross-reacted strongly in Western blots with the subunit proteins of CFA/I, CS1 and CS2. Similarly, CFA/I fimbriae prime and boost immune responses against CS4 and *vice versa* (Rudin & Svennerholm, 1994). This suggests that these proteins have a common epitope that is not exposed on the surface. Cross-reactions between ETEC strains of heterologous serotypes that produce CFA/I of CFA/II fimbriae were observed in one volunteer experiment (Evans *et al.*, 1988). MAbs against dissociated CFA/I sub-units cross-react with CS1, CS2, CS4, PCFO166 and CS17 fimbriae (Rudin *et al.*, 1994). These MAbs also inhibit haemagglutination by strains that express CFA/I, CS1 and CS4 fimbriae and the binding to Caco-2 cells of strains that produce CFA/I, CS2, CS4 and PCFO166.

The architecture of fimbrial adhesins

The location of the receptor-binding sites on fimbriae varies. In some ETEC fimbriae, such as K88, K99, 987P and CFA/I, the adhesive properties are associated with the major fimbrial subunit. In this group, K88 and K99 fimbriae are multivalent in the sense that the receptor-binding site of the individual major subunits is exposed on the fimbrial surface and is available for multiple interactions with host tissues. CFA/I fimbriae are monovalent and only the major subunit at the tip has an exposed receptor site. In type-1, P- and S-fimbriae, minor fimbrial subunits at the tip of the fimbrial structure are responsible for interaction with the host tissue. In some cases, multivalent interactions between fimbriae and host tissue result from the sparse presence of these tip proteins at locations along the major fimbrial structure.

Though some fimbriae have adhesive tip proteins that differ from their major subunit, this does not mean that fimbriae with major adhesive subunits do not have tip proteins. For example, K88 fimbriae have at their tip a minor fimbrial subunit, FaeC, that does not have adhesive proper-ties.

The general concept that arises from these observations is that the adhesive properties of fimbriae can be associated with major or minor fimbrial components and that they are located either exclusively at the tip, or along the length of the fimbrial structure. Multivalent receptor binding may enhance the affinity of bacterial cells for host tissue.

Differences in the molecular architecture of fimbriae are not restricted to the presence and location of minor fimbrial components but are also obvious from their morphological appearance. Fimbriae with specialised adhesin molecules, such as type-1 or S-fimbriae, are rigid 7-nm diameter rod-like structures embedded in the polysaccharide capsule, of which only the distal parts are accessible for receptor recognition. Fimbriae with major adhesive subunits (K88, K99) appear to be much more flexible fibrillar 2- to 4-nm diameter structures that surround the bacteria in a capsule-like fashion, as has been shown for the CS31A antigen.

Host cell receptors

ETEC colonise the mucosal surface of the intestinal tract by adhering to mucus and/or epithelial brush border membranes. Such colonisation can be considered as a two-step process in which initial colonisation and growth in mucus is followed by an interaction with the epithelial cells.

Fimbriae generally interact with glycolipids and/or glycoproteins in a lectin-like fashion. Various glyco-conjugates, present in mucus or brush borders, probably share similar oligosaccharide moieties that are recognised by the fimbrial adhesin. In a model of bacterial adherence, a receptor epitope is formed by an oligosaccharide core that may be part of a much larger projecting oligosaccharide exposed in such a way that it fits with the receptor-binding site of the bacterial adhesin (lectin). Conformational predictions have shown that the carbohydrate residues involved in specific adhesin binding are located in a fixed spatial orientation that is accessible to the adhesin ligand. Eukaryotic cell membranes carry an abundance of glyco-conjugates and an enormous diversity of oligosaccharide sequences. The species, tissue and cell distribution of these oligosaccharides is not uniform, which explains the preference of various pathogens for particular host tissues. Successful colonisation of the intestinal mucus and, eventually, adherence to the epithelial cell layer indicate that the rate of bacterial growth is faster in mucus than is the rate at which they are sloughed off into the intestinal lumen. This hypothesis is supported by the observation that *E. coli* can utilise, for growth, lipids present in the caecal mucus layer. In this situation in particular it has been observed that phosphatidylserine can serve as the sole carbon and nitrogen source for *E. coli* and salmonellaes (Krivan *et al.*, 1992).

The K88 receptor

The existence of three serological variants of K88 fimbriae has been explained as an attempt by *E. coli* to exploit antigenic variation as an escape from the host immune system. At the molecular level, the differences between the K88 variants can be ascribed exclusively to a small number of mutations in the fimbrial subunit gene *faeG* that results in a limited number of amino-acid substitutions. The other genes in the three *fae* operons are identical (Bakker *et al.*, 1992a). The common 'a' epitopes are the most relevant epitopes for the induction of protective immunity. On the other hand, only MAbs against subspecies-specific epitopes prevent binding of fimbriate bacteria to epithelial cells (van Zijderveld *et al.*, 1990). A probable explanation for the existence of three K88 variants may, therefore, be genetic drift to adapt further to specific receptors on particular host tissues or a broadening in the variety of glyco-conjugates that have to be recognised. Serotype-associated variation in tissue tropism is supported by the fact that the three K88 subtypes have different haemagglutination patterns and differ in their ability to adhere to the brush border membranes of up to five different pig phenotypes (Bijlsma *et al.*, 1982; Bakker *et al.*, 1992a).

Not all pigs are susceptible to infections by K88-positive ETEC. Resistant pigs do not have the K88 receptor, which is inherited in a simple Mendelian manner involving a single locus with two alleles; the 'adhesive' allele is dominant over the 'non-adhesive' allele (Rutter *et al.*, 1975). This points to a single glyco-conjugate as the predominant K88 receptor, but the existence of five different pig phenotypes may reflect small differences in the glyco-conjugate receptor as a result of evolutionary changes.

Though glycolipids that carry Gal-(1→3)-Gal residues have been implicated as possible receptors for K88 fimbriae (de Graaf & Mooi, 1986), it is now thought that glycoproteins present in mucus and/or epithelial cell membranes are the true receptors for these fimbriae (Erickson *et al.*, 1992).

The K99 and CFA/I receptor

A receptor for K99 fimbriae was first isolated from horse erythrocytes and identified as Neu5Glcα-(2→3)-Gal$p$β-(1→4)-Glc$p$β-(1→1)-ceramide (Smit *et al.*, 1984). This glycolipid, also known as hematoside, is an abundant ganglioside in the glycolipid fraction of these erythrocytes. The specificity of the K99 receptor for a variety of sialic acids and their derivatives has been shown to be for the *N*-glycolyl group. Substitution of this group with an *N*-acetyl group abolishes binding of K99 fimbriae. Substitution of the C4 hydroxyl group for an *O*-acetyl group also strongly diminishes K99 receptor activity (Ono *et al.*, 1989). Though the terminal NeuGlc is crucial for K99 recognition, hydrophobic interactions with the ceramide moiety also play a role (Lindahl *et al.*, 1987).

Experiments *in vitro* with purified gangliosides confirmed others with

purified gangliosides, when it was observed that the acid glycolipids
N-glycolyl-GM3 and N-glycolylsialoparagloboside isolated from piglet
intestinal mucosa have a high binding affinity for K99 (Kyogashima *et al.*,
1989). N-Glycolylsialyl residues are present in glycoproteins and
glycolipids of piglets, calves and lambs, but not in human glyco-
conjugates, which explains the host-specificity of infections with K99-
fimbriate ETEC.

The binding of *E. coli* K99 is not restricted to glycolipids. Pig intestinal
mucus glycopeptides with carbohydrate chains similar to those observed
on glycolipids also bind to K99-fimbriate ETEC (Lindahl & Carlstedt,
1990).

CFA/I fimbriae bind to sialic-acid-containing glyco-conjugates, such as
ganglioside GM2. Similarly, a 26-kDa sialoglycoprotein, from human
erythrocyte membranes, binds to CFA/I-positive bacteria but not to
CFA/I-negative cells. CS1, CS2, CS3 and CS4 bind to the asi-
aloganglioside GM1 (Orø *et al.*, 1990). The use of different receptors by
the different fimbriae of human ETEC is also evident from the fact that
the binding to Caco-2 cells of ETEC that produce CFA/I, CFA/II and
CFA/III is inhibited only if the Caco-2 cells had previously been incubated with homologous, but not with heterologous, fimbriae (Darfeuille-
Michaud *et al.*, 1990).

Age-dependent receptors of the small intestine

Newborn animals are the most sensitive to ETEC infections. Resistance
develops with age, sometimes within a few days, as can be observed for
infections with K99-positive *E. coli*. A sudden temporary increase in
susceptibility may occur as a post-weaning phenomenon, similar to that
documented for K88-associated infections. This age-dependent susceptibility has been accounted for in a number of ways. These include, firstly,
the high relative permeability of the intestinal mucosa in neonatal
animals, secondly, the high relative gastric pH in newborn animals, which
allows the passage of bacteria through the stomach, thirdly, the rapid
change in intestinal conditions and redifferentiation of the ileal epithelium immediately after weaning, fourthly, the developing immune
system of the host and, finally, the age-dependent presence of intestinal
receptors.

The amount of K88 receptor in the ileal mucus of seven-week-old pigs
is 16 times that in neonatal piglets, and is sufficient to prevent adhesion to
the epithelial cells (Conway *et al.*, 1990). In neonatal piglets, however,

K88-positive *E. coli* cannot be sufficiently contained within the mucus layer. This allows the bacteria to pass across this layer and bind to the epithelial cells, where toxin is released and diarrhoea follows. The mucus of six-month-old pigs no longer has K88 receptors. In contrast, the presence of receptors in the brush-border fraction is independent of age (Willemsen & de Graaf, 1992).

A similar situation has been observed for *E. coli* that carry 987P fimbriae, which adhere equally well to isolated intestinal epithelial brush borders from neonatal and older pigs. They are, however, associated *in vivo* with mucus-like material in the bowel of older pigs, while in neonatal piglets they are associated with the epithelium (Dean *et al.*, 1989). Resistance is apparently due to the inability of bacteria to reach the epithelial cells because of their association with intestinal mucus and not because of the absence of receptors. Furthermore, differences have been observed between receptors for 987P fimbriae, present in brush border membranes of sensitive neonatal and resistant older animals, and in the receptor present in the mucus fraction of older pigs (Dean, 1990). Only trace amounts of the latter receptor were found in 987P-susceptible animals.

In contrast, isolated intestinal epithelial cells from older animals do not interact with K99-fimbriate bacteria, which indicates a loss of receptor material with ageing. Comparison of glycolipids from small intestinal mucosal scrapings of newborn and adult pigs for their ability to recognise K99-fimbriate bacteria showed that material from older pigs does not bind these organisms (Teneberg *et al.*, 1990). Analysis of the isolated glycolipids showed that the *N*-glycolyl groups disappeared with age and there was an increase in *N*-acetyl groups. Age-dependent O-acetylation of sialic acid in the mucosa is also said to contribute to age-dependent susceptibility (Lindahl *et al.*, 1987). Evidence for the existence of adhesive and non-adhesive pig phenotypes has been presented (Seignole *et al.*, 1991). The glycolipids of piglets of the K99-susceptible phenotype were richer in gangliosides with *N*-glycolyl groups than were those of the K99-resistant phenotype in which *N*-acetyl groups were predominant.

Structure–function relationships

As we have seen, the differences between the nucleotide sequence of the various K88 operons are confined to the gene that encodes the major fimbrial subunit FaeG (Bakker *et al.*, 1992a). Treatment of K88 fimbriae with 2 M urea at 55°C removes all the minor fimbrial subunits without affecting their adhesive properties (Bakker *et al.*, 1992b). The differences in haemagglutination pattern observed for the K88 subtypes can, therefore, be ascribed to differences in the primary structure of FaeG. Amino-acid substitutions in FaeG by site-directed mutagenesis and the construction of hybrid proteins in which various parts of the K88ab and K88ac fimbrial subunit were exchanged show that a limited number of amino-acid residues are responsible for subspecies-specific haemagglutination. There is a clear correlation between the receptor-binding site and the serotype-specific antigenic determinants (Bakker *et al.*, 1992a). The receptor-binding site is composed of two amino-acid residues with a phenylalanine or leucine hydrophobic side chain in combination with one or more charged residues. The FaeG domains involved in subunit–subunit interactions and in the interaction of FaeG and other components of the K88 excretion pathway have been detected by a similar approach (Bakker *et al.*, 1991; Pedersen, 1991).

Small peptides, derived from the K88 fimbrial subunit, that contain a phenylalanine residue inhibit haemagglutination by purified fimbriae and the adherence of the latter to intestinal brush borders (Jacobs *et al.*, 1987c). Mutation of phenylalanine-150 abolishes the adhesive capacity of the fimbriae (Jacobs *et al.*, 1987a). Knowledge of the conserved and variable regions in the K88 fimbrial subunit has made possible the insertion of foreign epitopes into particular regions of the FaeG sequence and an immune response to the foreign determinant is induced on immunisation (Thiry *et al.*, 1989; Bakker *et al.*, 1990).

Comparison of the primary structure of the K99 fimbrial subunit with the primary structure of other adhesins that recognise sialic-acid-containing receptors, such as CFA/I subunits, the SfaS adhesin of S-fimbriae and the β-subunits of heat-labile (LT) and cholera toxin (CT) enterotoxins revealed a homologous sequence that is probably involved in receptor binding. Alteration of lysine-132 or arginine-136 of the K99 fimbrial subunit and of lysine-116 or arginine-118 in the SfaS adhesin abolishes the adhesive properties of these fimbriae (Jacobs *et al.*, 1987b; Morschhäuser *et al.*, 1990).

Biosynthesis of fimbriae

In general terms, fimbrial gene clusters encode: (i) regulatory proteins, (ii) proteins involved in the transport of fimbrial subunits across the bacterial cell envelope, and (iii) minor and major fimbrial subunits. Most minor fimbrial subunits are structurally related to the major fimbrial subunit and much evidence indicates that they play a role in the initiation, elongation and termination of the assembly of major fimbrial subunits at the cell surface.

All of the fimbrial gene clusters so far studied, except the CFA/I and CS1 gene cluster, encode a periplasmic chaperon and a high-molecular-weight protein associated with the outer membrane. The three-dimensional structure of one of the fimbrial chaperones, PapD, is known (Holmgren & Bränden, 1989). The molecule has a boomerang shape and consists of two globular immunoglobulin-type domains oriented towards one another (see Chapter 8). Comparison of the primary structures of a variety of periplasmic chaperons from different fimbrial systems has revealed a high degree of structural relationship. Superimposition of their amino-acid sequences on the three-dimensional structure of PapD shows that the immunoglobulin-like fold of the PapD protein is present in all chaperons (Holmgren *et al.*, 1992). In contrast to PapD, a monomeric protein, the chaperon protein of the K88 operon (FaeE) is a dimer (Mol *et al.*, 1994) but the reason for this difference is not clear. As compared with PapD, the FaeE protein has a carboxyl-terminal extension of nine amino-acid residues that may be involved in the dimerisation of FaeE.

An important difference between periplasmic chaperons involved in fimbrial biosynthesis and cytoplasmic chaperons like SecB is that fimbrial subunits, when bound to periplasmic chaperons, maintain their native configuration (Bakker *et al.*, 1991), while proteins bound to the chaperons of the general secretion pathway of *E. coli* are partially unfolded.

The fimbrial operons of human ETEC appear to be simpler and to contain fewer genes than those of animal ETEC. The CFA/I operon does not have a gene that encodes a protein with the features of a chaperon-like protein (Jordi *et al.*, 1992b). It is at present unknown whether a similar function is carried out by one of the other proteins encoded by the operon or whether another chaperon protein, present in *E. coli* but not actually belonging to this operon, is involved. The operons that encode fibrillar adhesion antigens like CS3 and CS6 do, however, contain a gene for a protein with structural features similar to the PapD and FaeE proteins (Jalajakumari *et al.*, 1990).

Little is known about the high-molecular-weight proteins involved in the translocation of fimbrial subunits across the outer membrane. The number of K88 fimbriae per cell is directly related to the amount of the FaeD protein in the outer membrane. The subcellular localisation of the FaeD protein is evidence of an association with the outer membrane, but some FaeD protein is also found in association with the cytoplasmic membrane (van Doorn *et al.*, 1982). On the basis of computer predictions, it is assumed that these proteins contain a limited number of transmembrane sequences but are not integral outer-membrane proteins such as OmpA. The high-molecular-weight 'assembly platforms' for fimbrial biosynthesis are conserved in all systems. The primary structure of members of this protein family shows a fair degree of homology. It is probable that the 'assembly platforms' assist in the ordered assembly of fimbrial subunits in a process which requires: (i) the recognition of a chaperon–fimbrial subunit complex, (ii) the release of the chaperon and (iii) addition of the fimbrial subunit to the growing fimbriae. In this model the 'assembly platform' accommodates a binding site for chaperon-subunit complexes and an anchor site for growing fimbriae. Ordered assembly of major and various minor fimbrial subunits in the ultimate fimbrial structure may be guided by the relative concentrations of the different subunits in the periplasm, differences in affinity between various types of subunits, and/or differences in affinity of the chaperon–subunit complexes for their binding site on the assembly platform.

The regulation of fimbrial biosynthesis

Growth conditions

The biosynthesis of fimbriae is regulated by a number of environmental factors. In steady-state chemostat cultures fimbrial biosynthesis correlates with the specific growth rate (van Verseveld *et al.*, 1985; van der Woude *et al.*, 1989). The highest production is found at the maximal growth rate, while at lower growth rates production gradually decreases.

The biosynthesis of all fimbrial adhesins, other than type-1 fimbriae, is repressed below 37°C. Thermoregulation and growth-rate-dependent production of fimbriae affect the level of transcription, probably by controlling promoter activity (van der Woude *et al.*, 1990).

The effect of carbohydrates and amino-acids on production of fimbriae has been studied in detail for K99 fimbriae. Early experiments showed that the synthesis of these fimbriae is subject to glucose-induced catabolite repression. Production of K99 was repressed in a *cya* mutant and was restored on addition of exogenous cAMP (Isaacson, 1983). Catabolite repression appears to depend on the host strain and is restricted to the synthesis of fimbrial subunits, but the assembly of the fimbriae is not affected. Catabolite repression also plays a role in the synthesis of CFA/I and CFA/II fimbriae (Evans *et al.*, 1991; Karjalainen *et al.*, 1991).

Expression of fimbriae by human ETEC depends on the composition of the growth medium, and addition of bile salts to CFA agar improves the production of these fimbriae.

The expression of K99 fimbriae is repressed by low concentrations of alanine or leucine (de Graaf *et al.*, 1980; Girardeau *et al.*, 1982) and studies of the effect of the leucine-responsive regulatory protein (Lrp) on K99 biosynthesis has provided an insight into the mechanism by which these amino-acids affect K99 production (Braaten *et al.*, 1992). Lrp is a global regulator that controls the transcription of several genes in *E. coli* positively or negatively for fimbrial biosynthesis (Willins *et al.*, 1991; Ernsting *et al.*, 1992). Exogenous leucine affects expression by some members of the *lrp* regulon. The *pap* operon, which encodes P-fimbriae, and the *fan* operon, which encodes K99 fimbriae, are positively controlled by Lrp and mutants defective in Lrp show a greater than 200-fold reduction in the expression of K99 fimbriae. Lrp binds to a DNA fragment that contains the major promoter for the *fan* operon (Braaten *et al.*, 1992), and alanine and leucine are said to affect the affinity of Lrp for the *fan* regulatory DNA, so reducing its positive effect on K99 expression.

Regulatory proteins encoded by fimbrial operons

Most fimbrial operons contain a regulatory region that encodes the major promoter of the operon and two regulatory genes. In the case of the K88 operon the regulatory genes are separated by two insertion sequence 1 (IS1) elements. The effect of the regulatory proteins on fimbrial expression has been investigated by the construction of mutations in the respective genes. Except for FaeA (Huisman *et al.*, 1994), all regulatory proteins have a positive effect on transcription (Göransson *et al.*, 1989; Roosendaal *et al.*, 1989; Schmoll *et al.*, 1990). Control of expression by operon-specific regulators is, however, not as strict as that observed for global regulators, such as Lrp, or other regulatory proteins involved in thermoregulation. It is possible that operon-specific regulators lower in the hierarchy enable bacteria to fine-tune the production of fimbriae within limits set by regulators further up the hierarchy.

Another type of regulation is found in the biosynthesis of 987P fimbriae and for a number of fimbriae present on human ETEC. Here, production of fimbriae depends entirely on an operon-specific regulator that depends on the otherwise silent promoter of these operons (Caron *et al.*, 1989; Klaasen & de Graaf, 1990; Willshaw *et al.*, 1991). These regulators are basic proteins with a helix-turn-helix motif found in many DNA-binding proteins and they belong to the so-called AraC family of regulatory proteins. The positive regulator for CFA/I expression (CfaD) is not required in strains with a mutation in the histone-like protein H-NS (Jordi *et al.*, 1992a). This suggests that H-NS acts as a repressor or silencer of transcription of the CFA/I operon. At low temperatures H-NS is thought to bind to the promoter region of the CFA/I operon. This binding is too strong to be countered by the CfaD protein, expression of which is itself temperature regulated. At higher temperatures the binding of H-NS to the CFA/I promoter becomes less efficient, and CfaD can replace H-NS. Binding of CfaD to the promoter changes the DNA topology in such a way that stronger promoter activity is obtained. Experiments with fragments of the CFA/I promoter region introduced into H-NS-positive and H-NS-negative strains, in the presence or absence of CfaD, indicate that H-NS and CfaD do not bind to the same DNA sequence in the promoter region (Jordi *et al.*, 1992a). In bacteria, a cluster of genes necessary for a certain function is usually organised in a polycistronic operon, like the fimbrial operons. This enables the bacterium to co-ordinate the expression of all the genes involved, by regulating the activity of a single promoter. Usually, however, different amounts of the various gene products of the operon are needed. In the case of the CFA/I operon, the differential expression of the various genes is regulated by transcriptional termination and differential stability of mRNA segments (Jordi *et al.*, 1993).

Various mechanisms have apparently evolved to control the expression of fimbriae in relation to environmental conditions. Some regulatory phenomena are reasonably well understood but it is to be expected that several components of the regulatory networks have yet to be discovered.

References

Anderson, D. G. & Moseley, S. L. (1988). The *Escherichia coli* F41 adhesin: genetic organization, nucleotide sequence, and homology with the K88 determinant. *Journal of Bacteriology*, **170**, 4890–96.

Bakker, D., Vader, C. E. M., Roosendaal, B., Mooi, F. R., Oudega, B. & de Graaf, F. K. (1991). Structure and function of periplasmic chaperone-like proteins involved in the biosynthesis of K88 and K99 fimbriae in entero-toxigenic *Escherichia coli*. *Molecular Microbiology*, **5**, 875–86.

Bakker, D., Van Zijderveld, F. G., van der Veen, S., Oudega, B. & de Graaf, F. K. (1990). K88 fimbriae as carriers of heterologous antigenic determi-nants. *Microbial Pathogenesis*, **8**, 343–52.

Bakker, D., Willemsen, P. T. J., Simons, L. H., van Zijderveld, F. G. & de Graaf, F. K. (1992a). Characterization of the antigenic and adhesive properties of FaeG, the major subunit of K88 fimbriae. *Molecular Microbiology*, **6**, 247–55.

Bakker, D., Willemsen, P. T. J., Willems, R. H., Huisman, T. T., Mooi, F. R., Oudega, B., Stegehuis, F. & de Graaf, F. K. (1992b). Identification of minor fimbrial subunits involved in biosynthesis of K88 fimbriae. *Journal of Bacteriology*, **174**, 6350–8.

Bijlsma, I. G. W., de Nijs, A., van der Meer, C. & Frik, J. F. (1982). Different pig phenotypes affect adherence of *Escherichia coli* to jejunal brush borders by K88ab, K88ac, and K88ad antigens. *Infection and Immunity*, **37**, 891–4.

Braaten, B. A., Platko, J. V., van der Woude, M. W., Simons, B. H., de Graaf, F. K., Calvo, J. M. & Low, D. A. (1992). Leucine-responsive regulatory protein controls the expression of both the *pap* and *fan* pili operons in *Escherichia coli*. *Proceedings of the National Academy of Science, USA*, **89**, 4250–4.

Caron, J., Coffield, L.M. & Scott, J. R. (1989). A plasmid encoded regulatory gene rns, required for expression of the CS1 and CS2 adhesins of enterotoxigenic *Escherichia coli*. *Proceedings of the National Academy of Science, USA*, **86**, 963–7.

Conway, P. L., Welin, A. & Cohen, P. S. (1990). Presence of K88-specific receptors in porcine ileal mucus is age dependent. *Infection and Immunity*, **58**, 3178–82.

Darfeuille-Michaud, A., Aubel, D., Chauviere, G., Rich, C., Bourges, M., Servin, A. & Joly, B. (1990). Adhesion of enterotoxigenic *Escherichia coli* to the human colon carcinoma cell line Caco-2 in culture. *Infection and Immunity*, **58**, 893–902.

Dean, E. A. (1990). Comparison of receptors for 987P pili of enterotoxigenic *Escherichia coli* in the small intestines of neonatal and older pigs. *Infection and Immunity*, **58**, 4030–5.

Dean, E. A., Whipp, S. C. & Moon, H. W. (1989). Age-specific colonization of porcine intestinal epithelium by 987P-piliated enterotoxigenic *Escherichia coli*. *Infection and Immunity*, **57**, 82–7.

Erickson, A. K., Willgohs, J. A., McFarland, S. Y., Benfield, D. A. & Francis, D. H. (1992). Identification of two porcine brush border glycoproteins that bind the K88ac adhesin of *Escherichia coli* and correlation of these glycoproteins with the adhesive phenotype. *Infection and Immunity*, **60**, 983–8.

Ernsting, B. R., Atkinson, M. R., Ninfa, A. J. & Matthews, R. G. (1992). Characterization of the regulon controlled by the leucine-responsive regulatory protein in *Escherichia coli*. *Journal of Bacteriology*, **174**, 1099–118.

Evans, D. G., Evans, D. J. Jr., Karjalainen, T. K. & Lee, C.-H. (1991). Production of Colonization factor antigen II of enterotoxigenic *Escherichia coli* is subject to catabolite repression. *Current Microbiology*, **23**, 71–4.

Evans, D. G., Evans, D. J. Jr., Opekun, A. R. & Graham, D. Y. (1988). Non-replicating oral whole cell vaccine protective against *Escherichia coli* (ETEC) diarrhea: stimulation of anti-CFA (CFA/I) and anti-enterotoxin (anti-LT) intestinal IgA and protection against challenge with ETEC belonging to heterologous serotypes. *FEMS Microbiology and Immunology*, **47**, 117–26.

Faris, A., Lindahl, M. & Wadström, T. (1980). GM2-like glycoconjugate as possible erythrocyte receptor for the CFA/I and K99 haemagglutinins of enterotoxigenic *Escherichia coli*. *FEMS Microbiology Letters*, **7**, 265–9.

Girardeau, J. P., Bertin, Y., Martin, C., Der Vartanian, M. & Boeuf, C. (1991). Sequence analysis of the *clpG* gene, which codes for surface antigen CS31A subunit: evidence of an evolutionary relationship between CS31A, K88 and F41 subunit genes. *Journal of Bacteriology*, **173**, 7673–83.

Girardeau, J. P., Dubourguier, H. C. & Gouet, P. (1982). Inhibition of K99 antigen synthesis by L-alanine in enterotoxigenic *Escherichia coli*. *Journal General Microbiology*, **128**, 463–70.

Göransson, M., Forsman, K., Nilsson, P. & Uhlin, B. E. (1989). Upstream activating sequences that are shared by two divergently transcribed operons mediate cAMP–CRP regulation of pilus-adhesin in *Escherichia coli*. *Molecular Microbiology*, **3**, 1557–65.

de Graaf, F. K., Klaasen-Boor, P. & van Hees, J. E. (1980). Biosynthesis of the K99 surface antigen is impaired by alanine. *Infection and Immunity*, **30**, 125–8.

de Graaf, F. K. & Mooi, F. R. (1986). The fimbrial adhesins of *Escherichia coli*. *Advances in Microbial Physiology*, **28**, 65–143.

Holmgren, A. & Bränden, C.-I. (1989). Crystal structure of chaperone protein PapD reveals an immunoglobulin fold. *Nature*, **342**, 248–51.

Holmgren, A., Kuehn, M. J., Bränden, C.-I. & Hultgren, S. J. (1992). Conserved immunoglobulin-like features in a family of periplasmic pilus chaperones in bacteria. *EMBO Journal*, **11**, 1617–22.

Huisman, T. T., Bakker, D., Klaasen, P. & de Graaf, F. K. (1994). Leucine-responsive regulatory protein, IS*1* insertions, and the negative regulator FaeA control the expression of the *fae* (K88) operon in *Escherichia coli*. *Molecular Microbiology*, **11**, 525–36.

Isaacson, R. E. (1983). Regulation of expression of *Escherichia coli* pilus K99. *Infection and Immunity*, **40**, 633–9.

Jacobs, A. A. C., Roosendaal, B., van Breemen, J. F. L. & de Graaf, F. K. (1987a). Role of phenylalanine 150 in the receptor-binding domain of the K88 fibrillar subunit. *Journal of Bacteriology*, **169**, 4907–11.

Jacobs, A. A. C., Simons, B. H. & de Graaf, F. K. (1987b). The role of lysine-132 and arginine-136 in the receptor-binding domain of the K99 fibrillar subunit. *EMBO Journal*, **6**, 1805–8.

Jacobs, A. A. C., Venema, J., Leeven, R., van Pelt-Heerschap, H. & de Graaf, F. K. (1987c). Inhibition of adhesive activity of K88 fibrillae by peptides derived from the K88 adhesin. *Journal of Bacteriology*, **169**, 735–41.

Jalajakumari, M. B., Thomas, C. J., Halter, R. & Manning, P. A. (1990). Genes for biosynthesis and assembly of CS3 pili of CFA/II enterotoxigenic *Escherichia coli*: novel regulation of pilus production by bypassing an amber codon. *Molecular Microbiology*, **3**, 1685–95.

Jordi, B. J. A. M., Dagberg, B., de Haan, L. A. M., Hamers, A. M., van der Zeijst, B. A. M., Gaastra, W. & Uhlin, B. E. (1992a). The positive regulator CfaD overcomes the repression mediated by histone-like protein H-NS (H1) in the CFA/I fimbrial operon of *Escherichia coli*. *EMBO Journal*, **11**, 2627–32.

Jordi, B. J. A. M., Op den Camp, I. E. L., de Haan, L. A. M., van der Zeijst, B. A. M. & Gaastra, W. (1993). Differential decay of RNA of the CFA/I fimbrial operon and the control of relative gene expression. *Journal of Bacteriology*, **175**, 7976–81.

Jordi, B. J. A. M., Willshaw, G. A., van der Zeijst, B. A. M. & Gaastra, W. (1992b). The complete nucleotide sequence of region 1 of the CFA/I fimbrial operon of human enterotoxigenic *Escherichia coli*. *DNA Sequences*, **2**, 257–63.

Karjalainen, T. K., Evans, D. G., Evans, D. J. Jr., Graham, D. Y. & Lee, C.-H. (1991). Catabolite repression of the colonization factor antigen I (CFA/I) operon of *Escherichia coli*. *Current Microbiology*, **23**, 307–13.

Klaasen, P. & de Graaf, F. K. (1990). Characterization of FapR, a positive regulator of expression of the 987P operon in enterotoxigenic *Escherichia coli*. *Molecular Microbiology*, **4**, 1779–83.

Klemm, P. & Mikkelsen, L. (1982). Prediction of antigenic determinants and secondary structures of the K88 and CFA/I fimbrial proteins from enterotoxigenic *Escherichia coli*. *Infection and Immunity*, **38**, 41–5.

Krivan, H. C., Franklin, D. P., Wang, W., Laux, D. C. & Cohen, P. S. (1992). Phosphatidylserine found in intestinal mucus serves as a sole source of carbon and nitrogen for *Salmonellae* and *Escherichia coli*. *Infection and Immunity*, **60**, 3943–6.

Kyogashima, M., Ginsburg, V. & Krivan, H. C. (1989). *Escherichia coli* K99 binds to *N*-glycolylsialoparagloboside and *N*-glycolyl-GM3 found in piglet small intestine. *Archives of Biochemistry and Biophysics*, **270**, 392–7.

Lindahl, M., Brossmer, R. & Wadström, T. (1987). Carbohydrate receptor specificity of K99 fimbriae of enterotoxigenic *Escherichia coli*. *Glycoconjugate Journal*, **4**, 51–18.

Lindahl, M. & Carlstedt, I. (1990). Binding of K99 fimbriae of enterotoxigenic *Escherichia coli* to pig small intestinal mucin glycopeptides. *Journal General Microbiology*, **136**, 1609–14.

McConnell, M. M., Chart, H. & Rowe, B. (1989). Antigenic homology within human enterotoxigenic *Escherichia coli* fimbrial colonization factor antigens: CFA/I, coli-surface associated antigens (CS)1, CS2, CS4 and CS17. *FEMS Microbiology Letters*, **61**, 105–8.

Mol, O., Visschers, R. W., de Graaf, F. K. & Oudega, B. (1994). *Escherichia coli* periplasmic chaperone–FaeE is a homodimer and the chaperone-K88 subunit complex is a heterotrimer. *Molecular Microbiology*, **11**, 391–402.

Morschhäuser, J., Hoschützky, H., Jann, K. & Hacker, J. (1990). Functional analysis of the sialic acid-binding adhesin SfaS and pathogenic *Escherichia coli* by site-specific mutagenesis. *Infection and Immunity*, **58**, 2133–8.

Ono, E., Abe, K., Nakazawa, M. & Naiki, M. (1989). Ganglioside epitope recognized by K99 fimbriae from enterotoxigenic *Escherichia coli*. *Infection and Immunity*, **57**, 907–11.

Orø, H. S., Kolstø, A.-B., Wennerås, C. & Svennerholm, A.-M. (1990). Identification of asialo GM1 as a binding structure for *Escherichia coli* colonization factor antigens. *FEMS Microbiology Letters*, **72**, 289–92.

Pedersen, P. A. (1991). Structure–function analysis of the K88ab fimbrial subunit protein from porcine eneterotoxigenic *Escherichia coli*. *Molecular Microbiology*, **5**, 1073–80.

Roosendaal, B., Damoiseaux, J., Jordi, W. & de Graaf, F. K. (1989). Transcriptional organization of the DNA region controlling expression of the K99 gene cluster. *Molecular and General Genetics*, **215**, 250–6.

Rudin, A., McConnel, M. M. & Svennerholm, A.-M. (1994). Monoclonal antibodies against enterotoxigenic *Escherichia coli* Colonization Factor Antigen I (CFA/I) that cross-react immunologically with heterologous CFAs. *Infection and Immununity*, **62**, 4339–46.

Rudin, A. & Svennerholm, A.-M. (1994). Colonization factor antigens (CFAs) of enterotoxigenic *Escherichia coli* can prime and boost immune responses against heterologous CFAs. *Microbial Pathogenesis*, **16**, 131–9.

Rutter, J. M., Burrows, M. R., Sellwood, R. & Gibbons, R. A. (1975). A genetic basis for resistance to enteric disease caused by *E. coli*. *Nature*, **257**, 135–6.

Schmoll, T., Morschhäuser, J., Ott, M., Ludwig, B., van Die, I. & Hacker, J. (1990). Complete genetic organization and functional aspects of the *Escherichia coli* S fimbrial adhesin determinants: nucleotide sequence of the genes *sfaB, C, D, E, F*. *Microbial Pathogenesis*, **9**, 331–43.

Seignole, D., Mouricout, M., Duval-Iflah, Y., Quintard, B. & Julien, R. (1991). Adhesion of K99 fimbriated *Escherichia coli* to pig intestinal epithelium: correlation of adhesive and non-adhesive phenotypes with the sialoglycolipid content. *Journal of General Microbiology*, **137**, 1591–601.

Smit, H., Gaastra, W., Kamerling, J. P., Vliegenthart, J. F. G. & de Graaf, F. K. (1984). Isolation and structural characterization of the equine erythrocyte receptor for enterotoxigenic *Escherichia coli* K99 fimbrial adhesin. *Infection and Immunity*, **46**, 578–84.

Teneberg, S., Willemsen, P., de Graaf, F. K. & Karlsson, K.-A. (1990). Receptor-active glycolipids of epithelial cells of the small intestine of young and adult pigs in relation to susceptibility to infection with *Escherichia coli* K99. *FEBS Letters*, **263**, 10–14.

Thiry, G., Clippe, A., Scarcez, T. & Petre, J. (1989). Cloning of DNA sequences encoding foreign peptides and their expression in the K88 pili. *Applied and Environmental Microbiology*, **55**, 984–93.

Van Doorn, J., Oudega, B., Mooi, F. R. & de Graaf, F. K. (1982). Sub-cellular localization of polypeptides involved in the biosynthesis of K88ab fimbriae. *FEMS Microbiology Letters*, **13**, 99–104.

Van Verseveld, H. W., Bakker, P., van der Woude, T., Terleth, C. & de Graaf, F. K. (1985). Production of fimbrial adhesins K99 and F41 by enterotoxigenic *Escherichia coli* as a function of growth-rate domain. *Infection and Immunity*, **49**, 159–63.

Van der Woude, M. W., Arts, P. A., Bakker, D., van Verseveld, H. W. & de Graaf, F. K. (1990). Growth-rate dependent synthesis of K99 fimbrial sub-units is regulated at the level of transcription. *Journal of General Microbiology*, **136**, 897–903.

Van der Woude, M. W., de Graaf, F. K. & van Verseveld, H. W. (1989). Production of the fimbrial adhesin 987P by enterotoxigenic *Escherichia coli* during growth under controlled conditions in a chemostat. *Journal of General Microbiology*, **135**, 3421–9.

Van Zijderveld, F. G., Anakotta, J., Brouwers, R. A. M., van Zijderveld, A. M., Bakker, D. & de Graaf, F. K. (1990). Epitope analysis of the F4 (K88) fimbrial antigen complex of enterotoxigenic *Escherichia coli* by using monoclonal antibodies. *Infection and Immunity*, **58**, 1870–8.

Van Zijderveld, F. G., Westenbrink, F., Anakotta, J., Brouwers, R. A. M. & van Zijderveld, A. M. (1989). Characterization of the F41 fimbrial antigen of enteropathogenic *Escherichia coli* by using monoclonal antibodies. *Infection and Immunity*, **57**, 1192–9.

Willemsen, P. T. J. & de Graaf, F. K. (1992). Age and serotype dependent binding of K88 fimbriae to porcine intestinal receptors. *Microbial Pathogenesis*, **12**, 367–75.

Willins, D. A., Ryan, C. W., Platko, J. V. & Calvo, J. M. (1991). Characterization of Lrp, and *Escherichia coli* regulatory protein that mediates a global response to leucine. *Journal of Biological Chemistry*, **266**, 10768–74.

Willshaw, G. A., Smith, H. R., McConnell, M. M. & Rowe, B. (1991). Cloning of regulator genes controlling fimbrial production by enterotoxigenic *Escherichia coli. FEMS Microbiology Letters*, **82**, 125–30.

Worobec, E. A., Shastry, P., Smart, W., Bradley, R., Singh, B. & Paranchych, W. 1983). Monoclonal antibodies against colonization factor antigen I pili from enterotoxigenic *Escherichia coli. Infection and Immunity*, **41**, 1296–301.

8

Assembly of adhesive virulence-associated pili in Gram-negative bacteria

K. W. DODSON, F. JACOB-DUBUISSON,
R. T. STRIKER and S. J. HULTGREN

Many infections, including urinary tract infections, are initiated by molecular interactions between bacterial adhesins and specific complementary molecules on host cells called receptors. Bacteria have developed complex mechanisms to present their adhesins to eukaryotic receptors that promote binding and determine whether extracellular colonisation, internalisation or other cellular responses will occur (Beachey et al., 1988; Jones et al., 1992). Three basic molecular mechanisms for presenting hundreds of different kinds of adhesive proteins and organelles have been described for Gram-negative bacteria; the chaperone/usher pathway that will be discussed in detail below, the general assembly pathway (type-IV pili), and the extracellular nucleation/precipitation pathway (curli) (Hultgren et al., 1995; Pugsley, 1993).

The chaperon/usher-dependent pathway is present in all Enterobacteriaceae and other Gram-negative bacteria (Hultgren et al., 1995) and is probably the best understood of all of the assembly mechanisms. The bacterial adhesins assembled by the chaperone/usher-dependent pathway are frequently located in adhesive fibres called pili or fimbriae and mediate the colonisation of mucosal surfaces through high-affinity binding to specific cell surface glycolipid and glycoprotein architectures (Normark et al., 1986; Williams et al., 1988; Stromberg et al., 1992). The recognition of host receptor structures by pilus adhesins is extremely finely tuned and allows for selective interactions with the host that partly account for the restricted range of hosts, tissues and cell types that a pathogen is able to colonise (Hultgren et al., 1993a). This phenomenon is referred to as tropism. Host and tissue tropism of pathogenic microorganisms restricts the search for receptor molecules to a specific set of tissues, as is illustrated by the clinical features of a given infection.

Microbial infections are often accompanied by an immediate and intense inflammatory reaction with a significant impact on the survival of the pathogen and on the severity of the disease. In some cases the inflammatory response is the result of an interaction between pilus-associated adhesins and complementary receptors on inflammatory cells, such as mast cells, neutrophils and macrophages (see Chapter 19). These adhesin–receptor interactions induce the release of significant amounts of histamine, leukotrienes (LTB_4), and various cytokines including tumour necrosis factor α (TNF-α) (Malaviya *et al.*, 1996). Thus, in addition to the role of bacterial adhesins in mediating microbial colonisation of mucosal surfaces and the initiation of infections, they also induce an inflammatory response that results in the clinical manifestations of disease. In this chapter uropathogenic bacteria will be considered as the model for an understanding of the molecular basis of the function of bacterial adhesins, their assembly by the chaperone/usher-dependent pathway and the mechanisms by which the structural pilus subunits are assembled into adhesive pili.

Urinary tract infections

Urinary tract infection is a major cause of morbidity, particularly in females. Up to 20 per cent of American women receive medical attention for a urinary tract infection at least once and almost three per cent have more than one infection a year (Patton *et al.*, 1991; Ronald & Pattullo, 1991). In pre-school children urinary tract infection can lead to renal scarring.

Escherichia coli is the most common Gram-negative organism to cause urinary tract infection and is responsible for 85 per cent of community-acquired and 25 per cent of nosocomial urinary tract infections. It is also responsible for about six per cent of hospital-acquired septicaemia, much of which is related to a primary urinary tract infection. Urinary tract infections are considered in detail in Chapter 18.

Some five to ten per cent of human faecal strains of *E. coli* and up to 90 per cent of those isolated from the urinary tract of children with acute pyelonephritis possess genes involved in the biosynthesis and expression of functional P-pili, which allow these organisms to bind to and colonise the host tissue.

The composite structure of P-pili

The architecture of P-pili reveals both singular and general features for pilus assembly in Gram-negative bacteria. Most adhesive fibres assembled by the chaperone/usher-dependent pathway adopt one of two basic morphologies, as seen by low resolution electron microscopy. These are, rod-like helical fibres with a diameter of 5–10 nm (Brinton, 1965; Gong & Makowski, 1992), or flexible, thin fibrillae with a diameter of 2–5 nm (Duguid *et al.*, 1955, 1979; Brinton, 1959; Duguid & Old, 1980; de Graaf *et al.*, 1986). The S-, 987P-, CFA/I-, CS1-, CS2-, and F17-pili of *E. coli* appear to have a rod-like architecture similar to that of the closely related type-1 and P-pili (de Graaf *et al.*, 1986). In contrast, other pili, such as those that facilitate intestinal colonisation and those associated with enterotoxin-producing *E. coli*, K88-, K99-, F41- and CS3-pili (fibrillae), appear to have an open helical structure without an axial hole and consequently, are much thinner and less rigid structures (de Graaf *et al.*, 1981, 1986). Another group of adhesive organelles assembled by the chaperone/usher-dependent pathway are less than 2 nm in diameter and tend to coil up into a fuzzy adhesive mass on the surface of the bacterium that is sometimes called a capsular antigen or thin aggregative pili. There are also many examples of adhesins that are not part of any known oligomeric structures. These adhesins are typically referred to as non-pilus associated adhesins (Jones *et al.*, 1995a; Hung *et al.*, 1996.

The two *pap* gene clusters of a urinary isolate of *E. coli* (J96) that encode for P-pili have been cloned (Hull *et al.*, 1981), sequenced and characterised by linker insertion mutagenesis (Hultgren *et al.*, 1991a,b, 1993a; Jones *et al.*, 1992). The *pap* gene cluster contains 11 genes (Plate 1). Together these encode the regulatory, assembly and structural proteins necessary to form an adhesive composite structure on the surface of *E. coli*. *PapA* encodes the major subunit which, when polymerised, forms a stiff right-handed helical rod extending from the surface of bacteria. By means of genetic methods and high-resolution freeze-etch electron microscopy it was shown that P-pili are composite structures in which PapK, PapE, PapF and PapG form a flexible adhesive fibrillum that is joined to the distal end of the pilus rod (Kuehn *et al.*, 1992) (Plate). The PapG adhesin is localised at the distal end of the tip fibrillae which are composed mostly of repeating PapE subunits. Examination of purified type-1 pili of clinical isolates of *E. coli*, *Enterobacter cloacae*, *Citrobacter freundii*, and *Klebsiella pneumoniae* and S-fimbriae from a meningitis isolate of *E. coli* showed that these structures are also composite fibres with tip fibrillae joined end-to-end to pilus rods (Jones *et al.*, 1995b). Type-1 tip fibrillae are composed of FimH, the mannose-binding adhesin, and at least one of the minor pilus proteins, FimG. The location of the adhesins PapG and FimH in flexible tip structures may represent an evolutionary selection to present the adhesins in the best possible position for binding to their respective receptors on eukaryotic epithelial tissues. The presence of the rigid helical rods may position the adhesin away from the interference of lipopolysaccharide and other bacterial cell surface components, while the flexible tip fibrillum allows the adhesin maximum steric freedom to recognise and bind to receptors on the host epithelium.

A three-dimensional reconstruction of the P-pilus rod has been described by Bullitt & Makowski (1995). The pilus rod is a right-handed helix (3.3 subunits per turn), 68 Å (6.8 nm) in diameter and approximately 1 mm in length. In addition, the pilus rod has a 15 Å (1.5 nm) helical cavity that winds through it with a set of radial channels that allow access to the external environment. From the reconstruction it was inferred that PapA subunits interact in at least four ways in the rod. Two of the interactions are best described as head-to-tail between neighbouring subunits and define the fibrillar PapA polymer. The other two interactions result in the transition from the thin fibrillar conformation of the PapA polymer to the right-handed helical rod.

Bacteria that possess P-pili are resistant to displacement from the uroepithelium by bulk fluid flow. Bullit & Makowski (1995) presented a 'bungee cord' model to account for this resistance to shear force and the observation of stretched out pili and sharp bends in pili when viewed by electron microscopy after normal preparation protocols. They suggested that the rod-forming interactions might be perturbed by bulk fluid flow in the urinary tract resulting in the pili reverting to a linear polymer conformation. It is of interest that the extended segments of the PapA polymer resemble tip fibrillae and have an open helical structure and dimensions similar to those of tip fibrillae. This model suggests that transition of the PapA polymer from the helical to the fibrillar conformation provides a degree of flexibility that allows bacteria to adhere and colonise tissues in the urinary tract.

The assembly proteins

Pili assembled by the chaperone/usher-dependent pathway have diverse molecular architectures and possess different adhesins that recognise a wide range of receptors (Hultgren *et al.*, 1995). In each case a member of the chaperone family of proteins is required in the periplasm to escort each structural subunit from the inner membrane to a member of the usher family of proteins in the outer membrane. Here the chaperone is dissociated from the subunit, which is then correctly positioned in the final pilus structure. The ordered progression of protein–protein recognition events required for the growth of virulence-associated pili therefore represents a common theme in Gram-negative pathogens. A better understanding of these common processes will provide a basis to study and test means of interrupting these processes and so facilitate the design of novel anti microbial compounds for the treatment and prevention of infections due to diverse Gram-negative bacterial pathogens.

The chaperone family

The assembly of adhesive pili requires specialised periplasmic chaperones to ensure that correct assembly predominates over non-productive interactions (Hultgren *et al.*, 1993a). Periplasmic chaperones function to cap and partition interactive pilin subunits imported into the periplasmic space into assembly-competent complexes (Kuehn *et al.*, 1991). More than 30 members of the periplasmic chaperone family are recognised. They can be divided into two subfamilies based on the clustering of subfamily-specific conserved residues in a region that in the PapD chaperone is critical for subunit binding. One subfamily assembles rod-like pili, while the other assembles non-pilus organelles that have an atypical morphology. PapD, the P pilus chaperone, is the prototype member of the periplasmic chaperone family (Hung *et al.*, 1996). PapD is a classical example of a molecular chaperone. Its function is to bind related proteins (PapA, PapK, PapE, PapF, and the adhesin PapG) and escort them from the cytoplasmic membrane to an outer-membrane assembly site that consists of PapC, to allow the correct folding and assembly of the various components into pili without the chaperone itself becoming a part of the final structures. Most molecular chaperone proteins, such as GroEL and Hsp70, appear to bind a diverse group of target proteins in a sequence-independent manner and maintain them in semi-unfolded conformations (Hemmingsen *et al.*, 1988; Crooke *et al.*,

1988a,b; Lecker *et al.*, 1989, 1990; Ostermann, 1990; Ellis & van der Vies, 1991; Flynn *et al.*, 1991; Grimm *et al.*, 1991), but the molecular details of how chaperones recognise the diverse target proteins remain unclear. PapD is unique among these general cellular chaperones in that it appears to maintain its bound target in a folded conformation (Kuehn *et al.*, 1991). The structure of PapD has been shown to be an immunoglobulin-like fold (Holmgren & Brändén, 1989), a structure that specialises in protein–protein recognition events (Hultgren *et al.*, 1993b). PapD consists of two immunoglobulin-like domains oriented in a boomerang shape so that a cleft is formed (Holmgren & Brändén, 1989). Unlike binding paradigms used by other proteins with immunoglobulin domains, PapD recognises and binds subunits by its highly conserved cleft (Slonim *et al.*, 1992; Kuehn *et al.*, 1993).

The chaperone recognition paradigm

It has been shown that the extreme carboxyl-terminus of the pap subunits forms part of the recognition domain for PapD (Kuehn *et al.*, 1993). Most pilin subunits have a conserved pattern of carboxyl-terminal alternating hydrophobic residues. In addition, many pilin subunits have a penulti- mate tyrosine and a glycine 14 residues from their carboxyl-terminus. In PapG this region is important for chaperone binding, since deletion of the last 14 residues abolishes the formation of a PapD–PapG complex *in vivo* (Hultgren *et al.*, 1989). Peptides have been synthesised that correspond to the last 19 amino acids of the P-pilus subunits, and the ability of PapD to bind the carboxyl-terminal peptides was tested by ELISA. PapD binds best to the peptide that corresponds to the carboxyl-terminus of PapG (Kuehn *et al.*, 1993). In addition, the PapG peptide blocks the binding of PapD to PapG *in vitro*, which suggests that the interaction was biolog- ically relevant. The X-ray crystal structure of the PapD–PapG peptide complex shows that the carboxyl-terminus of the peptide is anchored in the bottom of the PapD cleft by hydrogen bonds between the carboxyl group of the peptide and the invariant arginine 8 and lysine 112 residues of PapD (Plate 1). The positioning of the peptide along the exposed edge of the G1 β-strand of PapD is mostly the result of backbone hydrogen bonds. In addition, the alternating hydrophobic residues in the peptide are in register with corresponding hydrophobic residues in the G1 strand of PapD, which allows hydrophobic interactions to take place. The bound peptide forms a parallel β-strand so that the β-sheet of domain 1 in PapD is extended into the peptide. This chaperone-binding paradigm is, there-

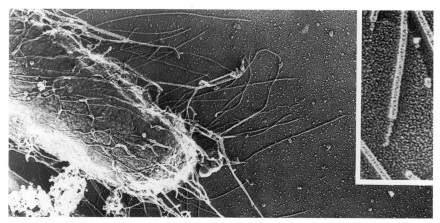

Plate 1 [A] Electron micrograph of a P-piliated bacterium. The inset is a freeze-etch electron micrograph (courtesy of J. Heuser) showing the composite nature of P-pili, which are composed of a thin flexible tip fibrillum joined end-to-end to a rigid helical rod.

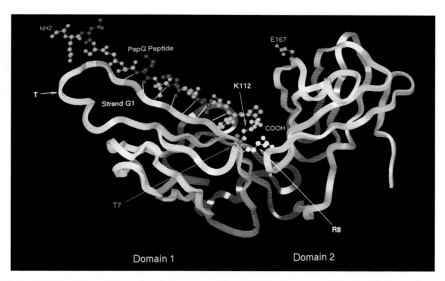

[B] Model of the three-dimensional structure of PapD (ribbon) co-crystallised with the carboxyl-terminal G1-19 peptide shown in ball and stick (Kuehn *et al.*, 1993). The PapG peptide is bound in an extended conformation to the G1 strand of PapD, with the carboxyl-terminus of the peptide anchored in the cleft by interactions with the Arg-8 (R8) and Lys-112 (K112) of PapD. The hydrogen bonds between main chain atoms in the peptide and PapD are shown with white lines.

I	B	A	H	C	D	J	K	E	F	G
		Major pilus rod protein	Minor pilin - pilus anchor	Outer-membrane usher	Periplasmic chaperone		Minor pilin -adaptor/ initiator	Major tip compo- nent	Minor pilin - adaptor/ initiator	Galα (1-4) Gal-binding adhesin

[C] Representation of the genetic organisation of the *pap* gene cluster. Proposed functions for the gene products are shown below the genes.

see facing page 218

fore, referred to as a β-zipper and the carboxyl-terminal motif of subunits recognised by PapD is referred to as a β-zipper motif. Site-directed mutations in the anchoring residues of the chaperone (arginine 8 and lysine 112) abolish the ability of PapD to bind to subunits and mediate their assembly into pili. Based on these and other studies it is proposed that immunoglobulin-like chaperones bind to their subunits by a β-zipper recognition paradigm.

A second site on PapG critical for recognition by PapD has been identified by Zu *et al.* (1995). Binding studies *in vitro* and *in vivo* with a series of gene fusions that encode differing lengths of the carboxyl-terminus of PapG and *papG* truncates show that a second site in PapG, between residues 175 and 190, is critical for a stable interaction with PapD. Further detailed investigation of the two interaction sites of PapG with PapD and of folding and assembly will lead to a more detailed understanding of the role of the PapD chaperone in pilus assembly.

Chaperone–subunit complexes

Chaperone–subunit complexes are stable and can be purified. This has been done for the PapD–PapG, PapD–PapK, PapD–PapE and PapD–PapA complexes (Hultgren *et al.*, 1989; Lindberg *et al.*, 1989; Striker *et al.*, 1994). In addition, a stable PapD–(PapA)$_2$ complex has been isolated and shown to consist of a PapA–PapA dimer bound to PapD. In the absence of the chaperone the subunits cannot be incorporated into pili because they aggregate prematurely and/or are degraded by periplasmic proteases such as DegP (Bakker *et al.*, 1991; C. H. Jones & S. J. Hultgren, unpublished). When bound to the chaperone, the subunits are maintained in native conformations; the disulphide bonds of the subunits in their complexes are formed, the PapG adhesin can bind its glycolipid receptor, and PapA can interact in a stable manner with another PapA (Hultgren *et al.*, 1989; Kuehn *et al.*, 1991; Striker *et al.*, 1994).

The usher family

The conversion of the chaperone–subunit complexes into pili depends on PapC, since it does not occur in its absence (Norgren *et al.*, 1987). Studies *in vitro* by Dodson *et al.* (1993) suggest that PapC may regulate the ordered targeting of chaperone–subunit complexes to the outer membrane-assembly site, where the chaperone is dissociated from the respective subunit to allow its polymerisation into pili. PapC is referred to as a molecular 'usher' (Jones *et al.*, 1992; Dodson *et al.*, 1993), because, like a human usher, PapC can distinguish between 'ticket holders' and allow them entry into the pilus structure only at the proper time and place. PapC is a representative member of a growing family of more than 30 (Lombardo & S. J. Hultgren, unpublished) outer-membrane proteins from a variety of Gram-negative bacteria that are required for pilus assembly in these organisms (for examples see Orndorff & Falkow, 1984; Mooi *et al.*, 1986; Jalajakumari *et al.*, 1989; Roosendaal & de Graaf, 1989; Lintermans, 1990; Rioux *et al.*, 1990; Schmoll *et al.*, 1990; Allen *et al.*, 1991; Karlyshev *et al.*, 1992; Locht *et al.*, 1992; Watson *et al.*, 1994). It is likely that all these proteins have similar usher functions that act in concert with their respective chaperone partners (Holmgren *et al.*, 1992; Jacob-Dubuisson *et al.*, 1993b; Hung *et al.*, 1996). The interaction of the chaperone–subunit complex with the usher results in the dissociation of the chaperone and the subsequent assembly of subunits into ordered adhesive structures. It is of interest that a chromosomally located homologue of PapC (HtrE) has been characterised (Raina *et al.*, 1993). Transposon insertion mutations within *htrE* result in a temperature-sensitive growth phenotype, which raises the possibility that homologues of the pilus ushers may have wider roles in cellular maintenance.

Subunit contacts and models of assembly

PapD forms two distinct periplasmic complexes with the major pilin subunit PapA (Striker *et al.*, 1994). One is a 1:1 PapD–PapA complex, while the other is a 1:2 PapD–(PapA)$_2$ complex. The latter can be dissociated with sodium dodecyl sulphate into PapD and a PapA–PapA dimer, which suggests that the 1:2 complex contains stable PapA–PapA interactions. PapA also forms higher order oligomers in the periplasm, as does the only other fibre-forming subunit PapE, but PapA is the only subunit that can associate with PapD as a dimer. All of the other chaperone–subunit complexes are thought to exist in a 1:1 stoichiometry. Subunits that do not make homopolymeric interactions, such as PapK, do not form oligomers in the periplasm (Striker *et al.*, 1994).

The 1:1 PapD–PapA complex is a true assembly intermediate, because its depletion from the periplasm shows the same first-order kinetics as the incorporation of PapA into pili. The role of the PapD–(PapA)$_2$ complex is not clear at present. While it seems that most PapA subunits are

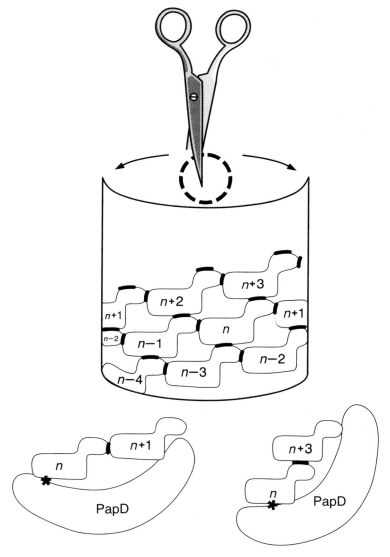

Fig. 8.1. Model of P-pilus structure. Reconstruction of the P-pilus by Bullitt & Makowski (1995) by electron microscopy shows that a PapA subunit in the pilus makes contacts not only with the subunits that are direct linear neighbours ($n\pm1$), but also with the subunits one turn ahead and one turn behind in the helical pilus rod ($n\pm3$). The PapA–PapA contact in the PapD–(PapA)$_2$ complex most probably represents either a $n\pm1$ or $n\pm3$ contact.

incorporated into the final pilus structure from the 1:1 PapD–PapA complex, and not from the 1:2 PapD–(PapA)$_2$ complex, it is possible that the latter plays a role in nucleating the assembly of PapA subunits into the thick helical fimbrial shaft that follows the linear polymerisation of PapE in the tip fibrillum (Striker *et al.*, 1994). The PapA–PapA interaction in the PapD–(PapA)$_2$ complex is assembly-competent, at least *in vitro*, because repeated freezing and thawing of purified PapD–(PapA)$_2$ leads to the dissociation of PapD and the formation of short rods virtually identical to pili in dimension and ultrastructure (Bullit *et al.*, 1996). The interactions between the two PapA subunits in the PapD–(PapA)$_2$ complex probably, therefore, represent one of the two PapA contacts found in the pilus (see Figure 8.1). Further work should elucidate the nature of the PapA–PapA interactions in the PapD-(PapA)$_2$ complex and in the pilus, and give a better insight into the extremely stable nature of the fimbrial structure.

The assembly of protein polymers has been characterised as following one of two different mechanisms. One is linear growth, where the addition of each subunit occurs at the same rate throughout assembly. The other is nucleated growth, in which a small number of subunits polymerise at a relatively slow rate to form a nucleation centre. Once nucleus formation is complete, polymerisation of additional subunits is a rapid and co-operative process. The latter mechanism occurs in most well-studied systems, such as actin and microtubule assembly, sickle-cell haemoglobin aggregation, and amyloid deposition (Jarrett & Lansbury, 1993). Whether PapA and PapE oligomers present in the periplasmic space are true intermediates has important implications for which model is correct for pilus assembly.

A system has been developed for the reconstitution *in vitro* of the two major sub-assemblies of virulence-associated P-pili (Bullit *et al.*, 1996), by dissociating the PapD chaperone from purified chaperone–subunit complexes. Excess PapD blocks the formation of pilus subassemblies, which suggests that it binds competitively to an interactive surface of the subunit involved in subunit–subunit interactions. The fate of each pilus subunit type after chaperone dissociation *in vitro* is the same as its fate *in vivo*: PapA forms rod-like subassemblies, PapE forms fibrillum-like subassemblies and PapK does not form any observable complexes at all after chaperone uncapping. The rapid formation of pilus sub-assemblies after chaperone uncapping illustrates the important role of PapD *in vivo*. The carboxyl-terminal β-zipper motif which is bound by PapD is also important in subunit–subunit interaction. This explains how the PapD chaperone controls the development of pilus fibres by capping subunit interaction sites.

Why are chaperones and ushers necessary?

The two-part subunit escorting system that involves PapD and PapC helps to ensure that the interactions between the subunits occur at the correct time and place in the cell. If PapD is not present, the subunits aggregate in the periplasmic space, either by specific interactions between the subunits or by non-specific interactions between 'sticky' uncapped regions on the subunits and other cellular components. Subsequently, these aggregates are degraded by periplasmic proteases, including DegP (Bakker *et al.*, 1991; C. H. Jones & S. J. Hultgren unpublished). If PapC is not present, the chaperone–subunit complexes are not converted into pili and, thus, chaperone–subunit complexes accumulate in the periplasm.

The problem of regulating stable protein–protein interactions is common to many cellular processes, including membrane assembly, protein secretion, organelle assembly and filament and cytoskeletal assembly. In each of these systems incorrect inter- and intra-molecular protein interactions must be prevented. Methods for regulating protein interactions include protein conformational changes, covalent modifications and differential nucleotide binding. Other mechanisms for the facilitation of ordered protein–protein interactions include physical or temporal separation and auxiliary protein binding to shield potential interactive sites from each other (for examples see Randall *et al.*, 1987; Wickner, 1989; Gething & Sambrook, 1992; Mukherjee *et al.*, 1993). Pilus assembly has evolved to use the last approach. After entry of each subunit into the periplasm, the chaperone PapD binds to and forms a stable complex with each subunit, so preventing its premature aggregation. Inherent in regulated assembly systems must be not only the ability to block interactions, but also the ability to unblock or promote correct protein–protein interactions in appropriate places at appropriate times. This might be achieved by a conformational change and/or the removal of a covalent modification or the cleavage of a nucleotide, the localisation at the same time of two interactive proteins within the same compartment of the cell, or the dissociation of an auxiliary protein to allow the creation or exposure of an interactive surface. If the mechanism for removal of the assembly block is localised in one portion of the cell, this also ensures that the assembly is spatially regulated. This appears to be the case for pilus assembly. PapC appears to be necessary for the removal of PapD from the subunits, so allowing polymerisation of the subunits to form the pilus. Localisation of PapC to the outer membrane may play a role in ensuring that the removal of PapD and subunit polymerisation are concomitant with the extrusion of the pilus through the outer membrane.

The ordering of assembly

The biogenesis *in vivo* of the final highly ordered P-pilus structure from the stable periplasmic chaperone–subunit intermediate complexes requires a regulated series of protein–protein interactions and the function of the PapC usher protein. Jacob-Dubuisson *et al.* (1993a) showed that subunit polymerisation into wild-type P-fimbriae takes place in the sequence PapG, PapF, PapE, PapK and PapA. The mechanism by which this final sequence is achieved can only be elucidated when the following two basic questions have been answered. Firstly, how are the pairwise contacts between subunits regulated and, secondly, what starts polymerisation? In answering the first question Jacob-Dubuisson *et al.* (1993a) showed that the most efficient pairwise subunit–subunit interactions are PapG–PapF, PapF–PapE, PapE–PapE, PapE–PapK, PapK–PapA and finally PapA–PapA. Insertion mutations in the *papF* gene abolish or greatly reduces the correct incorporation of the PapG adhesin into pili and also result in fewer pili being produced. This suggests that PapF is the only subunit able to join PapG efficiently to the rest of the tip fibrillum. Insertion mutations in the *papE* gene result in a dramatic reduction in the length of adhesive tip fibrillae joined to PapA pilus rods, since repeating subunits of PapE constitute the bulk of the tip fibrillae (Kuehn *et al.*, 1992). PapK is apparently able to substitute for PapE in binding to PapF, thus maintaining the ability to produce adhesive fimbriae in the absence of PapE. Similarly, the ability to produce adhesive fimbriae in the absence of PapK shows that PapE has a complementary surface that can substitute for the ability of PapK to attach to the PapA rod. In a *papK*⁻ background, however, an increased number of PapE subunits is incorporated to make the tip fibrillae approximately five times longer than in the wild-type. This suggests that the 'fit' between PapE and PapA is imperfect, resulting in additional rounds of PapE incorporation in the absence of PapK before formation of the pilus rod is initiated. When PapK is overproduced in the presence of the other tip components, extremely short adhesive tips are formed, which suggests a role for PapK in regulating the length of the tip fibrillum. In the absence of the tip fibrillar genes, P-pilus rods are not assembled, which suggests that fibrillum assembly is a prerequisite for rod assembly. It is of interest that PapK was the only tip subunit able to initiate pilus rod assembly in the absence of all other tip components. This suggests that part of the role of PapK in wild-type assembly is to terminate growth of the tip fibrillum and initiate growth of the pilus rod. Taken together, these observations show that, while the tip subunits to some extent have interchangeable activities, they each appear to be adapted for a specific role in pilus biogenesis, in this way ensuring the normal order of subunit incorporation into the pilus structure.

An insight into the mechanism that ensures that each pilus rod is joined end-to-end to an adhesive tip fibrillum was provided by Dodson *et al.* (1993), who identified and characterised specific interactions between chaperone–fimbrial protein complexes and PapC. They showed that PapD–PapG, PapD–PapF and PapD–PapE complexes can bind to PapC *in vitro*, while neither PapD–PapK nor PapD–PapA were able to bind. Moreover, PapD–PapG has a greater affinity for PapC than either PapD–PapF or PapD–PapE. It was proposed, therefore, that tip fibrillum assembly starts with PapG, because the PapD–PapG complex has the highest affinity for PapC and would be the first to bind to the assembly site (Figure 8.2). Tip assembly then proceeds with the subsequent binding of PapD–PapF, the removal of the chaperone and the joining of PapF to PapG, followed by multiple rounds of PapD–PapE binding and PapE incorporation. It was proposed that the growing tip fibrillum, in the context of PapC, then provides a site for PapD–PapK binding and PapK incorporation, which terminates growth of the tip fibrillum and allows initiation of pilus rod assembly. This is then followed by multiple rounds of PapD–PapA binding and PapA rod formation. The inability of PapD-PapK or PapD–PapA to bind to PapC alone may have been a mechanism selected in evolution to ensure the presence of an adhesive tip fibrillum at the distal end of each fimbria.

Energy

As we have seen, the assembly of P-pili takes place at the outer membrane and proceeds from chaperone–subunit periplasmic intermediates. Several events can be distinguished in the assembly of pili. Firstly, the proper targeting of chaperone–subunit complexes to the outer membrane usher protein. Secondly, dissociation of the chaperone–subunit complexes at the assembly site and release of the chaperone. Thirdly, polymerisation of one subunit with another; and, finally, physical

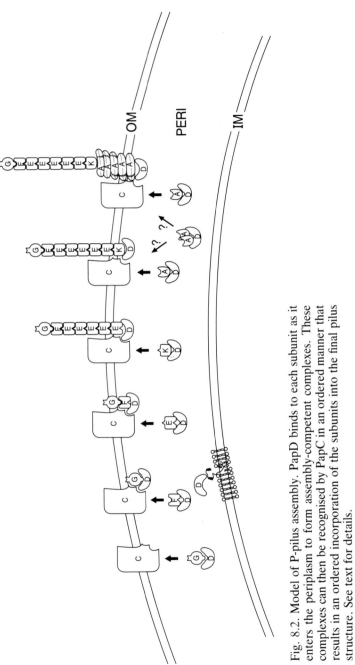

Fig. 8.2. Model of P-pilus assembly. PapD binds to each subunit as it enters the periplasm to form assembly-competent complexes. These complexes can then be recognised by PapC in an ordered manner that results in an ordered incorporation of the subunits into the final pilus structure. See text for details.

extrusion of the growing polymer. It is not known whether energy is required for any of these events, and no obvious source of energy is available in the periplasmic space or in the outer membrane. Furthermore, in contrast to cytoplasmic and intra-organelle chaperones, bacterial periplasmic chaperones do not appear to have ATP-binding sites.

In the search for an energy source, *in vivo* experiments were performed to follow the assembly of pili under various conditions, and the effect of *tonA* and *tonB* mutants on pilus assembly was investigated. TonB transmits the energy of the electrochemical potential generated across the cytoplasmic membrane to the outer membrane by means of conformational changes in order to trigger certain transport processes (Hannavy *et al.*, 1990). The function of TolA may be related to that of TonB. P-pilus assembly was unaffected in *tonB* or *tolA* null mutants (Jacob-Dubuisson *et al.*, 1995), which suggests that these proteins are not involved as an energy source for assembly, or that an as yet unidentified pilus-specific TonB-like protein may be required for assembly. In favour of the former hypothesis is the fact that inhibition of the proton-motive force with carbonylcyanide-*m*-chlorophenylhydrazone (CCCP), an inhibitor of oxidative phosphorylation, does not affect fimbrial assembly.

A pulse-chase system was established *in vivo*, in which the expression of PapC was regulated independently from that of the rest of the operon. Induction of the expression of the subunits and the chaperone, followed by a pulse labelling resulted in the accumulation of radioactively labelled chaperone–subunit complexes in the periplasm. These complexes were converted into pili during the chase only after the induction and synthesis of PapC. A lag that corresponded to the time required to synthesise and translocate PapC to the outer membrane, was followed by a net incorporation of PapE and PapA over a few minutes (Jacob-Dubuisson *et al.*, 1995). The rate of subunit incorporation was restricted by the limiting amount of PapC. In this system, the addition of CCCP just after the beginning of fimbrial assembly did not affect the incorporation of the subunits into fimbriae (Figure 8.3).

It is unlikely that there is an electrochemical gradient across the outer membrane of *E. coli*, but this has been proposed as a possible motor of protein secretion in another Gram-negative organism (Wong & Buckley, 1989). Adjustment of the external medium pH from pH 7 to pH 5 should decrease the magnitude of the proposed gradient, but this does not affect subunit incorporation into pili, which suggests that the energy from a possible electrochemical gradient across the outer membrane is not necessary for pilus assembly.

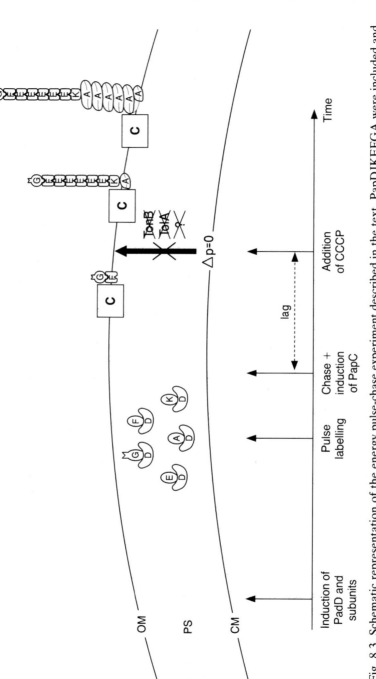

Fig. 8.3. Schematic representation of the energy pulse-chase experiment described in the text. PapDJKEFGA were included and pulse-labelled before the induction of PapC. Pilus assembly was synchronised by the induction of PapC at the beginning of the chase period. CCCP (75 μM) was added four minutes after the induction of PapC. This allowed sufficient time for PapC to reach the outer membrane (OM) and attain and functional conformation capable of initiating pilus assembly. The addition of CCCP did not affect pilus assembly, which suggests that the electro-chemical gradient across the cytoplasmic membrane (CM) was not necessary for this process.

What other energy sources may be available in the periplasm and the outer membrane? Many enzymes, toxins and adhesins are secreted by Gram-negative bacteria into the medium and serve as virulence factors, but the mechanisms that govern their secretion across the outer membrane are poorly understood. A group of proteins, collectively referred to as the general secretion pathway, function in Gram-negative organisms to translocate secretory proteins from the periplasmic space into the medium (Pugsley, 1993). One protein of the general secretory pathway, located on the cytoplasmic side of the cytoplasmic membrane, possesses an ATP-binding motif, and mutations in that nucleotide-binding site abolish protein secretion (Turner *et al.*, 1993). Assembly of type-IV pili, for which no periplasmic intermediate of assembly has been described, also require a homologous nucleotide-binding protein and certain other proteins of the general secretion pathway. Gene clusters that code for proteins homologous to the general secretion pathway proteins are also required for the secretion of certain toxins (Jiang & Howard, 1992). The apparatus that secretes proteins that do not have a detectable periplasmic intermediate, such as HlyA of *E. coli*, also includes an ATP-binding protein and proton-motive force is required in the early steps of their translocation (Koronakis *et al.*, 1991). Finally, the translocation of exported proteins across the cytoplasmic membrane by the *sec* system uses the energy of ATP hydrolysis and/or that of the proton-motive force (Bakker & Randall, 1984; Driessen, 1992). In the above examples a clear energy requirement has been demonstrated for the translocation of proteins across the cytoplasmic membrane. In contrast, the role of the ATP-binding component of the general secretory pathway in the secretion of proteins across the outer membrane has not, as yet, been clarified. It may be involved indirectly by participating in the assembly of a porthole composed of the fimbrial subunit-like proteins assembled between the two membranes, a structure that may be necessary for outer membrane secretion (Pugsley, 1993), but this has not been confirmed (Pugsley & Possot, 1994).

Secretory proteins with a periplasmic intermediate have, in most cases, achieved a substantial level of folding before translocation across the outer membrane, and some oligomeric toxins are even assembled before they are secreted (Hirst & Holmgren, 1987). Pilus subunits in pre-assembly complexes with a chaperone also appear essentially to have completed their folding, their disulphide bonds are formed, they possess a high content of secondary structure, and the adhesin has achieved its receptor-binding properties (Hultgren *et al.*, 1989; Kuehn *et al.*, 1991).

From this stage, the conversion of pilus subunits into supramolecular assemblies probably involves limited structural change. Therefore, a net energy gain derived from the folding process probably does not assist secretion. However, the association of the P-pilus subunits with a periplasmic chaperone cannot substitute for all quaternary interactions present in the final structure. Pili are very stable assemblies and the free energy difference of a subunit bound to a chaperone and a subunit incorporated into the pilus may drive assembly thermodynamically. This 'spontaneous' assembly of pili may, however, require the environment of the outer membrane and the presence of PapC. It may be a co-operative process, but it is at present not possible to measure the rate of assembly of individual PapA subunits in order to compare the incorporation of the first helical turn of PapA into that of the rest of the helix. The only rate that has been measured is the global rate of PapA incorporation into pili. Comparison of the individual rate constants with those of known co-operative processes would make it possible to define the assembly pathway better and to determine the degree of co-operativity of the process. There are other unexplored possibilities, such as the involvement of the outer membrane phosphodiesterase in providing energy for assembly. A defined *in vitro* assembly system would help to clarify the trigger for chaperone dissociation and the function of PapC in the assembly process.

Conclusions

How a diverse group of Gram-negative pathogens assemble adhesive fimbrial structures on their surfaces has been considered. The study of pilus assembly has provided valuable insights into the basic mechanisms by which cells regulate the protein–protein interactions required for protein folding, secretion and macromolecular assembly. PapD represents a large family of periplasmic chaperone proteins in Gram-negative bacteria that probably all contain an immunoglobulin-fold structure that bind to and regulates the interactions of diverse fimbrial subunits. Similarly, PapC represents a large family of outer-membrane proteins in Gram-negative bacteria that are required for the conversion of the chaperone–subunit complexes into ordered adhesive structures. The pilus subunits, while homologous to each other, have unique roles in the assembly process, including initiation and termination. Structural details of the components necessary to present adhesive pili in pathogenic bacteria are revealing opportunities for the exploitation of bacterial adhesins as new targets for multi-component vaccines against many bacterial infections. An understanding of the molecular details of the protein–protein interactions in the development of pili may make it possible to design assembly inhibitors for these structures that might be used to treat or prevent a bacterial infection by specifically inhibiting the colonisation of mucosal surfaces by pathogenic bacteria.

References

Allen, B. L., Gerlach, G. F. & Clegg, S. (1991). Nucleotide sequence and functions of *mrk*determinants necessary for expression of type 3 fimbriae in *Klebsiella pneumoniae*. *Journal of Bacteriology*, **173**, 916–20.

Bakker, E. & Randall, L. (1984). The requirement for energy during export of β-lactamase in *Escherichia coli* is fulfilled by the total proton-motive force. *EMBO Journal*, **3**, 895–900.

Bakker, D., Vader, C. E., Roosendaal, B., Mooi, F. R., Oudega, B. & de Graaf, F. K. (1991). Structure and function of periplasmic chaperone-like proteins involved in the biosynthesis of K88 and K99 fimbriae in enterotoxigenic *Escherichia coli*. *Molecular Microbiology*, **5**, 875–86.

Beachey, E. H., Giampapa, C. S. & Abraham, S. N. (1988). Adhesin receptor-mediated attachment of pathogenic bacteria to mucosal surfaces. *Mexican Review of Respiratory Disease*, **138**, S45–S48.

Brinton, C. C. (1959). Non-flagellar appendages of bacteria. *Nature* **183**, 782–6.

Brinton, C. C. Jr. (1965). The structure, function, synthesis, and genetic control of bacterial pili and a model for DNA and RNA transport in Gram-negative bacteria. *Transactions of the New York Academy of Sciences*, **27**, 1003–165.

Bullit, E., Jones, C. H., Striker, R., Sato, G., Jacob-Dubuisson, F., Pinkner, J., Wick, M. J., Makowski, L. & Hultgren, S. J., (1996). Development of pilus organelle sub-assemblies *in vitro* depends on chaperone uncapping of a beta zipper. *Proceedings of the National Academy of Sciences, USA*, in press.

Bullit, E. & Makowski, L. (1995). Structural polymorphism of bacterial adhesive pili. *Nature*, **373**, 164–7.

Crooke, E., Brundage, L., Rice, M. & Wickner, W. (1988a). Pro OmpA spontaneously folds into a membrane assembly competent state which trigger factor stabilizes. *EMBO Journal*, **7**, 1831–5.

Crooke, E., Guthrie, B., Lecker, S., Lil, R. & Wickner, W. (1988b). Pro OmpA is stabilized for membrane translocation by either purified *E. coli* trigger factor or canine signal recognition particle. *Cell*, **54**, 1003–11.

Dodson, K. W., Jacob-Dubuisson, F., Striker, R. T. & Hultgren, S. J. (1993). Outer membrane PapC usher discriminately recognizes periplasmic chaperone–pilus subunit complexes. *Proceedings of the National Acadamy of Sciences, USA*, **90**, 3670–4.

Driessen, A. (1992). Precursor protein translocation by the *E. coli* translocase is directed by the proton motive force. *EMBO Journal*, **11**, 847–53.

Duguid, J. P., Clegg, S. & Wilson, M. I. (1979). The fimbrial and non-fimbrial haemagglutinins of *Escherichia coli*. *Journal of Medical Microbiology*, **12**, 213–27.

Duguid, J. P. & Old, D. C. (1980). Adhesive properties of Enterobacteriacae. In *Bacterial Adherence Receptors and Recognition*, ed. E. H. Beachey, pp. 186–217. London: Chapman & Hall.

Duguid, J. P., Smith, I. W., Dempster, G. & Edmunds, P. N. (1955). Non-flagellar filamentous appendages ('fimbriae') and hemagglutinating activity in *bacterium coli*. *Journal of Pathology and Bacteriology*, **70**, 335–48.

Ellis, R. J. & van der Vies, S. (1991). Molecular chaperones. *Annual Review of Biochemistry*, **60**, 321–47.

Flynn, G. C., Pohl, J., Flocco, M. T. & Rothman, J. E. (1991). Peptide-binding specificity of the molecular chaperone BiP. *Nature*, **353**, 726–30.

Gething, M.-J. & Sambrook, J. (1992). Protein folding in the cell. *Nature*, **355**, 33–45.

Gong, M. & Makowski, L. (1992). Helical Structure of Pap adhesion pili from *Escherichia coli*. *Journal of Molecular Biology*, **228**, 735–42.

de Graaf, F. K., Klemm, P. & Gaastra, W. (1981). Purification, characterization and partial covalent structure of *Escherchia coli* adhesive antigen K99. *Infection and Immununity*, **33**, 877–83.

de Graaf, F. K. & Mooi, F. R. (1986). The fimbrial adhesins of *Escherichia coli*. *Advances in Microbial Physiology*, **28**, 65–143.

Grimm, R., Speth, V. Gatenby, A. A. & Schafer, E. (1991). GroEL-related molecular chaperones are present in the cytosol of oat cells. *FEBS Letters*, **286**, 155–8.

Hannavy, K., Baar, G., Dorman, C., Adamson, J., Mazengera, L., Gallagher, M., Evans, J., Levine, B., Trayer, I. & Higgins, C. (1990). TonB protein of *Salmonella typhimurium*: a model for signal transduction between membranes. *Journal of Molecular Biology*, **216**, 897–910.

Hemmingsen, S. M., Woolford, C., van der Vies, S. M., Tilly, K., Dennis, D. T., Georgopoulos, C. P., Hendrix, R. W. & Ellis, R. J. (1988). Homologous plant and bacterial proteins chaperone oligomeric protein assembly. *Nature*, **333**, 330–4.

Hirst, T. & Holmgren, J. (1987). Conformation of proteins secreted across bacterial outer membranes: a study of enterotoxin translocation from *Vibrio cholerae*. *Proceedings of the National Academy of Sciences, USA*, **84**, 7418–22.

Holmgren, A. & Brändén, C. (1989). Crystal structure of chaperone protein PapD reveals an immunoglobulin fold. *Nature*, **342**, 248–51.

Holmgren, A., Kuehn, M. J., Brändén, C.-I. & Hultgren, S. J. (1992). Conserved imunoglobulin-like features in a family of periplasmic pilus chaperones in bacteria. *EMBO Journal*, **11**, 1617–22.

Hull, R. A., Gill, R. E., Hsu, P., Minshaw, B. H. & Falkow, S. (1981). Construction and expression of recombinant plasmids encoding type 1 and D-mannose-resistant pili from a urinary tract infection *Escherichia coli* isolate. *Infection and Immunity*, **33**, 933–8.

Hultgren, S. J., Abraham, S. N., Caparon, M., Falk, P., St. Geme, J. W., III & Normark, S. (1993a). Pilus and non-pilus bacterial adhesins: assembly and function in cell recognition. *Cell*, **73**, 887–901.

Hultgren, S. J., Jacob-Dubuisson, F., Jones, C. H. & Brändén, C.-I. (1993b). PapD and superfamily of periplasmic immunoglobulin-like pilus chaperones. *Advances in Protein Chemistry*, **44**, 99–123

Hultgren, S. J., Jones, C. H. & Normark, S. (1996). Bacterial adhesins and their assembly. *In* Escherichia coli and Salmonella typhimurium, pp. 2370–56. Washington DC: American Society for Microbiology.

Hultgren, S. J., Lindberg, F., Magnusson, G., Kihlberg, J., Tennent, J. M. & Normark, S. (1989). The PapG adhesin of uropathogenic *Escherichia coli* contains separate regions for receptor binding and for the incorporation into the pilus. *Procceedings of the National Acadamy of Sciences, USA*, **86**, 4357–61.

Hultgren, S. J. & Normark, S. (1991a). Biogenesis of the bacterial pilus. *Current Opinion in Genetics and Development*, **1**, 313–18.

Hultgren, S. J., Normark, S. & Abraham, S. N. (1991b). Chaperone-assisted assembly and molecular architecture of adhesive pili. *Annual Review of Microbiology*, **45**, 383–415.

Hung, D. L., Knight, S. D., Woods, R. M., Pinkner, J. S. & Hultgren, S. J. (1996). Molecular basis of two subfamilies of immunoglobulin-like chaperones. *EMBO Journal*. **15**, 3792–805.

Jacob-Dubuisson, F., Heuser, J., Dodson, K., Normark, S. & Hultgren, S. J. (1993a). Initiation of assembly and association of the structural elements of a bacterial pilus depend on two specialized tip proteins. *EMBO Journal*, **12**, 837–47.

Jacob-Dubuisson, F., Kuehn, M. & Hultgren, S. J. (1993b). A novel secretion apparatus for the assembly of adhesive bacterial pili. *Trends in Microbiology*, **1**, 50–5.

Jacob-Dubuisson, F., Striker, R. & Hultgren, S. J. (1994). Chaperone-assisted self-assembly of pili independent of cellular energy. *Journal of Biological Chemistry*, **269**, 12447–55.

Jalajakumari, M. B., Thomas, C. J., Halter, R. & Manning, P. A. (1989). Genes for biosynthesis and assembly of CS3 pili of CFA/II enterotoxigenic *Escherichia coli*: novel regulation of pilus production by bypassing an amber codon. *Molecular Microbiology*, **3**, 1685–95.

Jarrett, J. & Lansbury, P. (1993). Seeding 'one dimensional crystallization' of amyloid: a pathogenic mechanism in Alzheimer's disease and scrapie? *Cell*, **73**, 1055–8.

Jiang, B. & Howard, S. (1992). The *Aeromonas hydrophila exeE* gene, required both for protein secretion and normal outer membrane biogenesis, is a member of the general secretion pathway. *Molecular Microbiology*, **6**, 1351–61.

Jones, C. H., Dodson, K. W. & Hultgren, S. J. (1995a). Structure, function and assembly of adhesive p pili. In *Urinary Tract Infection: Molecular Pathogenesis to Clinical Management*, pp. 175–219. Washington DC: American Society for Microbiology.

Jones, C. H., Jacob, D. F., Dodson, K., Kuehn, M., Slonim, L., Striker, R. & Hultgren, S. J. (1992). Adhesin presentation in bacteria requires molecular chaperones and ushers. *Infection and Immunity*, **60**, 4445–51.

Jones, C. H., Pinkner, J. S., Roth, R., Heuser, J., Nicholes, A. V., Abraham, S. N. & Hultgren, S. J. (1995b). Fim H adhesin of type 1 pili is assembled into a fibrillar tip structure in the Enterobacteriaceae. *Proceedings of the National Academy of Sciences, USA*, **92**, 2081–85.

Karlyshev, A., Galyov, E., Smirnov, O., Guzayev, A., Abramov, V. & Zav'yalov, V. (1992). A new gene of the *f1* operon of *Y. pestis* involved in the capsule biogenesis. *FEBS Letters*, **297**, 77–80.

Koronakis, V., Hughes, C. & Koronakis, E. (1991). Energetically distinct early and late stages of HlyB/HlyD-dependent secretion across *Escherichia coli* membranes. *EMBO Journal*, **10**, 3263–72.

Kuehn, M. J., Heuser, J., Normark, S. & Hultgren, S. J. (1992). P pili in uropathogenic *E. coli* are composite fibres with distinct fibrillar adhesive tips. *Nature*, **356**, 252–5.

Kuehn, M. J., Normark, S. & Hultgren, S. J. (1991). Immunoglobulin-like PapD chaperone caps and uncaps interactive surfaces of nascently translocated pilus subunits. *Proceedings of the National Academy of Sciences, USA*, **88**, 10586–90.

Kuehn, M. J., Ogg, D. J., Kihlberg, L. N., Flemmer, K., Bergfors, T. & Hultgren, S. J. (1993). Structural basis of pilus subunit recognition by the PapD chaperone. *Science*, **262**, 1234–41.

Lecker, S., Driessen, A. J. M. & Wickner, W. (1990). ProOmpA contains secondary and tertiary structure prior to translocation and is shielded from aggregation by association with SecB. *EMBO Journal*, **9**, 2309–14.

Lecker, S., Lill, R., Ziegelhoffer, T., Georgopoulos, C., Bassford, P. J., Kumamoto, C. A. & Wickner, W. (1989). Three pure chaperone proteins of *Escherichia coli* SecB, trigger factor and GroEL–form soluble complexes with precursor proteins *in vitro*. *EMBO Journal*, **8**, 2703–9.

Lindberg, F., Tennant, J. M., Hultgren, S. J., Lund, B. & Normark S. (1989). PapD, a periplasmic transport protein in P-pilus biogenesis. *Journal of Bacteriology*, **171**, 6052–8.

Lintermans, P. (1990). Characterization of the F17 and F111 fimbriae on *Escherichia coli* and genetic analysis of the F17 gene cluster. PhD Thesis, Rijksuniversiteit Ghent, Belgium.

Locht, C., Geoffroy, M.-C. & Renauld, G. (1992). Common accessory genes for the *Bordetella pertussis* filamentous hemagglutinin and fimbriae share sequence similarities with the *papC* and *papD* gene families. *EMBO Journal*, **11**, 3175–83.

Malaviya, R., Ikeda, T., Ross, E. & Abraham, S. N. (1996). Mast cell modulation of neutrophil influx and bacterial clearance at sites of infection through TNF-α. *Nature, London*, **381**, 77–80.

Mooi, F. R., Claassen, I., Bakker, D., Kuipers, H. & de Graaf, F. K. (1986). Regulation and structure of an *Escherichia coli* gene coding for an outer membrane protein involved in export of K88ab fimbrial subunits. *Nucleic Acids Research*, **14**, 2443–57.

Mukherjee, A., Dai, K. & Lutkenhaus, J. (1993). *Escherichia coli* cell division protein FtsZ is a guanine nucleotide binding protein. *Proceedings of the National Academy of Sciences USA*, **90**, 1053–7.

Norgren, M., Baga, M., Tennent, J. M. & Normark, S. (1987). Nucleotide sequence, regulation and functional analysis of the *papC* gene required for cell surface localization of Pap pili of uropathogenic *Escherichia coli*. *Molecular Microbiology*, **1**, 169–78.

Normark, S., Baga, M., Goransson, M., Lindberg, F. P., Lund, B., Norgren, M. & Uhlin, B. E. (1986). Genetics and biogenesis of *Escherichia coli* adhesins. In *Microbial Lectins and Agglutinins*, ed. D. Mirelman, pp. 113–143. New York: Wiley Interscience.

Orndorff, P. E. & Falkow, S. (1984). Organization and expression of genes responsible for type 1 piliation in *Escherichia coli*. *Journal of Bacteriology*, **159**, 736–44.

Patton, J. P., Nash, D. B. & Abrutyn, E. (1991). Urinary tract infection: economic considerations. *Medical Clinics of North America*, **75**, 495–513.

Pugsley, A. (1993). The complete general secretory pathway in Gram negative bacteria. *Microbiological Reviews*, **57**, 50–108.

Pugsley, A. & Possot, G. (1994). The general secretory pathway of *Klebsiella oxytoca*: No evidence for relocalization or assembly of pilin-like PulG protein into a multiprotein complex. *Molecular Microbiology*, **10**, 665–74.

Raina, S., Missiakas, D., Baird, L., Kumar, S. & Georgopoulos, C. (1993). Identification and transcriptional analysis of the *Escherichia coli htrE* operon which is homologous to pap and related pilin operons. *Journal of Bacteriology*, **175**, 5009–21.

Randall, L. L., Hardy, S. J. S. & Thom, J. R. (1987). Export of protein: a biochemical view. *Annual Review of Microbiology*, **41**, 507–41.

Rioux, C. R., Friedrich, M. J. & Kadner, R. J. (1990). Genes on the 90-kilobase plasmid of *Salmonella typhimurium* confer low-affinity cobalamin transport: relationship to fimbria biosynthesis genes. *Journal of Bacteriology*, **172**, 6217–22.

Ronald, A. R. & Pattullo, A. L. (1991). The natural history of urinary infection in adults. *Medical Clinics of North America*, **75**, 299–312.

Roosendaal, B. & de Graaf, F. (1989). The nucleotide sequence of the *fanD* gene encoding the large outer membrane protein involved in the biosynthesis of K99 fimbiae. *Nucleic Acids Research*, **17**, 1263.

Schmoll, T., Morschhauser, J., Ott, M., Ludwig, B., van Die, I. & Hacker, J. (1990). Complete genetic organization and functional aspects of the *Escherichia coli* S fimbrial adhesion determinant: nucleotide sequence of the genes *sfa* B, C, D, E, F. *Microbial Pathogenesis*, **9**, 331–43.

Slonim, L. N., Pinkner, J. S., Branden, C. I. & Hultgren, S. J. (1992). Interactive surface in the PapD chaperone cleft is conserved in pilus chaperone superfamily and essential in subunit recognition and assembly. *EMBO Journal*, **11**, 4747–56.

Striker, R., Jacob-Dubuisson, F., Frieden, C. & Hultgren, S. J. (1994). Stable fiber forming and non-fiber forming chaperone-subunit complexes in pilus biogenesis. *Journal of Biological Chemistry*, **269**, 12233–9.

Stromberg, N., Hultgren, S. J., Russell, D. G. & Normark, S. (1992). Microbial attachment, molecular mechanisms. In *Encyclopedia of Microbiology*, vol. 3, ed. J. Lederberg, pp. 143–58. San Diego: Academic Press.

Turner, L., Lara, J., Nunn, D. & Lory, S. (1993). Mutations in the consensus ATP-binding sites of XcpR and PilB eliminate extracellular protein secretion and pilus biogenesis in *Pseudomonas aeruginosa*. *Journal of Bacteriology*, **175**, 4962–9.

Watson, W. J., Gilsdorf, J. R., Tucci, M. A., McCrea, K. W., Forney, L. J. & Marrs, C. F. (1994). Identification of a gene essential for piliation in *Haemophilus influenzae* type b with homology to the pilus assembly platform genes of Gram-negative bacteria. *Infection and Immunity*, **62**, 468–75.

Wickner, W. 1989. Secretion and membrane assembly. *Trends in Biological Sciences*, **14**, 280–5.

Williams, P. H., Roberts, M. & Hinson, G. (1988). Stages in bacterial invasion. *Journal of Applied Bacteriology, Symposium Supplement*, **17**, 131–47S.

Wong, K. & Buckley, J. (1989). Proton motive force involved in protein transport across the outer membrane of *Aeromonas salmonicida*. *Science*, **246**, 654–6.

Xu, Z., Jones, C. H., Haslam, D., Pinkner, J. S., Dodson, K., Kihlberg, J. & Hultgren, S. J. (1995). Molecular dissection of PapD interaction with PapG reveals two chaperone binding sites. *Molecular Microbiology*, **16**, 1011–20.

9

The heat-labile and heat-stable enterotoxins of *Escherichia coli*

G. B. NAIR and Y. TAKEDA

Recent estimates indicate that 3.2 million of the 12.9 million deaths of children under five years of age in developing countries are due to diarrhoea (WHO, 1992). It is the high incidence of diarrhoea, with rates of about ten episodes per year per child in some settings (Snyder & Merson, 1983; Guerrant *et al.*, 1990), rather than the death-to-case ratio that makes diarrhoea one of the three commonest causes of death in most developing countries (Tulloch & Richards, 1993). The most important causes of bacterial diarrhoea in early childhood are enterotoxigenic *Escherichia coli (ETEC), Shigella* and *Campylobacter jejuni* (Huilan *et al.*, 1991) and, in addition, ETEC is responsible for more than half of the cases of travellers' diarrhoea (Shore *et al.*, 1974; Gorbach *et al.*, 1975). ETEC strains are non-invasive and cause a highly secretory kind of diarrhoea by producing a heat-labile enterotoxin and/or a heat-stable enterotoxin. These enterotoxins have been the subject of intense research during the last decade.

Heat-labile enterotoxin

Classification

The heat-labile enterotoxins (LT) of *E. coli* are a family of multimeric protein toxins that are related to each other in structure and function. LT can be classified into two types, type I (LTI) and type II (LTII), and antisera against the one toxin do not neutralise the other (Holmes *et al.* 1986; Pickett *et al.*, 1986, 1987, 1989; Finkelstein *et al.*, 1987). LTI can be further divided into LTh-I and LTp-I; these are antigenically cross-reacting variants of LTI produced, respectively, by *E. coli* strains from humans and pigs (Honda *et al.*, 1981; Dallas, 1983). LTII also has two antigenic variants, designated as LTIIa and LTIIb (Guth *et al.*, 1986b; Pickett *et al.*, 1986; Holmes *et al.*, 1988; Pickett *et al.*, 1989) and strains of ETEC that produce LTII have been isolated from water-buffalo, cattle, pigs and foods but they are rarely isolated from humans (Guth *et al.*, 1986a; Seriwatana *et al.*, 1988).

Type-I heat-labile enterotoxin (LTI)

Certain strains of *E. coli*, which do not belong to the classical entero-pathogenic *E. coli* (EPEC) serotypes, produce a diarrhoeagenic toxin (De *et al.*, 1956). During the cholera season of 1968 these findings were confirmed in Calcutta by the isolation from human cases of diarrhoea of *E. coli* strains that produced heat-labile, non-dialysable toxins that caused fluid accumulation in rabbit ileal loops (Sack *et al.*, 1971). These strains were called 'enterotoxigenic *E. coli*' because they did not belong to the recognised serotypes of EPEC. Subsequent investigations have shown that ETEC are prevalent in almost all areas of the world and are amongst the most important causative agents of travellers' diarrhoea (Merson *et al.*, 1976).

LTI is a plasmid-encoded periplasmic protein very similar to the cholera toxin (CT) produced by toxigenic *Vibrio cholerae*. The native toxin consists of one catalytic A subunit (240 amino-acids, 27 kDa) and five identical B subunits (103 amino acids, 11.4 kDa). The enzymatic activity of the toxin resides in the A subunit, while the five B subunits mediate binding of the toxin to intestinal epithelial cells and are primarily responsible for its immunogenicity. The A subunit undergoes post-translational processing to generate two peptides, A1 and A2, that are linked to each other by a single disulphide bond (Lai *et al.*, 1976; Gill & Richardson, 1980). The A1 peptide possesses the enzymatic activity, while A2 peptide is thought to function in toxin internalisation into the target cell. The three-dimensional crystal structure of LTI reveals a remarkable structure that consists of a wedge-shaped A subunit of which the carboxyl-terminus enters the pore formed by a doughnut-shaped ring of five B subunits. The A subunit interacts with the B pentamer at the inlet of the pore by means of a number of polar and charged residues (Sixma *et al.*, 1991, 1992).

Although LTh-I and LTp-I share immunological and physico-chemical similarities, LTh-I is distinct from LTp-I in its isoelectric point, elec-trophoretic mobility (Tsuji *et al.*, 1982) and immunological properties (Kunkel & Robertson, 1979; Honda *et al.*, 1981; Clements *et al.*, 1982;

Geary *et al.*, 1982; Takeda *et al.*, 1983b). The amino-acid sequences of LTI and CT are largely conserved, with differences scattered throughout the sequence, except for the region around the cleavage site between the A1 and A2 subunits, where the homology is only 33 per cent (Spangler, 1992). The amino-acid sequence of the B subunits of LTh-I more closely resembles that of the B subunit of CT than that of LTp-I (Yamamoto *et al.*, 1984).

Type-II heat-labile enterotoxin (LTII)

The second group in the LT family, LTII, has a protein structure and mechanism of action similar to that of LTI, but is different in respect of its immunoreactivity and ganglioside-binding capacity (Pickett *et al.*, 1987; Fukuta *et al.*, 1988). LTIIa has been purified from an *E. coli* strain isolated from a water-buffalo in Korat, Thailand (Mosely *et al.*, 1982; Green *et al.*, 1983). The other toxin, LTIIb, which has also been purified, has several properties that distinguish it from LTIIa, including partial antigenic identity, differences in isoelectric point (LTIIa pI = 6.8; LTIIb pI = 5.4), a lower specific toxicity for Y1 adrenal cells and greater activation after treatment with trypsin (Guth *et al.*, 1986b). LTIIa and LTIIb also differ from each other and from LTh-I in their specificity for the kind of oligosaccharide moieties of particular ganglioside receptors (Fukuta *et al.*, 1988). It should be emphasised that the role of LTIIa and LTIIb in the pathogenesis of disease due to *E. coli* has not so far clearly been established.

Genetics of LTI and LTII

The structural genes for LTI are carried by plasmids (Gyles *et al.*, 1974), while those for LTII are chromosomal (Green *et al.*, 1983). The genes that encode the A and B polypeptide of LTh-I, LTp-I, LTIIa and LTIIb have been cloned and sequenced (Dallas & Falkow, 1980; Yamamoto *et al.*, 1984; Leong *et al.*, 1985; Pickett *et al.*, 1987). At the nucleotide level, the A and B cistrons of the LTI and CT operons, respectively, show 75 and 77 per cent homology (Dallas & Falkow, 1980; Mekalanos *et al.*, 1983). Pickett *et al.*(1989) demonstrated that the A subunit genes for LTI and LTII represent distinct branches of an evolutionary tree and that the divergence between the A subunit genes of LTIIa and LTIIb is greater than that between CT and LTI, but it was not possible to demonstrate an evolutionary relationship between the B subunits of LTI and LTII. The apparent lack of homology between the B subunits of LTI and LTII is consistent with their different ganglioside-binding specificities, and the limited homology between the A2 fragments of LTI and LTII may reflect co-evolution of the A2 polypeptide with the specific B polypeptides to which they bind (Holmes *et al.*, 1990).

Holotoxin assembly

The individual A and B subunits of LTI are produced as leader peptide-containing precursors that are translocated across the cytoplasmic membrane of *E. coli*. After removal of the signal peptides, the mature subunits are released into the periplasm where they assemble non-covalently into AB_5 complexes (Hirst *et al.*, 1984; Hofstra & Witholt, 1985). The 14 carboxyl-terminal amino-acids of the A subunit consist of two functional domains that differentially affect oligomerisation and holotoxin stability. The last four residues of the A subunit act as an 'anchoring' sequence responsible for maintaining the stability of A/B subunit interaction during holotoxin assembly (Streatfield *et al.*, 1992). Chemical modification and mutant analysis have shown that a single amino-acid alanine-64 from the amino-terminus, is critical for the native B subunit to form an oligomer structure and express its functions (Iida *et al.*, 1989).

Hybrid toxins between CT and LTI have been produced by denaturation and subsequent renaturation *in vitro* of mixtures of their A and B polypeptides, and the toxicities of these hybrids are comparable with those of their native toxins (Takeda *et al.*, 1981; Hardy *et al.*, 1988). Similarly, hybrid toxins of LTIIa and LTIIb have been produced, but the toxicity of the hybrids is usually lower than that of the wild-type holotoxin (Cornell & Holmes, 1992). It has also been shown that all homologous and heterologous combinations of A and B polypeptides from LTI and LTII can assemble *in vivo* into active holotoxins, but not with equal efficiency (Cornell & Holmes, 1992).

Membrane receptor of the LT family

As in the case of CT, the membrane receptor of the LTI family has been identified as GM_1 ganglioside. Early work showed that the activity of LTI on vascular permeability and ileal loops is inhibited by GM_1 ganglioside, although the affinity of the binding of LT to GM_1 ganglioside was much less than that of CT (Holmgren, 1973). LT can also bind to GM_2 (asialo-GM_1) and to glycoprotein (Griffiths *et al.*, 1986; Fukuta *et al.*, 1988).

Chemical modification has revealed that the trypophan-88 (Mullin *et al.*, 1976; de Wolf *et al.*, 1981) and the glycine-33 from the amino-terminus of the B subunit (Tsuji *et al.*, 1985) are important for binding the B subunit to its ganglioside receptor. LTIIa binds with greatest affinity to ganglioside GD_{1b}, while LTIIb binds preferentially to ganglioside GD_{1a} (Fukuta *et al.*, 1988).

Mode of action of LT

The export, host-cell binding and mode of action of LT have recently been intensively studied and the understanding of these mechanisms has been greatly aided by detailed knowledge of the three-dimensional structure of LT.

Since the first description of ETEC by De *et al.* (1956), it was thought that the mode of action of *E. coli* enterotoxin was similar to that of *V. cholerae* enterotoxin. That this was so, was first demonstrated by Bywater (1970) in Thiry-Vella loops of calf small intestine, an observation that was supported by Pierce & Wallace (1972) who showed that *E. coli* enterotoxin does not alter the rate of jejunal fluid accumulation in dogs after the maximum secretory rate had been induced by CT. These experiments were usually carried out with crude toxin preparations and, as a result, it was not clear whether LT or ST was responsible for the observed phenomena.

The observation that, as in the case of CT, accumulation of intestinal fluid due to *E. coli* LT is due to activation of adenylate cyclase by the enterotoxin was made by Evans *et al.* (1972), using rabbit ileal mucosal cells and isolated rat adipocytes. Guerrant *et al.* (1973) then showed that *E. coli* LT also activates adenylate cyclase in the jejunum of dogs. Subsequently it was shown that activation of adenylate cyclase by LT, followed by an increase in the accumulation of intracellular cAMP, can be observed in various tissues and cells, including thyroid slices (Mashiter *et al.*, 1973), rabbit intestinal mucosa (Kantor *et al.*, 1974), rat fat cells (Hewlett *et al.*, 1974), cultured human embryonic intestinal epithelial cells (Kantor *et al.*, 1974), mouse thymocytes (Zenser & Metzger, 1974) and cat myocardial tissue (Dorner & Mayer, 1975).

The A subunit of LT is activated, by tryptic activity in the bowel or within the target cell into the A1 and A2 fragments which are then held together by a disulphide bridge. Reduction of the disulphide bridge within the cell releases A1, which activates plasma membrane adenylate cyclase by catalysing ADP–ribosylation of the regulatory protein Gsα.

The biological effects of LT are mediated by an increase in the concentration of cAMP in the target cells, but cAMP-independent effects of enterotoxins that may be mediated by prostaglandins, eicosanoids or by cross-linking of gangliosides in plasma membranes have also been described (Peterson & Ochoa, 1989; Francis *et al.*, 1990)

Heat-stable enterotoxin

Classification

The heat-stable enterotoxins (ST) are a family of closely related peptides that induce secretory diarrhoea in humans and animals. The STs of ETEC are classified into two structurally, functionally and immunogenically unrelated types, namely, STa and STb (Burgess *et al.*, 1978; Weikel & Guerrant, 1985), which, respectively, are also known as STI and STII. STa includes methanol-soluble infant mouse-active peptide toxins, while STb is methanol-insoluble and active in weaned pigs, but inactive in infant mice. The toxic activity of STa is resistant to protease (Staples *et al.*, 1980; Dreyfus *et al.*, 1984), while that of STb is inactivated by treatment with trypsin (Whipp, 1987).

Several enteric bacteria produce structurally homologous and antigenically cross-reacting STa enterotoxins. The STa family consists of at least eight distinct types, including two different STa enterotoxins from strains of *E. coli* of human (STh) and porcine (STp) origin (So & McCarthy, 1980; Mosely *et al.*, 1983), NAG-ST from *V. cholerae* non-O1 (Arita *et al.*, 1986; Yoshimura *et al.*, 1986), H-ST from Hakata strains of *V. cholerae* non-O1 (Arita *et al.*, 1991a), M-ST from *V. mimicus* (Arita *et al.*, 1991b), Y-ST from *Yersinia enterocolitica* (Takao *et al.*, 1984, 1985), and C-ST from *Citrobacter freundii* (Guarino *et al.*, 1987, 1989a). The most recent addition to the family is O1-ST, which was detected in a CT-gene-positive strain of *V. cholerae* O1 (Takeda *et al.*, 1991). Other enteric bacteria such as *Klebsiella* have also been reported to produce a STa-like toxin (Klipstein *et al.*, 1983; Guarino *et al.*, 1989b).

The biochemical, physiological and immunological properties and amino-acid composition of the various STa enterotoxins characterised so far are remarkably similar. They have a common, highly conserved region with ten amino-acids, including six Cys residues, located in the same relative positions and linked intramolecularly by three disulphide bonds, which suggests that these enterotoxins have similar tertiary structures (Shimonishi *et al.*, 1987), and the secretory potency and heat-stability of the STa enterotoxins are determined by the conserved core sequence (Yoshimura *et al.*, 1985, 1986; Shimonishi *et al.*, 1987).

Type-I heat-stable enterotoxin (STI or STa)

As we have seen, two classes of *E. coli* STh enterotoxin, ST_h and STp, are recognised. Purification of STp was first accomplished by Alderete & Robertson (1978) from an ETEC strain of porcine origin. The toxin was purified by column chromatography and the molecular weight was estimated as approximately 5 kDa. So & McCarthy (1980) then cloned a gene from an *E. coli* strain of bovine origin that encodes STp. The amino-acid sequence deduced from the nucleotide sequence showed that the whole STI molecule is synthesised as a 72-residue precursor. Similarly, Aimoto *et al.* (1982) determined the amino-acid sequence of STh purified from an ETEC strain isolated from a human patient with diarrhoea. The sequence of STh was different from that deduced from the nucleotide STp but it was identical to the carboxyl-terminal sequence of 19 amino-acids deduced from the nucleotide sequence of the ST gene reported by Moseley *et al.* (1983). It is now known that STp and STh are extracellular enterotoxins of 18 and 19 amino-acids, respectively, that result from two independent proteolytic cleavages of a 72-amino-acid precursor (pre-pro-STp or STh). The first cleavage yields a periplasmic 53-amino-acid pro-STp or STh that is extracellularly processed to the mature STp or STh (Rasheed *et al.*, 1990). A synthetic, fully toxic analogue of STp has been crystallised, and X-ray diffraction analysis of STp has revealed that it has a right-handed spiral structure that consists of three β-turns fixed by three disulphide linkages. Part of the toxin surface is amphiphilic, which is important for its receptor binding activity (Ozaki *et al.*, 1991)

STh and STp are heat stable and cause fluid accumulation in the suckling mouse even after they have been heated at 100°C for 30 minutes (Smith & Gyles, 1970). Heating STh at 100°C for ten minutes at a concentration of 30 ng/ml inactivates the toxin, but heating at a higher concentration (60 ng/ml) under the same conditions does not affect its activity (Takeda *et al.*, 1979). Reducing agents such as β-mercaptoethanol and dithiothreitol inactivate *E. coli* STa enterotoxins (Dreyfus *et al.*, 1984) by reduction of disulphide bonds (Eldeib *et al.*, 1986).

Escherichia coli STa enterotoxins are poorly immunogenic. However, high-titre polyclonal anti-ST antibodies can be obtained by conjugation of the toxin with an appropriate protein carrier, such as bovine IgG (Gianella *et al.*, 1981), bovine serum albumin or haemocyanin (Frantz &

Robertson, 1981), or by polymerisation with toluene 2,4-di-isocyanate (Okamoto *et al.*, 1983). Antisera against *E. coli* STh and STp are cross-neutralising (Takeda *et al.*, 1983a). Moreover, antibodies against *E. coli*-STa cross-react with Y-ST (Okamoto *et al.*, 1983).

The preparation of monoclonal antibody (MAb) against STa has been attempted by several investigators. Hemelhof *et al.* (1984) prepared a MAb against STh, while Brandwein *et al.* (1985) isolated a clone that produces a MAb antibody against STp. Svennerholm *et al.* (1986) prepared several MAbs against STh and used these to develop an ST GM_1-ELISA. The antigenic determinants of STh have been extensively analysed with a combination of MAb prepared against STh and short, chemically synthesised analogues of various STa enterotoxins. Three distinct antigenic sites of STh sufficiently separated from each other have been recognised, one near the amino-terminus, another in the core functional region of the toxin and the third in the carboxyl-terminal region (Takeda *et al.*, 1993). Characterisation of the various epitopes has revealed that the MAbs that recognise the amino-terminal residues, which are not essential for toxic activity, have a potent protective capacity (Takeda *et al.*, 1993).

Structure–activity relationship of Escherichia coli STa

Chemically synthesised STh and STp have been used to study the structure-activity relationship of *E. coli* STa enterotoxins. Comparison of the nuclear magnetic resonance spectra of synthetic and native ST has shown that synthetic STh and STp have the same tertiary structure as native ST (Ikemura *et al.*, 1984; Yoshimura *et al.*, 1984). Synthetic STh and STp are as heat stable as the native STa enterotoxins and, respectively, produce fluid accumulation in suckling mice at doses of 0.8 ng (Ikemura *et al.*, 1984) and 1.5–2.0 ng (Yoshimura *et al.*, 1984), which are similar to the effective doses of the respective native STa enterotoxins. Synthetic analogues of the 13-amino-acid peptide sequence of STh and STp from the Cys near the amino-terminus to the Cys at the carboxyl-terminus (STh 6–18 and STp 5–17) with three disulphide bonds have the same physiological and immunological properties as the respective native STh and STp. It may, therefore, be concluded that the essential structure for the activity of STh and STp resides in this sequence of 13 amino-acids, which has six Cys residues linked by three intramolecular disulphide bonds (Yoshimura *et al.*, 1985).

Which of these three intramolecular disulphide bonds is important for the spatial structure of STh and for expression of toxicity was investigated by Yamasaki *et al.*(1988). They found that peptides with only one disulphide bond are not biologically active, but peptides with a disulphide bond between the Cys-7 and Cys-15 and one other disulphide bond had distinct activity; a peptide that lacks a disulphide bond between Cys-7 and Cys-15 is not toxic. Clearly, the latter disulphide bond and another between Cys-6 and Cys-11 or between Cys-10 and Cys-18, which stabilise the spatial structure of STh, are necessary for STh toxicity.

Receptor for Escherichia coli STa in intestinal tissues

The first step in the biological action of STI is its interaction with specific high-affinity receptors. Binding of STI to the epithelial cell membranes of rabbits (Field *et al.*, 1978; Rao *et al.*, 1980) and rats (Guerrant et al., 1980; Gianella *et al.*, 1983; Dreyfus & Robertson, 1984) stimulates membrane-bound guanylate cyclase, which leads to an increase in the intracellular concentration of guanosine 3′,5′-cyclic monophosphate (cGMP), followed by activation of cGMP-dependent protein kinase (de Jonge & Lohmann, 1985; Hirayama *et al.*, 1989). This culminates in inhibition of Na^+ absorption and stimulation of Cl^- secretion (Field *et al.*, 1978). The superficial similarity between STa, CT and LT is an increase in the short-circuit current across rabbit intestinal membranes (Field *et al.*, 1978). However, the effect of STI appears to be tissue-specific, whereas *E. coli* LT and CT can affect many different tissues.

Gianella *et al.*(1983) showed that ^{125}I-labelled STh binds to rat jejunal and ileal epithelial cells. The binding was specific because it was inhibited by increasing concentrations of STh and STp, but not by LT or CT, but addition of excess unlabelled ST resulted in dissociation of the greater part of the ^{125}I-labelled ST. This suggests that there are two binding sites that counteract each other and Dreyfus & Robertson (1984) suggested that the binding component on brush border membranes is a protein. Further work has shown, however, that there may be multiple STh-binding proteins in the rat intestinal cell membrane. A specific, high-affinity STh receptor, which consists of three binding-domain proteins of 60 kDa, 68 kDa and 80 kDa respectively, has been demonstrated by affinity cross-labelling (Kuno *et al.*, 1986). Two other proteins of 57 kDa and 75 kDa have been identified as putative STh receptors by means of a photo-affinity STh analogue of a radioiodinated STh derivative with a benzoylbenzoate photo-reactive group (Gariepy & Schoolnik, 1987). Since then, two kinds of homodimer proteins of 135 kDa and 150 kDa have been reported as STh receptors, although only a single binding affinity was observed by Scatchard analysis (Ivens *et al.*, 1990).

Incubation of rat intestine cell membranes with a radioiodinated STh analogue, followed by photolysis, results in the specific and exclusive radiolabelling of a 70-kDa protein, with apparent labelling of additional minor protein bands of 45 kDa and 53 kDa on sodium dodecyl sulphate–polyacrylamide gel electrophoresis (Kubota *et al.*, 1989; Hirayama *et al.*, 1990b). *E. coli* STp and STh competitively inhibit the photo-affinity labelling of the 70-kDa protein, which suggests that they share a common receptor protein in the rat intestinal cell membrane (Kubota *et al.*, 1989). Furthermore, biologically active analogues of the ST of *Y. enterocolitica* and *V. cholerae* non-O1 also completely inhibit the photo-affinity labelling of the 70-kDa protein (Hirayama *et al.*, 1990b). It has been shown, with synthetic analogues of STh, that a disulphide bond between Cys-7 and Cys-15 are important for the binding of STh to the 70 kDa protein. (Yamasaki *et al.*, 1988).

The STp-binding protein from the rat intestinal brush border membrane (apparent molecular weight of 100 kDa) has been solubilised and purified by its affinity for a Con-Sepharose column (Robertson & Jaso-Friedman, 1988). Two glycoprotein STh receptors, STR-200R and STR-200B, can be separated by ConA column chromatography (Hirayama *et al.*, 1990a). STR-200A is a peptide of 70 kDa with a single binding domain, whereas STR-200B has two binding domains of 53 kDa and 77 kDa. By means of a specific glycosidase, Hirayama *et al.* (1990a) showed that the binding-domain peptide contains N-linked mannose-rich and hybrid-type oligosaccharides that do not appear to contribute to the binding specificity. They also reported that the 53-kDa STR-200B protein is devoid of sialic acid.

Type-II heat-stable enterotoxin

Much less is known about the heat-stable enterotoxin STb (STII), as compared with the type-I STa enterotoxins. STb consists of 71 amino-acids, of which the 23 amino-terminal amino-acids comprise the signal peptide; the mature STb secreted by the organism, therefore, consists of 48 amino-acids (Lee *et al.*, 1983; Picken *et al.*, 1983). STb was purified to homogeneity by Fujii *et al.* (1991) who showed that the purified enterotoxin was composed of 48 amino-acids with an isoelectric point of 9.7 (Fujii *et al.*, 1994). Its amino-acid sequence was identical to that of the 48 carboxyl-terminal amino-acids of STb predicted from the DNA sequence

(Lee *et al.*, 1983). STb has four cysteine residues that form two intra-molecular disulphide bonds (Fujii *et al.*, 1991), and there is no amino-acid sequence homology between STa and STb. A single processing event on precursor pre-STb (M^r 8100) yields a transient periplasmic species that, without further apparent modification, becomes the mature extracellular 48-amino-acid STb (Kupersztoch *et al.*, 1990). The nucleotide sequence of the gene that encodes STb is totally different from those that code for LT and STa, although STb is also encoded on a plasmid (Lee *et al.*, 1983; Picken *et al.*, 1983; Betley *et al.*, 1986) but the gene for STb can be associated with a 9-kb transposable element (Betley *et al.*, 1986).

Until recently it has been possible to demonstrate the biochemical activity of STb only in pigs (Kennedy *et al.*, 1984), but, by using a trypsin inhibitor to block intestinal protease activity, Whipp (1990) was able to obtain an intestinal response to STb in mice, rats, rabbits and calves. The mode of action of STb differs from those of STa and CT (Hitotsubashi *et al.*, 1992). STb does not alter cGMP or cAMP levels in the intestinal mucosa, but it increases the level of prostaglandin E_2. This implicates prostaglandin E_2 in the mechanism of action of STb (Hitotsubashi *et al.*, 1992). Site directed mutagenesis has shown that substitution of nine basic amino-acid residues reduced toxicity, particularly if the lysine at positions 22 and 23 was altered (Fujii *et al.*, 1994).

STb is mainly associated with ETEC isolated from diarrhoea in swine, and the gene that encodes this toxin is the most common of the toxin genes in porcine ETEC (Moon *et al.*, 1986; Monckton & Hasse, 1988). By means of an STb probe and an immunoassay, Lortie *et al.* (1991) showed that STb enterotoxin can also be detected in strains of *E. coli* isolated from humans with diarrhoea and restriction endonuclease analysis has shown that the STb gene from human isolates is similar to the STb gene of porcine strains. Recently, STb-producing strains have been isolated from patients with travellers' diarrhoea (Okamoto *et al.*, 1993).

References

Aimoto, S., Takao, T., Shimonishi, Y., Hara, S., Takeda, T., Takeda Y. & Miwatani, T. (1982). Amino-acid sequence of a heat-stable enterotoxin produced by human enterotoxigenic. *Escherichia coli. European Journal of Biochemistry*, **129**, 257–63.

Alderate, J. F. & Robertson, D. C. (1978). Purification and chemical characterisation of the heat-stable enterotoxin produced by porcine strains of enterotoxigenic *Escherichia coli. Infection and Immunity*, **19**, 1021–30.

Arita, M., Honda, T., Miwatani, T., Ohmori, K., Takao, T. & Shimonishi, Y. (1991a). Purification and characterisation of a new heat-stable enterotoxin produced by *Vibrio cholerae* non-O1 serogroup Hakata. *Infection and Immunity*, **59**, 2186–8.

Arita, M., Honda, T., Miwatani, T., Takeda, T., Takao, T. & Shimonishi, Y. (1991b). Purification and characterisation of a heat-stable enterotoxin of *Vibrio mimicus*. *FEMS Microbiology Letters*, **79**, 105–10.

Arita, M., Takeda, T., Honda, T. & Miwatani, T. (1986). Purification and characterisation of *Vibrio cholerae* non-O1 heat-stable enterotoxin. *Infection and Immunity*, **52**, 45–9.

Betley, M. J., Miller, V. L. & Mekalanos, J. J. (1986). Genetics of bacterial enterotoxins. *Annual Reviews of Microbiology*, **40**, 577–605.

Brandwein, H., Deutsch, A., Thompson, M. & Gianella, R. (1985). Production of neutralising monoclonal antibodies to *Escherichia coli* heat-stable enterotoxin. *Infection and Immunity*, **47**, 242–6.

Burgess, M. N., Bywater, R. J., Corley, C. M., Mullan, M. N. & Newsome, P. M. (1978). Biological evaluation of a methanol soluble, heat-stable *Escherichia coli* enterotoxin in infant mice, pigs, rabbits, and calves. *Infection and Immunity*, **21**, 526–31.

Bywater, R. J. (1970). Some effects of *Escherichia coli* enterotoxin on net fluid, glucose and electrolyte transfer in calf small intestine. *Journal of Comparative Pathology*, **80**, 565–73.

Clements, J. D., Flint, D. C. & Klipstein, F. A. (1982). Immunological and physiochemical characterisation of heat-labile enterotoxins isolated from two strains of *Escherichia coli*. *Infection and Immunity*, **38**, 806–9.

Cornell, T. D. & Holmes, R. K. (1992). Characterisation of hybrid toxins produced in *Escherichia coli* by assembly of A and B polypeptides from type I and type II heat-labile enterotoxins. *Infection and Immunity*, **60**, 1653–61.

Dallas, W. S. (1983). Conformity between heat-labile toxin genes from human and porcine enterotoxigenic *Escherichia coli*. *Infection and Immunity*, **40**, 647–52.

Dallas, W. S. & Falkow, S. (1980) Amino acid sequence homology between cholera toxin and *Escherichia coli* heat-labile toxin. *Nature (London)*, **288**, 499–501.

De, S. N., Bhattacharya, K. & Sarkar, J. K. (1956). A study of the pathogenicity of strains of *Bacterium coli* from acute chronic enteritis. *Journal of Pathology and Bacteriology*, **71**, 201–9.

Dorner, F. & Mayer, P. (1975). *Escherichia coli* enterotoxin: stimulation of adenylate cyclase in broken-cell preparation. *Infection and Immunity*, **11**, 429–35.

Dreyfus, L. A., Jaso-Friedman, L. & Robertson, D. C. (1984). Characterisation of the mechanism of action of *Escherichia coli* heat-stable enterotoxin. *Infection and Immunity*, **44**, 493–501.

Dreyfus, L. A. & Robertson, D. C. (1984). Solubilisation and partial characterization of the intestinal receptor for *Escherichia coli* heat-stable enterotoxin. *Infection and Immunity*, **46**, 537–43.

Eldeib, M. M. R., Dove, C. R., Parker, C. D., Veum, T. L., Zinn, G. M. & White, A. A. (1986). Reversal of the biological activity of *Escherichia coli* heat-stable enterotoxin by disulphide reducing agents. *Infection and Immunity*, **51**, 24–30.

Evans, D. J. Jr., Chan, L.C., Curlin, G. T. & Evans, D. J. (1972). Stimulation of adenyl cyclase by *Escherichia coli* enterotoxin. *Nature (London)*, **236**, 137–8.

Field, M. J., Graf, L. H. Jr., Laird, W. J. & Smith, P. L. (1978). Heat-stable enterotoxin of *Escherichia coli*: *in vitro* effects on guanylate cyclase activity, cyclic GMP concentration, and ion transport in small intestine. *Proceedings of the National Academy of Science USA*, **75**, 2800–4.

Finkelstein, R. A., Burks, M. F., Zupan, A., Dallas, W. S., Jacob, C. O. & Ludwig, D. S. (1987). Antigenic determinants of the cholera/*E. coli* family of enterotoxins. *Reviews of Infectious Disease*, **9**, S490-S502.

Francis, M. L., Moss, J., Fitz, T. A. & Mond, J. J. (1990). cAMP-independent effects of cholera toxin on B cell activation. I. A possible role for cell surface ganglioside GM_1 in B cell activation. *Journal of Immunology*, **145**, 3162–9.

Frantz, J. C. & Robertson, D. C. (1981). Immunological properties of *Escherichia coli* heat-stable enterotoxins: development of a radioimmunoassay specific for heat-stable enterotoxins with suckling mouse activity. *Infection and Immunity*, **33**, 193–8.

Fujii, Y., Hayashi, M., Hitotsubashi, S., Fuke, Y., Yamanabe, H. & Okamoto, K. (1991). Purification and characterization of *Escherichia coli* heat-stable enterotoxin II. *Journal of Bacteriology*, **173**, 5516–22.

Fujii, Y., Okamoto, Y., Hitotsubashi, S., Saito, A., Akashi, N. & Okamoto, K. (1994). Effect of alterations of basic amino acid residues of *Escherichia coli* heat-stable enterotoxin II on enterotoxicity. *Infection Immunity*, **62**, 2295–301.

Fukuta, S., Magnani, J. L., Twiddy, E. M., Holmes, R. K. & Ginsburg, V. (1988). Comparison of the carbohydrate-binding specificities of cholera toxin and *Escherichia coli* heat-labile enterotoxins LTh-I, LT-IIa, and LT-IIb. *Infection and Immunity*, **56**, 1748–53.

Gariepy, J. & Schoolnik, G. K. (1987). Design of a photoreactive analogue of the *Escherichia coli* heat-stable enterotoxin STb: Use in identifying its receptor on rat brush border membrane. *Proceedings of the National Academy of Science, USA*, **83**, 483–7.

Geary, S. J., Marchlewicz, B. A. & Finkelstein, R. A. (1982). Comparison of heat-labile enterotoxins from porcine and human strains of *Escherichia coli*. *Infection and Immunity*, **36**, 215–20.

Giannella, R. A., Drake, K. W. & Luttrell, M. (1981). Development of radioimmunoassay for *Escherichia coli* heat-stable enterotoxin: comparison with the suckling mouse bioassay. *Infection and Immunity*, **33**, 186–92.

Gianella, R. A., Luttrell, M. & Thompson, M. (1983). Binding of *Escherichia coli* heat-stable enterotoxin to receptors on rat intestinal cells. *American Journal of Physiology*, **245**, 492–8.

Gill, D. M. & Richardson, R. H. (1980). Adenosine diphosphate-ribosylation of adenylate cyclase catalyzed by heat-labile enterotoxin of *Escherichia coli*. *Journal of Infectious Diseases*, **141**, 64–70.

Gorbach, S. L., Kean B. H., Evans, D. G., Evans, D. J. Jr & Bessudo, D. (1975). Traveller's diarrhea and toxigenic *Escherichia coli*. *New England Journal of Medicine*, **292**, 933–6.

Green, B. A., Neill, R. J., Ruyechan, W. T. & Holmes, R. K. (1983). Evidence that a new enterotoxin of *Escherichia coli* which activates adenylate cyclase in eukaryotic target cells is not plasmid mediated. *Infection and Immunity*, **41**, 383–90.

Griffiths, S. L., Finkelstein, R. A. & Critchery, D. R. (1986). Characterization of the receptor for cholera toxin and *Escherichia coli* heat-labile toxin in rabbit intestinal brush border. *Biochemistry Journal*, **238**, 313–22.

Guarino, A., Capano, G., Malamisura, B., Alessio, M., Guandalini, S. & Rubino, A. (1987). Production of *Escherichia coli* STa-like heat-stable enterotoxin by *Citrobacter freundii* isolated from humans. *Journal of Clinical Microbiology*, **25**, 110–14.

Guarino, A., Giannella, R. & Thompson, M. R. (1989a). *Citrobacter freundii* produces an 18-amino-acid heat-stable enterotoxin identical to the 18-amino-acid *Escherichia coli* heat-stable enterotoxin (STIa). *Infection and Immunity*, **57**, 649–52.

Guarino, A., Guandalini, S., Akssio, M., Gentile, F., Tarollo, L., Capano, G., Migliavacca, M. & Rubino, A. (1989b). Characteristics and mechanism of action of a heat-stable enterotoxin produced by *Klebsiella pneumoniae* from infants with secretory diarrhoea. *Pediatric Research*, **25**, 514–18.

Guerrant, R. L., Ganguly, U., Casper, A. G. T., Moore, E. J., Pierce, N. F. & Carpenter, C. C. J. (1973). Effects of *Escherichia coli* on fluid transfer across canine small bowel: mechanism and time-course with enterotoxin and whole bacterial cell. *Journal of Clinical Investigation*, **52**, 1707–14.

Guerrant, R., Hughes, J. M., Chang, B., Robertson, D. C. & Marad, F. (1980). Activation of intestinal guanylate cyclase by heat-stable enterotoxin of *Escherichia coli*: studies on tissue specificity, potential receptors, and intermediates. *Journal of Infectious Diseases*, **142**, 220–8.

Guerrant, R. L., Hughes, J. M., Lima, N. L. & Crane, J. (1990). Diarrhoea in developed and developing countries: magnitude, special settings and etiologies. *Reviews of Infectious Diseases*, 12, S41-S50.

Guth, B. E., Pickett, C. L., Twiddy, E. M., Holmes, R. K., Gomes, T. A., Lima, A. A., Guerrant, R. L., Francs, B. D. & Trabulsi, L. R. (1986a). Production of type II heat-labile enterotoxin by *Escherichia coli* isolated from food and human feces. *Infection and Immunity*, **54**, 587–9.

Guth, B. E., Twiddy, E. M., Trabulsi, L. R. & Holmes, R. K. (1986b). Variation in chemical properties and antigenic determinants among type II heat-labile enterotoxins of *Escherichia coli*. *Infection and Immunity*, **54**, 529–36.

Gyles, C. L., So, M. & Falkow, S. (1974). The enterotoxin plasmids of *Escherichia coli*. *Journal of Infectious Diseases*, **130**, 40–9.

Hardy, S. J., Holmgren, J., Johanssan, S., Scanchez, J. & Hirst, T. R. (1988). Coordinated assembly of multisubunit proteins: oligomerization of bacterial enterotoxins *in vivo* and *in vitro*. *Proceedings of the National Academy of Science, USA*, **85**, 7109–13.

Hemelhof, W., Retore, P., De Mol, P., Butzler, J. P., Takeda, T., Miwatani, T. & Takeda, Y. (1984). Production of a monoclonal antibody against heat-stable enterotoxin produced by human strain of enterotoxigenic *Escherichia coli*. *Lancet*, **1**, 1011–12.

Hewlett, E. L., Guerrant, R. L., Evans, D. J. Jr. & Greenough, W. B. III. (1974) Toxins of *Vibrio cholerae* and *Escherichia coli* stimulate adenyl cyclase in rat fat cells. *Nature (London)*, **249**, 371–3.

Hirayama, T., Ito, H. & Takeda, Y. (1989). Inhibition by the protein kinase inhibitors, isoquinolinosulfonamides, of fluid accumulation induced by *Escherichia coli* heat-stable enterotoxin, 8-bromo-cGMP and 8-bromo-cAMP in suckling mice. *Microbial Pathogenesis*, **7**, 255–61.

Hirayama, T., Oku, Y., Takeda, Y., Iwata, N., Aimoto, S., & Shimonishi, Y. (1990b). Photoaffinity labeling of receptors of *Escherichia coli* heat-stable enterotoxin on cell membrane of rat intestine. In *Advances in Research on Cholera and Related Diarrhoeas*, eds. R. B. Sack & Y. Zinnaka, pp. 105–112. Tokyo: KTK Publishers.

Hirayama, T., Shimonishi, Y. & Takeda, Y. (1990a). Glycoprotein receptors for heat-stable enterotoxin produced by *Escherichia coli*. In *Advances in Second Messenger and Phosphoprotein Research*, **24**, 51.

Hirst, R., Sanchez, J., Kaper, J. B., Hardy, S. J. & Holmgren, J. (1984). Mechanism of toxin secretion by *Vibrio cholerae* investigated in strains harboring plasmids that encode heat-labile enterotoxins of *Escherichia coli*. *Proceedings of the National Academy of Science, USA*, **81**, 7752–6.

Hitotsubashi, S., Fujii, Y., Yamanaka, H. & Okamoto, K. (1992). Some properties of purified *Escherichia coli* heat-stable enterotoxin II. *Infection and Immunity*, **60**, 4468–74.

Hofstra, H. & Witholt, B. (1985). Heat-labile enterotoxin in *Escherichia coli*. Kinetics of association of subunits into periplasmic holotoxin. *Journal of Biological Chemistry*, **260**, 16037–44.

Holmes, R. K., Pickett, C. L. & Twiddy, E. M. (1988). Genetic and biochemical studies of type II heat-labile enterotoxins of *Escherichia coli*. *Zentralblat für Bakteriologie, Supplement*, **17**, 187–94.

Holmes, R. K., Twiddy, E. M. & Pickett, C. L. (1986). Purification and characterization of type II heat-labile enterotoxin of *Escherichia coli*. *Infection and Immunity*, **53**, 464–73.

Holmes, R. K., Twiddy, E. M., Pickett, C. L., Marcus, H., Jobling, M. G. & Petitjean, F. M. J. (1990). The *Escherichia coli-Vibrio cholerae* family of enterotoxins. In *Symposium on Molecular Mode of Action of Selected Microbial Toxins in Foods and Feeds*, eds. A. E. Pohland, V. R. Dowell, Jr. & J. L. Richard, pp. 91–102. New York: Plenum Press.

Holmgren, J. (1973). Comparison of the tissue receptors for *Vibrio cholerae* and *Escherichia coli* enterotoxins by means of ganglioside and natural cholera toxoid. *Infection and Immunity*, **8**, 851–9.

Honda, T., Tsuji, T., Takeda, Y. & Miwatani, T. (1981). Immunological non-identity of heat-labile enterotoxins from human and porcine enterotoxigenic *Escherichia coli*. *Infection and Immunity*, **34**, 337–40.

Hulian, S., Zhen, L. G. & Mathan, M. M. (1991). Etiology of acute diarrhoea among children in developing countries: a multicentric study in five countries. *Bulletin of World Health Organization*, **69**, 549–55.

Iida, T., Tsuji, T., Miwatani, T., Wakabayashi, S., Wada, K. & Matsubara, H. (1989). A single amino-acid substitution in B subunit of *Escherichia coli* enterotoxin affects its oligomer formation. *Journal of Biological Chemistry*, **264**, 14065–70.

Ikemura, H., Watanabe, H., Aimoto, S., Shimonishi, Y., Hara, S., Takeda, T., Takeda, Y. & Miwatani, T. (1984). Heat-stable enterotoxin (STh) of human enterotoxigenic *Escherichia coli* (strain SK-1). Structure–activity relationship. *Bulletin of the Chemical Society of Japan*, **57**, 2550–6.

Ivens, K., Gazzano, H., O'Henly, P. & Waldmann, S. A. (1990). Heterogeneity of intestinal receptors for *Escherichia coli* heat-stable enterotoxin. *Infection and Immunity*, **58**, 1817–20.

de Jonge, H. & Lohmann, S. M. (1985). Mechanism by which cyclic nucleotide and other intracellular mediators regulate secretion. *CIBA Foundation Symposium*, **112**, 116–38.

Kantor, H. S., Tao, P. & Wisdom, C. (1974). Action of *Escherichia coli* enterotoxin: adenylate cyclase behavior of intestinal epithelial cells in culture. *Infection and Immunity*, **9**, 1003–10.

Kennedy, D. J., Greenberg, R. N., Dunn, J. A., Abernathy, R., Ryerse, J. S. & Guerrant, R. L. (1984). Effects of *Escherichia coli* heat-stable enterotoxin b on intestine of mice, rats, rabbits, and piglets. *Infection and Immunity*, **46**, 639–43.

Klipstein, F. A., Engert, R. F. & Houghten, R. A. (1983). Immunological properties of *Klebsiella pneumonia* heat-stable enterotoxin. *Infection and Immunity*, **42**, 838–41.

Kubota, H., Hidaka, Y., Ozaki, H., Hirayama, T., Takeda, Y. & Shimonishi, Y. (1989). A long-acting heat-stable enterotoxin analog of enterotoxigenic *Escherichia coli* with a single D-amino acid. *Biochemical and Biophysical Research Communications*, **161**, 229–35.

Kunkel, S. V & Robertson, D. C. (1979). Purification and chemical characterization of the heat-labile enterotoxin produced by enterotoxigenic *Escherichia coli*. *Infection and Immunity*, **25**, 586–96.

Kuno, T., Kamisaki, Y., Waldman, S. A., Gariepy, J., Schoolnik, G. & Murad, F. (1986). Characterization of the receptor for heat-stable enterotoxin for *Escherichia coli* in rat intestines. *Journal of Biological Chemistry*, **261**, 1470–6.

Kupersztoch, Y. M., Tachias, K., Mooman, C. R., Dreyfus, L. A., Urban, R., Slaughter, C. & Whipp, S. (1990). Secretion of methanol-insoluble heat-stable enterotoxin (STb): energy- and *sec*A-dependent conversion of pro-STb to an intermediate indistinguishable from the extracellular toxin. *Journal of Bacteriology*, **172**, 2427–32.

Lai, C. Y., Mendez, E. & Chang, D. (1976). Chemistry of cholera toxin: the subunit structure. *Journal of Infectious Diseases*, **133**, S23-S30.

Lee, C. H., Moseley, S. L., Moon, H. W., Whipp, S. C., Gyles, C. L. & So, M. (1983). Characterization of the gene encoding heat-stable toxin II and the preliminary molecular epidemiological studies of enterotoxigenic *Escherichia coli* heat-labile toxin II. *Infection and Immunity*, **42**, 264–8.

Leong, J., Vinal, A. C. & Dallas, W. S. (1985). Nucleotide sequence comparison between B-subunit cistrons from *Escherichia coli* of a human and porcine origin. *Infection and Immunity*, **48**, 73–7.

Lortie, L. A., Dubreuil, J. D. & Hard, J. (1991). Characterization of *Escherichia coli* strains producing heat-labile toxin b (STb) isolated from humans with diarrhea. *Journal of Clinical Microbiology*, **29**, 656–9.

Mashiter, K., Mashiter, G. D., Hauger, R. L. & Field, J. B. (1973). Effects of cholera and *E. coli* enterotoxin on cyclic adenosine-3'5'-monophosphate levels and intermediary metabolism in the thyroid. *Endocrinology*, **92**, 541–9.

Mekalanos, J. J., Swartz, G. D., Pearson, N., Harford, N., Groyne, F. & Wilde, M. (1983). Cholera toxin genes: nucleotide sequence, deletion analysis and vaccine development. *Nature (London)*, **306**, 551–7.

Merson, M. H., Morris, G. K., Sack, D. A., Wells, J. G., Feeley, J. C., Sack, R. B., Kapikian, A. Z., & Gangarosa, E. J. (1976). Travellers' diarrhoea in Mexico: a prospective study of physicians and family members attending a congress. *New England Journal of Medicine*, **294**, 1299–305.

Monckton, R. P. & Hasse, D. (1988). Detection of enterotoxigenic *Escherichia coli* in piggeries in Victoria by DNA hybridization using K88, LT, ST1 and ST2 probes. *Veterinary Microbiology*, **16**, 273–81.

Moon, H. W., Schneider, R. A. & Moseley, S. L. (1986). Comparative prevalence of four enterotoxin genes among *Escherichia coli* isolated from swine. *American Journal of Veterinary Research*, **47**, 210–12.

Moseley, S. L., Echevarria, P., Seriwatana, J., Tirapat, C., Chaicumpa, W., Sakuldaipeara, T. & Falkow, S. (1982). Identification of enterotoxigenic

Escherichia coli by colony hybridization using three enterotoxin gene probes. *Journal of Infectious Diseases*, **145**, 863–9.

Moseley, S. L., Hardy, J. M., Huq, M. I., Echevarria, P. & Falkow, S. (1983). Isolation and nucleotide sequence determination of a gene encoding a heat-stable enterotoxin of *Escherichia coli*. *Infection and Immunity*, **39**, 1167–74.

Mullin, B. R., Alog, S. M., Fishman, P. H., Lee, G., Kohn, L. D. & Brady, R. O. (1976). Cholera toxin interactive with thyrotropin receptors on thyroid plasma membranes. *Proceedings of the National Academy of Science, USA*, **73**, 1679–83.

Okamoto, K., Fujii, Y., Akashi, N., Hitotsubashi, S., Kurazono, H., Karasawa, T. & Takeda, Y. (1993). Identification and characterization of heat-stable enterotoxin II-producing *Escherichia coli* from patients with diarrhea. *Microbiology and Immunology*, **37**, 411–4.

Okamoto, K., Miyama, A., Takeda, T., Takeda, Y. & Miwatani, T. (1983). Cross-neutralization of heat-stable enterotoxin activity of enterotoxigenic *Escherichia coli* and of *Yersinia enterocolitica*. *FEMS Microbiology Letters*, **16**, 85–7.

Ozaki, H., Sato, T., Kubota, Y., Hata, Y., Katsube, Y. & Shimonishi, Y. (1991). Molecular structure of the toxic domain of heat-stable enterotoxin produced by a pathogenic strain of *Escherichia coli*. *Journal of Biological Chemistry*, **266**, 5934–41.

Peterson, J. W. & Ochoa, L. G. (1989). Role of prostaglandins and cAMP in the secretory effects of cholera toxin. *Science*, **245**, 857–9.

Picken, R. N., Mazaitis, A. J., Maas, W. K., Rey, M. & Heyneker, H. (1983). Nucleotide sequence of the gene for heat-stable enterotoxin II of *Escherichia coli*. *Infection and Immunity*, **42**, 269–75.

Pickett, C. L., Twiddy, E. M., Belisie, B. W. & Holmes, R. K. (1986). Cloning of genes that encode a new heat-labile enterotoxin of *Escherichia coli*. *Journal of Bacteriology*, **165**, 348–52.

Pickett, C. L., Twiddy, E. M., Coker, C. & Holmes, R. K. (1989). Cloning, nucleotide sequence, and hybridization studies of the type IIb heat-labile enterotoxin gene of *Escherichia coli*. *Journal of Bacteriology*, **171**, 4945–52.

Pickett, C. L., Weinstein, D. L. & Holmes, R. K. (1987). Genetics of type IIa heat-labile enterotoxin of *Escherichia coli*: operon fusions, nucleotide sequence, and hybridization studies. *Journal of Bacteriology*, **169**, 5180–9.

Pierce, N. F. & Wallace, C. K. (1972). Stimulation of jejunal secretion by a crude *Escherichia coli* enterotoxin. *Gastroenterology*, **63**, 439.

Rao, M. C., Guandalini, S., Smith, P. L. & Field, M. (1980). Mode of action of heat-stable *Escherichia coli* enterotoxin: tissue and subcellular specificities and role of cyclic GMP. *Biochimica et Biophysica Acta*, **632**, 35–46.

Rasheed, K., Guzman-Verduzio, L. M. & Kupersztoch, Y. M. (1990). Two precursors of the heat-stable enterotoxin of *Escherichia coli*: evidence of extracellular processing. *Molecular Microbiology*, **4**, 265–74.

Robertson, D. C. & Jaso-Friedmann, L. (1988). Partial purification and characterization of the intestinal receptor for *Escherichia coli* enterotoxin (STa). In *Advances in Cholera Related Diarrhea*, vol. 4, eds. S. Kuwahara & N. F. Pierce, pp 167–79. Tokyo: KTK Scientific Publishers.

Sack, R. B., Gorbach, S. L., Banwell, J. G., Jacobs, B., Chatteryee, B. D. & Mitra, R. C. (1971). Enterotoxigenic *Escherichia coli* isolated from patients with severe cholera-like disease. *Journal of Infectious Diseases*, **123**, 378–85.

Seriwatana, J., Echevarria, P., Taylor, D. N., Rasirinaul, L., Brown, J. E., Peiris, J. S. & Clayton, C. L. (1988). Type II heat-labile enterotoxin-producing *Escherichia coli* isolated from animals and humans. *Infection and Immunity*, **56**, 1158–61.

Shore, E. G., Dean, A. G., Holik, K. J. & Davis, B. R. (1974). Enterotoxin producing *Escherichia coli* in adult travellers: a prospective study. *Journal of Infectious Diseases*, **129**, 577–82.

Shimonishi, Y., Hidaka, Y., Kaiumi, M., Hane, M., Aimoto, S., Takeda, T., Miwatani, T. & Takeda, Y. (1987). Mode of disulphide bond formation of a heat-stable enterotoxin (STh) produced by a human strain of enterotoxigenic *Escherichia coli*. *FEBS Letters*, **215**, 165–70.

Sixma, T. K., Pronk, S. E., Kalk, K. H., Wartna, E. S., van Zanten, B. A. M., Witholt, B. & Hol, W. G. J. (1991). Crystal structure of a cholera toxin related heat-labile enterotoxin from *E. coli*. *Nature (London)*, **351**, 371–7.

Sixma, T. K., Pronk, S. E., Kalk, K. H., Wartna, E. S., van Zanten, B. A. M., Witholt, B. & Hol, W. G. J. (1992). Lactose binding to heat-labile enterotoxin revealed by x-ray crystallography. *Nature (London)*, **355**, 561–4.

Smith, H. W. & Gyles, C. L. (1970). The relationship between two apparently different enterotoxins produced by enteropathogenic strains of *Escherichia coli* of porcine origin. *Journal of Medical Microbiology*, **3**, 387–401.

Snyder, J. H. & Merson, M. H. (1982). The magnitude of the global problem of acute diarrhoeal diseases: a review of active surveillance data. *Bulletin of the World Health Organization*, **60**, 605–13.

So, M. & McCarthy, B. J. (1980). Nucleotide sequence of transposon Tn1681 encoding a heat-stable toxin (ST) and its identification in enterotoxigenic *Escherichia coli* strains. *Proceedings of the National Academy of Science, USA*, **77**, 4011–15.

Spangler, B. D. (1992). Structure and function of cholera toxin and the related *Escherichia coli* heat-labile enterotoxin. *Microbiological Reviews*, **56**, 647–62.

Staples, S. J., Asher, S. E. & Giannella, R. A. (1980). Purification and characterization of heat-stable enterotoxin produced by a strain of *E. coli* pathogenic for man. *Journal of Biological Chemistry*, **255**, 4716–21.

Streatfield, S. J., Scandkvist, M., Sixma, T., Bagdasarian, M., Hol, W. G. J. & Hirst, T. R. (1992). Intermolecular interactions between the A and B subunits of heat-labile enterotoxin from *Escherichia coli* promote holotoxin assembly and stability *in vivo*. *Proceedings of the National Academy of Science, USA*, **89**, 12140–4.

Svennerholm, A. M., Wikstrom, M., Lindbald, M. & Holmgren, J. (1986). Monoclonal antibodies against *Escherichia coli* heat-stable toxin (STa) and their use in a diagnostic ST ganglioside GM1-enzyme-linked immunosorbent assay. *Journal of Clinical Microbiology*, **24**, 585–90.

Takao, T., Shimonishi, Y., Kobayashi, M., Nishimura, O., Arita, M., Takeda, T., Honda, T. & Miwatani, T. (1985). Amino acid sequence of heat-stable enterotoxin produced by *V. cholerae* non-O1. *FEBS Letters*, **193**, 250–4.

Takao, T., Tominaga, N., Shimonishi, Y., Hara, S., Inoue, T. & Miyama, A. (1984). Primary structure of heat-stable enterotoxin produced by *Yersinia enterocolitica*. *Biochemical and Biophysical Research Communications*, **125**, 845–51.

Takao, T., Tominaga, N., Yoshimura, Y., Shimonishi, Y., Hara, S., Inoue, T. & Miyama, A. (1985). Isolation, primary structure and synthesis of heat-stable enterotoxin produced by *Yersinia enterocolitica*. *European Journal of Biochemistry*, **152**, 199–206.

Takeda, T., Nair, G. B., Suzuki, K., Zhe, H. X., Yokoo, Y., De Mol, P., Hemelhof, W., Butzler, J. P., Takeda, Y. & Shimonishi, Y. (1993). Epitope mapping and characterization of antigenic determinants of heat-stable enterotoxin (STh) of enterotoxigenic *Escherichia coli* by using monoclonal antibodies. *Infection and Immunity*, **61**, 289–94.

Takeda, T., Penia, Y., Ogawa, A., Dohi, S., Abe, H., Nair, G. B. & Pal, S. C. (1991). Detection of heat-stable enterotoxin in a cholera toxin gene-positive strain of *Vibrio cholerae* O1. *FEMS Microbiology Letters*, **80**, 23–8.

Takeda, T., Takeda, Y., Aimoto, S., Takao, T., Ikemura, H., Shimonishi, Y. & Miwatani, T. (1983a). Neutralization of activity of two different heat-stable enterotoxins (STh and STp) of enterotoxigenic *Escherichia coli* by homologous and heterologous antisera. *FEMS Microbiology Letters*, **20**, 357–9.

Takeda, Y., Honda, T., Sima, H., Tsuji, T. & Miwatani, T. (1983b) Analysis of antigenic determinants in cholera enterotoxin and heat-labile enterotoxins from human and porcine enterotoxigenic *Escherichia coli*. *Infection and Immunity*, **41**, 50–53.

Takeda, Y., Honda, T., Taga, S. & Miwatani, T. (1981). *In vitro* formation of hybrid toxins between subunits of *Escherichia coli* heat-labile enterotoxin and those of cholera toxin. *Infection and Immunity*, **34**, 341–6.

Takeda, Y., Takeda, T., Yano, T., Yamamoto, K. & Miwatani, T. (1979). Purification and partial characterization of heat-stable enterotoxin of enterotoxigenic *Escherichia coli*. *Infection and Immunity*, **25**, 978–85.

Tsuji, T., Honda, T., Miwatani, T., Wakabayashi, S. & Matsubara, H. (1985). Analysis of receptor-binding site in *Escherichia coli* enterotoxin. *Journal of Biological Chemistry*, **260**, 8552–8.

Tsuji, T., Taga, S., Honda, T., Takeda, Y. & Miwatani, T. (1982). Molecular heterogeneity of heat-labile enterotoxin from human and porcine enterotoxigenic *Escherichia coli*. *Infection and Immunity*, **38**, 444–8.

Tulloch, J. & Richards, L. (1993). Childhood diarrhoea and acute respiratory infections in developing countries. *Medical Journal of Australia*, **159**, 46–51.

Weikel, C. S. & Guerrant, R. L. (1985). STb enterotoxin of *Escherichia coli*: cyclic nucleotide independent secretion. *CIBA Foundation Symposium*, **112**, 94–114.

Whipp, S. C. (1987). Protease degradation of *Escherichia coli* heat-stable, mouse-negative, pig-positive enterotoxin. *Infection and Immunity*, **55**, 2057–60.

Whipp, S. C. (1990). Assay for enterotoxigenic *Escherichia coli* heat-stable enterotoxin in rats and mice. *Infection and Immunity*, **58**, 930–4.

de Wolf, M. J. S., Friedkin, M., Epstein, M. M. & Kohn, L. D. (1981). Structure-function studies of cholera toxin and its A promoters and B promoters-modification of tryptophan residues. *Journal of Biological Chemistry*, **256**, 5481–8.

World Health Organization, 45th World Health Assembly (1992). *Implementation of the global strategy for all by the year 2000*. Second evolution, and eighth report of the World Health Situation. Geneva: WHO, 145/3.

Yamamoto, T., Nakazawa, T., Miyata, T., Kaji, A. & Yokota, T. (1984) Evolution and structure of two ADP-ribosylation enterotoxins, *Escherichia coli* heat-labile toxin and cholera toxin. *FEBS Letters*, **169**, 241–6.

Yamasaki, S., Hidaka, Y., Ito, H., Takeda, Y. & Shimonishi, Y. (1988). Structure requirements for the spatial structure and toxicity of heat-stable enterotoxin (STh) of enterotoxigenic *Escherichia coli*. *Bulletin of the Chemical Society of Japan*, **61**, 1701–6.

Yamasaki, S., Sato, T., Hidaka, Y., Ozaki, H., Ito, H., Hirayama, T., Takeda, Y., Sugimura, T., Tai, A. & Shimonishi, Y. (1990). Structure–activity relationship of *Escherichia coli* heat-stable enterotoxin: role of Ala residue at position 14 in toxin–receptor interaction. *Bulletin of the Chemical Society of Japan*, **63**, 2063–70.

Yoshimura, S., Ikemura, H., Watanabe, H., Aimoto, S., Shimonishi, Y., Hara, S., Takeda, T., Miwatani, T. & Takeda, Y. (1985). Essential structure for full enterotoxigenic activity of heat-stable enterotoxin produced by enterotoxigenic *Escherichia coli*. *FEBS Letters*, **181**, 138–42.

Yoshimura, S., Miki, M., Ikemura, H., Aimoto, S., Shimonishi, Y., Takeda, T., Takeda, Y. & Miwatani, T. (1984). Chemical synthesis of a heat-stable enterotoxin produced by enterotoxigenic *Escherichia coli* 18B. *Bulletin of the Chemical Society of Japan*, **57**, 125–133.

Yoshimura, S., Takano, T., Shimonishi, Y., Arita, M., Takeda, T., Imaishi, H., Honda, T. & Miwatani, T. (1986). A heat-stable enterotoxin of *Vibrio cholerae* non-O1: chemical synthesis, and biological and physicochemical properties. *Biopolymers*, **25**, 69–83.

Zenser, T. V. & Metzger, J. F. (1974). Comparison of the action of *Escherichia coli* enterotoxin on the thymocyte adenylate cyclase–cyclic adenosine monophosphate system to that of cholera toxin and prostaglandin E_1. *Infection and Immunity*, **10**, 503.

10

Vero cytotoxins

S. M. SCOTLAND and H. R. SMITH

Vero-cytotoxin- (VT-) producing strains of *Escherichia coli* (VTEC) are a cause of diarrhoeal disease in humans and animals (see Chapter 15). In particular, they are associated with haemolytic-uraemic syndrome in humans, which is characterised by kidney failure and microangiopathic anaemia, and with oedema disease of pigs. In both of these infections the central nervous system may be affected. Circulating VT may be directly responsible for systemic effects by causing vascular endothelial damage or the induction of platelet aggregation. Less direct roles for VT have, however, also been proposed, as summarised in the reviews by Cleary (1988), Obrig (1992) and Pickering *et al*. (1994). For example, damage to the intestine may allow bacterial products, such as endotoxin, to trigger a Shwartzman-like reaction. Alternatively, damage to the vascular endothelium by VT may contribute to existing congenital or acquired defects in the coagulation mechanism. Attempts to evaluate the role of VT have been hampered by the lack of an animal model that adequately reproduces the disease seen in humans.

Vero cytotoxin, or verotoxin, was first described by Konowalchuk *et al*. (1977), who noted the cytotoxic effect on Vero cells (African Green monkey kidney cells) of culture supernatants of some strains of *E. coli*. These included strains H19 and H30, both of serotype O26:H11, and strain H.I.8, of serogroup O128, from a case of infant diarrhoea and strain E57, of serogroup O138. The latter had been isolated from porcine oedema disease (Erskine *et al*., 1957). An antiserum raised against the toxin produced by H30 did not neutralise the toxins of strains H.I.8 or E57. Konowalchuk & Speirs (1979) noted that VT produced by strain H30 had some cytotoxic activity on HeLa cells but that the toxins of strains H.I.8 and E57 did not. Since this pioneering work it has been recognised that the toxins produced by these strains belong to a family of

Table 10.1. *Genes that encode Shiga toxin and Vero cytotoxins*

Gene product (gene) and synonyms	(stx)	Source	Host strain	Reference
Shiga toxin		Human	3818T, *Sh. dysenteriae* type 1	Strockbine *et al.* (1988)
VT1	SLTI(*slt*-I)	Human	H19,O26:H11	Scotland *et al.* (1983, 1985)
VT2	SLTII(*slt*-II)	Human	933,O157:H7	O'Brien *et al.* (1984)
VT2v	SLTIIc(*slt*-IIc)	Human	E32511,O157:H⁻	Scotland *et al.* (1985) Schmitt *et al.* (1991)
VT2vha(*vtx*2ha), VT2v-a	SLTIIvha	Human	B2F1,O91:H21	Ito *et al.* (1990)
VT2vhb(*vtx*2hb), VT2v-b	SLTIIvhb	Human	B2F1,O91:H21	Ito *et al.* (1990)
VT2e, VTe, VT2vp, VT2vpl	SLTIIv(*slt*-IIv)	Pig	S1191,O139 412,O139:H1	Weinstein *et al.* (1988) Gyles *et al.* (1988)
VT2ev, VTev, VT2vp2	SLTIIva(*slt*-IIva) SLTIIvhc(*slt*-IIvhc)	Human Human	H.1.8,O128:H⁻ 7279,O157:H7	Gannon *et al.* (1990) Meyer *et al.* (1992)
VT2v(pKTN1054)		Bovine	KY-O19,O22:H⁻	Lin *et al.* (1993b)
VT2v(pKTN1050)	SLTIIc(*slt*-IIc)	Human Meat	TK-O51,O157:H7 LM76, *C. freundii*	Lin *et al.* (1993b) Schmidt *et al.* (1993)
	SLTII-OX3	Human	OX3:H21	Paton *et al.* (1992)

related toxins that includes Shiga toxin produced by *Shigella dysenteriae* type 1.

O'Brien & LaVeck (1983) purified the toxin from strain H30 and showed that it possessed many of the properties of Shiga toxin and for this reason they called the new toxin Shiga-like toxin (SLT). The abbreviations VT and SLT are now both in common use. In the light of their similarity, it may be possible to relate much of the work on Shiga toxin to that on VT, but consideration of this topic is beyond the scope of this discussion and reference should be made to the reviews of Acheson *et al.* (1991), O'Brien & Holmes (1987) and Jackson & O'Brien (1994).

Two major classes of VT have been proposed, based on toxin neutralisation and DNA hybridisation tests (Scotland *et al.*, 1985). The first, termed VT1, is neutralised by antibodies to Shiga toxin but the second, termed VT2, is not. The VT1 class, which includes the toxins produced by strains H19 and H30, is very homogeneous, whereas there are several variant forms of VT2, as judged by neutralisation tests, comparison of activity on different cell lines and, more recently, DNA sequencing (see below). These variants include VT2e produced by strains of porcine origin, such as E57, and VT2ev produced by strain H.I.8; both strains were included in the original study of Konowalchuk *et al.* (1977). Some of the synonyms in the increasingly complex VT2 nomenclature are listed in Table 10.1 and for consistency and clarity in the present discussion, the first designation listed for each toxin in the table will be used below. A proposal for the rationalisation of the nomenclature has been made by O'Brien *et al.* (1994). All the VT2s are neutralised to some extent by polyclonal antiserum raised against another VT2 but the titres against heterologous toxins may not be as high as against the homologous toxin (Gannon *et al.*, 1990; Hii *et al.*, 1991).

VTEC may produce either VT1 or VT2, or both toxins (Scotland *et al.*, 1985, 1987; Newland & Neill, 1988; Dickie *et al.*, 1989; Willshaw *et al.*, 1992). Strains have been described that possess genes for more than one form of VT2 (Ito *et al.*, 1990; Schmitt *et al.*, 1991). Some VTEC from animal sources, but so far not from human disease, also produce heat-labile or heat-stable enterotoxins (Kashiwazaki *et al.*, 1981; Gannon *et al.*, 1988; Smith *et al.*, 1988).

Purification

Although VT may, in some strains, be cell-associated, sufficient toxin is liberated into liquid culture media for most test purposes. To obtain optimal yields, toxin can, however, be released by treatment in a French press, by sonication or by brief incubation in the presence of mitomycin or polymyxin (O'Brien & LaVeck, 1983; Noda *et al.*, 1987; Petric *et al.*, 1987; Head *et al.*, 1988). For VT1, but not VT2, yields are increased by growth in media depleted of iron, by treatment with the chelating resin iminodiacetic acid (Chelex) (O'Brien & LaVeck, 1983) or the presence of the iron chelator, desferrioxamine mesylate (Desferal) (Chart *et al.*, 1989).

High yields of biologically active purified Shiga toxin, VT1 and VT2 (Donohue-Rolfe *et al.*, 1989), and VT2e and VT2vh (Acheson *et al.*, 1993) have been obtained by affinity chromatography with the VT-binding glycoproteins present in partially purified sheep hydatid cyst fluid. Milligram amounts of the B subunit were obtained by Calderwood *et al.* (1990) by a similar method. Others have used antibodies raised against the toxins for affinity chromatography (Kongmuang *et al.*, 1987; Downes *et al.*, 1988; MacLeod & Gyles, 1990).

Structure

Shiga toxin, VT1 and VT2 are proteins composed of an enzymatically active A subunit and multiple receptor-binding B subunits. X-ray crystallography of the B oligomer revealed a five-sided assembly of six-stranded anti-parallel β-sheets (Stein *et al.*, 1992). The similarity of this structure to the B pentamer of heat-labile enterotoxin was noted and it was suggested that this structure indicates a distant evolutionary relationship between the two groups of toxins, but there is no sequence conservation. The structure of one A subunit to five B subunits may be the most favourable energetic conformation to allow association of the subunits. The 38 carboxyl-terminal amino acids of the A subunit are crucial for the formation of the holotoxin and they stabilise the interaction between the A and B subunits (Austin *et al.*, 1994).

Genetics

Genetic control of VT production

In several *E. coli* strains VT production is encoded by lysogenic phages, as was first demonstrated for strain H19 (Scotland *et al.*, 1983; Smith *et al.*, 1983). VT phages have also been isolated from strains of serogroups O26, O29, O111, O119, O128 and particularly O157 (Smith *et al.* 1983; O'Brien *et al.* 1984; Smith *et al.* 1984; Karch *et al.*, 1987; Willshaw *et al.*, 1987; Rietra *et al.* 1989; Thomas *et al.*, 1993).

VT phages can be divided into two morphological types, those with elongated hexagonal heads and non-contractile flexible tails and those with regular hexagonal heads and shorter contractile tails (O'Brien *et al.*, 1984; Smith *et al.*, 1984; Willshaw *et al.*, 1987; Rietra *et al.*, 1989). Phages that encode VT1 in strains of serogroup O26, including H19, are of the first type, whereas the VT phages detected in strains of serogroups O29 and O157 belong to the second morphological type. Strains of O157 VTEC that produce VT1 and VT2, including strain 933, carry two morphologically similar phages that respectively encode VT1 and VT2 production (Rietra *et al.*, 1989). Analysis of restriction enzyme digests in the latter study showed that two phages from a wild-type strain were closely related, apart from the VT genes, and that they were distinguishable from the phage from strain H19. The results obtained by O'Brien *et al.* (1984) agreed with respect to a VT2-encoding phage (933W) from strain 933, but the VT1-encoding phage (933J) was virtually identical to that from strain H19 (H19J). Later O'Brien *et al.* (1989) re-examined their original results and concluded that H19J and 933J were in fact the same phage and they were unable to detect a VT1-encoding phage in strain 933. In the light of this, all references in the literature to 933J, and its derivatives, should be considered as being references to H19J.

Strains of porcine origin that produce VT2e have also been examined for phages that determine VT production, but there was no evidence for lysogenic conversion and it was concluded that VT2e genes are chromosomally located (Smith *et al.*, 1983; Marques *et al.*, 1987; Rietra *et al.* 1989).

Cloning of VT genes

The genes of VT1 and VT2 have been cloned in *E. coli* K-12, from phages isolated from strains of serogroups O26 and O157 (Newland *et al.*, 1985; Willshaw *et al.*, 1985; Huang *et al.*, 1986; Newland *et al.*, 1987; Willshaw *et al.*, 1987). The VT1 gene, cloned from strain H19, was very similar to the VT1 gene cloned from strain E30480 of serotype O157:H7 (Willshaw *et al.*, 1987). Comparison of cloned VT1 and VT2 genes did not show similarities in their restriction maps but under conditions of 'reduced stringency' there was weak hybridisation (Newland *et al.*, 1985; Willshaw *et al.*, 1985; Newland *et al.*, 1987; Willshaw *et al.*, 1987). The structural genes for VT2e and a number of other VT2 variants have been cloned and are summarised in Table 10.1.

Table 10.2. *DNA homology between different VT2 genes*

Gene	VT2		VT2v		vtx2ha[a]		VT2e	
	A	B	A	B	A	B	A	B
VT2	*100*		99.7	95	99	96	94	79
VT2v	99.7	95	*100*		99	100	94	83
vtx2ha	99	96	99	100	*100*		95	83
VT2e	94	79	94	83	95	83	*100*	
VT2ev	70	78	–	–	–	–	71	98
slt-IIvhc	99	95	–	–	–	–	95	81
sltII-OX3	96	86	–	–	96	89	92	80
VT2v(pKTN1054)	99	95	–	–	–	–	–	–
VT2v(pKTN1050)	99	96	–	–	–	–	–	–
C. freundii slt-IIc	99	96	99	99	99	99	–	–

[a] *vtx*2ha has 99.3% and 98.9% homology with the A and B subunit genes of *vtx*2hb respectively (Ito *et al.*, 1990).

Sequencing of VT genes

All the VT genes described above have now been sequenced and this has allowed detailed comparisons of homology between genes and particularly between variants of the VT2 gene. The nucleotide homologies between the different VT2 variants are summarised in Table 10.2. There are only a few nucleotide differences between the genes that encode Shiga toxin and VT1 toxins from several different wild-type strains, so that the toxins are identical (Takao *et al.*, 1988) or differ only by one or two amino acids in the A subunit (Strockbine *et al.*, 1988; Paton *et al.*, 1993a). There is homology of about 58 per cent between VT1 and VT2 and this is distributed throughout the A and B subunit genes (Jackson *et al.*, 1987).

The A and B genes are organised in tandem, with the A subunit gene coming first and separated from the B subunit gene by a 12-bp gap for VT1 and by 14 bp in the case of VT2 (Jackson *et al.*, 1987). Both open reading frames are preceded by ribosome-binding sites. The A and B genes appear to be transcribed as a single operon from a promoter that maps about 100 bp upstream from the start of the A subunit. A sequence that may be the termination codon for the operon has been identified 279 bp downstream from the end of the 3′ end of the B subunit gene. Translation of the mRNA to yield one A and five B subunits is most

Table 10.2. *cont.*

VT2ev		*slt*-IIvhc		*slt*II-OX3		VT2v (pKTN1054)		VT2v (pKTN1050)		*C. freundii* *slt*-IIc	
A	B	A	B	A	B	A	B	A	B	A	B
70	78	99	95	96	86	99	95	99	96	99	96
–	–	–	–	–	–	–	–	–	–	99	99
–	–	–	–	96	89	–	–	–	–	99	99
71	98	95	81	92	80	–	–	–	–	–	–
	100	–	–	–	–	–	–	–	–	–	–
–	–	*100*		96	89	–	–	–	–	99.6	100
–	–	96	89	*100*		–	–	–	–	–	–
–	–	–	–	–	–	*100*		–	–	–	–
–	–	–	–	–	–	–	–	*100*		–	–
–	–	99.6	100	–	–	–	–	–	–	*100*	

probably achieved by more efficient initiation of the translation of the B subunit. Analysis of sequence data has revealed three regions of limited homology between the A subunit of all VT genes and the gene that encodes the toxin ricin, derived from beans of the castor plant (Calderwood *et al.*, 1987; De Grandis *et al.*, 1987; Yamasaki *et al.*, 1991).

Regulation of VT production by iron

The production of Shiga toxin is repressed by high levels of iron and this has also been demonstrated for VT1 (O'Brien & Holmes, 1987). Production of VT2 and VT2e is not, however, affected by iron (Chart *et al.*, 1989; Sung *et al.*, 1990). The promoters for VT1, VT2 and VT2e have been mapped and sequenced and the data show a region of dyad symmetry for VT1 and also for the Shiga toxin gene *stx* (Betley *et al.*, 1986; De Grandis *et al.*, 1987). This arrangement is also found in promoters of other iron-repressed genes (see Chapter 12). The VT1 gene is regulated by the product of the *fur* gene, a DNA-binding protein that complexes with iron and blocks transcription. The VT2 and VT2e promoters lack the *fur* operator sequence (Sung *et al.*, 1990).

Biological activity

Enzymatic activity

The biological activities of VTs, Shiga toxin and ricin in eukaryotic cells are the result of the irreversible inhibition of protein synthesis. At the molecular level, the toxins cleave a specific N-glycosidic bond at site 4324 in the 28S ribosomal RNA of the 60S ribosomal subunit. This results in the release of a single adenine residue and the failure of elongation-factor-1-dependent binding of aminoacyl–tRNA to ribosomes. So far, all the different forms of VT appear to have the same enzymatic activity (Igarashi *et al.*, 1987; Endo *et al.*, 1988; Furutani *et al.*, 1990).

One of the gene sequences conserved in Shiga toxin, VT and ricin has been shown, by site-directed mutagenesis, to be an active site. The conservative change of glutamic acid to aspartic acid at site 167 in the VT1 A subunit, or the equivalent site 166 in the VT2 A subunit, reduced enzymatic activity and Vero cell toxicity at least 100-fold, and this was not due to any conformational derangement (Hovde *et al.*, 1988; Jackson *et al.*, 1990a). Similar effects were observed when leucine was substituted for arginine at site 170 in the VT1 A subunit (Yamasaki *et al.*, 1991). The mutant VT1 toxins had similar antigenic properties to those of the wild-type toxin, and these mutant toxins may be candidate toxoids to protect against VT1-mediated diseases (Takeda *et al.*, 1993).

Binding affinity

Toxin subunit B binds to cell glycolipids that have a Galα-(1→4)-Gal moiety, which is regarded as the functional receptor on cells. A possible binding site has been located by X-ray crystallography in a cleft formed by β-sheet interactions (Stein *et al.*, 1992) and this accords well with regions of conserved amino-acid residues in the B subunit (Jackson *et al.*, 1990b).

The various VTs are not identical in binding tests *in vitro*. VT1 and VT2, like Shiga toxin, bind preferentially to Gb$_3$ [Galα-(1→4)-Galβ-(1→4)-GlcCeramide] in which the galactose disaccharide is terminal (Lingwood *et al.*, 1987; Waddell *et al.*, 1988; Brown *et al.*, 1991; Tesh *et al.*, 1993). Although VT2e and VT2vha to some extent bind to Gb$_3$, binding is preferentially to Gb$_4$ [GalNAcβ-(1→3)Galα-(1→4)-Galβ-(1→4)-GlcCeramide] in which the disaccharide is internal (Samuel *et al.*, 1990).

There may also be binding to other glycolipids. Thus, Boyd &

Lingwood (1989) demonstrated the binding of VT1 to Gb_3 derived from the medulla and cortex of human kidneys, but there was also significant binding to another unidentified glycolipid which, unlike Gb_3 was present only in some kidneys. VT1 also binds to Gb_3, which is present in the gastro-intestinal tract and lung tissue of rabbits, but the VT receptor in the central nervous system appeared to be a glycolipid distinct from Gb_3 (Zoja *et al.*, 1992).

Gb_3 and related glycolipids are present on erythrocytes and there are differences in their levels between P blood group types. It has been suggested that the binding of VT to erythrocytes affects the severity of the disease in VTEC infections (Lingwood *et al.*, 1987; Taylor *et al.*, 1990). Newburg *et al.* (1993) demonstrated that lower levels of Gb_3 were associated with haemolytic-uraemic syndrome. The binding of different VTs to human erythrocytes has been confirmed *in vitro* and the binding correlates with P blood group antigens (Bitzan *et al.*, 1994). However, a role for the binding of VT to erythrocytes in pathogenesis remains to be established (Lingwood, 1994).

The level of Gb_3 expression by glomerular endothelial cells is increased by the effect of cytokines, tumour necrosis factor-α and interleukin-1 (van der Kar *et al.*, 1992). These cytokines are induced by the action of VT, and also endotoxin, on macrophages and monocytes (Tesh *et al.*, 1994).

Activity against continuous cell lines in vitro

The cytotoxic effect of VT was first observed in relation to Vero cells. The sensitivity to VT of HeLa cells differs with lines maintained in different laboratories. Thus, VT2e and VT2ev were not active on the HeLa cells used by Konowalchuk & Speirs (1979). On the other hand, Samuel *et al.* (1990) reported that, while VT1 and VT2 were only ten-fold more toxic for Vero cells than for HeLa cells, VT2e and VT2vha, respectively, were 10,000-fold and 1000-fold more toxic for Vero cells. It could not be shown that these HeLa cells expressed Gb_4. However, the HeLa 229 cell line used by Acheson *et al.* (1993) was only fivefold less sensitive to VT2e or VT2vh than Vero cells. Both Gb_3 and Gb_4 were present in the two cell lines, but Vero cells contained about twice as much Gb_4 as the HeLa cells. The cytotoxicity of VT2ev was 125-fold greater on Vero cells than HeLa 229 cells (Gannon *et al.*, 1990).

Activity on primary cell material in vitro

There is some correlation between damage to the vascular endothelial cells *in vivo* and test results *in vitro*. The cytotoxicity of VT for human umbilical cord cells (Obrig *et al.*, 1987), human saphenous vein cells (Tesh *et al.*, 1991) and porcine aortic cells (Kavi *et al.*, 1987) has been shown. In some tests cytotoxicity was most apparent on young, proliferating cells. A significant advance in the study of VT and Shiga toxin on vascular endothelial cells is the availability of human glomerular microvascular endothelial cells. These are much more sensitive to cytotoxic effects because of a 50- to 150-fold higher level of Gb_3 than is present on other endothelial cells (Obrig *et al.*, 1993).

Tests in vivo

Several animals have been tested for their susceptibility to VT and experimental infection with VTEC; the most commonly used are rabbits, pigs, mice and calves (Gyles, 1994).

Porcine oedema disease is characterised by anorexia and oedema of the eyelids and intestinal sites, though there may not be diarrhoea (see Chapter 2). Usually there are neurological signs, such as staggering and paralysis, and a neurotoxin, termed the *edema disease principle* (EDP), is considered to be the cause of the disease. Much work suggests that EDP and VT2e are identical. This was confirmed by comparing preparations from an *E. coli* K-12 strain carrying VT2e genes, cloned from a wild-type strain associated with oedema disease, and preparations from a K-12 strain that differed only in carrying inactivated VT2e genes (Gannon *et al.*, 1989). The latter preparations had no effect but typical oedema disease symptoms were reproduced in weaned pigs by intravenous injection of preparations produced by the VT2e-producing strain. Some differences were seen between the lesions in the brain and intestine and those in natural or experimental infections with VTEC, and it was suggested that this may have been due to the different routes by which toxin was administered. Similar results had been obtained in earlier experiments in which VT2e genes were transferred to *E. coli* K-12 by conjugation (Smith *et al.*, 1983).

It has been more difficult to establish that VT is responsible for the pathological effects seen during VTEC infection of humans. The pig has been suggested as a useful model because, unlike other animals such as rabbits, VT-binding sites are present in kidney tissue. Neurological effects and brain lesions, similar to those caused by VT2e, were seen when VT2vha from strain B2F1 and VT1 from a K-12 strain that carries VT1 genes cloned from strain H19 were injected intravenously in pigs (Gannon *et al.*, 1989). In this animal model VT1 and VT2vh differed from VT2e in that they caused lesions in the kidney but failed to cause intestinal damage.

O'Brien & LaVeck (1983) showed that VT1 shares with Shiga toxin the ability to cause fluid accumulation in the rabbit ileal loop test (RILT) and hind leg paralysis and subsequently death when injected intraperitoneally into mice. Neutralisation of the toxin by a monoclonal antibody that binds to the B subunit prevents all these biological effects (Strockbine *et al.*, 1985). Other VTs have been shown to have similar effects in the RILT and to be lethal for mice. Significant differences in the LD_{50} for mice have been observed with different toxins, ranging from 2000 ng for VT1 to 0.9 pg for VT2e (O'Brien & LaVeck 1983; Kongmuang *et al.*, 1987; Noda *et al.*, 1987; Yutsudo *et al.*, 1987; Oku *et al.*, 1989; MacLeod & Gyles, 1990; Tesh *et al.*, 1993). It has recently been shown that VT2 and VT2vhb are equally toxic for mice but the latter is some 100-fold less active than VT2 on Vero cells (Lindgren *et al.*, 1994). The lower cytotoxic activity of VT2vhb is due to the amino-acid at position 16 of the B subunit.

Intravenous administration to rabbits of VT1 or VT2 (Head *et al.*, 1988; Richardson *et al.*, 1992; Zoja *et al.*, 1992) or of VT2 by continuous perfusion into the peritoneal cavity (Barrett *et al.*, 1989) results in anorexia, diarrhoea and neurological symptoms. In two studies (Head *et al.*, 1988; Richardson *et al.*, 1992) diarrhoeal faeces contained blood and mucus. The symptoms correlated with oedema and mucosal petechiae or colonic haemorrhages and pathological lesions in the brain and spinal cord but other tissues, including the kidneys, were normal. Binding of toxin to tissues has been shown directly by immunofluorescence and ^{125}I-labelling (Richardson *et al.*, 1992) and this correlated with the sites of lesions and the location of glycolipid VT receptors. When corrected for differences in blood flow, the greatest accumulations of ^{125}I-labelled VT1 were in the spinal cord, followed by brain tissue, colon and small intestine. Binding of VT1 to the central nervous system and intestines of immune animals was negligible.

Tests for Vero cytotoxin

Cell tests

The cytotoxic effect of VT can be detected on monolayers of Vero cells grown in tissue culture. The production of VT1 or VT2 or both can be distinguished by means of neutralisation tests with polyclonal antisera (Scotland *et al.*, 1987). For routine purposes, bacteria are grown in a medium such as trypticase soy broth and the toxin is assayed in filtrates of culture supernatants. Free VT present in material such as faeces can be detected by similar methods.

Vero cells are extremely sensitive to VT with a 50 per cent cytotoxic dose of about 1 pg (Downes *et al.*, 1988; Dickie *et al.*, 1989). Consequently, it has proved difficult to develop tests, such as those described in the following sections, with comparable sensitivity.

Enzyme-linked immunosorbent assays (ELISA)

ELISAs for VT can be divided into those that depend on a monoclonal anti-VT antiserum to bind the toxin (Downes *et al.*, 1989) and those in which a glycolipid or glycoprotein receptor is used (Ashkenazi & Cleary, 1989; Acheson *et al.*, 1990). Bound toxin is then detected with monoclonal or polyclonal anti-VT antisera followed by the appropriate enzyme-labelled immunoglobulin and enzyme substrates. Most of these assays, although simple to carry out, have a sensitivity 70- to 2000-fold less than the Vero cell test.

An ELISA for VT1 has been described in which the receptor is lyso-Gb_3, a more polar form of Gb_3 obtained by de-*N*-acylation (Basta *et al.*, 1989). The sensitivity of this modified receptor test was stated to be at least equal to the Vero cell test.

The heterogeneity of VTs, particularly VT2, makes it necessary to take care in the selection and evaluation of ELISA reagents, so that the types of toxin detected are known.

Colony blot assays

Tests for the production of VT by agar-grown bacterial colonies can be carried out after the transfer of growth to nitrocellulose filters. After lysis and unbound sites have been blocked, VT can be detected with specific antibodies similar to those described above for ELISAs. Toxin yields can be increased with agar media that contain trimethoprim-sulphamethoxazole (Karch *et al.*, 1986) or mitomycin (Hull *et al.*, 1993). In the latter case a monoclonal antibody was used that recognises epitopes in the B subunits of both VT1 and VT2. The treatment of colonies with polymyxin B can result in the release of larger amounts of toxin (Jackson *et al.*, 1990b).

Tests for Vero cytotoxin genes

Hybridisation

Polynucleotide probes specific for VT1 and VT2 genes have been developed from cloned VT sequences (Willshaw *et al.*, 1987; Newland & Neill, 1988). To permit further subdivision of VT genes, oligonucleotide probes have been synthesised, and these can also be used to confirm the identify of polymerase chain reaction (PCR) products (Karch & Meyer, 1989; Hii *et al.*, 1991; Thomas *et al.*, 1993)

Amplification of the polymerase chain reaction

The first PCR for VT genes made use of 'degenerated' primers that permitted amplification of VT1, VT2 and VT2 variant genes (Karch & Meyer, 1989). The products were identified with specific VT1 or VT2 oligonucleotide probes, but the VT2 probe did not hybridise with the amplified product from a VT2e gene. The VT2 probe did, however, hybridise with the product from a VT2v gene. These two genes were, therefore, not distinguishable by this PCR system. Lin *et al.* (1993a) described a set of primers that amplified VT1 and five different VT2 sequences. Another approach to the use of PCR has been the development of primers, as defined by sequence analysis, for each different type of VT gene (Pollard *et al.*, 1990a). The primers and products for PCR tests are summarised in Table 10.3.

Primers from the VT1 sequence amplified DNA from strains of *Shigella dysenteriae* type 1 and VT1-producing *E. coli*. It was possible to distinguish between the two with primers from the promoter region of VT1, which did not amplify the corresponding sequence of the Shiga toxin gene (Pollard *et al.*, 1990b). Two sets of primers have been described to differentiate VT2 from VT2v and VT2vha/vhb. Restriction enzyme digestion of the 285-bp product obtained with primers VT2-c and VT2-d allowed VT2 or the variant genes to be identified (Tyler *et al.*, 1991). With primers VT2v-1 and VT2v-2, amplification takes place only with the VT2 variant genes, *vtx*2ha and *vtx*2hb, but not with VT2. It is possible to use two sets of primers in a single PCR, but this 'multiplex' PCR method requires optimisation of the conditions for the different primer sets (Cebula *et al.*, 1995).

Table 10.3. *Identification of VT genes by polymerase chain reaction*

Gene	Primers (5'→3')[a]	Product (bp)	Reference
VT1-a	1191–1210	130	Pollard *et al.* (1990a)
VT1-b	1301–1320		
SLTI-F	938–957	614	Gannon *et al.* (1992)
SLTI-R	1520–1539		
5'I	691–715	370	Brian *et al.* (1992)
3'I	1033–1057		
VT1-c	31–50	140	Pollard *et al.* (1990b);
VT1-d	151–170		Strockbine *et al.* (1988)
VT2-a	426–445	346	Jackson *et al.* (1987)
VT2-b	752–771		Pollard *et al.* (1990a)
VT2-c[b]	1210–1229	285	Jackson *et al.* (1987); Tyler *et al.* (1991);
VT2-d	1475–1494		Gannon *et al.* (1992)
SLTII-F[c]	624–644	779	Gannon *et al.* (1992)
SLTII-R	1384–1403		
5'II	691–715	283	Brian *et al.* (1992)
3'II	950–973		
VT2v-1[d]	1319–1338	385	Ito *et al.* (1990); Tyler *et al.* (1991)
VT2v-2	1684–1703		
VT2e-a	217–236	230	Gyles *et al.* (1988); Johnson *et al.* (1990);
VT2e-b	427–446		Weinstein *et al.* (1988)
VT2ev-a	290–309	490	Gannon *et al.* (1990);
VT2ev-b	760–779		Johnson *et al.* (1991)

[a] The primers refer to the sequences published in the references.
[b] These primers also amplify a 285-bp fragment in VT2v genes.
[c] These primers also amplify the VT2 variant genes *slt*-IIv, *slt*-IIva, *vtx*2ha and *vtx*2hb.
[d] Analysis of the product by restriction enzyme digestion allows subdivision into VT2v-a or VT2v-b.

Conclusions

Animal experiments have provided support for the hypothesis that VT causes vascular damage and loss of the functional integrity of the vessel wall resulting in oedema or haemorrhage. The unequal distribution of toxin-binding sites in the tissues of different animals may in part be responsible for the different effects of VT that have been reported. Levels of VT receptors in tissues may also change with age, as in the intestine of rabbits in which the level of Gb_3 reached a maximum at 24 days (Mobassaleh *et al.*, 1988; Lingwood, 1994). The targeting of organs rich in receptor sites has been clearly shown in the experiments of Richardson *et al.* (1992) and Zoja *et al.* (1992). The role of other host factors in the response to infection has yet to be evaluated, including the immunological response. In particular, the factors responsible for the progression from diarrhoea to the haemolytic-uraemic syndrome are poorly understood.

Physiological effects may also be affected by differences in the binding affinities of toxins. The effects may be complex, and Tesh *et al.* (1993) have suggested that VT1 may bind preferentially to tissues, such as the colonic epithelium, that express low levels of Gb_3 while VT2 with a lower binding affinity for Gb_3 may be free to enter the circulation and bind to other tissues with higher levels of Gb_3. The route by which a toxin is administered to animals may also affect the outcome.

It is now possible to characterise more fully the classes of VT, especially VT2, produced by VTEC and the polymerase chain reaction technique seems particularly valuable for this purpose (Tyler *et al.*, 1991). Alterations in the sequences of the VT2 B subunit can result in changes in the preferred receptor, and this may have important consequences in terms of the type of host affected and the progression of an infection. For example, production of VT2e is predominant in porcine oedema strains, and the binding properties of this toxin are different from those of VT2. Though less well documented, minor changes to the A subunit may affect enzymatic activity. Thus, Paton *et al.* (1993b) noted that a single amino-acid difference in the VT2 A subunits of two toxins resulted in a fourfold difference in their cytotoxicity.

The intestinal damage caused by some VTEC has been related to their ability to cause attaching and effacing lesions of the microvillus structure, since diarrhoeal symptoms may be seen in animals fed VTEC variants that lack the ability to produce VT (see Chapter 2). The production of enterohaemolysin, haemolysin and fimbriae has also been described for VTEC (see Chapters 7 and 11). The involvement of these various virulence properties, together with VT production on pathogenic effects, in the gastro-intestinal tract and in the circulation, needs further study.

Some alterations in VT sequence may be minor but may still be very useful for typing VT genes for epidemiological purposes. Thus, Thomas *et al.* (1993) showed that O157 VTEC, assigned to a single type by the O157 phage typing scheme, could be differentiated further by the classes of their VT genes.

Finally, improved tests for VT and VT genes are necessary to make it possible to identify VTEC more easily and with greater sensitivity. Since at present the emphasis is on the identification of O157 VTEC, the role of VTEC of other serogroups may be underestimated.

References

Acheson, D. W. K., Donohue-Rolfe, A. & Keusch, G. T. (1991). The family of Shiga and Shiga-like toxins. In *Sourcebook of Bacterial Protein Toxins*, eds. J. E. Alouf & J. H. Freer, pp. 415–33. London: Academic Press.

Acheson, D. W. K., Jacewicz, M., Kane, A. V., Donohue-Rolfe, A. & Keusch, G. T. (1993). One step high yield affinity purification of shiga-like toxin II variants and quantitation using enzyme linked immunosorbent assays. *Microbial Pathogenesis*, **14**, 57–66.

Acheson, D. W. K., Keusch, G. T., Lightowlers, M. & Donohue-Rolfe, A. (1990). Enzyme-linked immunosorbent assay for Shiga toxin and Shiga-like toxin II using P_1 glycoprotein from hydatid cysts. *Journal of Infectious Diseases*, **161**, 134–7.

Ashkenazi, S. & Cleary, T. G. (1989). Rapid method to detect Shiga toxin and Shiga-like toxin I based on binding to globotriosyl ceramide (Gb_3), their natural receptor. *Journal of Clinical Microbiology*, **27**, 1145–50.

Austin, P. R., Jablonski, P. E., Bohach, G. A., Dunker, A. K. & Hovde, C. J. (1994). Evidence that the A2 fragment of Shiga-like toxin type I is required for holotoxin integrity. *Infection and Immunity*, **62**, 1768–75.

Barrett, T. J., Potter, M. E. & Wachsmuth, I. K. (1989). Continuous peritoneal infusion of Shiga-like toxin II (SLT II) as a model for SLTII induced diseases. *Journal of Infectious Diseases*, **159**, 774–7.

Basta, M., Karmali, M. & Lingwood, C. (1989). Sensitive receptor-specified enzyme-linked immunosorbent assay for *Escherichia coli* Verocytotoxin. *Journal of Clinical Microbiology*, **27**, 1617–22.

Betley, M. J., Miller, V. L. & Mekalanos, J. J. (1986). Genetics of bacterial enterotoxins. *Annual Review of Microbiology*, **40**, 577–605.

Bitzan, M. J., Richardson, S., Huang, C., Boyd, B., Petric, M. & Karmali, M. A. (1994). Evidence that Verotoxins (Shiga-like toxins) from *Escherichia coli* bind to P blood group antigens of human erythrocytes *in vitro*. *Infection and Immunity*, **62**, 3337–47.

Boyd, B. & Lingwood, C. (1989). Verotoxin receptor glycolipid in human renal tissue. *Nephron*, **51**, 207–10.

Brian, M. J., Frosolono, M., Murray, B. E., Miranda, A., Lopez, E. L., Gomez, H. F. & Cleary, T. G. (1992). Polymerase chain reaction for diagnosis of haemorrhagic *Escherichia coli* infection and hemolytic-uremic syndrome. *Journal of Clinical Microbiology*, **30**, 1801–6.

Brown, J. E., Echeverria, P. & Lindberg, A. A. (1991). Digalactosyl-containing glycolipids as cell surface receptors for Shiga toxin of *Shigella dysenteriae* 1 and related cytotoxins of *Escherichia coli*. *Reviews of Infectious Diseases*, **13**, Supplement 4, S298–S303.

Calderwood, S. B., Acheson, D. W. K., Goldberg, M. B., Boyko, S. A. & Donohue-Rolfe, A. (1990). A system for production and rapid purification of large amounts of Shiga toxin/Shiga-like toxin I B subunit. *Infection and Immunity*, **58**, 2977–82.

Calderwood, S. B., Auclair, F., Donohue-Rolfe, A., Keusch, G. T. & Mekalanos, J. J. (1987). Nucleotide sequence of the Shiga-like toxin genes of *Escherichia coli*. *Proceedings of the National Academy of Sciences, USA*, **84**, 4364–8.

Cebula, T. A., Payne, W. L. & Feng, P. (1995). Simultaneous identification of strains of *Escherichia coli* serotype O157:H7 and their shiga-like toxin type by mismatch amplification assay – multiplex PCR. *Journal of Clinical Microbiology*, **33**, 248–50.

Chart, H., Scotland, S. M. & Rowe, B. (1989). Production of Vero cytotoxins by *Escherichia coli* and Shiga toxin by *Shigella dysenteriae* 1 as related to the growth medium and availability of iron. *Zentralblatt für Bakteriologie und Hygiene A*, **272**, 1–10.

Cleary, T. G. (1988). Cytotoxin-producing *Escherichia coli* and the hemolytic uremic syndrome. *New Topics in Pediatric Infectious Disease*, **35**, 485–501.

De Grandis, S., Ginsberg, J., Toone, M., Climie, S., Friesen, J. & Brunton, J. (1987). Nucleotide sequence and promoter mapping of the *Escherichia coli* Shiga-like toxin operon of bacteriophage H-19B. *Journal of Bacteriology*, **169**, 4319–9.

Dickie, N., Speirs, J. I., Akhtar, M., Johnson, W. M. & Szabo, R. A. (1989). Purification of an *Escherichia coli* serogroup O157:H7 verotoxin and its detection in North American hemorrhagic colitis isolates. *Journal of Clinical Microbiology*, **27**, 1973–8.

Donohue-Rolfe, A., Acheson, D. W. K., Kane, A. V. & Keusch, G. T. (1989). Purification of Shiga toxin and Shiga-like toxins I and II by receptor analog affinity chromatography with immobilized P1 glycoprotein and production of cross-reactive monoclonal antibodies. *Infection and Immunity*, **57**, 3888–93.

Downes, F. P., Barrett, T. J., Green, J. H., Aloisio, C. H., Spika, J. S., Strockbine, N. A. & Wachsmuth, I. K. (1988). Affinity purification and characterization of Shiga-like toxin II and production of toxin-specific monoclonal antibodies. *Infection and Immunity*, **56**, 1926–33.

Downes, F. P., Green, J. H., Greene, K., Strockbine, N., Wells, J. G. & Wachsmuth, I. K. (1989). Development and evaluation of enzyme-linked immunosorbent assays for detection of Shiga-like toxin I and Shiga-like toxin II. *Journal of Clinical Microbiology*, **27**, 1292–7.

Endo, Y., Tsurugi, K., Yutsudo, T., Takeda, Y., Ogasawara, T. & Igarashi, K. (1988). Site of action of a Vero toxin (VT2) from *Escherichia coli* O157:H7 and of Shiga toxin on eukaryotic ribosomes: RNA *N*-glycosidase activity of the toxins. *European Journal of Biochemistry*, **171**, 45–50.

Erskine, R. G., Sojka, W. J. & Lloyd, M. K. (1957) The experimental reproduction of a syndrome indistinguishable from oedema disease. *Veterinary Record*, **69**, 301–3.

Furutani, M., Ito, K., Oku, Y., Takeda, T. & Igarashi, K. (1990). Demonstration of RNA *N*-glycosidase activity of a Vero toxin (VT2 variant) produced by *Escherichia coli* O91:H21 from a patient with the hemolytic uremic syndrome. *Microbiology and Immunology*, **34**, 387–92.

Gannon, V. P. J., Gyles, C. L. & Friendship, R. W. (1988). Characteristics of verotoxigenic *Escherichia coli* from pigs. *Canadian Journal of Veterinary Research*, **52**, 331–7.

Gannon, V. P. J., Gyles, C. L. & Wilcock, B. P. (1989). Effects of *Escherichia coli* Shiga-like toxins (verotoxins) in pigs. *Canadian Journal of Veterinary Research*, **53**, 306–12.

Gannon, V. P. J., King, R. K., Kim, J. Y. & Thomas, E. J. G. (1992). Rapid and sensitive method for detection of Shiga-like toxin-producing *Escherichia coli* in ground beef using the polymerase chain reaction. *Applied and Environmental Microbiology*, **58**, 3809–15.

Gannon, V. P. J., Teerling, C., Masri, S. A. & Gyles, C. J. (1990). Molecular cloning and nucleotide sequence of another variant of the *Escherichia coli* Shiga-like toxin II family. *Journal of General Microbiology*, **136**, 1125–35.

Gyles, C. L. (1994). VT toxemia in animal models. In *Recent Advances in Vero Cytotoxin-Producing Escherichia coli Infections*, eds. M. A. Karmali & A. G. Goglio, pp. 233–40. Amsterdam: Elsevier.

Gyles, C. L., De Grandis, S. A., MacKenzie, C. & Brunton, J. L. (1988). Cloning and nucleotide sequence analysis of the genes determining vero-cytotoxin production in a porcine edema disease isolate of *Escherichia coli*. *Microbial Pathogenesis*, **5**, 419–26.

Head, S. C., Petric, M., Richardson, S., Roscoe, M. & Karmali, M. A. (1988). Purification and characterization of verocytotoxin 2. *FEMS Microbiology Letters*, **51**, 211–16.

Hii, J. H., Gyles, C., Morooka, T., Karmali, M. A., Clarke, R., De Grandis, S. & Brunton, J. L. (1991). Development of Verotoxin 2- and Verotoxin 2 variant (VT2v)-specific oligonucleotide probes on the basis of the nucleotide sequence of the B cistron of VT2v from *Escherichia coli* E32511 and B2F1. *Journal of Clinical Microbiology*, **29**, 2704–9.

Hovde, C. J., Calderwood, S. B., Mekalanos, J. J. & Collier, R. J. (1988). Evidence that glutamic acid 167 is an active-site residue of Shiga-like toxin I. *Proceedings of the National Academy of Sciences, USA*, **85**, 2568–72.

Huang, A., De Grandis, S., Friesen, J., Karmali, M., Petric, M., Congi, R. & Brunton, J. L. (1986). Cloning and expression of the genes specifying Shiga-like toxin production in *Escherichia coli* H19. *Journal of Bacteriology*, **166**, 375–9.

Hull, A. E., Acheson, D. W. K., Echeverria, P., Donohue-Rolfe, A. & Keusch, G. T. (1993). Mitomycin immunoblot colony assay for detection of Shiga-like toxin-producing *Escherichia coli* in fecal samples: comparison with DNA probes. *Journal of Clinical Microbiology*, **31**, 1167–72.

Igarashi, K., Ogasawara, T., Ito, K., Yutsudo, T. & Takeda, Y. (1987). Inhibition of elongation factor 1-dependent aminoacyl-tRNA binding to ribosomes by Shiga-like toxin I (VT1) from *Escherichia coli* O157:H7 and Shiga toxin. *FEMS Microbiology Letters*, **44**, 91–4.

Ito, H., Terai, A., Kurazono, H., Takeda, Y. & Nishibuchi, M. (1990). Cloning and nucleotide sequencing of Vero toxin 2 variant genes from *Escherichia coli* O91:H21 isolated from a patient with the hemolytic uremic syndrome. *Microbial Pathogenesis*, **8**, 47–60.

Jackson, M. P., Deresiewicz, R. L. & Calderwood, S. B. (1990a). Mutational analysis of the Shiga toxin and Shiga-like toxin II enzymatic subunits. *Journal of Bacteriology*, **172**, 3346–50.

Jackson, M. P., Neill, R. J., O'Brien, A. D., Holmes, R. K. & Newland, J. W. (1987). Nucleotide sequence analysis and comparison of the structural genes for Shiga-like toxin I and Shiga-like toxin II encoded by bacteriophages from *Escherichia coli* 933. *FEMS Microbiology Letters*, **44**, 109–14.

Jackson, M. P. & O'Brien, A. D. (1994). Structure–function relationships of Shiga toxin and Shiga-like toxins to bacterial enterotoxins and ribosome-inactivating proteins. In *Recent Advances in Vero Cytotoxin-Producing Escherichia coli Infections*, eds. M. A. Karmali & A. G. Goglio, pp. 123–30. Amsterdam: Elsevier.

Jackson, M. P., Wadolkowski, E. A., Weinstein, D. I., Holmes, R. K. & O'Brien, A D. (1990b). Functional analysis of the Shiga toxin and Shiga-like toxin type-II variant binding subunits by using site-directed mutagenesis. *Journal of Bacteriology*, **172**, 653–8.

Johnson, W. M., Pollard, D. R., Lior, H., Tyler, S. D. & Rozee, K. R. (1990). Differentiation of genes coding for *Escherichia coli* Verotoxin 2 and the Verotoxin associated with porcine edema disease (VTe) by the polymerase chain reaction *Journal of Clinical Microbiology*, **28**, 2351–3.

Johnson, W. M., Tyler, S. D., Wang, G. & Lior, H. (1991). Amplification by the polymerase chain reaction of a specific target sequence in the gene coding for *Escherichia coli* verotoxin (VTe variant). *FEMS Microbiology Letters*, **84**, 227–30.

Karch, H., Heesemann, J. & Laufs, R. (1987). Phage-associated cytotoxin production by and enteroadhesiveness of enteropathogenic *Escherichia coli* isolated from infants with diarrhea in West Germany. *Journal of Infectious Diseases*, **155**, 707–15.

Karch, H. & Meyer, T. (1989). Single primer pair for amplifying segments of distinct Shiga-like toxin genes by polymerase chain reaction. *Journal of Clinical Microbiology*, **27**, 2751–7.

Karch, H., Strockbine, N. A. & O'Brien, A. D. (1986). Growth of *Escherichia coli* in the presence of trimethoprim-sulfamethoxazole facilitates detection of Shiga-like toxin producing strains by colony blot assay. *FEMS Microbiology Letters*, **35**, 141–5.

Kashiwazaki, M., Ogawa, T., Nakamura, K., Isayama, Y., Tamura, K. & Sakazaki, R. (1981). Vero cytotoxin produced by *Escherichia coli* strains of animal origin. *National Institute of Animal Health Quarterly (Japan)*, **21**, 68–72.

Kavi, J., Chant, I., Maris, M. & Rose, P. E. (1987). Cytopathic effect of verotoxin in endothelial cells. *Lancet*, **ii**, 1035.

Kongmuang, U., Honda, T. & Miwatani, T. (1987). A simple method for purification of Shiga or Shiga-like toxin from *Shigella dysenteriae* and *Escherichia coli* O157:H7 by immunoaffinity column chromatography. *FEMS Microbiology Letters*, **48**, 379–83.

Konowalchuk, J. & Speirs, J. I. (1979). Response of various cell lines to *Escherichia coli* toxic products. *Canadian Journal of Microbiology*, **25**, 335–9.

Konowalchuk, J., Spiers, J. I. & Stavric, S. (1977). Vero response to a cytotoxin of *Escherichia coli*. *Infection and Immunity*, **18**, 775–9.

Lin, Z., Kurazano, H., Yamasaki, S. & Takeda, Y. (1993a). Detection of various variant Verotoxin genes in *Escherichia coli* by polymerase chain reaction. *Microbioloty and Immunology*, **37**, 543–8.

Lin, Z., Yamasaki, S., Kurazono, H., Ohmura, M., Karasawa, T., Inoue, T., Sakamoto, S., Suganami, T., Takeoka, T., Taniguchi, Y. & Takeda, Y. (1993b). Cloning and sequencing of two new Verotoxin 2 variant genes of *Escherichia coli* isolated from cases of human and bovine diarrhea. *Microbiology and Immunology*, **37**, 451–9.

Lindgren, S. W., Samuel, J. E., Schmitt, C. K. & O'Brien, A. D. (1994). The specific activities of Shiga-like toxin type II (SLT-II) and SLTII-related toxins of enterohemorrhagic *Escherichia coli* differ when measured by Vero cell cytotoxicity but not by mouse lethality. *Infection and Immunity*, **62**, 623–31.

Lingwood, C. A. (1994). Verotoxin recognition of its glycolipid receptor, globotriaosylceramide: role in pathogenesis. In *Recent Advances in Vero Cytotoxin-Producing Escherichia coli Infections*, eds. M. A. Karmali & A. G. Goglio, pp. 131–7. Amsterdam: Elsevier.

Lingwood, C. A., Law, H., Richardson, S., Petric, M., Brunton, J. L., De Grandis, S. & Karmali, M. (1987). Glycolipid binding of purified and recombinant *Escherichia coli* produced verotoxin *in vitro*. *Journal of Biological Chemistry*, **262**, 8834–9.

MacLeod, D. L. & Gyles, C. L. (1990). Purification and characterization of an *Escherichia coli* Shiga-like toxin II variant. *Infection and Immunity*, **58**, 1232–9.

Marques, L. R. M., Peiris, J. S. M., Cryz, S. J. & O'Brien, A. D. (1987). *Escherichia coli* strains isolated from pigs with edema disease produce a variant of Shiga-like toxin II. *FEMS Microbiology Letters*, **44**, 33–8.

Meyer, T., Karch, H., Hacker, J., Bocklage, H. & Heesemann, J. (1992). Cloning and sequencing of a Shiga-like toxin II-related gene from *Escherichia coli* O157:H7 strain 7279. *Zentralblatt für Bakteriologie und Hygiene A*, **276**, 176–88.

Mobassaleh, M., Donohue-Rolfe, A., Jacewicz, M., Grand, R. J. & Keusch, G. T. (1988). Pathogenesis of *Shigella* diarrhea: evidence for a developmentally regulated glycolipid receptor for Shigella toxin involved in the fluid secretory response of rabbit small intestine. *Journal of Infectious Diseases*, **157**, 1023–31.

Newburg, D. S., Chaturvedi, P., Lopez, E. L., Devoto, S., Fayed, A. & Cleary, T. G. (1993). Susceptibility to hemolytic-uremic syndrome relates to erythrocyte glycosphingolipid patterns. *Journal of Infectious Diseases*, **168**, 476–9.

Newland, J. W. & Neill, R. J. (1988). DNA probes for Shiga-like toxins I and II and for toxin-converting bacteriophages. *Journal of Clinical Microbiology*, **26**, 1292–7.

Newland, J. W., Strockbine, N. A., Miller, S. F., O'Brien, A. D. & Holmes, R. K. (1985). Cloning of Shiga-like toxin structural genes from a toxin converting phage of *Escherichia coli*. *Science*, **230**, 179–81.

Newland, J. W., Strockbine, N. A. & Neill, R. J. (1987). Cloning of genes for production of *Escherichia coli* Shiga-like toxin type II. *Infection and Immunity*, **55**, 2675–80.

Noda, M., Yutsudo, T., Nakabayashi, N., Hirayama, T. & Takeda, Y. (1987). Purification and some properties of Shiga-like toxin from *Escherichia coli* O157:H7 that is immunologically identical to Shiga toxin. *Microbial Pathogenesis*, **2**, 339–49.

O'Brien, A. D. & Holmes, R. K. (1987). Shiga and Shiga-like toxins. *Microbiological Reviews*, **51**, 206–20.

O'Brien, A. D., Karmali, M. A. & Scotland, S. M. (1994). A proposal for rationalizing the nomenclature of the *Escherichia coli* cytotoxins. In *Recent Advances in Vero Cytotoxin-Producing Escherichia coli Infections*, eds. M. A. Karmali & A. G. Goglio, pp. 147–49. Amsterdam: Elsevier.

O'Brien, A. D. & LaVeck, G. D. (1983). Purification and characterization of a *Shigella dysenteriae* 1-like toxin produced by *Escherichia coli*. *Infection and Immunity*, **40**, 675–83.

O'Brien, A. D., Marques, L. R. M., Kerry, C. F., Newland, J. W. & Holmes, R. K. (1989). Shiga-like toxin converting phage of enterohemorrhagic *Escherichia coli* strain 933. *Microbial Pathogenesis*, **6**, 381–90.

O'Brien, A. D., Newland, J. W., MIller, S. F., Holmes, R. K., Smith, H. W. & Formal, S. B. (1984). Shiga-like toxin-converting phages from *Escherichia coli* strains that cause hemorrhagic colitis or infantile diarrhea. *Science*, **226**,694–6.

Obrig, T. G. (1992). Pathogenesis of Shiga toxin (verotoxin)-induced endothelial cell injury. In *Haemolytic uremic syndrome and thrombotic thrombocytopenic purpura*. eds. B. S. Kaplan, R. S. Trompeter & J. L. Moake, pp. 405–19. New York: Marcel Dekker.

Obrig, T. G., Louise, C. B., Lingwood, C. A., Boyd, B., Barley-Moloney, L. & Daniel, T. O. (1993). Endothelial heterogeneity in Shiga toxin receptors and responses. *Journal of Biological Chemistry*, **268**, 154–8.

Obrig, T. G., del Vecchio, P. J., Karmali, M. A., Petric, M., Moran, T. P. & Judge, T. K. (1987). Pathogenesis of haemolytic uraemic syndrome. *Lancet*, **ii**, 687.

Oku, Y., Yutsudo, T., Hirayama, T., O'Brien, A. D. & Takeda, Y. (1989). Purification and some properties of a Vero toxin from a human strain of *Escherichia coli* that is immunologically related to Shiga-like toxin II (VT2). *Microbial Pathogenesis*, **6**, 113–22.

Paton, A. W., Paton, J. C., Goldwater, P. N., Heuzenroeder, M. W. & Manning, P. A. (1993a). Sequence of a variant Shiga-like toxin type I operon of *Escherichia coli* O111:H-. *Gene*, **129**, 87–92.

Paton, A. W., Paton, J. C., Heuzenroeder, M. W., Goldwater, P. N. & Manning, P. A. (1992). Cloning and nucleotide sequence of a variant Shiga-like toxin II gene from *Escherichia coli* O3:H21 isolated from a case of Sudden Infant Death Syndrome. *Microbial Pathogenesis*, **13**, 225–36.

Paton, A. W., Paton, J. C. & Manning, P. A. (1993b). Polymerase chain reaction amplification, cloning and sequencing of variant *Escherichia coli* Shiga-like toxin type II operons. *Microbial Pathogenesis*, **15**, 77–82.

Petric, M., Karmali, M. A., Richardson, S. & Cheung, R. (1987). Purification and biological properties of *Escherichia coli* verocytotoxin. *FEMS Microbiology Letters*, **41**, 63–8.

Pickering, L. K., Obrig, T. G. & Stapleton, F. B. (1994). Hemolytic-uremic syndrome and enterohemorrhagic *Escherichia coli*. *Pediatric Infectious Disease Journal*, **13**, 459–76.

Pollard, D. R., Johnson, W. M., Lior, H., Tyler, S. D. & Rozee, K. R. (1990a). Rapid and specific detection of Verotoxin genes in *Escherichia coli* by the polymerase chain reaction. *Journal of Clinical Microbiology*, **28**, 540–5.

Pollard, D. R., Johnson, W. M., Lior, H., Tyler, S. D. & Rozee, K. R. (1990b). Differentiation of Shiga toxin and Vero cytotoxin type 1 genes by polymerase chain reaction. *Journal of Infectious Diseases*, **162**, 1195–8.

Richardson, S. E., Rotman, T. A., Jay, V., Smith, C. R., Becker, L. E., Petric, M., Olivieri, N. F. & Karmali, M. A. (1992). Experimental vero-cytotoxemia in rabbits. *Infection and Immunity*, **60**, 4154–67.

Rietra, P. J. G. M., Willshaw, G. A., Smith, H. R., Field, A. M., Scotland, S. M. & Rowe, B. (1989). Comparison of Vero-cytotoxin-encoding phages from *Escherichia coli* of human and bovine origin. *Journal of General Microbiology*, **135**, 2307–18.

Samuel, J. E., Perera, L. P., Ward, S., O'Brien, A. D., Ginsburg, V. & Krivan, H. C. (1990). Comparison of the glycolipid receptor specificities of Shiga-like toxin type II and Shiga-like toxin type II variants. *Infection and Immunity*, **58**, 611–18.

Schmidt, H., Montag, M., Bockemühl, J., Heesemann, J. & Karch, H. (1993). Shiga-like toxin II-related cytotoxins in *Citrobacter freundii* strains from humans and beef samples. *Infection and Immunity*, **61**, 534–43.

Schmitt, C. K., McKee, M. L. & O'Brien, A. D. (1991). Two copies of Shiga-like toxin II-related genes common in enterohemorrhagic *Escherichia coli* strains are responsible for the antigenic heterogeneity of the O157:H- strain E32511. *Infection and Immunity*, **59**, 1065–73.

Scotland, S. M., Smith, H. R. & Rowe, B. (1985). Two distinct toxins active on Vero cells from *Escherichia coli* O157. *Lancet*, **ii**, 885–6.

Scotland, S. M., Smith, H. R., Willshaw, G. A. & Rowe, B. (1983). Vero cytotoxin production in strain of *Escherichia coli* is determined by genes carried on bacteriophage. *Lancet*, **ii**, 216.

Scotland, S. M., Willshaw, G. A., Smith, H. R. & Rowe, B. (1987). Properties of strains of *Escherichia coli* belonging to serogroup O157 with special reference to production of Vero cytotoxins VT1 and VT2. *Epidemiology and Infection*, **99**, 613–24.

Smith, H. R., Day, N. P., Scotland, S. M., Gross, R. J. & Rowe, B. (1984). Phage-determined production of Vero cytotoxin in strains of *Escherichia coli* serogroup O157. *Lancet*, **i**, 1242–3.

Smith, H. R., Scotland, S. M., Willshaw, G. A., Wray, C., McLaren, I. M., Cheasty, T. & Rowe, B. (1988). Vero cytototoxin production and presence of VT genes in *Escherichia coli* strains of animal origin. *Journal of General Microbiology*, **134**, 829–34.

Smith, H. W., Green, P. & Parsell, Z. (1983). Vero cell toxins in *Escherichia coli* and related bacteria: transfer by phage and conjugation and toxic action in laboratory animals, chickens and pigs. *Journal of General Microbiology*, **129**, 3121–37.

Stein, P. F., Boodhoo, A., Tyrrell, G., Brunton, J. L. & Read, R. J. (1992). Crystal structure of the cell binding B oligomer of Verotoxin-1 from *E. coli*. *Nature*, **355**, 748–50.

Strockbine, N. A., Jackson, M. P., Sung, L. M., Holmes, R. K. & O'Brien, A. D. (1988). Cloning and sequencing of the genes for Shiga toxin from *Shigella dysenteriae* type 1. *Journal of Bacteriology*, **170**, 1116–22.

Strockbine, N. A., Marques, L. R. M., Holmes, R. K. & O'Brien, A. D. (1985). Characterization of monoclonal antibodies against Shiga-like toxin from *Escherichia coli*. *Infection and Immunity*, **50**, 695–700.

Sung, L. M., Jackson, M. P., O'Brien, A. D. & Holmes, R. K. (1990). Transcription of the Shiga-like toxin type II and Shiga-like toxin type II variant operons of *Escherichia coli*. *Journal of Bacteriology*, **172**, 6386–95.

Takao, T., Tanabe, T., Hong, Y.-M., Shimonishi, Y., Kurazono, H., Yutsudo, T., Sasakawa, C., Yoshikawa, M. & Takeda, Y. (1988). Identity of molecular structure of Shiga-like toxin I (VT1) from *Escherichia coli* O157:H7 with that of Shiga toxin. *Microbial Pathogenesis*, **5**, 357–69.

Takeda, Y., Kurazono, H. & Yamasaki, S. (1993). Vero toxins (Shiga-like toxins) produced by enterohemorrhagic *Escherichia coli* (Verocytotoxin-producing *E. coli*). *Microbiology and Immunology*, **37**, 591–9.

Taylor, C. M., Milford, D. V., Rose, P. E., Roy, T. C. F. & Rowe, B. (1990). The expression of blood group P1 in post-enteropathic haemolytic uraemic syndrome. *Pediatric Nephrology*, **4**, 59–61.

Tesh, V. L., Burris, J. A., Owens, J. W., Gordon, V. M., Wadolkowski, E. A., O'Brien, A. D. & Samuel, J. E. (1993). Comparison of the relative toxicities of Shiga-like toxin type I and type II for mice. *Infection and Immunity*, **61**, 3392–402.

Tesh, V. L., Ramegowda, B. & Samuel, J. E. (1994). Purified Shiga-like toxins induce expression of proinflammatory cytokines from murine peritoneal macrophages. *Infection and Immunity*, **62**, 5085–94.

Tesh, V. L., Samuel, J. E., Perera, L. P., Sharefkin, J. B. & O'Brien, A. D. (1991). Evaluation of the role of Shiga and Shiga-like toxins in mediating direct damage to human vascular endothelial cells. *Journal of Infectious Diseases*, **164**, 344–52.

Thomas, A., Smith, H. R. & Rowe, B. (1993). Use of digoxigenin-labelled oligonucleotide DNA probes for VT2 and VT2 human variant genes to differentiate Vero cytotoxin-producing *Escherichia coli* strains of serogroup O157. *Journal of Clinical Microbiology*, **31**, 1700–3.

Tyler, S. D., Johnson, W. M., Lior, H., Wang, G. & Rozee, K. R. (1991). Identification of Verotoxin type 2 variant B subunit genes in *Escherichia coli* by the polymerase chain reaction and restriction fragment length polymorphism analysis. *Journal of Clinical Microbiology*, **29**, 1339–43.

Van der Kar, N. C. A. J., Monnens, L. A. H., Karmali, M. A. & Hinsbergh, V. W. M. (1992). Tumor necrosis factor and interleukin-1 induce expression of the verocytotoxin receptor globotriosylceramide on human endothelial cells: implications for the pathogenesis of the hemolytic uremic syndrome. *Blood*, **80**, 2755–64.

Waddell, T., Head, S., Petric, M., Cohen, A. & Lingwood, C. (1988). Globotriosyl ceramide is specifically recognized by the *Escherichia coli* verocytotoxin 2. *Biochemical and Biophysical Research Communications*, **152**, 674–9.

Weinstein, D. L., Jackson, M. P., Samuel, J. E., Holmes, R. K. & O'Brien, A. D. (1988). Cloning and sequencing of a Shiga-like toxin type II variant from an *Escherichia coli* strain responsible for edema disease of swine. *Journal of Bacteriology*, **170**, 4223–30.

Willshaw, G. A., Scotland, S. M., Smith, H. R. & Rowe, B. (1992). Properties of Vero cytotoxin-producing *Escherichia coli* of human origin of O-serogroups other than O157. *Journal of Infectious Diseases*, **166**, 797–802.

Willshaw, G. A., Smith, H. R., Scotland, S. M., Field, A. M. & Rowe, B. (1987). Heterogeneity of *Escherichia coli* phages encoding Vero cytotoxins: comparison of cloned sequences determining VT1 and VT2 and development of specific gene probes. *Journal of General Microbiology*, **133**, 1309–17.

Willshaw, G. A., Smith, H. R., Scotland, S. M. & Rowe, B. (1985). Cloning of genes determining the production of Vero cytotoxin by *Escherichia coli*. *Journal of General Microbiology*, **131**, 3047–53.

Yamasaki, S., Furutani, M., Ito, K., Igarashi, K., Nishibuchi, M. & Takeda, Y. (1991). Importance of arginine at position 170 of the A subunit of Vero toxin 1 produced by enterohemorrhagic *Escherichia coli* for toxin activity. *Microbial Pathogenesis*, **11**, 1–9.

Yutsudo, T., Nakabayashi, N., Hirayama, T. & Takeda, Y. (1987). Purification and some properties of a Vero toxin from *Escherichia coli* O157:H7 that is immunologically unrelated to Shiga toxin. *Microbial Pathogenesis*, **3**, 21–30.

Zoja, C., Corna, D., Farina, C., Sacchi, G., Lingwood, C., Doyle, M. P., Padhye, V. V., Abbate, M. & Remuzzi, G. (1992). Verotoxin glycolipid receptors determine the localization of microangiopathic process in rabbits given verotoxin-1. *Journal of Laboratory and Clinical Medicine*, **120**, 229–38.

11

Haemolysins of *Escherichia coli*

A. LUDWIG and W. GOEBEL

Haemolysins are produced by a variety of Gram-positive and Gram-negative bacteria and, in most cases, epidemiological and experimental evidence suggest that they are involved in the pathogenesis of disease. Of these toxins, the α-haemolysin of *Escherichia coli* is the most extensively studied. Haemolysis, that is the lysis of erythrocytes, may be brought about by the enzymatic activities of some species of bacteria, such as phospholipase C of *Pseudomonas aeruginosa*. The α-haemolysin of *E. coli*, however, and most other protein haemolysins act by forming pores in the cytoplasmic membrane of erythrocytes. In hypotonic media, pore formation leads to a net influx of water followed by cell swelling and ultimately osmotic lysis. In spite of its classical designation as a 'haemolysin', the pore-forming activity of *E. coli* α-haemolysin is not restricted to erythrocytes, but extends to a wide range of other mammalian and human cell types. This toxin is, therefore, more appropriately designated as a cytolysin.

The introduction of recombinant DNA techniques has made possible analysis of the genes and gene products involved in the synthesis and secretion of active α-haemolysin and this, in turn, has facilitated study of the specific functions and activities of this toxin. In addition, use of the cloned α-haemolysin determinant in animal models and studies *in vitro* with isolated target cells have confirmed the contribution of α-haemolysin to the multifactorial virulence of *E. coli* strains that cause extra-intestinal infections, particularly those of the urinary tract.

The molecular analysis of the determinants that encode cytolytic toxins in other bacterial species has revealed that *E. coli* α-haemolysin is a member of a family of related haemolysins and leucotoxins widely disseminated in Gram-negative bacteria. All these 'RTX toxins' are secreted from their cells by a highly conserved transport system. In

E. coli, α-haemolysin is one of the few known proteins that is truly secreted into the extracellular environment.

In this chapter the genetics and secretion of *E. coli* α-haemolysin and recent advances in the biochemical and functional characterisation of this toxin will be considered. The significance of α-haemolysin as a virulence factor in the pathogenesis of extra-intestinal *E. coli* infections will also be discussed. Also included are sections that deal with bacterial proteins related to α-haemolysin and with *E. coli* haemolysins that differ from α-haemolysin.

Significance of *Escherichia coli* α-haemolysin as a virulence factor

Strains of *E. coli* with extracellular haemolytic activity (i.e. strains producing α-haemolysin) were first described by Kayser in 1903. Subsequently, several investigators recognised the association between α-haemolysin production and the virulence of *E. coli* strains that cause human extra-intestinal infections, particularly urinary tract infections (UTI), peritonitis, appendicitis, septicaemia and neonatal meningitis. Numerous epidemiological surveys have shown that about 35–60 per cent of the *E. coli* strains isolated from all kinds of UTI produce α-haemolysin. The prevalence of α-haemolysin-positive *E. coli* strains in normal human faeces and in the stool of patients suffering from diarrhoeal diseases is significantly lower, varying in different studies from 3 to 27 per cent (Dudgeon *et al.*, 1921; Cooke & Ewins, 1975; Minshew *et al.*, 1978; DeBoy *et al.*, 1980; Evans *et al.*, 1981; Green & Thomas, 1981; Hughes *et al.*, 1982; van den Bosch *et al.*, 1982b; Hacker *et al.*, 1983b; Hughes *et al.*, 1983; Caprioli *et al.*, 1987; Johnson *et al.*, 1988; Brauner *et al.*, 1990; Opal *et al.*, 1990; Cosar, 1991; Stapleton *et al.*, 1991; Tullus *et al.*, 1991; Blanco *et al.*, 1992; Siitonen, 1992). The prevalence of α-haemolysin production in *E. coli* isolated from patients with sepsis or septicaemia, is about 30–50 per cent (DeBoy *et al.*, 1980; Evans *et al.*, 1981; Blanco *et al.*, 1990, 1992). This has led to the conclusion that α-haemolysin production is an important virulence factor in the pathogenesis of extra-intestinal *E. coli* infections. Several experiments *in vivo* have confirmed this hypothesis. Fried *et al.* (1971) showed that the renal virulence of α-haemolytic wild-type *E. coli* strain injected intravenously into mice or rats is considerably greater than that of a non-haemolytic mutant of the same strain. Similar results were obtained by Smith and Huggins (1985), who also reported that culture supernatants of α-haemolysin-producing

E. coli strains given intravenously are toxic and lethal for mice. It has also been shown that an *E. coli* strain with α-haemolysin production encoded on a plasmid is nephropathogenic for mice, and elimination of the plasmid results in loss of virulence (Waalwijk *et al.*, 1982). Several other animal models also support the assumption that α-haemolysin is a virulence factor in extra-intestinal *E. coli* infections (Minshew *et al.*, 1978; Hull *et al.*, 1982; Van den Bosch *et al.*, 1981, 1982a,b; O'Hanley *et al.*, 1991).

Direct evidence for the importance of α-haemolysin in the pathogenesis of extra-intestinal *E. coli* infections has been provided by recombinant DNA techniques. It has been shown, with an experimental rat peritonitis model, that the cloned α-haemolysin determinant from a uropathogenic *E. coli* isolate confers strong virulence to a previously non-haemolytic avirulent faecal *E. coli* strain (Welch *et al.*, 1981). When the cloned *hly* determinant was inactivated by a Tn1 insertion, the recombinant faecal *E. coli* strain remained avirulent. Other experimental infections of mice and rats with isogenic *E. coli* strains, with and without cloned haemolysin genes, have also confirmed that α-haemolysin determinants from various *E. coli* isolates markedly increase the virulence of *E. coli* (Hacker *et al.*, 1983a; Marre *et al.*, 1986). These studies also demonstrated that chromosomally inherited α-haemolysin determinants contribute to the virulence of *E. coli* to a greater extent than plasmid-encoded determinants. This may be due to differences in the level of expression of the haemolysin genes (Welch & Falkow, 1984), and to qualitative differences that result from amino-acid substitutions in the α-haemolysins of different origin (Hacker *et al.*, 1983a; Ludwig *et al.*, 1987). Moreover, it has been shown *in vivo* that expression of α-haemolysin is not itself sufficient to confer full virulence on *E. coli*. It is now well established that the pathogenicity of *E. coli* in extra-intestinal infections is determined by a combination of virulence factors, none of which alone is sufficient for full virulence. Apart from two toxins, that is α-haemolysin and cytotoxic necrotising factor type 1, these virulence factors include fimbrial adhesins that mediate binding to host cell surfaces, as well as serum resistance and iron-uptake substances. In addition, the types of lipopolysaccharide (O-antigen) (see Chapter 5) and capsule (K-antigen) (see Chapter 4) play an important role in the pathogenicity of extra-intestinal *E. coli* strains (reviewed by Johnson, 1991).

In contrast to its importance in extra-intestinal infections, α-haemolysin appears not to play a significant role in the pathogenesis of diarrhoea caused by *E. coli* in humans and animals (Smith & Linggood, 1971; DeBoy *et al.*, 1980; Giaffer *et al.*, 1992).

The precise function of *E. coli* α-haemolysin in the pathogenesis of extra-intestinal infections is still unclear and may be multifactorial. The α-haemolysin lyses erythrocytes from a wide range of species including sheep, cow, rabbit, mouse, horse and human (Rennie & Arbuthnott, 1974). Quantitative studies have shown that the binding of a low number of toxin molecules to an erythrocyte is sufficient to evoke haemolysis (Eberspächer *et al.*, 1989). It has been suggested that the lysis of erythrocytes may stimulate bacterial growth in the infected organism by increasing the level of available iron. This is consistent with the observation that the virulence of non-haemolytic mutants of extra-intestinal *E. coli* isolates can be raised by pre-treating the host with haemoglobin or ferrous sulphate. In other words, α-haemolysin production can apparently to some extent be substituted for by administration of iron compounds (Linggood & Ingram, 1982; Waalwijk *et al.*, 1983; Smith & Huggins, 1985). However, making iron available for bacterial growth is probably only one of the functions of *E. coli* α-haemolysin. Indeed, α-haemolysin efficiently lyses erythrocytes only when applied in relatively high concentrations; at significantly lower concentrations it affects a wide range of nucleated host cells. Indeed, it is the most potent known leucocidal toxin. The cytotoxic effect of α-haemolysin is due to pore formation in the cytoplasmic membrane of target cells, followed by a rapid and irreversible depletion of cellular ATP (Bhakdi & Tranum-Jensen, 1988; Bhakdi *et al.*, 1990; Jonas *et al.*, 1993). Polymorphonuclear leucocytes, monocytes and peripheral human T lymphocytes have been identified as preferred targets for *E. coli* α-haemolysin (Cavalieri & Snyder, 1982a,b; Gadeberg *et al.*, 1983; Gadeberg & Ørskov, 1984; Bhakdi *et al.*, 1989, 1990; Gadeberg & Mansa, 1990; Jonas *et al.*, 1993). These cells are killed by α-haemolysin at concentrations far lower than those that cause erythrocyte lysis. The capacity of α-haemolysin to kill polymorphonuclear and mononuclear phagocytes as well as peripheral T lymphocytes efficiently probably provides a mechanism by which extra-intestinal *E. coli* strains impair and resist the host immune defences. In addition to its leucotoxic activity, *E. coli* α-haemolysin displays a marked cytotoxic and cytolytic effect on endothelial cells (Seeger *et al.*, 1989; Grimminger *et al.*, 1990a,b; Suttorp *et al.*, 1990), on mouse fibroblasts and chick embryo fibroblasts (Chaturvedi *et al.*, 1969; Cavalieri & Snyder, 1982c) and on proximal renal tubular epithelial cells (Keane *et al.*, 1987; Mobley *et al.*, 1990; Kreft *et al.*, 1992). In acute pyelonephritis, the most serious form of a urinary tract infection, killing of renal tubular cells may allow bacterial penetration through the kidney epithelium and colonisation of the kidney parenchyma. In a mouse pyelonephritis model, the production of α-haemolysin has been shown to correlate with renal parenchymal damage (O'Hanley *et al.*, 1991).

The activity of *E. coli* α-haemolysin is not, however, restricted to the killing and lysis of target cells. There is convincing evidence that very low, non-lytic concentrations of α-haemolysin modulate the normal functions of several types of host cells, thereby increasing the probability that *E. coli* can establish and maintain an infection. Sub-nanomolar concentrations of *E. coli* α-haemolysin increase the membrane permeability of polymorphonuclear granulocytes, which results in granule exocytosis and loss of phagocytic killing capacity (Bhakdi *et al.*, 1989). Furthermore, very low concentrations of α-haemolysin induce an oxidative burst in these phagocytic cells, of which the hallmark is production of superoxide anions. It is interesting that this reaction appears to precede trans-membrane pore formation and to be independent of it. The exidative burst may be triggered by the initial interaction of the toxin with cell surface receptor molecules (Cavalieri & Snyder, 1982b; Bhakdi & Martin, 1991).

Sub-lytic concentrations of *E. coli* α-haemolysin induce the formation of large amounts of specific leukotrienes in human polymorphonuclear leucocytes and monocytes by activating lipoxygenase-controlled arachidonic acid metabolism and they trigger the release of pre-formed histamine from human basophils and rat mast cells (Scheffer *et al.*, 1985,1986; König *et al.*, 1986, 1994; Steadman *et al.*, 1990; Grimminger *et al.*, 1991a). In human platelets, very low concentrations of the toxin specifically stimulate the release of pre-formed serotonin from dense granules, the *de novo* generation and release of 12-hydroxyeicosatetraenoic acid (12-HETE) and dose-dependent platelet aggregation (König *et al.*, 1990, 1994; König & König, 1993b). Leukotrienes, 12-HETE, histamine and serotonin are important mediators of inflammatory reactions that lead to the enhancement of vascular permeability, neutrophil and eosinophil chemotaxis, chemoaggregation, lysosomal enzyme release and smooth muscle contraction. The release of these mediators may facilitate bacterial invasion and spread within the inflamed tissue. Serotonin and histamine are vasoactive and cause vasoconstriction and vasodilation, while leukotrienes and 12-HETE are potently chemotactic for polymorphonuclear granulocytes and may mediate leucocyte diapedesis. Furthermore, 12-HETE induces the expression of heat-shock proteins by human leucocytes, which may alter the responses of neutrophils to bacterial products. In addition, platelet-derived 12-HETE can be rapidly incorporated into bystander cells, such as human leucocytes, and thereby function as a transcellular signal (Köller & König, 1991; König *et al.*, 1994).

Cellular responses to low concentrations of α-haemolysin are probably mediated by a defined signal transduction cascade. The trans-membrane pores formed by the toxin probably act as non-physiological gates that cause the passive influx of Ca^{2+} ions. The increased intracellular Ca^{2+} concentration may then initiate secondary Ca^{2+}-dependent reactions in the target cell (Bhakdi & Tranum-Jensen, 1988; Suttorp *et al.*, 1990). In addition to Ca^{2+}, the activation of protein kinase C and the G protein system, as well as phosphatidylinositol hydrolysis, seem to be involved in the signal transduction pathway (König *et al.*, 1990; König & König, 1991, 1993b; Grimminger *et al.*, 1991b).

In cultured pulmonary artery endothelial cells the α-haemolysin-mediated Ca^{2+}-influx leads to stimulation of arachidonate metabolism that results in the production of prostacyclin. Furthermore, Ca^{2+}-influx appears to cause alterations in the cytoskeleton that lead to endothelial cell contraction, thereby damaging the barrier function of endothelial cell monolayers (Suttorp *et al.*, 1990). A similar susceptibility of pulmonary endothelial cells to *E. coli* α-haemolysin was observed in isolated, blood-free, buffer-perfused rabbit lungs (Seeger *et al.*, 1989, 1991; Grimminger *et al.*, 1990a,b; Ermert *et al.*, 1992). The intravascular application of very low doses of α-haemolysin or α-haemolysin-secreting *E. coli* cells to the isolated lungs resulted in events typical of the development of acute respiratory distress syndrome (ARDS), that is thromboxane-mediated pulmonary hypertension and sustained vascular leakage with progressive development of lung oedema. These biophysical alterations were preceded by a marked production of inflammatory lipid mediators, predominantly leukotrienes and hydroxyeicosatetraenoic acid (HETE) (Grimminger *et al.*, 1990a,b). Thus, *E. coli* α-haemolysin may directly contribute to the pathogenesis of respiratory failure associated with sepsis or pneumonia.

It is not clear at present whether low doses of *E. coli* α-haemolysin stimulate or inhibit the release of cytokines from leucocytes. Investigations to settle this matter have led to contradictory results (Bhakdi *et al.*, 1990; König & König, 1993a; König *et al.*, 1994).

In addition to the activities described above, α-haemolysin apparently contributes to the resistance of *E. coli* to the bactericidal activity of human serum and to phagocytosis and intracellular killing in polymorphonuclear leucocytes and monocytes. The explanation for these effects is unknown (Gadeberg *et al.*, 1989; Siegfried *et al.*, 1992).

The genes that determine α-haemolysin production

Smith and Halls (1967) first observed that the genes that encode α-haemolysin production by *E. coli* may be extra-chromosomal. They noted that the haemolytic phenotype of some isolates can be transferred by conjugation with non-haemolytic *E. coli* K-12 cells and concluded that, in these strains, the α-haemolysin determinant is probably located on a plasmid. Subsequently, several investigators showed that the α-haemolysin determinant in most haemolytic *E. coli* strains of mammalian faecal origin is located on large, conjugative plasmids varying in size between 50 and 160 kb (Goebel & Schrempf, 1971; Goebel *et al.*, 1974; Monti-Bragadin *et al.*, 1975; Royer-Pokora & Goebel, 1976; de la Cruz *et al.*, 1979; Prada *et al.*, 1991). These Hly plasmids belong to different incompatibility groups, predominantly *inc*I2, *inc*FIII, *inc*FIV and *inc*FVI (Monti-Bragadin *et al.*, 1975; de la Cruz *et al.*, 1979, 1980). However, most haemolytic strains of *E. coli* isolated from urinary tract infections and other extra-intestinal infections in humans, and also from normal human faeces, carry the haemolysin determinant on their chromosomes (Welch *et al.*, 1981; Berger *et al.*, 1982; Hull *et al.*, 1982; de la Cruz *et al.*, 1983; Müller *et al.*, 1983; Welch *et al.*, 1983). Apparently, Hly plasmids occur only rarely in uropathogenic or human faecal *E. coli* strains (Höhne, 1973; Tschäpe & Rische, 1974; de la Cruz *et al.*, 1980; Waalwijk *et al.*, 1982; Grünig *et al.*, 1987; Grünig & Lebek, 1988).

The genetic determinant for the synthesis and secretion of active α-haemolysin was first cloned from Hly plasmid pHly152 (Goebel & Hedgpeth, 1982). Construction of transposon mutants and deletion mutants of the cloned sequence and complementation of these mutants with sub-cloned fragments of the sequence showed that the α-haemolysin determinant of *E. coli* consists of four structural genes, arranged in the sequence *hlyC, hlyA, hlyB* and *hlyD*. These studies also showed that *hlyC* and *hlyA* are necessary for the synthesis of active α-haemolysin, while *hlyA* is the structural gene that encodes the haemolysin protein (HlyA) (Noegel *et al.*, 1979, 1981; Goebel & Hedgpeth, 1982). The genes *hlyB* and *hlyD* encode proteins necessary for the transport of α-haemolysin across both membranes of the *E. coli*

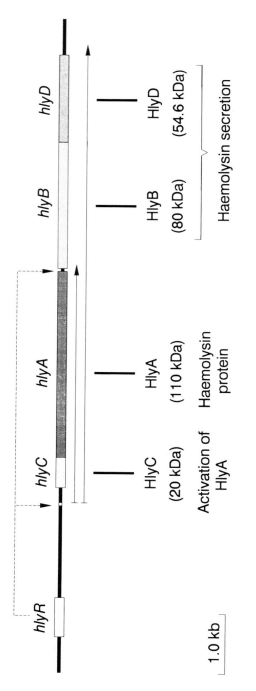

Fig. 11.1. Structure of the α-haemolysin determinant of pHly152. The transcriptional organisation of the *hly* operon is indicated by arrows.

cell (Noegel *et al.*, 1979, 1981; Wagner *et al.*, 1983). Hybridisation of other Hly plasmids or chromosomal DNA from uropathogenic haemolytic *E. coli* with the cloned *hly* genes revealed extensive homology between the different α-haemolysin determinants (de la Cruz *et al.*, 1980, 1983; Müller *et al.*, 1983). This homology was further confirmed by cloning and mapping of a variety of these determinants (Berger *et al.*, 1982; Stark & Shuster, 1982, 1983; Welch *et al.*, 1983; Mackman & Holland, 1984b; Waalwijk *et al.*, 1984; Mackman *et al.*, 1985a).

Direct evidence for the existence of the four structural *hly* genes was provided by the nucleotide sequence of a plasmid-encoded and a chromosomal α-haemolysin determinant (Felmlee *et al.*, 1985b; Hess *et al.*, 1986). In the plasmid-encoded *hly* determinant of pHly152, the genes have open reading frames (ORF) of 510 bp (*hlyC*), 3072 bp (*hlyA*), 2121 bp (*hlyB*) and 1434 bp (*hlyD*) and encode proteins of 20 kDa (HlyC), 110 kDa (HlyA), 80 kDa (HlyB) and 54.6 kDa (HlyD), respectively (Figure 11.1). The nucleotide sequence further confirmed extensive homology within the structural genes of plasmid-encoded and chromosomal *hly* determinants (more than 95 per cent identity) but only little homology is found in the 5' and 3' non-coding regions that flank the structural genes (Felmlee *et al.*, 1985b; Hess *et al.*, 1986). However, even these flanking regions are remarkably conserved in many haemolysin plasmids. The 5' non-coding region of several plasmid-encoded α-haemolysin determinants contains an insertion sequence element, IS2 (Knapp *et al.*, 1985). In addition, IS91-like elements were identified in several Hly plasmids (Zabala *et al.*, 1982), and in pHly152 the α-haemolysin determinant is flanked by a direct repetition of IS91-like elements (Zabala *et al.*, 1984). Such mobile genetic elements at both ends of the *hly* determinant may have allowed the transfer of the *hly* genes on a transposon-like structure and this again may explain the presence of homologous *hly* determinants on a large number of different plasmids (Zabala *et al.*, 1984). IS elements have not been found in the *hly* region upstream of chromosomal determinants (Knapp *et al.*, 1985).

Several copies of the *hly* determinant have been identified on the chromosomes of some uropathogenic *E. coli* isolates. For example, in *E. coli* 536, two *hly* determinants are located on large 'pathogenicity islands' (Pai) of 70 kb and 190 kb, respectively. Both of these are flanked by short direct repeats and, under normal cultural conditions, delete spontaneously at a rate of 10^{-3} to 10^{-4}, by homologous recombination of the repeat sequences (Knapp *et al.*, 1984, 1986; Hacker *et al.*, 1992). Interestingly, the various α-haemolysin determinants on the chromosomes of uropathogenic *E. coli* may be part of larger 'virulence gene blocks', that is, they may be physically linked to other genes involved in virulence, such as the *prf* gene cluster that encodes P-related fimbriae or the genes that encode cytotoxic necrotising factor type 1 (High *et al.*, 1988; Hacker *et al.*, 1990; Falbo *et al.*, 1992). In *E. coli* 536, for example, the deletion of the 190-kb pathogenicity island eliminates the *hly* determinant and the *prf* determinant. In addition, this deletion inhibits the expression of S-fimbrial adhesins, even though the *sfa* genes that encode these adhesins are still present on the chromosome, which suggests a *trans* regulatory effect of a gene product encoded by the *prf* determinant on the expression of the *sfa* genes (Hacker *et al.*, 1992).

Expression of the α-haemolysin genes

The genes *hlyC*, *hlyA*, *hlyB* and *hlyD* are organised in an operon that is transcribed from a promoter region upstream of *hlyC* (Noegel *et al.*, 1979, 1981; Wagner *et al.*, 1983; Juarez *et al.*, 1984; Mackman *et al.*, 1985a,b; Koronakis & Hughes, 1988; Welch & Pellett, 1988). S1 mapping and primer extension experiments led to the identification of different transcriptional start sites in plasmid-encoded and chromosomally encoded α-haemolysin determinants. In the plasmid-encoded *hly* determinant of pHly152, the transcriptional start site was found at a position 264 bp proximal to the ATG start codon of *hlyC*. In the chromosomal *hly* determinant of the urinary tract infection isolate *E. coli* J96, on the other hand, transcription apparently starts 462 and 464 nucleotides upstream of the *hlyC* initiation codon (Welch & Pallett, 1988). In both determinants, transcription from the promoter region upstream of *hlyC* results in the generation of two types of mRNA. The major product is a 4.0-kb *hlyCA* transcript that ends at a *rho*-independent terminator located between *hlyA* and *hlyB*. The minor 8.0-kb transcript comprises *hlyCABD* and terminates at a putative *rho*-independent signal downstream of *hlyD* (Welch and Pellett, 1988).

Transcription of the haemolysin genes is significantly affected by sequences located further upstream in the 5' non-coding region of various *hly* determinants. In the plasmid-encoded determinant of pHly152, the *hlyC*-proximal, non-coding region stimulates the initiation of transcription about three-fold but, more importantly, it suppresses transcription termination (i.e. it causes antitermination) at the *rho*-

independent termination signal located between *hlyA* and *hlyB*, which allows the efficient transcription of *hlyB* and *hlyD* (Koronakis *et al.*, 1988, 1989a). Consequently, the presence of this activating sequence results in a 50- to 100-fold increase in the amount of extracellular α-haemolysin (Gonzalez-Carrero *et al.*, 1985; Ludwig *et al.*, 1987; Vogel *et al.*, 1988). The latter authors narrowed down the activating region to a sequence of about 650 bp, termed *hlyR*, located 1.8 kb upstream of the *hlyC* initiation codon (Figure 11.1). The *hlyR* sequence is active only in *cis* and only in one orientation. In addition, it does not contain an ORF large enough to encode a regulatory protein. Therefore, it is assumed that *hlyR* increases the expression of the *hly* genes by binding one or more bacterial regulatory proteins, since *hlyR* contains sequence motifs that may function as regulatory protein binding sites (Vogel *et al.*, 1988). DNA bending may also be involved to bring the putative regulatory proteins in close contact with transcription initiation and termination sites.

Transcription anti-termination mediated by *hlyR* appears to be peculiar to exponentially growing cells and ceases as the cells enter the stationary phase. The loss of the full-length *hlyCABD* transcript accounts for the decline of α-haemolysin secretion observed when the bacteria enter the stationary phase (Koronakis *et al.*, 1989a).

An activator sequence homologous to *hlyR* has not been detected in chromosomally encoded *hly* determinants. However, a distinct 1.1-kb *Taq*I restriction fragment located 1 kb upstream of *hlyC* appears to activate the transcription of a chromosomal determinant in *cis*, in a manner similar to that observed with *hlyR*, though the effect is not as marked as in the plasmid-encoded *hly* determinant. In addition, this chromosomal sequence appears to activate the *hlyB/hlyD*-dependent secretion of α-haemolysin in *trans*, probably at the post-transcriptional level (Cross *et al.*, 1990). The activating sequence is highly conserved in chromosomal *hly* determinants from uropathogenic *E. coli* of various serotypes. Recent results indicate some similarity between this sequence and *hlyR*, which supports the view that different *E. coli* α-haemolysin determinants are regulated by similar mechanisms, although there are differences in detail (Bailey *et al.*, 1992).

Interestingly, Bailey *et al.* (1992) identified a chromosomal gene, *hlyT*, the product of which appeared to activate the transcription of *hlyA* in plasmid-encoded and chromosomal *hly* determinants. This gene is allelic with *rfaH* (*sfrB*), which is required for the transcription of the genes that encode synthesis of the sex pilus of *E. coli* and lipopolysaccharide (LPS) of *E. coli* and *Salmonella typhimurium*. Recent data obtained by Wandersman & Letoffe (1993) suggest that *hlyT* is not necessary for the expression of *hlyA* but that it is indirectly involved in α-haemolysin secretion (see below).

Another chromosomal locus apparently involved in α-haemolysin expression has been identified by Nieto *et al.* (1987, 1991). This locus, termed *hha*, encodes a polypeptide of 8.6 kDa that exhibits strong homology to the YmoA protein involved in the thermoregulation of various *Yersinia enterocolitica* virulence genes. The Hha protein appears to decrease the expression of α-haemolysin at the transcriptional level. However, the inactivation of this gene not only leads to an increased synthesis of α-haemolysin, but it also affects the expression of other heterologous proteins cloned into *E. coli*. In addition, the enhancement is evident only in the absence of *hlyR*. The *hha* mutation, therefore, seems to compensate for a missing *hlyR*, but it may not play a central role in the specific regulation of α-haemolysin expression. Evidence presented by Carmona *et al.* (1993) suggests that the *hha* mutation increases α-haemolysin expression through changes in the DNA topology. Recently, a 200-bp region ('*hlyM*') has been identified within the *hlyC* gene that appears to modulate the transcription of the *hly* operon. It was speculated that the Hha protein may decrease the expression of α-haemolysin by directly or indirectly interacting with this sequence (Jubete *et al.*, 1995).

In some *E. coli* strains the expression of the *hly* genes is regulated by iron in the growth medium. In these cases, an increase in extracellular iron concentration results in a decline of α-haemolysin synthesis and secretion. In the presence of iron chelators, on the other hand, α-haemolysin production increases significantly (Waalwijk *et al.*, 1983; Lebek & Grünig, 1985; Grünig *et al.*, 1987; Grünig & Lebek, 1988). Grünig *et al.* (1987) demonstrated that the iron-controlled expression of *hly* genes is mediated by the Fur protein, which, on binding of Fe^{2+}, also represses the transcription of other iron-regulated genes of *E. coli*. However, the consensus sequence that allows binding of the Fur repressor has not been identified in the promoter region of several sequenced *hly* determinants. Iron may serve as an environmental factor in humans and mammals, which have a very low level of available iron, to signal to the bacterium that successful infection has occurred.

Data recently obtained by Blight *et al.* (1995) suggest that expression of of HlyB is regulated at the level of translation, in addition to the tight regulation at the transcriptional level.

Secretion of *Escherichia coli* α-haemolysin

α-Haemolysin is secreted directly across both the inner and the outer membrane of *E. coli* without accumulating in the periplasmic space (Gray *et al.*, 1986; Mackman *et al.*, 1986; Felmlee & Welch, 1988; Koronakis *et al.*, 1989). Secretion is independent of the signal-peptide-dependent general export pathway. Indeed, HlyA does not contain the conventional transport signal sequence at the amino-terminus, which is usually found in proteins translocated across the cytoplasmic membrane via the SecA/Y pathway and proteolytic processing of HlyA does not occur during transport (Härtlein *et al.*, 1983; Felmlee *et al.*, 1985a). It has also been shown that the secretion of α-haemolysin is independent of SecA and SecY (Gray *et al.*, 1989; Gentschev *et al.*, 1990).

Three proteins, HlyB, HlyD and TolC, have been identified as being essential for the transport of α-haemolysin into the medium (Wagner *et al.*, 1983; Wandersman & Delepelaire, 1990). HlyB and HlyD, which are encoded by genes immediately distal to the α-haemolysin gene *hlyA*, have been localised to the inner membrane of *E. coli* but, unlike classical inner membrane proteins, in some experiments HlyB and HlyD appeared in small but significant amounts in outer-membrane fractions (Mackman *et al.*, 1985b; Wang *et al.*, 1991; Juranka *et al.*, 1992). TolC, a 52-kDa protein which is encoded by a chromosomal gene not located in the *hly* gene cluster, is a minor *E. coli* outer-membrane protein (Morona *et al.*, 1983; Wandersman & Delepelaire, 1990). It is assumed that HlyB, HlyD and TolC form a trans-envelope complex that spans both membranes of *E. coli*, perhaps at sites of adhesion between the inner and the outer membrane, so allowing direct secretion of α-haemolysin into the medium (Figure 11.2). TolC may be necessary to allow interaction of the HlyB/HlyD complex with the outer membrane in a specific manner. It is interesting that recent investigations have shown that oligomers of TolC are able to form ion-permeable channels in artificial lipid membranes, which suggests that TolC acts *in vivo* as an outer-membrane channel (Benz *et al.*, 1993). In TolC⁻ strains, α-haemolysin does not accumulate in the periplasmic space, but is retained in the cytoplasm (Wandersman & Delepelaire, 1990).

The signal that allows the specific secretion of α-haemolysin by the HlyB/HlyD/TolC transport machinery is located at the carboxyl-terminal end of HlyA, which suggests that the transport of α-haemolysin is strictly post-translational. The first indication of this unusual location of the secretion signal resulted from the analysis of truncated HlyA

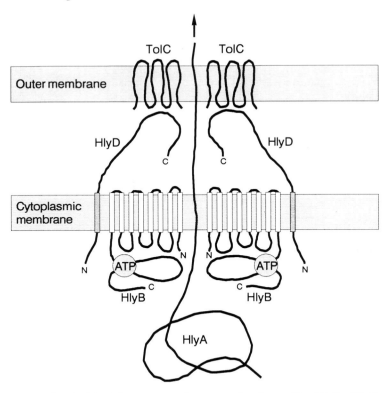

Fig. 11.2. Model of the transenvelope complex formed by HlyB, HlyD and TolC, which allows the specific secretion of *Escherichia coli* α-haemolysin.

derivatives that contained deletions of carboxyl-terminal sequences. Removal of 37 or 27 amino-acids from the carboxyl-terminus of HlyA blocked α-haemolysin secretion without affecting haemolytic activity (Gray *et al.*, 1986; Ludwig *et al.*, 1987). It has also been shown that carboxyl-terminal fragments of HlyA retain full secretion competence (Nicaud *et al.*, 1986; Mackman *et al.*, 1987). In an extensive analysis of carboxyl-terminal fragments of HlyA, the smallest transport-competent peptide capable of HlyB/HlyD/TolC-dependent secretion consisted of the carboxyl-terminal 62 amino-acids (Jarchau *et al.*, 1994). In addition, fusion proteins, consisting of non-transportable proteins and carboxyl-terminal sequences of HlyA, are secreted by the HlyB/HlyD/TolC transport system, though in some cases at a reduced efficiency (Mackman *et al.*, 1987; Gentschev *et al.*, 1990; Hess *et al.*, 1990; Kenny *et al.*, 1991; Hanke *et al.*, 1992; Gentschev *et al.*, 1992, 1994).

Recent results indicate that HlyB alone is able to recognise the carboxyl-terminal secretion signal of HlyA and to initiate the translocation of α-haemolysin across both membranes of *E. coli*. In a HlyB+/HlyD− mutant, the haemolysin protein is translocated into the cell envelope and part of HlyA is exposed on the cellular surface where it can be visualised by immunogold-labelled HlyA-specific antibodies (Oropeza-Wekerle *et al.*, 1990; Gentschev & Goebel, 1992). In HlyB−/HlyD− and HlyB−/HlyD+ mutants, HlyA is associated only with the inner membrane, showing that HlyA can, by itself, interact with the cytoplasmic membrane (Oropeza-Wekerle *et al.*, 1990).

HlyD is apparently not involved in the recognition of the secretion signal, but appears to be required to complete the translocation of α-haemolysin, by pulling it completely through the envelope and releasing it from the cell surface (Wagner *et al.*, 1983; Oropeza-Wekerle *et al.*, 1990). Based on computer-assisted predictions and results obtained with gene fusions of *bla* (β-lactamase), *lacZ* and *phoA* to *hlyD*, a topological model for HlyD has been proposed. According to this model, the 60 amino-terminal amino-acids are located in the cytoplasm, followed by a single trans-membrane segment from amino-acids 60 to 80 and a large periplasmic region extending from amino-acid 80 to the carboxyl-terminus (Wang *et al.*, 1991; Schülein *et al.*, 1992). The periplasmic domain of HlyD may anchor this translocator protein to the outer membrane, possibly to TolC (Schülein *et al.*, 1992). Thus, HlyD may form a bridge between the inner and the outer membrane of *E. coli* through which HlyA may cross the periplasmic space. It is of interest that the periplasmic domain of HlyD contains a region of 44 amino-acids which is highly conserved in the otherwise unrelated TolC protein, and it was shown that this sequence is important for the transport function of HlyD (Schülein *et al.*, 1994). In addition, the amino-acid sequence at the extreme carboxyl-terminus of HlyD, which is predicted to form a helix–loop–helix structure, is essential for the function of the secretion apparatus (Schülein *et al.*, 1994).

The correct incorporation of TolC into the outer membrane appears to depend on intact LPC (Wandersman & Letoffe, 1993). Mutations in the genes *rfaH* (= *hlyT*) and *galU*, which are necessary for LPS biosynthesis, lead to incomplete LPS and result in a significant reduction of the content of TolC in the outer membrane of *E. coli*. This, in turn, inhibits the secretion of α-haemolysin.

The ORF of *hlyB* predicts a gene product of 80 kDa, but a protein of this size has not been identified. Instead, two polypeptides, one of 66 kDa and a predominant one of 46 kDa, are consistently observed (Wang *et al.*, 1991; Gentschev & Goebel, 1992; Juranka *et al.*, 1992; Blight *et al.*, 1995). The presence of an apparent 66-kDa HlyB protein may be due to aberrant binding of SDS, which is often observed for integral membrane proteins (Blight & Holland, 1990). The smaller 46-kDa protein may be a HlyB derivative with unusual mobility characteristics, or more probably a degradation product of HlyB. It cannot represent the product of a reinitiation of translation at a potential AUG start codon within the *hlyB* mRNA, because the substitution of this internal methionine codon by a codon for valine or leucine did not abolish the appearance of the 46-kDa protein (Gentschev & Goebel, 1992).

The topology of HlyB within the cytoplasmic membrane has been studied by means of computer predictions, fusions between HlyB and β-lactamase and fusions between HlyB and LacZ or PhoA (Wang *et al.*, 1991; Gentschev & Goebel, 1992). The proposed models, though differing in their detailed structural predictions, suggest that HlyB is inserted into the cytoplasmic membrane by six to eight hydrophobic transmembrane segments in the amino-terminal domain. A relatively short sequence at the extreme amino-terminus and the carboxyl-terminal 240 amino-acids is located in the cytoplasm. This C-terminal cytoplasmic domain is rather hydrophilic and contains an ATP-binding sequence that spans approximately 200 amino-acids (Hyde *et al.*, 1990; Koronakis *et al.*, 1993, 1995).

In fact, HlyB is regarded as a member of the super-family of ATP-binding cassette (ABC) transporters, which includes prokaryotic and eukaryotic membrane proteins involved in the import and export of a variety of substrates, such as ions, peptides, large proteins and carbohydrates (Gerlach *et al.*, 1986; Higgins *et al.*, 1986; Rommens *et al.*, 1989; Hyde *et al.*, 1990; Monaco *et al.*, 1990; Fath & Kolter, 1993). Within this family, HlyB is especially related in structure and function to a group of export proteins sometimes referred to as the 'Mdr-like' sub-family, because one of its best-known members is the P-glycoprotein or Mdr protein, which pumps chemotherapeutic drugs out of human tumour cells and so mediates the multi-drug resistance phenotype of these cells. Other members of this sub-family include pfMdr, an Mdr homologue found in *Plasmodium falciparum*, which is also associated with drug resistance, the TAP peptide transporter encoded by the major histocompatibility locus and the cystic fibrosis transmembrane conductance regulator CFTR (Blight & Holland, 1990). As in the case of HlyB, all the latter proteins contain membrane-spanning domains and one or more highly conserved cytoplasmic nucleotide-binding domains. These are thought to bind and hydrolyse ATP, to provide the energy for translocation. Mdr and CFTR are generated by tandem duplications of *hlyB* gene homologues and, in the case of Mdr, it is known that the nucleotide-binding domains of both halves of the protein are required for drug export (Currier *et al.*, 1989). This suggests that two binding sites may also be needed in HlyB. Indeed, results obtained by Koronakis *et al.* (1993) indicate a dimeric structure for HlyB that is likely to be determined and/or stabilised by the amino-terminal integral membrane domain of HlyB.

The strong conservation of the primary sequence within the cytoplasmic nucleotide-binding domains of the HlyB homologues, in contrast to the more limited topological similarity of the membrane domains, has led to the assumption that the specificity for translocation resides within the membrane domains. Blight & Holland (1990) speculated that cytoplasmic loops of HlyB, within the amino-terminal membrane domain, are likely to be involved in the recognition of the HlyA secretion signal, while the periplasmic loops are more likely to be involved in the actual translocation step. In confirmation of this view, Zhang *et al.* (1993b) isolated several point mutations in HlyB that were able to suppress the transport-defective phenotype of a HlyA derivative that contains a deletion in the carboxyl-terminal secretion signal. All these point mutations were clustered in the amino-terminal multiple membrane-spanning domain of HlyB, on cytoplasmic loops close to the predicted transmembrane segments. On the other hand, Thomas *et al.* (1992) reported that the amino-terminal membrane domain of HlyB can be substituted by a foreign membrane domain, while the protein retains partial function in α-haemolysin secretion. However, α-haemolysin transport by the hybrid HlyB protein was only about ten per cent as efficient as the export in the presence of wild-type HlyB. It was not determined whether this residual secretion was dependent on the carboxyl-terminal transport signal of HlyA.

The ATP-binding cassette in the cytoplasmic domain of HlyB contains three prominent sequence motifs common to all ABC transporters: (i) the glycine-rich loop or 'Walker A' motif (GRSGSGKS), located at residues 502–509 in HlyB, is thought to be essential for nucleotide binding; (ii) the short linker peptide (LSGGQ) at position 606–610 in HlyB appears to be critical for the transmission of ATP-dependent signals, such as conformational change; and (iii) an aspartate residue at position 630, which is part of the 'Walker B' motif (ILIFD), is thought to be necessary for the co-ordination of Mg^{2+} (Walker *et al.*, 1982; Hyde *et al.*, 1990; Mimura *et al.*, 1991; Koronakis *et al.*, 1993, 1995). Koronakis *et al.* (1993) demonstrated that the cytoplasmic carboxyl-terminal domain of HlyB has a Mg^{2+}-dependent ATPase activity. They also showed that the hydrolysis of ATP bound to the cytoplasmic domain of HlyB is absolutely necessary to energise the export of α-haemolysin (Koronakis *et al.*, 1995). In particular, analysis of ABC-domain mutants of HlyB revealed that the protein exporter function of HlyB *in vivo* correlates directly with its ATPase activity *in vitro*. Mutations in residues that are invariant or highly conserved at the ATP-binding fold and in the linker peptide of prokaryotic and eukaryotic ABC transporters resulted in complete loss of the protein export function of HlyB and of its ATPase activity (Koronakis *et al.*, 1995). On the other hand, none of these mutations significantly reduced the binding of ATP by HlyB or ATP-induced conformational change in the HlyB protein (Koronakis *et al.*, 1995).

In addition to the hydrolysis of ATP, the HlyB/HlyD-dependent secretion of HlyA requires total proton-motive force (ΔP) at an early stage, probably during substrate association with the translocation machinery at the cytoplasmic membrane (Koronakis *et al.*, 1991). Subsequnt translocation of HlyA from the cytoplasmic to the outer membrane and beyond is independent of ΔP. This process may be driven directly by binding and hydrolysis of ATP by HlyB, but it is also possible that this is an energetically favourable transfer that does not require additional energy (Koronakis *et al.*, 1991). The available data actually suggest a requirement for ATP binding and hydrolysis at an early stage, before or during the association of HlyA with the inner membrane (Koronakis *et al.*, 1991). The precise role of ATP binding and hydrolysis by HlyB in the export of α-haemolysin is, however, unknown. Theoretically, the energy of ATP hydrolysis may be used to induce a translocation-competent folding state in the haemolysin protein or to strip it from bound chaperons on the cytoplasmic side of the membrane (Koronakis *et al.*, 1993).

It is interesting that the energy requirements of the HlyB/HlyD-dependent secretion of *E. coli* α-haemolysin are similar to those of other membrane translocation processes (Schiebel *et al.*, 1991; Driessen, 1992). The *sec*-dependent secretion of proteins, for example, also requires proton-motive force energy and the hydrolysis of ATP early in the process. Protein import into microsomes and mitochondria also requires ATP hydrolysis at an early stage.

The carboxyl-terminal targeting signal of HlyA has been studied intensively, but attempts to identify the exact structural features of the signal and its proximal boundary have provided conflicting results. As we will see below, several secreted proteins, with carboxyl-terminal secretion signals and that use a translocation system homologous to HlyB/HlyD/TolC, have recently been identified in closely and more distantly related Gram-negative bacteria. When expressed in *E. coli*, most of these proteins are secreted by the HlyB/HlyD/TolC transport machinery of α-haemolysin, though the efficiency of secretion is apparently reduced when compared with that achieved in the presence of their own transport proteins (Koronakis *et al.*, 1987; Chang *et al.*, 1989a; Delepelaire & Wandersman, 1990; Gygi *et al.*, 1990; Highlander *et al.*, 1990; Masure *et al.*, 1990; Guzzo *et al.*, 1991; Scheu *et al.*, 1992; Thompson & Sparling, 1993). The carboxyl-terminal targeting signals of these proteins, therefore, appear to share structural similarities. However, comparison of these carboxyl-terminal sequences revealed high primary sequence divergence and did not identify conserved primary or secondary structural features that might represent the targeting signal. The results of extensive site-directed mutagenesis analysis of the carboxyl-terminal targeting signal of HlyA suggested that the secretion signal is composed of a number of dispersed critical 'contact' residues, the side chains of which are required for recognition by the export proteins (Kenny *et al.*, 1992, 1994). It was suggested that alteration of some of these residues in the diverse carboxyl-terminal targeting signals, with compensatory changes in the signal recognition region of the corresponding translocation machineries, may explain the apparent absence of a conserved consensus signal.

Other investigators have, however, pointed out the significance of multiple secondary structural features, or even higher-order structures, within the carboxyl-terminal transport signal. It has been suggested that the carboxyl-terminal export signal of HlyA lies within the last 48 amino-acid residues and comprises three functional domains, namely a large amphipathic and charged helix of about 22 amino-acids, followed by a 13-amino-acid uncharged region and a hydroxylated tail of eight amino-acids at the extreme carboxyl-terminus. Analogous features were also found to some extent in the carboxyl-terminal sequences of other proteins secreted by HlyB/HlyD/TolC-like transport systems (Stanley *et al.*, 1991). On the other hand, Hess *et al.* (1990) and Jarchau *et al.* (1994) have shown that the last 60 to 62 amino-acids of HlyA are necessary and sufficient for the recognition of the secretion machinery. Analysis of mutations introduced within the carboxyl-terminal 60 amino-acids of HlyA suggested the presence of at least three functional regions. Region I, which consists of 21 amino-acids at the amino-terminus of the signal, is enriched in neutral polar amino-acids, and it was suggested that this region may represent a structure which exposes regions II (amino-acids 22–40) and III (amino-acids 41–60) at the end of the HlyA molecule. These may interact directly in a co-operative manner with HlyB, to allow α-haemolysin to bind to the translocator (Hess *et al.*, 1990). Zhang *et al.* (1993a) suggested that the transport signal of HlyA may be defined by structural motifs that consist of helix-turn-helix, followed by strand-loop-strand within the 58 carboxyl-terminal amino-acids.

Biochemical characterisation and structure–function relationships of α-haemolysin

The gene product of *hlyA* has been identified as a 107-kDa protein (Goebel & Hedgpeth, 1982; Welch *et al.*, 1983) that is secreted from actively growing *E. coli* cells and is associated with heat-labile haemolytic activity (Lovell & Rees, 1960; Springer & Goebel, 1980; Mackman & Holland, 1984a,b; Felmlee *et al.*, 1985a,b; Gonzalez-Carrero *et al.*, 1985; Nicaud *et al.*, 1985b; Wagner *et al.*, 1988). The HlyA protein itself is, however, haemolytically inactive. Early biochemical studies have suggested that, in the active toxin, the haemolysin protein HlyA may be associated with other non-protein components, particularly lipids (Cavalieri *et al.*, 1984; Bohach & Snyder, 1985, 1986). This view was confirmed by the observation that the haemolytic activity of *E. coli* α-haemolysin can be destroyed by ultrasonication or treatment with phospholipase C, without altering the molecular mass of the HlyA protein (Wagner *et al.*, 1988). The lability of the extracellular haemolytic activity seen under normal culture conditions is also not associated with proteolytic degradation of HlyA (Springer & Goebel, 1980; Wagner *et al.*, 1988; Oropeza-Wekerle *et al.*, 1989). This decline in haemolytic activity is, however, not obviously due to loss of a modifying component, but seems to be due to aggregation of α-haemolysin that is reversible in the presence of urea (Hardie *et al.*, 1991; Ostolaza *et al.*, 1991).

As we have seen, synthesis of active α-haemolysin depends on *hlyA* and *hlyC*, and it has been demonstrated that HlyA is activated in the cytoplasm by HlyC before export (Goebel & Hedgpeth, 1982; Welch *et al.*, 1983; Nicaud *et al.*, 1985a). HlyC has been identified as a cytoplasmic protein of 18–20 kDa (Noegel *et al.*, 1979; Härtlein *et al.*, 1983; Felmlee *et al.*, 1985b; Nicaud *et al.*, 1985a), but the physiologically active form may be a 40-kDa homodimer of HlyC (Hardie *et al.*, 1991).

Unactivated HlyA protein (proHlyA) cannot bind to erythrocyte membranes (Oropeza-Wekerle *et al.*, 1989; Boehm *et al.*, 1990b). However, even the unactivated proHlyA is able to form trans-membrane pores in artificial lipid bilayers, albeit at a very low frequency. These pores have characteristics similar to those formed by activated HlyA (see below), indicating that the pore-forming structure already exists in proHlyA (Ludwig *et al.*, 1996). The HlyC-mediated activation of pro-HlyA therefore appears only to be required to enhance the binding of α-haemolysin to the target cell membrane but not for pore formation.

Issartel *et al.* (1991) demonstrated that the activation of proHlyA by HlyC consists of post-translational, covalent and acyl-carrier-protein (ACP)-dependent fatty acid acylation of the haemolysin protein. This suggested that the activation facilitates the association of α-haemolysin with target cell membranes through lipid–hydrophobic interactions. In the activation process, HlyC seems to act as fatty acyl transferase, but its exact biochemical function is not completely understood. Comparison of the sequence of HlyC with that of known acyl transferases does not reveal any homology. HlyC may also be of structural importance in the activation process, because much more of this protein, that is amounts approximately equimolar to those of HlyA, is required for activation than would be expected for a merely catalytic function (Hardie *et al.*, 1991). *In vitro*, proHlyA can be acylated by a range of different fatty acids from C_{12} to C_{18}, with myristic acid (C_{14}) apparently the most active form (Issartel *et al.*, 1991). The resistance of the acylation to chemical treatments indicated that the linkage of the fatty acid group(s) to HlyA most probably occurs via an amide bond, and suggests that the acylated amino-acids are lysine residues (Issartel *et al.*, 1991). In fact, Stanley *et al.* (1994) reported that under *in vitro* conditions the haemolysin protein is acylated at two internal lysine residues (Lys 564 and Lys 690). These authors also reported that mutations of these two lysine residues result in a loss of haemolytic activity, which suggested that the fatty acid acylation may also occur *in vivo* at both sites. In agreement with this, Pellett *et al.* (1990) isolated a monoclonal antibody that binds exclusively to HlyC-activated α-haemolysin and neutralises it completely; its epitope has been mapped to the sequence between amino-acids 673 and 726 of HlyA, which contains one of the identified acylation sites (Rowe *et al.*, 1994). Recent investigations have confirmed that HlyC-mediated activation of proHlyA *in vivo* is accomplished by quantitative fatty acid acylation at the lysine residues Lys 564 and Lys 690 (Ludwig *et al.*, 1996).

Interestingly, Lys 564 and Lys 690 are located in the central region of HlyA that separates a hydrophobic region in the amino-terminal half of the protein from a pronounced repeat domain in the carboxyl-terminal half (Figure 11.3). These two structural domains are essential for the haemolytic activity of *E. coli* α-haemolysin.

It has long been known that haemolysis by α-haemolysin is Ca^{2+} dependent (Short & Kurtz, 1971; Rennie *et al.*, 1974) and recent investigations have made it evident that, in addition to the HlyC-mediated acylation of HlyA, Ca^{2+} is necessary to facilitate the interaction of α-haemolysin with erythrocyte membranes (Ludwig *et al.*, 1988; Boehm *et al.*, 1990a,b). HlyA binds Ca^{2+} in a manner that is independent of HlyC, but requires the repeat domain in the carboxyl-terminal half of the haemolysin protein. This domain contains 11 to 13 glycine-rich repeat units, each consisting of nine amino-acids with the consensus sequence X–Leu–X–Gly–Gly–X–Gly–Asn/Asp–Asp. The first two of the 13 repeat units each strongly diverge from the consensus sequence. At least one additional repeat unit is separated from the repeat domain and located more proximally in the HlyA sequence, between the two acylation sites. Binding of Ca^{2+} ions by the repeat units probably results in the formation and/or exposure of a structure in HlyA that may be required to recognise a so far unidentified receptor in the erythrocyte membrane. Structural considerations suggested that always three repeat units may form one octahedral Ca^{2+}-binding site, in which aspartate residues constitute the Ca^{2+} ligands (Ludwig *et al.*, 1988). The close proximity of the region that contains the modification sites to the repeat region suggests that these two regions constitute a large domain required for binding to the target membrane.

Pore formation in the target membrane is independent of the repeat domain, as well as of Ca^{2+}. α-Haemolysin derivatives with specific deletions in the repeat domain that are unable to bind to erythrocytes nevertheless efficiently form wild-type pores in artificial planar lipid bilayers (Ludwig *et al.*, 1988). In addition, wild-type α-haemolysin generates pores in these planar lipid membranes in the complete absence of Ca^{2+} (Benz *et al.*, 1989).

The actual pore-forming structure of *E. coli* α-haemolysin is provided by the amino-terminal half of HlyA. This region contains three markedly hydrophobic domains (DI, DII, DIII), although HlyA is otherwise a hydrophilic protein. Deletion of the hydrophobic sequences, or non-conservative amino-acid substitutions that alter their hydrophobicity entirely destroy the haemolytic and pore-forming activity without reducing α-haemolysin stability or secretion (Ludwig *et al.*, 1987, 1991). In addition, short synthetic peptides that represent regions of hydrophobic domain DII have been shown to exert haemolytic and pore-forming activity. This further confirms the importance of these hydrophobic sequences for the formation of the pore structure (Oropeza-Wekerle *et al.*, 1991, 1992). Computer-assisted analysis of the secondary structure of HlyA revealed four putative hydrophobic membrane-spanning α-helices of 21 amino-acids each within the three hydrophobic domains, one in DI, one in DII and two in DIII. Interestingly, the amino-acid sequences that flank the hydrophobic regions have amphipathic properties and may represent several additional trans-membrane domains that span the target membrane in the form of α-helices or β-strands (Ludwig *et al.*, 1991). Analysis of the biophysical characteristics of the pores generated by *E. coli* α-haemolysin in artificial lipid membranes has shown that the pores are cation-specific, hydrophilic and water-filled (Menestrina *et al.*, 1987; Benz *et al.*, 1989; Ropele & Menestrina, 1989; Menestrina *et al.*, 1990). Therefore, it was speculated that the putative amphipathic trans-membrane sequences may form the hydrophilic inner core of the channel, whereas the four hydrophobic α-helices are more probably located on the outside and form a sort of backbone that stabilises the pore structure and anchors it in the membrane (Ludwig *et al.*, 1991; Benz *et al.*, 1992).

Lysis protection experiments and artificial lipid membrane systems demonstrated that the pore generated by α-haemolysin has a diameter of 1–3 nm and a conductance of about 550 pS in the presence of 0.15M KCl (Bhakdi *et al.*, 1986; Benz *et al.*, 1989). This suggests that the trans-membrane domains of two or three HlyA molecules may be necessary to form a single pore. The instability of the α-haemolysin pore in planar lipid membranes, and the steep non-linear dependence of pore formation on the haemolysin concentration further argued for an unstable oligomerisation of HlyA molecules in the target membrane (Benz *et al.*, 1989). In addition, complementation analysis with specific α-haemolysin mutants affected in different regions confirmed that aggregation of at least two HlyA molecules takes place and that these aggregates are able to generate trans-membrane pores (Ludwig *et al.*, 1993). Our conclusion that *E. coli* α-haemolysin forms transient pores by means of unstable α-haemolysin oligomers is consistent with the results of electron micro-

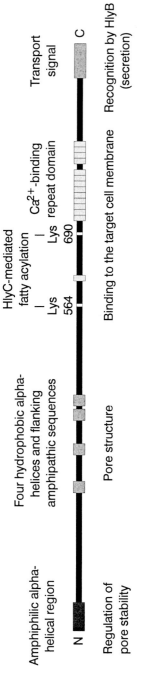

Fig. 11.3. Location of functional domains in the α-haemolysin protein (HlyA) of *Escherichia coli*.

scopy. In particular, target membranes treated with α-haemolysin did not have visible lesions, as has been documented for other cytolysins that form stable pores (Bhakdi & Tranum-Jensen, 1986).

The sequence at the extreme amino-terminus of HlyA is not directly involved in the generation of the pore structure, but seems to regulate the stability of the pore. This region has a putative amphiphilic α-helical structure that has been shown to be membrane-active (Erb *et al.*, 1987). However, as we have seen, it is not involved in the secretion of HlyA. In contrast, the amino-terminal amphiphilic portion of HlyA seems to prevent the stable insertion of the pore structure into the target membrane, resulting in the generation of typical transient pores with a limited life of about two and 30 seconds, respectively, for plasmid- and chromosomally encoded α-haemolysin. This may be due to competition for insertion into the membrane between the amino-terminal region of HlyA and the amphipathic pore-forming sequences (Ludwig *et al.*, 1991). The short life of the wild-type pore may have biological significance. While stable pores usually lead to target cell disruption, pores with a short life may trigger membrane-associated reactions that result in an alteration of normal host cell function, without necessarily causing cell lysis.

In conclusion, the cytolytic activity of *E. coli* α-haemolysin appears to be due to two distinct events, due to different domains of the haemolysin protein. Firstly, binding of the toxin to the target cell membrane requires the Ca^{2+}-binding repeat domain and modification (acylation) of HlyA, mediated by HlyC, in the region adjacent to the repeat domain and, secondly, pore formation depends on the trans-membrane sequences in the hydrophobic region of HlyA (Figure 11.3).

Nevertheless, in spite of the data described above, some authors doubt that the cytolytic activity of *E. coli* α-haemolysin is based on the formation of discrete-sized pores in the target cell membrane. Based on osmotic protection experiments, it has recently been suggested that α-haemolysin creates heterogeneous lesions in erythrocyte membranes, and that these lesions increase in size over time (Moayeri & Welch, 1994). Moreover, Ostolaza *et al.* (1993) reported that α-haemolysin-induced leakage of large unilamellar vesicles is the result of a detergent-like effect of the toxin, which disrupts the lipid bilayer.

Bacterial proteins related to *Escherichia coli* α-haemolysin

Nucleotide sequence analysis of various determinants that encode haemolysins and leucotoxins in several Gram-negative bacteria has revealed extensive homology with the *E. coli* α-haemolysin determinant. Indeed, α-haemolysin from *E. coli* is now regarded as the prototype of a family of structurally and functionally related RTX toxins produced by a variety of Gram-negative bacteria (Braun & Focareta, 1991; Ludwig & Goebel, 1991; Welch, 1991; Coote, 1992). Apart from *E. coli* α-haemolysin, the RTX toxins include haemolysins from *Proteus vulgaris*, *Morganella morganii* and *Enterobacter cloacae* (Koronakis *et al.*, 1987; Welch *et al.*, 1987; Eberspächer *et al.*, 1990; Prada & Beutin, 1991), haemolysins and cytotoxins from *Actinobacillus pleuropneumoniae*, *A. suis*, *A. equuli* and *A. liguieresii* (Chang *et al.*, 1989b; Frey *et al.*, 1991; Smits *et al.*, 1991; Burrows & Lo, 1992; Frey *et al.*, 1992; Gygi *et al.*, 1992; Macdonald & Rycroft, 1992; Frey *et al.*, 1993a,b; Jansen *et al.*, 1993; Macdonald & Rycroft, 1993), the leucotoxins from *Pasteurella haemolytica* and *Actinobacillus actinomycetemcomitans* (Lo *et al.*, 1987; Strathdee & Lo, 1987; Highlander *et al.*, 1989; Lally *et al.*, 1989; Strathdee & Lo, 1989; Guthmiller *et al.*, 1990a,b; Kraig *et al.*, 1990) and the bifunctional adenylate cyclase toxin of *Bordetella pertussis* (Glaser *et al.*, 1988a,b; Barry *et al.*, 1991; Hackett *et al.*, 1994). All these toxins are Ca^{2+}-dependent, pore-forming proteins, but they vary in target cell specificity. Some of these, for example *E. coli* α-haemolysin, are cytotoxic for a wide variety of eukaryotic cells, while others, such as the leucotoxins of *P. haemolytica* and *A. actinomycetemcomitans*, are active only against leucocytes from certain host species. In some of the haemolysins with a broad target cell spectrum, discrete separable regions have been identified that are apparently responsible for the specificity for erythrocytes or leucocytes (Forestier & Welch, 1991; McWhinney *et al.*, 1992). Interestingly, in the case of *E. coli* α-haemolysin, the erythrocyte specificity domain appears to be associated with the sequence between amino-acids 564 and 739, which includes both acylation sites (Lys 564 and Lys 690) (Forestier & Welch, 1991).

The most pronounced structural feature of the protein toxins related to *E. coli* α-haemolysin is the presence of a repetitive domain in the carboxyl-terminal region that contains a variable number of highly conserved glycine- and aspartate-rich repeat units, each of which consists of nine amino-acids. Based on this common structural feature, the term RTX (repeat toxins) has been proposed to designate toxins related to *E.*

coli α-haemolysin (Strathdee & Lo, 1989). All members of the RTX toxin family are synthesised as inactive precursor proteins and require post-translational activation by a *hlyC*-homologous protein encoded by a gene located immediately next to the toxin gene. In addition, the toxins of the RTX family are secreted across the double membrane of the Gram-negative bacterial cell by highly conserved transport machineries that consist of at least three proteins homologous to HlyB, HlyD and TolC of *E. coli*. As for *E. coli* α-haemolysin, this transport is independent of the general export pathway and involves an unprocessed carboxyl-terminal secretion signal in the toxins.

Recent investigations have also demonstrated the existence of several extracellular proteins in Gram-negative, mostly pathogenic bacteria, that are secreted by transport systems homologous to those of the repeat toxins, though they do not act as pore-forming toxins. These proteins include the metalloproteases A, B and C of *Erwinia chrysanthemi* (Delepelaire & Wandersman, 1989; Letoffe *et al.*, 1990; Delepelaire & Wandersman, 1990, 1991; Ghigo & Wandersman, 1992), the metal-loprotease SM of *Serratia marcescens* (Letoffe *et al.*, 1991), the alkaline protease of *Pseudomonas aeruginosa* (Guzzo *et al.*, 1991; Duong *et al.*, 1992), the nodulation protein NodO of *Rhizobium leguminosarum* (Economou *et al.*, 1990; Scheu *et al.*, 1992) and iron-regulated proteins produced by *Neisseria meningitidis* (Thompson *et al.*, 1993a,b). These proteins are only partially related to the RTX toxins, but they contain a tandem array of repeat units homologous to those of the RTX toxins and, as in the case of the RTX toxins, the secretion signal is at the carboxyl-terminal end of the proteins. Colicin V is also secreted by a transport system homologous to that of the RTX toxins, but the secretion signal of colicin V appears to be located at the amino-terminal end of the protein (Gilson *et al.*, 1990; Fath *et al.*, 1991).

The presence of homologous RTX toxin determinants in a wide spectrum of Gram-negative bacteria suggests that they have a common origin and that they may have spread among different species by horizon-tal gene transfer. Interestingly, DNA sequence analysis of the *E. coli* α-haemolysin determinant revealed a G+C content of only 40 per cent, which is ten per cent lower than the average for the *E. coli* genome (Felmlee *et al.*, 1985b; Hess *et al.*, 1986). In addition, several preferred *E. coli* codons are used only infrequently in the *E. coli* α-haemolysin determinant. These observations indicate that the *hly* genes have only recently been acquired by *E. coli* from another organism. In this respect it is remarkable that the genomic G+C content of *Actinobacillus* spp.,

Proteus vulgaris and *Pasteurella haemolytica*, which is about 40 per cent in each case, corresponds to that of the *E. coli* α-haemolysin determinant. Therefore, it has been suggested that the progenitor of the different determinants may have originated from one of these bacteria (Koronakis *et al.*, 1987; Strathdee & Lo, 1987; Welch, 1987). However, the G+C value of the adenylate cyclase toxin (*cya*) determinant of *Bordetella pertussis* (66 per cent) is similar to that of other genes of this organism, which suggests that the *cya* determinant was not a recent acquisition by *B. pertussis*. Welch (1991) speculated that the determinants of the RTX toxins and of the more distantly related proteins probably arose by combination of an ancient set of genes that encode HlyB-, HlyD- and TolC-like transport proteins and a progenitor of HlyA that contains a Ca^{2+}-binding element and a carboxyl-terminal secretion signal. The progenitor A protein then probably developed differently to acquire haemolytic, leucotoxic or proteolytic activities, while the HlyB-, HlyD- and TolC-like proteins were restrained by their secretion function. In the case of the adenylate cyclase toxin determinant of *B. pertussis*, an adenylate cyclase gene possibly of eukaryotic origin, this was most probably fused to the original toxin gene.

Escherichia coli haemolysins that differ from α-haemolysin

The production of different types of haemolysin by *E. coli* was first noted by Smith in 1963. In addition to the secreted α-haemolysin, he described a cell-associated lysin, termed β-haemolysin, which is produced by some *E. coli* strains, but little is known about this haemolysin. It produces clear zones of haemolysis on blood agar, as does α-haemolysin, but antiserum against α-haemolysin apparently did not neutralise β-haemolysin (Smith, 1963; Rennie & Arbuthnott, 1974). So far, the relationship between the two toxins has not been clarified but it has been suggested that β-haemolysin may be a cell-bound form of α-haemolysin (Rennie & Arbuthnott, 1974).

A third type of *E. coli* haemolysin, called γ-haemolysin, was identified by Walton & Smith (1969) in nalidixic-acid-resistant mutants *E. coli* K-12 strains. It appeared to be active against various mammalian red blood cells, but, in contrast to α- and β-haemolysins, not against those of humans or rabbits.

Another type of *E. coli* haemolysin was originally identified in some enteropathogenic and enterohaemorrhagic *E. coli* strains, predominantly of serogroups O26 and O111 (Beutin *et al.*, 1988, 1990). Because of its close association with strains that provoke enteric diseases, this haemolysin was designated 'enterohaemolysin' (Ehly). Early studies suggested that it is phenotypically, serologically and genetically different from α-haemolysin. In contrast to α-haemolysin, enterohaemolysin was detected only in cells grown to the stationary phase and it was not found in the culture medium. This was consistent with the observation that the zones caused by enterohaemolysin on blood agar are smaller and more turbid than those due to α-haemolysin. In colony immunoblots, entero-haemolytic *E. coli* O26 and O111 strains did not react with a monoclonal antibody against *E. coli* α-haemolysin, and DNA from enterohaemolysin-producing *E. coli* did not hybridise with an α-haemolysin-specific gene probe (Beutin *et al.*, 1988, 1990).

Beutin *et al.* (1990, 1993) and Stroeher *et al.* (1993) reported that enterohaemolysin production of *E. coli* O26 strains may be associated with temperate bacteriophages. In particular, they cloned two genetically different determinants from the temperate bacteriophages of two *E. coli* O26 isolates, which directed the expression of a putative enterohaemoly-tic phenotype when introduced into *E. coli* K-12. The determinant associated with the production of the putative enterohaemolysin 'Ehly 1' was assigned to a 2.15-kb restriction fragment (Beutin *et al.*, 1990). Nucleotide sequence analysis of this fragment revealed an ORF of 798 bp that encodes a protein of about 30 kDa (Stroeher *et al.*, 1993). It has been suggested that this protein may represent Ehly1, but this hypothesis was not confirmed by direct evidence. No significant homology was found between the amino-acid sequence of the 30-kDa protein and any known protein sequence (Stroeher *et al.*, 1993). The determinant directing the synthesis of the second putative enterohaemolysin ('Ehly2') was cloned on a 1.25-kb fragment. Sequencing of this fragment revealed three regions highly homologous to DNA sequences of bacteriophage λ, but without similarity to the Ehly1-associated sequence. Rather, the 1.25-kb fragment contained several overlapping ORFs that encoded proteins of about 9–22 kDa (Beutin *et al.*, 1993). The expression and function of these putative proteins have not been studied.

In DNA–DNA hybridisation experiments, various *E. coli* strains with an enterohaemolytic phenotype did not react with DNA probes isolated from the putative Ehly1-associated or Ehly2-associated sequences (Beutin *et al.*, 1993; Stroeher *et al.*, 1993). This suggested that, at least in these strains, the production of enterohaemolysin may be genetically independent of the cloned phage-encoded sequences. Indeed, it has recently been shown that the toxin responsible for the enterohaemolytic phenotype of enterohaemorrhagic *E. coli* (EHEC) O157:H7 is encoded on the 90-kb plasmid pO157 that is present in almost all clinical *E. coli* O157 isolates (Schmidt *et al.*, 1994). It is interesting that the pO157-encoded haemolysin, termed EHEC haemolysin or Ehx, belongs to the RTX family of pore-forming cytolysins and shares striking sequence homology with *E. coli* α-haemolysin (Schmidt *et al.*, 1994, 1995). Nucleotide sequence analysis of the EHEC haemolysin determinant revealed four genes in the order EHEC-*hlyC*, EHEC-*hylA*, EHEC-*hlyB* and EHEC-*hlyD*, which constitute a typical RTX operon (Schmidt *et al.*, 1995, 1996). The enterohaemolytic phenotype of EHEC O157:H7, which is characterised by the formation of small and turbid zones of lysis on blood agar, is due to the poor extracellular secretion of EHEC haemolysin. Since EHEC-HlyB and EHEC-HlyD have been shown to constitute a functionally active secretion system for the toxin, this may be due to low expression of the EHEC-*hly* (*ehx*) genes (Bauer & Welch, 1996). EHEC haemolysin is endowed with haemolytic and leucotoxic activity, but it appears to exhibit a greater target cell specificity than α-haemolysin (Bauer & Welch, 1996). The role of EHEC haemolysin in the virulence of EHEC O157:H7, which is the predominant cause of haemorrhagic colitis and haemolytic uraemic syndrome (HUS) in humans, has yet to be established. It has been shown that EHEC haemolysin induces a specific immune response in patients suffering from *E. coli* O157:H7-associated HUS, which indicates that the toxin is produced during the infection and suggests that it is of clinical importance (Schmidt *et al.*, 1995).

A novel haemolysin unrelated to α-haemolysin has recently been identified in *E. coli* K-12 (Ludwig *et al.*, 1995; Oscarsson *et al.*, 1996). It is not expressed in significant amounts under standard laboratory conditions. Its synthesis is, however, induced when the *slyA* gene of *Salmonella typhimurium* or *E. coli* that encodes a 17-kDa regulatory protein is introduced into *E. coli* K-12 on a plasmid. The available data indicate that this haemolysin is a cell-associated pore-forming protein (Ludwig *et al.*, 1995; Oscarsson *et al.*, 1996). The gene that encodes this cryptic *E. coli* haemolysin has yet to be characterised.

Conclusion

Extensive investigations in the past two decades have greatly increased our knowledge of the genetics, structure and activity of *E. coli* α-haemolysin. It has been unequivocally demonstrated that this toxin plays an important role in the pathogenicity of extra-intestinal *E. coli* strains. Identification and analysis of the specific α-haemolysin transport system has opened up the possibility of the secretion of heterologous proteins by *E. coli* by fusing these to the α-haemolysin secretion signal.

Several important questions about the activity of α-haemolysin and the toxin–target cell interaction remain. The precise mechanism of the HlyC-mediated activation of the α-haemolysin protein is still unclear. Moreover, very little is known about the α-haemolysin receptors on target cell membranes and about the features of HlyA that are responsible for its target cell specificity. Finally, although several distinctive effects of α-haemolysin on different cell types involved in host immune defence have been detected, it remains to be established how these activities co-operate to favour survival and growth of the α-haemolysin-producing bacteria in an infected host.

As compared with the many publications that deal with α-haemolysin, only little is known about the *E. coli* haemolysins that differ from α-haemolysin. Their biochemical analysis, characterisation of their cytolytic activity and target cell specificity, as well as determination of their possible role in pathogenesis are desirable.

References

Bailey, M. J. A., Koronakis, V., Schmoll, T. & Hughes, C. (1992). *Escherichia coli* HlyT protein, a transcriptional activator of haemolysin synthesis and secretion, is encoded by the *rfaH* (*sfrB*) locus required for expression of sex factor and lipopolysaccharide genes. *Molecular Microbiology*, **6**, 1003–12.

Barry, E. M., Weiss, A. A., Ehrmann, I. E., Gray, M. C., Hewlett, E. L. & Goodwin, M. St. M. (1991). *Bordetella pertussis* adenylate cyclase toxin and hemolytic activities require a second gene, *cyaC*, for activation. *Journal of Bacteriology*, **173**, 720–6.

Bauer, M. E. & Welch, R. A. (1996). Characterization of an RTX toxin from enterohemorrhagic *Escherichia coi* O157:H7. *Infection and Immunity*, **64**, 167–75.

Benz, R., Döbereiner, A., Ludwig, A.& Goebel, W. (1992). Haemolysin of *Escherichia coli*: comparison of pore-forming properties between chromosomal and plasmid-encoded haemolysins. FEMS *Microbiology Immunology*, **105**, 55–62.

Benz, R., Maier, E. & Gentschev, I. (1993). TolC of *Escherichia coli* functions as an outer membrane channel. *Zentralblatt für Bakteriologie*, **278**, 187–96.

Benz, R., Schmid, A., Wagner, W. & Goebel, W. (1989). Pore formation by the *Escherichia coli* hemolysin: evidence for an association–dissociation equilibrium of the pore-forming aggregates. *Infection and Immunity*, **57**, 887–95.

Berger, H., Hacker, J., Juarez, A., Hughes, C. & Goebel, W. (1982). Cloning of the chromosomal determinants encoding hemolysin production and mannose-resistant hemagglutination in *Escherichia coli*. *Journal of Bacteriology*, **152**, 1241–7.

Beutin, L., Bode, L., Özel, M. & Stephan, R. (1990). Enterohemolysin production is associated with a temperate bacteriophage in *Escherichia coli* serogroup O26 strains. *Journal of Bacteriology*, **172**, 6469–75.

Beutin, L., Prada, J., Zimmermann, S., Stephan, R., Ørskov, I. & Ørskov, F. (1988). Enterohemolysin, a new type of hemolysin produced by some strains of enteropathogenic *E. coli* (EPEC). *Zentralblatt für Bakteriologie und Hygiene A*, **267**, 576–88.

Beutin, L., Stroeher, U. H. & Manning, P. A. (1993). Isolation of enterohemolysin (Ehly2)-associated sequences encoded on temperate phages of *Escherichia coli*. *Gene*, **132**, 95–9.

Bhakdi, S., Greulich, S., Muhly, M., Eberspächer, B., Becker, H., Thiel, A. & Hugo, F. (1989). Potent leucocidal action of *Escherichia coli* hemolysin mediated by permeabilization of target cell membranes. *Journal of Experimental Medicine*, **169**, 737–54.

Bhakdi, S., Mackman, N., Nicaud, J.-M. & Holland, I. B. (1986). *Escherichia coli* hemolysin may damage target cell membranes by generating transmembrane pores. *Infection and Immunity*, **52**, 63–9.

Bhakdi, S. & Martin, E. (1991). Superoxide generation by human neutrophils induced by low doses of *Escherichia coli* hemolysin. *Infection and Immunity*, **59**, 2955–62.

Bhakdi, S., Muhly, M., Korom, S. & Schmidt, G. (1990). Effects of *Escherichia coli* hemolysin on human monocytes. Cytocidal action and stimulation of interleukin 1 release. *Journal of Clinical Investigation*, **85**, 1746–53.

Bhakdi, S. & Tranum-Jensen, J. (1986). Membrane damage by pore-forming bacterial cytolysins. *Microbial Pathogenesis*, **1**, 5–14.

Bhakdi, S. & Tranum-Jensen, J. (1988). Damage to cell membranes by pore-forming bacterial cytolysins. *Progress in Allergy*, **40**, 1–43.

Blanco, J., Alonso, M. P., Gonzalez, E. A., Blanco, M. & Garabal, J. I. (1990). Virulence factors of bacteraemic *Escherichia coli* with particular reference to production of cytotoxic necrotising factor (CNF) by P-fimbriate strains. *Journal of Medical Microbiology*, **31**, 175–83.

Blanco, J., Blanco, M., Alonso, M. P., Blanco, J. E., Gonzalez, E. A. & Garabal, J. I. (1992). Characteristics of haemolytic *Escherichia coli* with particular reference to production of cytotoxic necrotizing factor type 1 (CNF 1). *Research in Microbiology*, **143**, 869–78.

Blight, M. A. & Holland, I. B. (1990). Structure and function of haemolysin B, P-glycoprotein and other members of a novel family of membrane translocators. *Molecular Microbiology*, **4**, 873–80.

Blight, M. A., Menichi, B. & Holland, I. B. (1995). Evidence for posttranscriptional regulation of the synthesis of the *Escherichia coli* HlyB haemolysin translocator and production of polyclonal anti-HlyB antibody. *Molecular and General Genetics*, **247**, 73–85.

Boehm, D. F., Welch, R. A. & Snyder, I. S. (1990a). Calcium is required for binding of *Escherichia coli* hemolysin (HlyA) to erythrocyte membranes. *Infection and Immunity*, **58**, 1951–8.

Boehm, D. F., Welch, R. A. & Snyder, I. S. (1990b). Domains of *Escherichia coli* hemolysin (HlyA) involved in binding of calcium and erythrocyte membranes. *Infection and Immunity*, **58**, 1959–64.

Bohach, G. A. & Snyder, I. S. (1985). Chemical and immunological analysis of the complex structure of *Escherichia coli* alpha-hemolysin. *Journal of Bacteriology*, **164**, 1071–80.

Bohach, G. A. & Snyder, I. S. (1986). Composition of affinity-purified alpha-hemolysin of *Escherichia coli*. *Infection and Immunity*, **53**, 435–7.

Braun, V. & Focareta, T. (1991). Pore-forming bacterial protein hemolysins (cytolysins). *Critical Reviews in Microbiology*, **18**, 115–58.

Brauner, A., Katouli, M., Tullus, K. & Jacobson, S. H. (1990). Production of cytotoxic necrotizing factor, verocytotoxin and haemolysin by pyelonephritogenic *Escherichia coli*. *European Journal of Clinical Microbiology and Infectious Diseases*, **9**, 762–7.

Burrows, L. L. & Lo, R. Y. C. (1992). Molecular characterization of an RTX toxin determinant from *Actinobacillus suis*. *Infection and Immunity*, **60**, 2166–73.

Caprioli, A., Falbo, V., Ruggeri, F. M., Baldassarri, L., Bisicchia, R., Ippolito, G., Romoli, E. & Donelli, G. (1987). Cytotoxic necrotizing factor production by hemolytic strains of *Escherichia coli* causing extra-intestinal infections. *Journal of Clinical Microbiology*, **25**, 146–9.

Carmona, M., Balsalobre, C., Munoa, F., Mourino, M., Jubete, Y., De la Cruz, F. & Juarez, A. (1993). *Escherichia coli hha* mutants, DNA super-coiling and expression of the haemolysin genes from the recombinant plasmid pANN202-312. *Molecular Microbiology*, **9**, 1011–18.

Cavalieri, S. J., Bohach, G. A. & Snyder, I. S. (1984). *Escherichia coli* α-haemolysin: characteristics and probable role in pathogenicity. *Microbiological Reviews*, **48**, 326–43.

Cavalieri, S. J. & Snyder, I. S. (1982a). Effect of *Escherichia coli* alpha-hemolysin on human peripheral leukocyte viability *in vitro*. *Infection and Immunity*, **36**, 455–61.

Cavalieri, S. J. & Snyder, I. S. (1982b). Effect of *Escherichia coli* alpha-hemolysin on human peripheral leukocyte function *in vitro*. *Infection and Immunity*, **37**, 966–74.

Cavalieri, S. J. & Snyder, I. S. (1982c). Cytotoxic activity of partially purified *Escherichia coli* alpha-haemolysin. *Journal of Medical Microbiology*, **15**, 11–21.

Chang, Y.-F., Young, R., Moulds, T. L. & Struck, D. K. (1989a). Secretion of the *Pasteurella* leukotoxin by *Escherichia coli*. *FEMS Microbiology Letters*, **60**, 169–74.

Chang, Y.-F., Young, R. & Struck, D. K. (1989b). Cloning and character-ization of a hemolysin gene from *Actinobacillus (Haemophilus) pleuro-pneumoniae*. *DNA*, **8**, 635–47.

Chaturvedi, U. C., Mather, A., Khan, A. M. & Mehrotra, R. M. L. (1969). Cytotoxicity of filtrates of hemolytic *Escherichia coli*. *Journal of Medical Microbiology*, **2**, 211–18.

Cooke, E. M. & Ewins, S. P. (1975). Properties of strains of *Escherichia coli* isolated from a variety of sources. *Journal of Medical Microbiology*, **8**, 107–11.

Coote, J. G. (1992). Structural and functional relationships among the RTX toxin determinants of Gram-negative bacteria. *FEMS Microbiology Reviews*, **88**, 137–62.

Cosar, G. (1991). Antibiotic susceptibility, hemolysin production and haemag-glutinating activity of uropathogenic *Escherichia coli*. *Journal of Hygiene, Epidemiology, Microbiology and Immunology*, **35**, 303–7.

Cross, M. A., Koronakis, V., Stanley, P. L. D. & Hughes, C. (1990).
HlyB-dependent secretion of hemolysin by uropathogenic *Escherichia coli*
requires conserved sequences flanking the chromosomal *hly* determinant.
Journal of Bacteriology, **172**, 1217–24.

Currier, S. J., Ueda, K., Willingham, M. C., Pastan, I. & Gottesman, M. M.
(1989). Deletion and insertion mutants of the multidrug transporter.
Journal of Biological Chemistry, **264**, 14376–81.

DeBoy, J. M. II, Wachsmuth, I. K. & Davis, B. R. (1980). Hemolytic activity
in enterotoxigenic and non-enterotoxigenic strains of *Escherichia coli*.
Journal of Clinical Micribiology, **12**, 193–8.

De la Cruz, F., Müller, D., Ortiz, J. M. & Goebel, W. (1980). Hemolysis
determinant common to *Escherichia coli* hemolytic plasmids of different
incompatibility groups. *Journal of Bacteriology*, **143**, 825–33.

De la Cruz, F., Zabala, J. C. & Ortiz, J. M. (1979). Incompatibility among
α-haemolytic plasmids studied after inactivation of the α-haemolysin gene
by transposition of Tn802. *Plasmid*, **2**, 507–19.

De la Cruz, F., Zabala, J. C. & Ortiz, J. M. (1983). Hemolysis determinant
common to *Escherichia coli* strains of different O serotypes and origins.
Infection and Immunity, **41**, 881–7.

Delepelaire, P. & Wandersman, C. (1989). Protease secretion by *Erwinia
chrysanthemi*: proteases B and C are synthesized and secreted as
zymogens without a signal peptide. *Journal of Biological Chemistry*, **264**,
9083–9.

Delepelaire, P. & Wandersman, C. (1990). Protein secretion in Gram-negative
bacteria: the extracellular metalloprotease B from *Erwinia chrysanthemi*
contains a C-terminal secretion signal analogous to that of *Escherichia coli*
α-haemolysin. *Journal of Biological Chemistry*, **265**, 17118–25.

Delepelaire, P. & Wandersman, C. (1991). Characterization, localization and
transmembrane organization of the three proteins PrtD, PrtE and PrtF
necessary for protease secretion by the Gram-negative bacterium *Erwinia
chrysanthemi*. *Molecular Microbiology*, **5**, 2427–34.

Driessen, A. J. M. (1992). Precursor protein translocation by the *Escherichia
coli* translocase is directed by the proton motive force. *EMBO Journal*,
11, 847–53.

Dudgeon, L. S., Wordley, E. & Bawtree, F. (1921). On *Bacillus coli* infections
of the urinary tract especially in relation to haemolytic organisms. *Journal
of Hygiene, Cambridge*, **20**, 137–64.

Duong, F., Lazdunski, A., Cami, B. & Murgier, M. (1992). Sequence of a
cluster of genes controlling synthesis and secretion of alkaline protease in
Pseudomonas aeruginosa: relationships to other secretory pathways.
Gene, **121**, 47–54.

Eberspächer, B., Hugo, F. & Bhakdi, S. (1989). Quantitative study of the
binding and hemolytic efficiency of *Escherichia coli* hemolysin. *Infection
and Immunity*, **57**, 983–8.

Eberspächer, B., Hugo, F., Pohl, M. & Bhakdi, S. (1990). Functional
similarity between the haemolysins of *Escherichia coli* and *Morganella
morganii*. *Journal of Medical Microbiology*, **33**, 165–70.

Economou, A., Hamilton, W. D. O., Johnston, A. W. B. & Downie, J. A.
(1990). The *Rhizobium* nodulation gene *nodO* encodes a Ca^{2+}-binding
protein that is exported without N-terminal cleavage and is homologous to
haemolysin and related proteins. *EMBO Journal*, **9**, 349–54.

Erb, K., Vogel, M., Wagner, W. & Goebel, W. (1987). Alkaline phosphatase which lacks its own signal sequence becomes enzymatically active when fused to N-terminal sequences of *Escherichia coli* haemolysin (HlyA). *Molecular and General Genetics*, **208**, 88–93.

Ermert, L., Rousseau, S., Schütte, H., Birkemeyer, R. G., Grimminger, F., Bhakdi, S., Duncker, H. R. & Seeger, W. (1992). Induction of severe vascular leakage by low doses of *Escherichia coli* hemolysin in perfused rabbit lungs. *Laboratory Investigation*, **66**, 362–9.

Evans, D. J., Evans, D. G., Höhne, C., Noble, M. A., Haldane, E. V., Lior, H. & Young, L. S. (1981). Hemolysin and K antigens in relation to serotype and hemagglutination type of *Escherichia coli* isolated from extraintestinal infections. *Journal of Clinical Microbiology*, **13**, 171–8.

Falbo, V., Famiglietti, M. & Caprioli, A. (1992). Gene block encoding production of cytotoxic necrotizing factor 1 and hemolysin in *Escherichia coli* isolates from extraintestinal infections. *Infection and Immunity*, **60**, 2182–7.

Fath, M. J. & Kolter, R. (1993). ABC transporters: bacterial exporters. *Microbiological Reviews*, **57**, 995–1017.

Fath, M. J., Skvirsky, R. C. & Kolter, R. (1991). Functional complementation between bacterial MDR-like export systems: colicin V, alpha-hemolysin, and *Erwinia* protease. *Journal of Bacteriology*, **173**, 7549–56.

Felmlee, T., Pellett, S., Lee, E.-Y. & Welch, R. A. (1985a). *Escherichia coli* hemolysin is released extracellularly without cleavage of a signal peptide. *Journal of Bacteriology*, **163**, 88–93.

Felmlee, T., Pellett, S. & Welch, R. A. (1985b). Nucleotide sequence of an *Escherichia coli* chromosomal hemolysin. *Journal of Bacteriology*, **163**, 94–105.

Felmlee, T. & Welch, R. A. (1988). Alterations of amino acids repeats in the *Escherichia coli* hemolysin affect cytolytic activity and secretion. *Proceedings of the National Academy of Sciences, USA*, **85**, 5269–73.

Forestier, C. & Welch, R. A. (1991). Identification of RTX toxin target cell specificity domains by use of hybrid genes. *Infection and Immunity*, **59**, 4212–20.

Frey, J., Beck, M., Stucki, U. & Nicolet, J. (1993a). Analysis of hemolysin operons in *Actinobacillus pleuropneumoniae*. *Gene*, **123**, 51–8.

Frey, J., Bosse, J. T., Chang, Y.-F., Cullen, J. M., Fenwick, B., Gerlach, G. F., Gygi, D., Haesebrouck, F., Inzana, T. J., Jansen, R., Kamp, E. M., Macdonald, J., MacInnes, J. I., Mittal, K. R., Nicolet, J., Rycroft, A. N. Segers, R. P. A. M., Smits, M. A., Stenbaek, E., Struck, D. K., van den Bosch, J. F., Willson, P. J. & Young, R. (1993b). *Actinobacillus pleuropneumoniae* RTX-toxins: uniform designation of haemolysins, cytolysins, pleurotoxin and their genes. *Journal of General Microbiology*, **139**, 1723–8.

Frey, J., Meier, R., Gygi, D. & Nicolet, J. (1991). Nucleotide sequence of the hemolysin I gene from *Actinobacillus pleuropneumoniae*. *Infection and Immunity*, **59**, 3026–32.

Frey, J., Van den Bosch, H., Segers, R. & Nicolet, J. (1992). Identification of a second hemolysin (HlyII) in *Actinobacillus pleuropneumoniae* serotype 1 and expression of the gene in *Escherichia coli*. *Infection and Immunity*, **60**, 1671–6.

Fried, F. A., Vermeulen, C. W., Ginsburg, M. J. & Cone, C. M. (1971). Etiology of pyelonephritis: further evidence associating the production of experimental pyelonephritis with hemolysis in *Escherichia coli. Journal of Urology*, **106**, 351–4.

Gadeberg, O. V., Hacker, J. & Ørskov, I. (1989). Role of α-hemolysin for the *in vitro* phagocytosis and intracellular killing of *Escherichia coli. Zentralblatt für Bakteriologie und Hygiene*, **271**, 205–13.

Gadeberg, O. V. & Mansa, B. (1990). *In vitro* cytotoxic effect of alpha-hemolytic *Escherichia coli* on human blood granulocytes. Inhibition by alpha-hemolysin antibody. *International Journal of Medical Microbiology*, **273**, 492–500.

Gadeberg, O. V. & Ørskov, I. (1984). *In vitro* cytotoxic effect of α-hemolytic *Escherichia coli* on human blood granulocytes. *Infection and Immunity*, **45**, 255–60.

Gadeberg, O. V., Ørskov, I. & Rhodes, J. M. (1983). Cytotoxic effect of an alpha-hemolytic *Escherichia coli* strain on human blood monocytes and granulocytes. *Infection and Immunity*, **41**, 358–64.

Gentschev, I. & Goebel, W. (1992). Topological and functional studies on HlyB of *Escherichia coli. Molecular and General Genetics*, **232**, 40–8.

Gentschev, I., Hess, J. & Goebel, W. (1990). Change in the cellular localization of alkaline phosphatase by alteration of its carboxy-terminal sequence. *Molecular and General Genetics*, **222**, 211–16.

Gentschev, I., Mollenkopf, H.-J., Sokolovic, Z., Ludwig, A., Tengel, C., Gross, R., Hess, J., Demuth, A. & Goebel, W. (1994). Synthesis and secretion of bacterial antigens by attenuated *Salmonella* via the *Escherichia coli* hemolysin secretion system. *Behring Institute Research Communications*, **95**, 57–66.

Gentschev, I., Sokolovic, Z., Köhler, S., Krohne, G. F., Hof, H., Wagner, J. & Goebel, W. (1992). Identification of p60 antibodies in human sera and presentation of this listerial antigen on the surface of attenuated *Salmonellae* by the HlyB–HlyD secretion system. *Infection and Immunity*, **60**,5091–8.

Gerlach, J. H., Endicott, J. A., Juranka, P. F., Henderson, G., Sarangi, F., Deuchars, K. L. & Ling, V. (1986). Homology between P-glycoprotein and a bacterial haemolysin transport protein suggests a model for multi-drug resistance. *Nature*, **324**, 485–9.

Ghigo, J.-M. & Wandersman, C. (1992). Cloning, nucleotide sequence and characterization of the gene encoding the *Erwinia chrysanthemi* B374 PrtA metalloprotease: a third metalloprotease secreted via a C-terminal secretion signal. *Molecular and General Genetics*, **236**, 135–44.

Giaffer, M. H., Holdsworth, C. D. & Duerden, B. I. (1992). Virulence properties of *Escherichia coli* strains isolated from patients with inflammatory bowel disease. *Gut*, **33**, 646–50.

Gilson, L., Mahanty, H. K. & Kolter, R. (1990). Genetic analysis of an MDR-like export system: the secretion of colicin V. *EMBO Journal*, **9**, 3875–84.

Glaser, P., Ladant, D., Sezer, O., Pichot, F., Ullmann, A. & Danchin, A. (1988a). The calmodulin-sensitive adenylate cyclase of *Bordetella pertussis*: cloning and expression in *Escherichia coli. Molecular Microbiology*, **2**, 19–30.

Glaser, P., Sakamoto, H., Bellalou, J., Ullmann, A. & Danchin, A. (1988b). Secretion of cyclolysin, the calmodulin-sensitive adenylate cyclase-haemolysin bifunctional protein of *Bordetella pertussis*. *EMBO Journal*, **7**, 3997–4004.

Goebel, W. & Hedgpeth, J. (1982). Cloning and functional characterization of the plasmid-encoded hemolysin determinant of *Escherichia coli. Journal of Bacteriology*, **151**, 1290–8.

Goebel, W., Royer-Pokora, B., Lindenmaier, W. & Bujard, H. (1974). Plasmids controlling synthesis of hemolysin in *Escherichia coli*: molecular properties. *Journal of Bacteriology*, **118**, 964–73.

Goebel, W. & Schrempf, H. (1971). Isolation and characterization of super-coiled circular deoxyribonucleic acid from beta-hemolytic strains of *Escherichia coli. Journal of Bacteriology*, **106**, 311–17.

Gonzalez-Carrero, M. I., Zabala, J. C., De la Cruz, F. & Ortiz, J. M. (1985). Purification of α-hemolysin from an overproducing *E. coli* strain. *Molecular and General Genetics*, **199**, 106–10.

Gray, L., Baker, K., Kenny, B., Mackman, N., Haigh, R. & Holland, I. B. (1989). A novel C-terminal signal sequence targets *E. coli* haemolysin directly to the medium. *Journal of Cell Science, Supplement*, **11**, 45–57.

Gray, L., Mackman, N., Nicaud, J.-M. & Holland, I. B. (1986). The carboxy-terminal region of haemolysin 2001 is required for secretion of the toxin from *Escherichia coli. Molecular and General Genetics*, **205**, 127–33.

Green, C. P. & Thomas, V. L. (1981). Hemagglutination of human type O erythrocytes, hemolysin production, and serogrouping of *Escherichia coli* isolates from patients with acute pyelonephritis, cystitis, and asymptomatic bacteriuria. *Infection and Immunity*, **31**, 309–15.

Grimminger, F., Scholz, C., Bhakdi, S. & Seeger, W. (1991a). Subhemolytic doses of *Escherichia coli* hemolysin evoke large quantities of lipoxygenase products in human neutrophils. *Journal of Biological Chemistry*, **266**, 14262–9.

Grimminger, F., Sibelius, U., Bhakdi, S., Suttorp, N. & Seeger, W. (1991b). *Escherichia coli* hemolysin is a potent inductor of phosphoinositide hydrolysis and related metabolic responses in human neutrophils. *Journal of Clinical Investigation*, **88**, 1531–9.

Grimminger, F., Thomas, M., Obernitz, R., Walmrath, D., Bhakdi, S. & Seeger, W. (1990a). Inflammatory lipid mediator generation elicited by viable hemolysin-forming *Escherichia coli* in lung vasculature. *Journal of Experimental Medicine*, **172**, 1115–25.

Grimminger, F., Walmrath, D., Birkemeyer, R. G., Bhakdi, S. & Seeger, W. (1990b). Leukotriene and hydroxyeicosatetraenoic acid generation elicited by low doses of *Escherichia coli* hemolysin in rabbit lungs. *Infection and Immunity*, **58**, 2659–63.

Grünig, H.-M. & Lebek, G. (1988). Haemolytic activity and characteristics of plasmid and chromosomally borne *hly* genes isolated from *E. coli* of different origin. *Zentralblatt für Bakteriologie und Hygiene A*, **267**, 485–94.

Grünig, H.-M., Rutschi, D., Schoch, C. & Lebek, G. (1987). The chromosomal *fur* gene regulates the extracellular haemolytic activity encoded by certain Hly plasmids. *Zentralblatt für Bakteriologie und Hygiene A*, **266**, 231–8.

Guthmiller, J. M., Kolodrubetz, D., Cagle, M. P. & Kraig, E. (1990a). Sequence of the *lktB* gene from *Actinobacillus actinomycetemcomitans. Nucleic Acids Research*, **18**, 5291.

Guthmiller, J. M., Kraig, E., Cagle, M. P. & Kolodrubetz, D. (1990b). Sequence of the *lktD* gene from *Actinobacillus actinomycetemcomitans. Nucleic Acids Research*, **18**, 5292.

Guzzo, J., Duong, F., Wandersman, C., Murgier, M. & Lazdunski, A. (1991). The secretion genes of *Pseudomonas aeruginosa* alkaline protease are functionally related to those of *Erwinia chrysanthemi* proteases and *Escherichia coli* α-haemolysin. *Molecular Microbiology*, **5**, 447–53.

Gygi, D., Nicolet, J., Frey, J., Cross, M., Koronakis, V. & Hughes, C. (1990). Isolation of the *Actinobacillus pleuropneumoniae* haemolysin gene and the activation and secretion of the prohaemolysin by the HlyC, HlyB and HlyD proteins of *Escherichia coli*. *Molecular Microbiology*, **4**, 123–8.

Gygi, D., Nicolet, J., Hughes, C. & Frey, J. (1992). Functional analysis of the Ca^{2+}-regulated hemolysin I operon of *Actinobacillus pleuropneumoniae* serotype 1. *Infection and Immunity*, **60**, 3059–64.

Hacker, J., Bender, L., Ott, M., Wingender, J., Lund, B., Marre, R. & Goebel, W. (1990). Deletions of chromosomal regions coding for fimbriae and hemolysins occur *in vitro* and *in vivo* in various extraintestinal *Escherichia coli* isolates. *Microbial Pathogenesis*, **8**, 213–25.

Hacker, J., Hughes, C., Hof, H. & Goebel, W. (1983a). Cloned hemolysin genes from *Escherichia coli* that cause urinary tract infection determine different levels of toxicity in mice. *Infection and Immunity*, **42**, 57–63.

Hacker, J., Ott, M., Blum, G., Marre, R., Heesemann, J., Tschäpe, H. & Goebel, W. (1992). Genetics of *Escherichia coli* uropathogenicity: analysis of the O6:K15:H31 isolate 536. *Zentralblatt für Bakteriologie und Hygiene*, **276**, 165–75.

Hacker, J., Schröter, G., Schrettenbrunner, A., Hughes, C. & Goebel, W. (1983b). Hemolytic *Escherichia coli* strains in the human fecal flora as potential urinary pathogens. *Zentralblatt für Bakteriologie und Hygiene A*, **254**, 370–8.

Hackett, M., Guo, L., Shabanowitz, J., Hunt, D. F. & Hewlett, E. L. (1994). Internal lysine palmitoylation in adenylate cyclase toxin from *Bordetella pertussis*. *Science*, **266**, 433–5.

Hanke, C., Hess, J., Schumacher, G. & Goebel, W. (1992). Processing by OmpT of fusion proteins carrying the HlyA transport signal during secretion by the *Escherichia coli* hemolysin transport system. *Molecular and General Genetics*, **233**, 42–8.

Hardie, K. R., Issartel, J.-P., Koronakis, E., Hughes, C. & Koronakis, V. (1991). *In vitro* activation of *Escherichia coli* prohaemolysin to the mature membrane-targeted toxin requires HlyC and a low molecular-weight cytosolic polypeptide. *Molecular Microbiology*, **5**, 1669–79.

Härtlein, M., Schießl, S., Wagner, W., Rdest, U., Kreft, J. & Goebel, W. (1983). Transport of hemolysin by *Escherichia coli*. *Journal of Cellular Biochemistry*, **22**, 87–97.

Hess, J., Gentschev, I., Goebel, W. & Jarchau, T. (1990). Analysis of the haemolysin secretion system by PhoA-HlyA fusion proteins. *Molecular and General Genetics*, **224**, 201–8.

Hess, J., Wels, W., Vogel, M. & Goebel, W. (1986). Nucleotide sequence of a plasmid-encoded hemolysin determinant and its comparison with a corresponding chromosomal hemolysin sequence. *FEMS Microbiology Letters*, **34**, 1–11.

Higgins, C. F., Hiles, I. D., Salmond, G. P. C., Gill, D. R., Downie, J. A., Evans, I. J., Holland, I. B., Gray, L., Buckel, S. D., Bell, A. W. & Hermodson, M. A. (1986). A family of related ATP-binding subunits coupled to many distinct biological processes in bacteria. *Nature*, **323**, 448–50.

High, N. J., Hales, B. A., Jann, K. & Boulnois, G. J. (1988). A block of urovirulence genes encoding multiple fimbriae and hemolysin in *Escherichia coli* O4:K12:H⁻. *Infection and Immunity*, **56**, 513–17.

Highlander, S. K., Chidambaram, M., Engler, M. J. & Weinstock, G. M. (1989). DNA sequence of the *Pasteurella haemolytica* leukotoxin gene cluster. *DNA*, **8**, 15–28.

Highlander, S. K., Engler, M. J. & Weinstock, G. M. (1990). Secretion and expression of the *Pasteurella haemolytica* leukotoxin. *Journal of Bacteriology*, **172**, 2343–50.

Höhne, C. (1973). Hly-Plasmide in R-Plasmide tragenden Stämmen von *Escherichia coli*. *Zeitschrift für Allgemeine Mikrobiologie*, **13**, 49–53.

Hughes, C., Hacker, J., Roberts, A. & Goebel, W. (1983). Hemolysin production as a virulence marker in symptomatic and asymptomatic urinary tract infections caused by *Escherichia coli*. *Infection and Immunity*, **39**, 546–51.

Hughes, C., Phillips, R. & Roberts, A. P. (1982). Serum resistance among *Escherichia coli* strains causing urinary tract infection in relation to O type and the carriage of hemolysin, colicin, and antibiotic resistance determinants. *Infection and Immunity*, **35**, 270–5.

Hull, S. I., Hull, R. A., Minshew, B. H. & Falkow, S. (1982). Genetics of hemolysin of *Escherichia coli*. *Journal of Bacteriology*, **151**, 1006–12.

Hyde, S. C., Emsley, P., Hartshorn, M. J., Mimmack, M. M., Gileadi, U., Pearce, S. R., Gallagher, M. P., Gill, D. R., Hubbard, R. E. & Higgins, C. F. (1990). Structural model of ATP-binding proteins associated with cystic fibrosis, multidrug resistance and bacterial transport. *Nature*, **346**, 362–5.

Issartel, J.-P., Koronakis, V. & Hughes, C. (1991). Activation of *Escherichia coli* prohaemolysin to the mature toxin by acyl carrier protein-dependent fatty acylation. *Nature*, **351**, 759–61.

Jansen, R., Briaire, J., Kamp, E. M., Gielkens, A. L. J. & Smits, M. A. (1993). Structural analysis of the *Actinobacillus pleuropneumoniae*-RTX-toxin I (ApxI) operon. *Infection and Immunity*, **61**, 3688–95.

Jarchau, T., Chakraborty, T., Garcia, F. & Goebel, W. (1994). Selection for transport competence of C-terminal polypeptides derived from *Escherichia coli* hemolysin: the shortest peptide capable of autonomous HlyB/HlyD-dependent secretion comprises the C-terminal 62 amino acids of HlyA. *Molecular and General Genetics*, **245**, 53–60.

Johnson, J. R. (1991). Virulence factors in *Escherichia coli* urinary tract infection. *Clinical Microbiology Reviews*, **4**, 80–128.

Johnson, J. R., Moseley, S. L., Roberts, P. L. & Stamm, W. E. (1988). Aerobactin and other virulence factor genes among strains of *Escherichia coli* causing urosepsis: association with patient characteristics. *Infection and Immunity*, **56**, 405–12.

Jonas, D., Schultheis, B., Klas, C., Krammer, P. H. & Bhakdi, S. (1993). Cytocidal effects of *Escherichia coli* hemolysin on human T lymphocytes. *Infection and Immunity*, **61**, 1715–21.

Juarez, A., Hughes, C., Vogel, M. & Goebel, W. (1984). Expression and regulation of the plasmid-encoded hemolysin determinant of *Escherichia coli*. *Molecular and General Genetics*, **197**, 196–203.

Jubete, Y., Zabala, J. C., Juarez, A. & De la Cruz, F. (1995). *hly*M, a transcriptional silencer downstream of the promoter in the *hly* operon of *Escherichia coli*. *Journal of Bacteriology*, **177**, 242–6.

Jubete, Y., Zabala, J. C., Juarez, A. & De la Cruz, F. (1995). *hlyM*, a transcriptional silencer downstream of the promoter in the *hly* operon of *Escherichia coli*. *Journal of Bacteriology*, **177**, 242–6.

Juranka, P., Zhang, F., Kulpa, J., Endicott, J., Blight, M., Holland, I. B. & Ling, V. (1992). Characterization of the hemolysin transporter, HlyB, using an epitope insertion. *Journal of Biological Chemistry*, **267**, 3764–70.

Kayser, H. (1903). Ueber Bakterienhämolysine, im Besonderen das Colilysin. *Zeitschrift für Hygiene und Infektionskrankheiten*, **42**, 118–38.

Keane, W. F., Welch, R., Gekker, G. & Peterson, P. K. (1987). Mechanism of *Escherichia coli* alpha-hemolysin-induced injury to isolated renal tubular cells. *American Journal of Pathology*, **126**,350–7.

Kenny, B., Chervaux, C. & Holland, I. B. (1994). Evidence that residues −15 to −46 of the haemolysin secretion signal are involved in early steps in secretion, leading to recognition of the translocator. *Molecular Microbiology*, **11**, 99–109.

Kenny, B., Haigh, R. & Holland, I. B. (1991). Analysis of the haemolysin transport process through the secretion from *Escherichia coli* of PCM, CAT or β-galactosidase fused to the Hly C-terminal signal domain. *Molecular Microbiology*, **5**, 2557–68.

Kenny, B., Taylor, S. & Holland, I. B. (1992). Identification of individual amino acids required for secretion within the haemolysin (HlyA) C-terminal targeting region. *Molecular Microbiology*, **6**, 1477–89.

Knapp, S., Hacker, J., Jarchau, T. & Goebel, W. (1986). Large, unstable inserts in the chromosome affect virulence properties of uropathogenic *Escherichia coli* O6 strain 536. *Journal of Bacteriology*, **168**, 22–30.

Knapp, S., Hacker, J., Then, I., Müller, D. & Goebel, W. (1984). Multiple copies of hemolysin genes and associated sequences in the chromosomes of uropathogenic *Escherichia coli* strains. *Journal of Bacteriology*, **159**, 1027–33.

Knapp, S., Then, I., Wels, W., Michel, G., Tschäpe, H., Hacker, J. & Goebel, W. (1985). Analysis of the flanking regions from different haemolysin determinants of *Escherichia coli*. *Molecular and General Genetics*, **200**, 385–92.

Köller, M. & König, W. (1991). 12-Hydroxyeicosatetraenoic acid (12-HETE) induces heat shock proteins in human leukocytes. *Biochemical and Biophysical Research Communications*, **175**, 804–9.

König, B. & König, W. (1991). Roles of human peripheral blood leukocyte protein kinase C and G proteins in inflammatory mediator release by isogenic *Escherichia coli* strains. *Infection and Immunity*, **59**, 3801–10.

König, B. & König, W. (1993a). Induction and suppression of cytokine release (tumor necrosis factor-α; interleukin-6, interleukin-1β) by *Escherichia coli* pathogenicity factors (adhesions, α-haemolysin). *Immunology*, **78**, 526–33.

König, B. & König, W. (1993b). The role of the phosphatidylinositol turnover in 12-hydroxyeicosatetraenoic acid generation from human platelets by *Escherichia coli* α-haemolysin, thrombin and fluoride, *Immunology*, **80**, 633–9.

König, B., König, W., Scheffer, J., Hacker, J. & Goebel, W. (1986). Role of *Escherichia coli* alpha-hemolysin and bacterial adherence in infection: requirement for release of inflammatory mediators from granulocytes and mast cells. *Infection and Immunity*, **54**, 886–92.

König, B., Ludwig, A., Goebel, W. & König, W. (1994). Pore formation by the *Escherichia coli* alpha-hemolysin: role for mediator release from human inflammatory cells. *Infection and Immunity*, **62**, 4611–17.

König, B., Schönfeld, W., Scheffer, J. & König, W. (1990). Signal transduction in human platelets and inflammatory mediator release induced by genetically cloned hemolysin-positive and -negative *Escherichia coli* strains. *Infection and Immunity*, **58**, 1591–9.

Koronakis, E., Hughes, C., Milisav, I. & Koronakis, V. (1995). Protein exporter function and *in vitro* ATPase activity are correlated in ABC-domain mutants of HlyB. *Molecular Microbiology*, **16**, 87–96.

Koronakis, V., Cross, M. & Hughes, C. (1988). Expression of the *E. coli* hemolysin secretion gene *hlyB* involves transcript anti-termination within the *hly* operon. *Nucleic Acids Research*, **16**, 4789–800.

Koronakis, V., Cross, M. & Hughes, C. (1989a). Transcription antitermination in an *Escherichia coli* haemolysin operon is directed progressively by *cis*-acting DNA sequences upstream of the promoter region. *Molecular Microbiology*, **3**, 1397–1404.

Koronakis, V., Cross, M., Senior, B., Koronakis, E. & Hughes, C. (1987). The secreted hemolysins of *Proteus mirabilis*, *Proteus vulgaris*, and *Morganella morganii* are genetically related to each other and to the alpha-hemolysin of *Escherichia coli*. *Journal of Bacteriology*, **169**, 1509–15.

Koronakis, V. & Hughes, C. (1988). Identification of the promoters directing *in vivo* expression of hemolysin genes in *Proteus vulgaris* and *Escherichia coli*. *Molecular and General Genetics*, **213**, 99–104.

Koronakis, V., Hughes, C. & Koronakis, E. (1991). Energetically distinct early and late stages of HlyB/HlyD-dependent secretion across both *Escherichia coli* membranes. *EMBO Journal*, **10**, 3263–72.

Koronakis, V., Hughes, C. & Koronakis, E. (1993). ATPase activity and ATP/ADP-induced conformational change in the soluble domain of the bacterial protein translocator HlyB. *Molecular Microbiology*, **8**, 1163–75.

Koronakis, V., Koronakis, E. & Hughes, C. (1989b). Isolation and analysis of the C-terminal signal directing export of *Escherichia coli* hemolysin protein across both bacterial membranes. *EMBO Journal*, **8**, 595–605.

Kraig, E., Dailey, T. & Kolodrubetz, D. (1990). Nucleotide sequence of the leukotoxin gene from *Actinobacillus actinomycetemcomitans*: homology to the alpha-hemolysin/leukotoxin gene family. *Infection and Immunity*, **58**, 920–9.

Kreft, B., Carstensen, O., Straube, E., Bohnet, S., Hacker, J. & Marre, R. (1992). Adherence to and cytotoxicity of *Escherichia coli* for eukaryotic cell lines quantified by MTT (3-[4,5-dimethylthiazol-2-yl] -2,5-diphenyltetrazolium bromide). *International Journal of Medical Microbiology, Virology, Parasitology and Infectious Diseases*, **276**, 231–42.

Lally, E. T., Golub, E. E., Kieba, I. R., Taichman, N. S., Rosenbloom, J., Rosenbloom, J. C., Gibson, C. W. & Demuth, D. R. (1989). Analysis of the *Actinobacillus actinomycetemcomitans* leukotoxin gene. Delineation of unique features and comparison to homologous toxins. *Journal of Biological Chemistry*, **264**, 15451–6.

Lebek, G. & Grünig, H.-M. (1985). Relation between the hemolytic property and iron metabolism in *Escherichia coli*. *Infection and Immunity*, **50**, 682–6.

Letoffe, S., Delepelaire, P. & Wandersman, C. (1991). Cloning and expression in *Escherichia coli* of the *Serratia marcescens* metalloprotease gene: secretion of the protease from *E. coli* in the presence of the *Erwinia chrysanthemi* protease secretion functions. *Journal of Bacteriology*, **173**, 2160–6.

Linggood, M. A. & Ingram, P. L. (1982). The role of alpha haemolysin in the virulence of *Escherichia coli* for mice. *Journal of Medical Microbiology*, **15**, 23–30.

Lo, R. Y. C., Strathdee, C. A. & Shewen, P. E. (1987). Nucleotide sequence of the leukotoxin genes of *Pasteurella haemolytica* A1. *Infection and Immunity*, **55**, 1987–96.

Lovell, R. & Rees, T. A. (1960). A filterable haemolysin from *Escherichia coli*. *Nature*, **188**, 755–6.

Ludwig, A., Benz, R. & Goebel, W. (1993). Oligomerization of *Escherichia coli* haemolysin (HlyA) is involved in pore formation. *Molecular and General Genetics*, **241**, 89–96.

Ludwig, A., Garcia, F., Bauer, S., Jarchau, T., Benz, R., Hoppe, J. & Goebel, W. (1996). Analysis of the *in vivo* activation of hemolysin (HlyA) from *Escherichia coli*. *Journal of Bacteriology*, **178**, in press.

Ludwig, A. & Goebel, W. (1991). Genetic determinants of cytolytic toxins from Gram-negative bacteria. In *Sourcebook of Bacterial Protein Toxins*, eds. J. E. Alouf & J. H. Freer, pp. 117–46. London: Academic Press.

Ludwig, A., Jarchau, T., Benz, R. & Goebel, W. (1988). The repeat domain of *Escherichia coli* haemolysin (HlyA) is responsible for its Ca^{2+}-dependent binding to erythrocytes. *Molecular and General Genetics*, **214**, 553–61.

Ludwig, A., Schmid, A., Benz, R. & Goebel, W. (1991). Mutations affecting pore formation by haemolysin from *Escherichia coli*. *Molecular and General Genetics*, **226**, 198–208.

Ludwig, A., Tengel, C., Bauer, S., Bubert, A., Benz, R., Mollenkopf, H.-J. & Goebel, W. (1995). SlyA, a regulatory protein from *Salmonella typhimurium*, induces a haemolytic and pore-forming protein in *Escherichia coli*. *Molecular and General Genetics*, **249**, 474–86.

Ludwig, A., Vogel, M. & Goebel, W. (1987). Mutations affecting activity and transport of haemolysin in *Escherichia coli*. *Molecular and General Genetics*, **206**, 238–45.

Macdonald, J. & Rycroft, A. N. (1992). Molecular cloning and expression of *ptxA*, the gene encoding the 120-kilodalton cytotoxin of *Actinobacillus pleuropneumoniae* serotype 2. *Infection and Immunity*, **60**, 2726–32.

Macdonald, J. & Rycroft, A. N. (1993). *Actinobacillus pleuropneumoniae* haemolysin II is secreted from *Escherichia coli* by *A. pleuropneumoniae* pleurotoxin secretion gene products. *FEMS Microbiology Letters*, **109**, 317–22.

Mackman, N., Baker, K., Gray, L., Haigh, R., Nicaud, J.-M. & Holland, I. B. (1987). Release of a chimeric protein into the medium from *Escherichia coli* using the C-terminal secretion signal of haemolysin. *EMBO Journal*, **6**, 2835–41.

Mackman, N. & Holland, I. B. (1984a). Secretion of a 107 K Dalton polypeptide into the medium from a haemolytic *E. coli* K12 strain. *Molecular and General Genetics*, **193**, 312–15.

Mackman, N. & Holland, I. B. (1984b). Functional characterization of a cloned haemolysin determinant from *E. coli* of human origin, encoding information for the secretion of a 107 K polypeptide. *Molecular and General Genetics*, **196**, 129–34.

Mackman, N., Nicaud, J.-M., Gray, L. & Holland, I. B. (1985a). Genetical and functional organisation of the *Escherichia coli* haemolysin determinant 2001. *Molecular and General Genetics*, **201**, 282–8.

Mackman, N., Nicaud, J.-M., Gray, L. & Holland, I. B. (1985b). Identification of polypeptides required for the export of haemolysin 2001 from *E. coli*. *Molecular and General Genetics*, **201**, 529–36.

Mackman, N., Nicaud, J.-M., Gray, L. & Holland, I. B. (1986). Secretion of haemolysin by *Escherichia coli. Current Topics in Microbiology and Immunology*, **125**, 159–81.

Marre, R., Hacker, J., Henkel, W. & Goebel, W. (1986). Contribution of cloned virulence factors from uropathogenic *Escherichia coli* strains to nephropathogenicity in an experimental rat pyelonephritis model. *Infection and Immunity*, **54**, 761–7.

Masure, H. R., Au, D. C., Gross, M. K., Donovan, M. G. & Storm, D. R. (1990). Secretion of the *Bordetella pertussis* adenylate cyclase from *Escherichia coli* containing the hemolysin operon. *Biochemistry*, **29**, 140–5.

McWhinney, D. R., Chang, Y.-F., Young, R. & Struck, D. K. (1992). Separable domains define target cell specificities of an RTX hemolysin from *Actinobacillus pleuropneumoniae. Journal of Bacteriology*, **174**, 291–7.

Menestrina, G., Bashford, C. L. & Pasternak, C. A. (1990). Pore-forming toxins: experiments with *Staphylococcus aureus* alpha–toxin, *Clostridium perfringens* theta-toxin and *Escherichia coli* haemolysin in lipid bilayers, liposomes and intact cells. *Toxicon*, **28**, 477–91.

Menestrina, G., Mackman, N., Holland, I. B. & Bhakdi, S. (1987). *Escherichia coli* haemolysin forms voltage-dependent ion channels in lipid membranes. *Biochimica et Biophysica Acta*, **905**, 109–17.

Mimura, C. S., Holbrook, S. R. & Ames, G. F.-L. (1991). Structural model of the nucleotide-binding conserved component of periplasmic permeases. *Proceedings of the National Academy of Sciences, USA*, **88**, 84–8.

Minshew, B. H., Jorgensen, J., Counts, G. W. & Falkow, S. (1978). Association of hemolysin production, hemagglutination of human erythrocytes, and virulence for chicken embryos of extraintestinal *Escherichia coli* isolates. *Infection and Immunity*, **20**, 50–4.

Moayeri, M. & Welch, R. A. (1994). Effects of temperature, time, and toxin concentration on lesion formation by the *Escherichia coli* hemolysin. *Infection and Immunity*, **62**, 4124–34.

Mobley, H. L. T., Green, D. M., Trifillis, A. L., Johnson, D. E., Chippendale, G. R., Lockatell, C. V., Jones, B. D. & Warren, J. W. (1990). Pyelonephritogenic *Escherichia coli* and killing of cultured human renal proximal tubular epithelial cells: role of hemolysin in some strains. *Infection and Immunity*, **58**, 1281–9.

Monaco, J. J., Cho, S. & Attaya, M. (1990). Transport protein genes in the murine MHC: possible implications for antigen processing. *Science*, **250**, 1723–6.

Monti-Bragadin, C., Samer, L., Rottini, G. D. & Pani, B. (1975). The compatibility of Hly factor, a transmissible element which controls α-haemolysin production in *Escherichia coli. Journal of General Microbiology*, **86**, 367–9.

Morona, R., Manning, P. A. & Reeves, P. (1983). Identification and characterization of the TolC protein, an outer membrane protein from *Escherichia coli. Journal of Bacteriology*, **153**, 693–9.

Müller, D., Hughes, C. & Goebel, W. (1983). Relationship between plasmid and chromosomal hemolysin determinants of *Escherichia coli. Journal of Bacteriology*, **153**, 846–51.

Nicaud, J.-M., Mackman, N., Gray, L. & Holland, I. B. (1985a). Characterisation of HlyC and mechanism of activation and secretion of haemolysin from *E. coli* 2001. *FEBS Letters*, **187**, 339–44.

Nicaud, J.-M., Mackman, N., Gray, L. & Holland, I. B. (1985b). Regulation of haemolysin synthesis in *E. coli* determined by HLY genes of human origin. *Molecular and General Genetics*, **199**, 111–16.

Nicaud, J.-M., Mackman, N., Gray, L. & Holland, I. B. (1986). The C-terminal, 23 kDa peptide of *E. coli* haemolysin 2001 contains all the information necessary for its secretion by the haemolysin (Hly) export machinery. *FEBS Letters*, **204**, 331–5.

Nieto, J. M., Carmona, M., Bolland, S., Jubete, Y., De la Cruz, F. & Juarez, A. (1991). The *hha* gene modulates haemolysin expression in *Escherichia coli. Molecular Microbiology*, **5**, 1285–93.

Nieto, J. M., Tomas, J. & Juarez, A. (1987). Secretion of an *Aeromonas hydrophila* aerolysin by a mutant strain of *Escherichia coli. FEMS Microbiology Letters*, **48**, 413–17.

Noegel, A., Rdest, U. & Goebel, W. (1981). Determination of the functions of hemolytic plasmid pHly152 of *Escherichia coli. Journal of Bacteriology*, **145**, 233–47.

Noegel, A., Rdest, U., Springer, W. & Goebel, W. (1979). Plasmid cistrons controlling synthesis and excretion of the exotoxin α-haemolysin of *Escherichia coli. Molecular and General Genetics*, **175**, 343–50.

O'Hanley, P., Lalonde, G. & Ji, G. (1991). Alpha-hemolysin contributes to the pathogenicity of piliated digalactoside-binding *Escherichia coli* in the kidney: efficacy of an alpha-hemolysin vaccine in preventing renal injury in the BALB/c mouse model of pyelonephritis. *Infection and Immunity*, **59**, 1153–61.

Opal, S. M., Cross, A. S., Gemski, P. & Lyhte, L. W. (1990). Aerobactin and α-hemolysin as virulence determinants in *Escherichia coli* isolated from human blood, urine, and stool. *Journal of Infectious Diseases*, **161**,794–6.

Oropeza-Wekerle, R.-L., Kern, P., Sun, D., Muller, S., Briand, J. P. & Goebel, W. (1991). Characterization of monoclonal antibodies against alpha-hemolysin of *Escherichia coli. Infection and Immunity*, **59**, 1846–52.

Oropeza-Wekerle, R.-L., Müller, E., Kern, P., Meyermann, R. & Goebel, W. (1989). Synthesis, inactivation, and localization of extracellular and intracellular *Escherichia coli* hemolysins. *Journal of Bacteriology*, **171**, 2783–8.

Oropeza-Wekerle, R.-L., Muller, S., Briand, J. P., Benz, R., Schmid, A. & Goebel, W. (1992). Haemolysin-derived synthetic peptides with pore-forming and haemolytic activity. *Molecular Microbiology*, **6**, 115–21.

Oropeza-Wekerle, R.-L., Speth, W., Imhof, B., Gentschev, I. & Goebel, W. (1990). Translocation and compartmentalization of *Escherichia coli* hemolysin (HlyA). *Journal of Bacteriology*, **172**, 3711–17.

Oscarsson, J., Mizunoe, Y., Uhlin, B. E. & Haydon, D. J. (1996). Induction of haemolytic activity in *Escherichia coli* by the *slyA* gene product. *Molecular Microbiology*, **20**, 191–9.

Ostolaza, H., Bartolome, B., Ortiz de Zarate, I., De la Cruz, F. & Goñi, F. M. (1993). Release of lipid vesicle contents by the bacterial protein toxin α-haemolysin. *Biochimica et Biophysica Acta*, **1147**, 81–8.

Ostolaza, H., Bartolome, B., Serra, J. L., De la Cruz, F. & Goñi, F. M. (1991). α-Haemolysin from *E. coli*. Purification and self-aggregation properties. *FEBS Letters*, **280**, 195–8.

Pellett, S., Boehm, D. F., Snyder, I. S., Rowe, G. & Welch, R. A. (1990). Characterization of monoclonal antibodies against the *Escherichia coli* hemolysin. *Infection and Immunity*, **58**, 822–7.

Prada, J., Baljer, G., de Rycke, J., Steinrueck, H., Zimmermann, S., Stephan, R. & Beutin, L. (1991). Characteristics of alpha-hemolytic strains of *Escherichia coli* isolated from dogs with gastroenteritis. *Veterinary Microbiology*, **29**, 59–73.

Prada, J. & Beutin, L. (1991). Detection of *Escherichia coli* α-haemolysin genes and their expression in a human faecal strain of *Enterobacter cloacae*. *FEMS Microbiology Letters*, **79**, 111–14.

Rennie, R. P. & Arbuthnott, J. P. (1974). Partial characterisation of *Escherichia coli* haemolysin. *Journal of Medical Microbiology*, **7**, 179–88.

Rennie, R. P., Freer, J. H. & Arbuthnott, J. P. (1974). The kinetics of erythrocyte lysis by *Escherichia coli* haemolysin. *The Journal of Medical Microbiology*, **7**, 189–95.

Rommens, J. M., Ianuzzi, M. C., Kerem, B.-S., Drumm, M. L., Melmer, G., Dean, M., Rozmahel, R., Cole, J. L., Kennedy, D., Hidaka, N., Zsiga, M., Buchwald, M., Riordan, J. R., Tsui, L.-C. & Collins, F. S. (1989). Identification of the cystic fibrosis gene: chromosome walking and jumping. *Science*, **245**, 1059–65.

Ropele, M. & Menestrina, G. (1989). Electrical properties and molecular architecture of the channel formed by *Escherichia coli* hemolysin in planar lipid membranes. *Biochimica et Biophysica Acta*, **985**, 9–18.

Rowe, G. E., Pellett, S. & Welch, R. A. (1994). Analysis of toxinogenic functions associated with the RTX repeat region and monoclonal antibody D12 epitope of *Escherichia coli* hemolysin. *Infection and Immunity*, **62**, 579–88.

Royer-Pokora, B. & Goebel, W. (1976). Plasmids controlling synthesis of hemolysin in *Escherichia coli*. II. Polynucleotide sequence relationship among hemolytic plasmids. *Molecular and General Genetics*, **144**, 177–83.

Scheffer, J., König, W., Hacker, J. & Goebel, W. (1985). Bacterial adherence and hemolysin production from *Escherichia coli* induces histamine and leukotriene release from various cells. *Infection and Immunity*, **50**, 271–8.

Scheffer, J., Vosbeck, K. & König, W. (1986). Induction of inflammatory mediators from human polymorphonuclear granulocytes and rat mast cells by haemolysin-positive and -negative *E. coli* strains with different adhesins. *Immunology*, **59**, 541–8.

Scheu, A. K., Economou, A., Hong, G. F., Ghelani, S., Johnston, A. W. B. & Downie, J. A. (1992). Secretion of the *Rhizobium leguminosarum* nodulation protein NodO by haemolysin-type systems. *Molecular Microbiology*, **6**, 231–8.

Schiebel, E., Driessen, A. J. M., Hartl, F.-U. & Wickner, W. (1991). $\Delta\mu_H{}^+$ and ATP function at different steps of the catalytic cycle of preprotein translocase. *Cell*, **64**, 927–39.

Schmidt, H., Beutin, L. & Karch, H. (1995). Molecular analysis of the plasmid-encoded hemolysin of *Escherichia coli* O157:H7 strain EDL 933. *Infection and Immunity*, **63**, 1055–61.

Scheu, A. K., Economou, A., Hong, G. F., Ghelani, S., Johnston, A. W. B. & Downie, J. A. (1992). Secretion of the *Rhizobium leguminosarum* nodulation protein NodO by haemolysin-type systems. *Molecular Microbiology*, **6**, 231–8.

Schiebel, E., Driessen, A. J. M., Hartl, F.-U. & Wickner, W. (1991). $\Delta\mu_H^+$ and ATP function at different steps of the catalytic cycle of preprotein translocase. *Cell*, **64**, 927–39.

Schmidt, H., Beutin, L. & Karch, H. (1995). Molecular analysis of the plasmid-encoded hemolysin of *Escherichia coli* O157:H7 strain EDL 933. *Infection and Immunity*, **63**, 1055–61.

Schmidt, H., Karch, H. & Beutin, L. (1994). The large-sized plasmids of enterohemorrhagic *Escherichia coli* O157 strains encode hemolysins which are presumably members of the *E. coli* α-hemolysin family. *FEMS Microbiology Letters*, **117**, 189–96.

Schmidt, H., Kernbach, C. & Karch, H. (1996). Analysis of the EHEC *hly* operon and its location in the physical map of the large plasmid of enterohaemorrhagic *Escherichia coli* O157:H7. *Microbiology*, **142**, 907–14.

Schülein, R., Gentschev, I., Mollenkopf, H.-J. & Goebel, W. (1992). A topological model for the haemolysin translocator protein HlyD. *Molecular and General Genetics*, **234**, 155–63.

Schülein, R., Gentschev, I., Schlör, S., Gross, R. & Goebel, W. (1994). Identification and characterization of two functional domains of the hemolysin translocator protein HlyD. *Molecular and General Genetics*, **245**, 203–11.

Seeger, W., Obernitz, R., Thomas, M., Walmrath, D., Suttorp, N., Holland, I. B., Grimminger, F., Eberspächer, B., Hugo, F. & Bhakdi, S. (1991). Lung vascular injury after administration of viable hemolysin-forming *Escherichia coli* in isolated rabbit lungs. *American Review of Respiratory Diseases*, **143**, 797–805.

Seeger, W., Walter, H., Suttorp, N., Muhly, M. & Bhakdi, S. (1989). Thromboxane-mediated hypertension and vascular leakage evoked by low doses of *Escherichia coli* hemolysin in rabbit lungs. *Journal of Clinical Investigation*, **84**, 220–7.

Short, E. C. & Kurtz, H. J. (1971). Properties of the hemolytic activities of *Escherichia coli*. *Infection and Immunity*, **3**, 678–87.

Siegfried, L., Puzova, H., Kmetova, M. & Kerestesova, A. (1992). Killing of α-haemolytic and non-haemolytic *Escherichia coli* strains in human serum and polymorphonuclear leucocytes. *Journal of Medical Microbiology*, **37**, 3–7.

Siitonen, A. (1992). *Escherichia coli* in fecal flora of healthy adults: serotypes, P and type 1C fimbriae, non-P mannose-resistant adhesins, and hemolytic activity. *Journal of Infectious Diseases*, **166**, 1058–65.

Smith, H. W. (1963). The haemolysins of *Escherichia coli*. *Journal of Pathology and Bacteriology*, **85**, 197–211.

Smith, H. W. & Halls, S. (1967). The transmissible nature of the genetic factor in *Escherichia coli* that controls haemolysin production. *Journal of General Microbiology*, **47**, 153–61.

Smith, H. W. & Huggins, M. B. (1985). The toxic role of alpha-haemolysin in the pathogenesis of experimental *Escherichia coli* infection in mice. *Journal of General Microbiology*, **131**, 395–403.

Smith, H. W. & Linggood, M. A. (1971). Observations on the pathogenic properties of the K88, Hly and Ent plasmids of *Escherichia coli* with

Stanley, P., Packman, L. C., Koronakis, V. & Hughes, C. (1994). Fatty acylation of two internal lysine residues required for the toxic activity of *Escherichia coli* hemolysin. *Science*, **266**, 1992–6.

Stapleton, A., Moseley, S. & Stamm, W. E. (1991). Urovirulence determinants in *Escherichia coli* isolates causing first-episode and recurrent cystitis in women. *Journal of Infectious Diseases*, **163**, 773–9.

Stark, J. M. & Shuster, C. W. (1982). Analysis of hemolytic determinants of plasmid pHly185 by Tn5 mutagenesis. *Journal of Bacteriology*, **152**, 963–7.

Stark, J. M. & Shuster, C. W. (1983). The structure of cloned hemolysin DNA from plasmid pHly185. *Plasmid*, **10**, 45–54.

Steadman, R., Topley, N., Knowlden, J., Spur, B. & Williams, J. (1990). Leukotriene B_4 generation by human monocytes and neutrophils stimulated by uropathogenic strains of *Escherichia coli*. *Biochimica et Biophysica Acta*, **1052**, 264–72.

Strathdee, C. A. & Lo, R. Y. C. (1987). Extensive homology between the leukotoxin of *Pasteurella haemolytica* A1 and the alpha-hemolysin of *Escherichia coli*. *Infection and Immunity*, **55**, 3233–6.

Strathdee, C. A. & Lo, R. Y. C. (1989). Cloning, nucleotide sequence, and characterization of genes encoding the secretion function of the *Pasteurella haemolytica* leukotoxin determinant. *Journal of Bacteriology*, **171**, 916–28.

Stroeher, U. H., Bode, L., Beutin, L. & Manning, P. A. (1993). Characterization and sequence of a 33-kDa enterohemolysin (Ehly1)-associated protein in *Escherichia coli*. *Gene*, **132**, 89–94.

Suttorp, N., Flöer, B., Schnittler, H., Seeger, W. & Bhakdi, S. (1990). Effects of *Escherichia coli* hemolysin on endothelial cell function. *Infection and Immunity*, **58**, 3796–801.

Thomas, W. D., Wagner, S. P. & Welch, R. A. (1992). A heterologous membrane protein domain fused to the C-terminal ATP-binding domain of HlyB can export *Escherichia coli* hemolysin. *Journal of Bacteriology*, **174**, 6771–9.

Thompson, S. A. & Sparling, P. F. (1993). The RTX cytotoxin-related FrpA protein of *Neisseria meningitidis* is secreted extracellularly by *Meningococci* and by HlyBD+ *Escherichia coli*. *Infection and Immunity*, **61**, 2906–11.

Thompson, S. A., Wang, L. L. & Sparling, P. F. (1993a). Cloning and nucleotide sequence of *frpC*, a second gene from *Neisseria meningitidis* encoding a protein similar to RTX cytotoxins. *Molecular Microbiology*, **9**, 85–96.

Thompson, S. A., Wang, L. L., West, A. & Sparling, P. F. (1993b). *Neisseria meningitidis* produces iron-regulated proteins related to the RTX family of exoproteins. *Journal of Bacteriology*, **175**, 811–18.

Tschäpe, H. & Rische, H. (1974). Die Virulenzplasmide der Enterobacteriaceae. *Zeitschrift für Allgemeine Mikrobiologie*, **14**, 337–50.

Tullus, K., Jacobson, S. H., Katouli, M. & Brauner, A. (1991). Relative importance of eight virulence characteristics of pyelonephritogenic *Escherichia coli* strains assessed by multivariate statistical analysis. *Journal of Urology*, **146**, 1153–5.

Van den Bosch, J. F., Emödy, L. & Ketyi, I. (1982a). Virulence of haemolytic strains of *Escherichia coli* in various animal models. *FEMS Microbiology Letters*, **13**, 427–30.

Van den Bosch, J. F., Postma, P., de Graaff, J. & MacLaren, D. M. (1981). Haemolysis by urinary *Escherichia coli* and virulence in mice. *Journal of Medical Microbiology*, **14**, 321–31.

Van den Bosch, J. F., Postma, P., Koopman, P. A. R., de Graaff, J., MacLaren, D. M., van Brenk, D. G. & Guinee, P. A. M. (1982b). Virulence of urinary and faecal *Escherichia coli* in relation to serotype, haemolysis and haemagglutination. *Journal of Hygiene, Cambridge*, **88**, 567–77.

Vogel, M., Hess, J., Then, I., Juarez, A. & Goebel, W.(1988). Characterization of a sequence (*hlyR*) which enhances synthesis and secretion of hemolysin in *Escherichia coli*. *Molecular and General Genetics*, **212**, 76–84.

Waalwijk, C., de Graaff, J. & MacLaren, D. M. (1984). Physical mapping of hemolysin plasmid pCW2, which codes for virulence of a nephropathogenic *Escherichia coli* strain. *Journal of Bacteriology*, **159**, 424–6.

Waalwijk, C., MacLaren, D. M. & de Graaff, J. (1983). *In vivo* function of hemolysin in the nephropathogenicity of *Escherichia coli*. *Infection and Immunity*, **42**, 245–9.

Waalwijk, C., Van den Bosch, J. F., MacLaren, D. M. & de Graaff, J. (1982). Hemolysin plasmid coding for the virulence of a nephropathogenic *Escherichia coli* strain. *Infection and Immunity*, **35**, 32–7.

Wagner, W., Kuhn, M. & Goebel, W. (1988). Active and inactive forms of hemolysin (HlyA) from *Escherichia coli*. *Biological Chemistry Hoppe-Seyler*, **369**, 39–46.

Wagner, W., Vogel, M. & Goebel, W. (1983). Transport of hemolysin across the outer membrane of *Escherichia coli* requires two functions. *Journal of Bacteriology*, **154**, 200–10.

Walker, J. E., Saraste, M., Runswick, M. J. & Gray, N. J. (1982). Distantly related sequences in the α- and β-subunits of ATP synthase, myosin, kinases and other ATP-requiring enzymes and a common nucleotide binding fold. *EMBO Journal*, **1**, 945–51.

Walton, J. R. & Smith, D. H. (1969). New hemolysin (γ) produced by *Escherichia coli*. *Journal of Bacteriology*, **98**, 304–5.

Wandersman, C. & Delepelaire, P. (1990). TolC, an *Escherichia coli* outer membrane protein required for hemolysin secretion. *Proceedings of the National Academy of Sciences, USA*, **87**, 4776–80.

Wandersman, C. & Letoffe, S. (1993). Involvement of lipopolysaccharide in the secretion of *Escherichia coli* α-haemolysin and *Erwinia chrysanthemi* proteases. *Molecular Microbiology*, **7**, 141–50.

Wang, R., Seror, S. J., Blight, M., Pratt, J. M., Broome-Smith, J. K. & Holland, I. B. (1991). Analysis of the membrane organization of an *Escherichia coli* protein translocator, HlyB, a member of a large family of prokaryote and eukaryote surface transport proteins. *Journal of Molecular Biology*, **217**, 441–54.

Welch, R. A. (1987). Identification of two different hemolysin determinants in uropathogenic *Proteus* isolates. *Infection and Immunity*, **55**, 2183–90.

Welch, R. A. (1991). Pore-forming cytolysins of Gram-negative bacteria. *Molecular Microbiology*, **5**, 521–8.

Welch, R. A., Dellinger, E. P., Minshew, B. & Falkow, S. (1981). Haemolysin contributes to virulence of extra-intestinal *E. coli* infections. *Nature*, **294**, 665–7.

Welch, R. A. & Falkow, S. (1984). Characterization of *Escherichia coli* hemolysins conferring quantitative differences in virulence. *Infection and Immunity*, **43**, 156–60.

Welch, R. A., Hull R. & Falkow, S. (1983). Molecular cloning and physical characterization of a chromosomal hemolysin from *Escherichia coli*. *Infection and Immunity*, **42**, 178–86.

Welch, R. A. & Pellett, S. (1988). Transcriptional organization of the *Escherichia coli* hemolysin genes. *Journal of Bacteriology*, **170**, 1622–30.

Zabala, J. C., De la Cruz, F. & Ortiz, J. M. (1982). Several copies of the same insertion sequence are present in alpha-hemolytic plasmids belonging to four different incompatibility groups. *Journal of Bacteriology*, **151**, 472–6.

Zabala, J. C., Garcia-Lobo, J. M., Diaz-Aroca, E., De la Cruz, F. & Ortiz, J. M. (1984). *Escherichia coli* alpha-haemolysin synthesis and export genes are flanked by a direct repetition of IS91-like elements. *Molecular and General Genetics*, **197**, 90–7.

Zhang, F., Greig, D. I. & Ling, V. (1993a). Functional replacement of the hemolysin A transport signal by a different primary sequence. *Proceedings of the National Academy of Sciences, USA*, **90**, 4211–15.

Zhang, F., Sheps, J. A. & Ling, V. (1993b). Complementation of transport-deficient mutants of *Escherichia coli* α-hemolysin by second-site mutations in the transporter hemolysin B. *Journal of Biological Chemistry*, **268**, 19889–95.

12

Iron and the virulence of *Escherichia coli*

E. GRIFFITHS

The discovery that the genetic determinants for certain virulence charac-teristics, such as enterotoxin production and adhesiveness, can be carried by plasmids was a significant development in our understanding of *Escherichia coli* infections (Elwell & Shipley, 1980). However, the presence of a plasmid is not the only factor involved in virulence (Griffiths *et al.*, 1980). The pathogenicity of *E. coli*, as that of other pathogens, is now known to depend on a variety of bacterial properties, some chro-mosomally encoded and others plasmid mediated, rather than on any one trait. Thus, the ability of pathogenic *E. coli* to evade host defences, such as the bactericidal action of serum, the ability to adhere to specific tissues *in vivo*, as well as to invade certain host cells and to produce various toxins are all important factors that contribute to the capacity of this micro-organism to proliferate *in vivo* and to cause various diseases. These properties are not, however, sufficient in themselves for pathogenicity, and the ability of *E. coli* to multiply successfully in host tissues is also crucial (Griffiths, 1983). Factors that may be expected to affect bacterial multiplication *in vivo* include temperature, pH, oxygen tension and the availability of nutrients. One of the best understood aspects of the host environment and of its effect on bacterial growth concerns the availability of iron. It is evident that the restricted availability of iron *in vivo* not only presents microbial pathogens with the problem of acquiring sufficient iron for multiplication, but also constitutes a major environmental signal that regulates the expression of a number of virulence genes that are apparently unrelated to iron metabolism, including those that encode toxins (Griffiths, 1991).

Availability of iron

The ability of invading pathogens to multiply in host tissues has long been known to be markedly affected by the availability of iron. Animals injected with various forms of iron are far more susceptible to infection by a variety of bacteria, including *E. coli*, than are untreated controls (Bullen & Griffiths, 1987; Bullen *et al.*, 1991). Generally, iron affects the susceptibility of normal animals to infection by reducing the lethal dose of bacteria. For example, the lethal dose of *E. coli* O111 for normal guinea-pigs is about 10^8 cells whereas, for guinea-pigs injected with ferric ammonium citrate or haem compounds, this dose is reduced to about 10^3 cells, a 10^5-fold reduction (Bullen *et al.*, 1968). Only iron has been found to act in this way. Investigation of this phenomenon has led to an explanation of the changes in resistance that sometimes accompany clinical alterations in the iron status of the host. It has also greatly increased our understanding of the mechanisms involved in microbial pathogenicity (Bullen & Griffiths, 1987; Crosa, 1989; Weinberg, 1989; Martinez *et al.*, 1990; Williams & Griffiths, 1992; Wooldridge & Williams, 1993). Much of this new understanding of how pathogenic bacteria adapt to and grow in the iron-restricted extracellular environment of the host has come from studies of *E. coli*. For these purposes *E. coli* has provided an ideal experimental model; a great deal was already known about its biochemistry and genetics, and it is the cause of important infections in humans and animals. Studies of the growth of *E. coli in vitro* under conditions of iron restriction and *in vivo* during infection have established the principle that pathogenic bacteria are subject to considerable phenotypic changes in their metabolism and in the composition of their outer membranes. This information has served as a guide for the often more difficult investigation of other pathogens.

The importance of iron lies in its strictly limited availability in living tissues. Though iron is plentiful in the body fluids of humans and animals, the amount of free iron readily available to invading bacteria intracellularly is normally extremely small. Most of the iron in the body is found as ferritin, haemosiderin or haem, while extracellular iron in serum and other body fluids is fixed to high-affinity iron-binding glycoproteins, transferrin in blood and lymph and lactoferrin in external secretions and milk; a related protein called ovotransferrin is found in avian egg white (Bullen & Griffiths, 1987). These iron-binding proteins have molecular masses of about 80 kDa and each is capable of binding two ferric (Fe^{3+}) ions reversibly with the simultaneous incorporation of two bicarbonate ions. Since these proteins have association constants for iron of about 10^{36}, and are normally only partially saturated with iron, the amount of free iron in equilibrium with these iron-binding proteins at neutral pH is of the order of 10^{-18}M, which is far too low to support bacterial growth. The 'free iron' pool is kept so extremely small, because under physiological conditions ferric iron tends to oxidise, hydrolyse and polymerise, to form essentially insoluble ferric hydroxide and oxyhydroxide polymers (Griffiths, 1987a; Crichton & Ward, 1992); for this reason ferric iron must be maintained in a soluble form. Loosely bound iron is also toxic (Griffiths, 1987a). Moreover, lactoferrin binds iron under the more acidic conditions that often prevail at sites of inflammation. Iron binding by transferrin is reduced below pH 6, while lactoferrin binds iron until the pH falls below 4 (McClelland & van Furth, 1976; Ainscough *et al.*, 1980; Crichton & Ward, 1992). During infection the host further reduces the amount of iron bound to serum transferrin. This reduction is called the *hypoferraemia of infection*, and can be reproduced experimentally by the injection of small amounts of endotoxin (Kluger & Bullen, 1987; Konijn & Hershko, 1989).

Since all known bacterial pathogens require iron to multiply, it can be argued that they must be able to adapt to severely iron-restricted environments. In order to multiply successfully in normal body fluids, and to establish extracellular infections, bacteria possess mechanisms for assimilating protein-bound iron. Alternatively they can acquire it from other sources, such as free haem or haemoglobin. Little is known about the availability of iron within cells, but it seems likely that, in at least some cells, iron is more readily available (Lawlor *et al.*, 1987; Nassif *et al.*, 1987; Byrd & Horwitz, 1989). It is not known whether ferritin can act directly as an iron source for bacterial pathogens.

High-affinity iron-uptake systems

Under normal physiological conditions, bacteria can be expected to assimilate ferric iron (Fe^{3+}) bound by the high-affinity iron-binding glycoproteins of the host, by one of four mechanisms (Table 12.1). Little is known about mechanisms one and two, but much progress is being made at present in the understanding of mechanism three, which involves highly specific bacterial transferrin and lactoferrin receptors (Williams & Griffiths, 1992). *Escherichia coli* does not express such receptors, nor does it appear to have an extracellular iron reductase system (Table 12.1, mechanism two), but, when available, it can use ferrous iron (Fe^{2+}), for

Table 12.1. *Mechanisms used by pathogenic bacteria to assimilate iron bound to the host iron-binding proteins, transferrin and lactoferrin*

---

1.   Proteolytic cleavage of the iron-binding protein that results in disruption of the iron-binding properties of the molecule and the release of iron

2.   Reduction of the Fe^{3+}–protein complex to a Fe^{2+}–protein complex with the consequent release of ferrous iron

3.   Direct interaction between specific transferrin- or lactoferrin-specific receptors on the bacterial cell surface and the Fe^{3+}–protein complex

4.   Production of low-molecular-weight ferric-chelating compounds called siderophores that remove iron from the Fe^{3+}–protein complex and deliver it to the bacterial cell via specific ferric-siderophore receptors

---

example under anaerobic conditions (Hantke, 1987a). Many organisms, including *E. coli*, deal with the biological unavailability of iron in aerobic environments, in which iron exists in the ferric state (Fe^{3+}), by producing low-molecular-weight iron-chelating agents called siderophores (Raymond & Carrano, 1979; Neilands, 1981). Some of these siderophores can remove iron from iron-binding proteins and siderophore-mediated high-affinity iron uptake mechanisms are the best understood systems used by pathogenic bacteria to acquire iron from host iron-binding proteins and possibly other sources (Griffiths, 1987b; Crosa, 1989; Weinberg, 1989; Neilands, 1990; Wooldridge & Williams, 1993). Of these systems, perhaps the best characterised are those used by *E. coli*.

Siderophore-mediated iron uptake

Under conditions of iron restriction *in vitro*, *E. coli*, *Salmonella typhimurium* and *Klebsiella pneumoniae* produce the catecholate iron chelator enterobactin, which is also known as enterochelin (O'Brien & Gibson, 1970; Pollack & Neilands, 1970; Rogers, 1973; Rogers *et al.*, 1977; Rogers, 1983). This compound, which is the cyclic triester of 2,3-dihydroxy-*N*-benzoyl-L-serine (Figure 12.1), is synthesised only under conditions of iron restriction. It efficiently removes iron from the iron-binding proteins and delivers it into the bacterial cell (Rogers, 1973; Rogers *et al.*, 1977; Carrano & Raymond, 1979); the process is represented diagrammatically in Figure 12.2. Enterobactin acts as a hexadentate chelating agent that binds iron through its three catechol groups, which, when co-ordinating with ferric iron, act as a six-proton acid. At neutral pH the hexa co-ordinate complex carries three negative charges

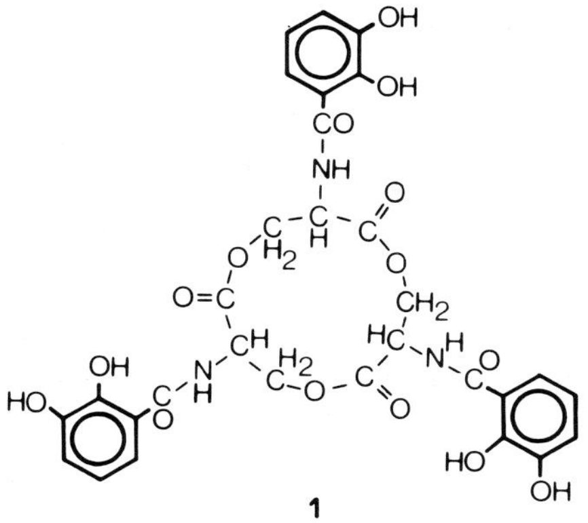

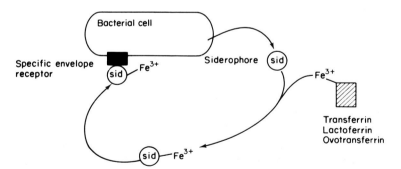

Fig. 12.1. Structure of enterobactin (1) and aerobactin (2)

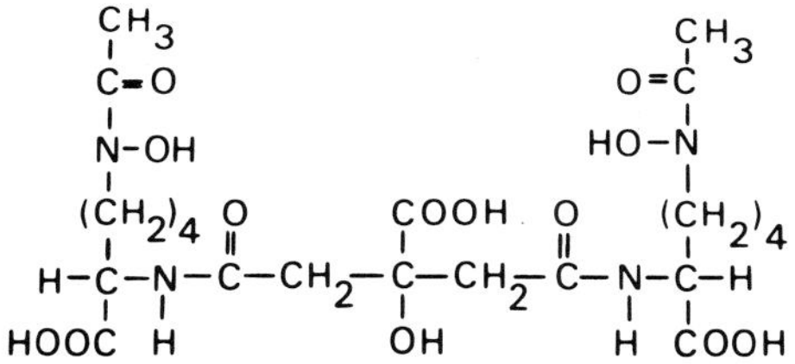

Fig. 12.2. Diagrammatic representaion of siderophore-mediated iron uptake in *Escherichia coli*.

$[\text{Fe(ent)}]^{3-}$ (Harris *et al.*, 1979a). The single most outstanding feature of siderophores is their extremely high affinity for ferric iron; the formation constant for ferric–enterobactin at neutral pH approaches 10^{52}. Until recently this was the highest known formation constant ever recorded for a ferric iron chelator (Harris *et al.*, 1979a,c), but a siderophore from a marine bacterium has recently been discovered which is said to have an affinity for iron close to that of enterobactin (Reid *et al.*, 1993). Organisms that use enterobactin-mediated iron uptake are, therefore, able to compete effectively for iron that is complexed to iron-binding proteins. The fact that an enterobactin-producing strain of *Salmonella* can obtain iron from transferrin when the protein is in a dialysis bag clearly shows that contact between the transferrin and the bacterial cell surface is not required for siderophore-mediated removal of iron (Tidmarsh & Rosenberg, 1981).

The synthesis of enterobactin in *E. coli* involves the products of seven genes, *entA* to *entG*, which are located in the enterobactin gene cluster at 13 minutes on the chromosome (Young *et al.*, 1971; Greenwood & Luke, 1976; Fleming *et al.*, 1985; Earhart, 1987; Liu *et al.*, 1989; Nahlik *et al.*, 1989; Ozenberg *et al.*, 1989). Synthesis begins with the conversion of chorismic acid, a central precursor of the aromatic amino-acid biosynthetic pathway (Figure 12.3), via isochorismate, into 2,3-dihydroxybenzoic acid (Liu *et al.*, 1990; Rusnak *et al.*, 1990). Adenosine triphosphate (ATP) is required for the assembly of 2,3-dihydroxybenzoic acid and L-serine into enterobactin, a process carried out by the products of genes *entD*, *entE*, *entF* and *entG*, which are believed to operate as a multienzyme complex (Armstrong *et al.*, 1989; Nahlik *et al.*, 1989; Rusnak *et al.*, 1989).

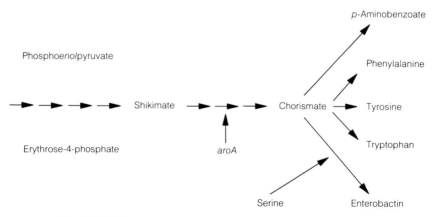

Fig. 12.3. Biosynthesis of enterobactin via the aromatic amino-acid biosynthetic pathway. Disruption of the *aroA* gene in the common pathway results in mutants which require aromatic amino-acids and *p*-aminobenzoate for growth and which are unable to produce enterobactin.

A given molecule of enterobactin is used only once to transport iron into the cell. The cyclic triester linkages of ferric–enterobactin are cleaved by a specific esterase upon entry into the cell, apparently in order to release the iron, ultimately to produce 2,3-dihydroxybenzoylserine, which is then discarded (Rosenberg & Young, 1974; Greenwood & Luke, 1978). It has been suggested that hydrolysis of the ester bonds is necessary because ferric–enterobactin has too low a reduction potential to be physiologically reducible. Consequently it must be hydrolysed to permit reduction with the resulting release of iron. Cleavage of the ester bonds certainly increases the redox potential of the enterobactin–ferric iron complex (Cooper *et al.*, 1978; Harris *et al.*, 1979; Raymond & Carrano, 1979). However, the fact that a carbocyclic analogue of enterobactin, which lacks the ester bonds, effectively supplies iron to an enterobactin-deficient strain of *E. coli* has raised questions about the exact role of the esterase, and these questions have yet to be satisfactorily answered (Hollifield & Neilands, 1978). The esterase of *E. coli* has recently been over-expressed and purified (Brickman & McIntosh, 1992), and there is evidence to support the notion that reduction of iron in enterobactin may depend upon, and take place subsequent to, esterase activity; the hydro-lysis of the cyclic platform of enterobactin appears to be independent of any reduction of the iron. A ferrous–enterobactin complex has been identified (Hider *et al.*, 1979), in which the metal is held much less tightly than in ferric–enterobactin. This complex could readily donate the iron to other co-ordinating ligands within the cell. Whatever the exact role of the esterase, it is clear that *fes* mutants of *E. coli*, which lack esterase activity, are unable to use the ferric–enterobactin complex as an iron source (Langman *et al.*, 1972; Rosenberg & Young, 1974). Such strains accumulate ferric–enterobactin with the result that a sedimented pellet of these cells is distinctly pink.

Enterobactin production by *E. coli in vitro* has usually been studied with *E. coli* K12, but it is known that pathogenic strains also produce this chelator under conditions of iron restriction. Indeed, virtually all wild-type and clinical isolates of *E. coli* produce enterobactin (Griffiths, 1987b). Furthermore, enterobactin is known to be produced *in vivo* during infection (Griffiths & Humphreys, 1980), since enterobactin and its degradation products have been detected in the peritoneal washings from guinea-pigs infected with *E. coli* O111. This supports the notion that the presence of iron-binding proteins in body fluids creates an iron-restricted environment *in vivo* and affects bacterial metabolism accord-ingly.

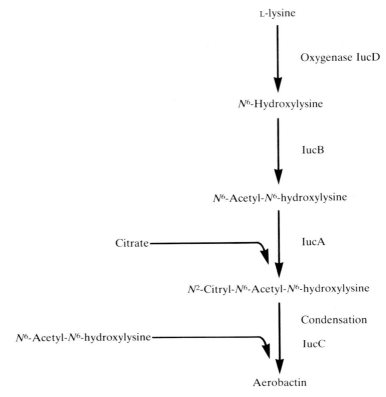

L-lysine

Oxygenase IucD

N^6-Hydroxylysine

IucB

N^6-Acetyl-N^6-hydroxylysine

Citrate ──────────   IucA

N^2-Citryl-N^6-Acetyl-N^6-hydroxylysine

Condensation

N^6-Acetyl-N^6-hydroxylysine ──────────   IucC

Aerobactin

Fig. 12.4. The biosynthetic pathway for aerobactin. The enzymes responsible are shown to the right of the arrows.

Although enterobactin appears to be the main endogenous siderophore produced by *E. coli* during conditions of iron restriction, several clinical isolates possess another high-affinity iron-uptake system mediated by the hydroxamate siderophore, aerobactin. In particular, many of the strains that cause septicaemia or other extra-intestinal infections produce aerobactin. The genes for the synthesis of aerobactin can be located on the chromosome or on a plasmid (Williams, 1979; Valvano *et al.*, 1986; Lafont *et al.*, 1987; Jacobson *et al.*, 1988; de Lorenzo & Martinez, 1988; Gadó *et al.*, 1989; Opal *et al.*, 1990). For example, *E. coli* strains that cause septicaemia in humans and animals carry aerobactin synthetic genes on the colicin V [pColV] and other plasmids (Williams, 1979; Williams & Warner, 1980; Crosa, 1987; Griffiths, 1987b; Gonzalo *et al.*, 1988; Crosa, 1989; Wooldridge &

Williams, 1993). Enteroinvasive strains of *E. coli*, which cause *Shigella*-like disease, and *Shigella flexneri* produce aerobactin (Payne *et al.*, 1983; Griffiths *et al.*, 1985b) but have chromosomally located aerobactin genes (Marolda *et al.*, 1987). The widespread distribution of the genes for the aerobactin-mediated iron-uptake system suggests that the aerobactin operon may be genetically mobile, and there is some evidence to support this view (de Lorenzo *et al.*, 1988a). The aerobactin operon in ColV-K30 is flanked by inverted IS1 (i.e. insertion sequence 1) elements (Lawlor & Payne, 1984; McDougall & Neilands, 1984; Perez-Casal & Crosa, 1984) and two distinct replication regions, REPI and REPII (Perez-Casal & Crosa, 1984). For a number of reasons (Waters & Crosa, 1986; Crosa, 1987), however, it seems doubtful whether the fragment between the two IS1 elements in pColV-K30, which contains the aerobactin genes, constitutes a true transposon. The chromosomal aerobactin operon of *E. coli* K1 contains neither IS1 sequences nor REPII-related sequences, but sequences upstream of the aerobactin genes show some homology with a subset of the REPI region (Valvano & Crosa, 1984; Crosa, 1987). Roberts *et al.* (1986) suggested that in some instances the sequences that surround the aerobactin genes may represent the remnants of an 'extinct transposon', and Waters & Crosa (1986) proposed that the region bounded by the IS1 elements is only part of a larger 'virulence factor replication unit', including the aerobactin genes and the REPI sequences. Whatever the true nature of the transposition events, it seems likely that the flanking IS1 sequences and the upstream REPI element have been instrumental in the past in spreading the aerobactin genes amongst different organisms.

Aerobactin is a member of the hydroxamic acid–citrate family of siderophores and was originally isolated from *Aerobacter aerogenes* (Gibson & Magrath, 1969). It is a conjugate of 6-(N-acetyl-N-hydroxyamino)-2-aminohexanoic acid and citric acid (Figur 12.1) and forms an octahedral ferric complex with the two bidentate hydroxamate groups, the central carboxylate and probably the citrate hydroxyl group (Harris *et al.*, 1979b). The biosynthesis of aerobactin involves a series of steps that are illustrated in Figure 12.4 (Neilands, 1991).

Although enterobactin and aerobactin are the only known siderophores produced by *E. coli* growing under conditions of iron restriction, the organism has a remarkable ability for obtaining iron by means of a variety of exogenous chelators produced by other micro-organisms (Leong & Neilands, 1976; Raymond & Carrano, 1979; Neilands, 1981; Hantke, 1983). Thus, *E. coli* can use the fungal hydroxamate chelators ferrichrome, coprogen and rhodotorulic acid (Leong & Neilands, 1976; Hantke, 1983). Unlike enterobactin, ferrichrome is not destroyed when transporting iron into *E. coli*, but it is acetylated at one of its hydroxy-lamino oxygens after the reductive separation of Fe^{3+} (Hartman & Braun, 1980). This seems to be an essential step in the ferrichrome-mediated iron-transport system. Recent studies indicate that some *E. coli* strains can also utilise ferrioxamine B as a source of iron (Nelson *et al.*, 1992). The latter is a hydroxamate-type siderophore made by *Streptomyces*, but a previous report suggested that *E. coli* was unable to use it as an iron source (Rabsch & Reissbrodt, 1988). Further work is necessary to establish whether this discrepancy is due to strain differences or to the concentration of chelator used in the two investigations. It is not known whether these exogenous siderophores can play any part in supplying iron to pathogenic *E. coli* during infection *in vivo*. Similarly, it is not known whether iron chelated to citrate can serve as a source of iron for *E. coli in vivo*. *E. coli* possesses a citrate-mediated iron-transport system that is induced when *E. coli* is grown in an iron-limited medium that contains citrate (Woodrow *et al.*, 1978; Hussain *et al.*, 1981; Zimmermann *et al.*, 1984). Most strains of *E. coli* seem not to utilise citrate as a carbon source, but it has been reported that strains of *E. coli* that carry H1 plasmids use citrate as a sole energy source (Smith *et al.*, 1978). By acting like a siderophore, dihydroxybenzoyl-serine, a breakdown product of enterobactin, can also stimulate the growth of *E. coli* under iron-limiting conditions (Hantke, 1990).

Ferric-siderophore receptors

The process of adapting for growth in an iron-restricted environment involves not only the expression of enzymes for siderophore synthesis, but also the production of membrane protein receptors and enzymes that are involved in the uptake and release of iron from the ferric-siderophore (Neilands, 1982; Griffiths, 1987b). The need for specific outer-membrane receptors is due in part to the fact that the molecular weights of the siderophores exceed the diffusion limit, about 600, of the small, water-filled pores of the outer membrane (Nikaido, 1979; Braun *et al.*, 1991). However, the molecular mass of the iron-dicitrate complex is probably no greater than 443 and the fact that there is also a specific receptor for this iron complex suggests that the iron requirements of the cell can be satisfied only by initial adsorption of the ferric-siderophore to surface receptors, where iron can be accumulated relative to the

Table 12.2. *Iron-regulated siderophore receptor proteins of the outer membrane of* Escherichia coli

Receptor	Apparent molecular weight (kDa)	Phage/colicin binding	Iron-uptake function
Cir	74	Colicin 1	Catecholate-mediated
FecA	80.5	–	Fe^{3+}–citrate
FepA	81	Colicin B	Fe^{3+}–enterobactin
FhuA	78	Phages T1, T5 Ø80, Colicin M	Ferrichrome
FhuE	76	–	Fe^{3+}–coprogen
Fiu	83	–	Catecholate-mediated
FoxB	66+26	–	Ferrioxamine B
IutA	74	Cloacin DF13	Fe^+–aerobactin
76 kDa	76	Cloacin DF13	Fe^{3+}–aerobactin in EIEC[a] and *Shigella flexneri*

[a] Enteroinvasive *E. coli*.

concentration in the growth medium. The strict requirement for a receptor for siderophore-mediated iron uptake is shown by the absence of transport activity by strains that lack such proteins, or which have receptors altered by insertion mutagenesis (Grewal *et al.*, 1982; Carmel *et al.*, 1990). Most of the siderophore receptors also act as receptors for bacteriophages and/or colicins (Table 12.2).

Several new outer membrane proteins are produced by *E. coli* during iron-restricted growth and some of these have been identified as ferric-siderophore receptors (Table 12.2). An 81-kDa protein, FepA, is the receptor for ferric–enterobactin and is the product of the *fep* gene that maps in the *ent fep fes* gene cluster at approximately 13 minutes on the *E. coli* chromosome (Neilands, 1982). This gene cluster controls the biosynthesis, uptake and hydrolysis of enterobactin, and expression of the various genes is tightly controlled by iron levels in the cell. A 78-kDa protein, FhuA, encoded by the *fhuA* gene, located at 3.5 minutes on the *E. coli* chromosome, functions as the receptor for ferrichrome (Neilands, 1982; Coulton *et al.*, 1983; Braun *et al.*, 1991). Ferric coprogen and ferric rhodotorulic acid also have their own receptor, FhuE (Hantke, 1983; Braun *et al.*, 1991), as does ferrioxamine B, for which the receptor is FoxB (Nelson *et al.*, 1992). Expression of FoxB appears to be regulated not only by iron, but also by the presence of ferriox-amine B. The ColV plasmid-encoded 74-kDa protein, IutA, functions as the aerobactin receptor in *E. coli* that harbour this plasmid (Bindereif *et al.*, 1982; Grewal *et al.*, 1982). In enteroinvasive strains of *E. coli*, however, the aerobactin receptor is a 76-kDa protein (Griffiths *et al.*, 1985b). Two other iron-regulated *E. coli* proteins, Fiu and the 74-kDa Cir protein, have for some time been recognised, but their functions unknown. It has recently been shown that a novel group of catechol-substituted β-lactam antibiotics, with a 100-fold higher antibiotic activity against *E. coli* and other Gram-negative bacteria than classical cephalosporins, are taken up into bacterial cells via the Cir and Fiu receptors. This suggests that both receptors play a part in the uptake of natural catecholate-type siderophores (Watanabe *et al.*, 1987; Curtis *et al.*, 1988). Indeed, Hantke (1990) showed that 2,3-dihydroxybenzoylserine, which can act as a weak siderophore for *E. coli*, is taken up by the bacterial cell via Fiu and Cir, and less effectively by FepA. Strains of *E. coli* that can use iron-dicitrate as an iron source, produce another outer-membrane protein, FecA, which is part of the citrate-mediated iron-transport system (Wagegg & Braun, 1981) and has an apparent molecular weight of about 81 kDa. It is expressed only by bacteria growing in iron-restricted media that contain citrate (Frost & Rosenberg, 1973; Hancock *et al.*, 1976; Zimmermann *et al.*, 1984; Pressler *et al.*, 1988). Although the siderophore-specific outer-membrane receptors are essential for siderophore-mediated iron uptake, other less specific inner or cytoplasmic membrane components are also necessary for iron transport. Hydroxamate siderophores use common inner-membrane transport functions specified by the *fhuC*, *fhuD* and *fhuB* genes (Hantke & Zimmermann, 1981; Coulton *et al.*, 1987; Köster & Braun, 1989, 1990a,b; Köster & Böhm, 1992). Similarly, enterobactin-mediated iron uptake across the periplasm and cyto-plasmic membrane requires the products of at least five additional genes, *fepB*, *fepC*, *fepD*, *fepE* and *fepG* (Ozenberger *et al.*, 1987; Elkins & Earhart, 1989; Chenault & Earhart, 1991; Shea & McIntosh, 1991). FepB is believed to be a periplasmic binding protein for ferric entero-bactin (Elkins & Earhart, 1989) but the other proteins are less well characterised. By analogy with other systems, it is thought likely that they are highly hydrophobic membrane proteins present in very small amounts.

Siderophore-mediated iron-uptake mechanisms differ from porin-mediated diffusion of solutes across the outer membrane, because of their high substrate specificities and their energy requirement. Processes of energy-coupled transport across the outer membrane depend crucially on a product of the *tonB* gene, the TonB protein (Postle, 1990a; Braun *et al.*, 1991; Köster, 1991). The TonB protein serves as an energy transducer that couples cytoplasmic membrane energy to high-affinity active transport of ferric-siderophores and vitamin B_{12} across the outer membrane. It is anchored in the cytoplasmic membrane, but is believed to span the periplasmic space (Postle & Skare, 1988; Hannavy *et al.*, 1990) and to interact directly with the outer-membrane receptor proteins (Brewer *et al.*, 1990; Postle, 1990a, Skare *et al.*, 1993). Common structures that may be recognised by TonB have been identified in these outer membrane receptor proteins; they are located close to the amino-termini of these proteins and are called the 'TonB box' (Postle, 1990a; Braun *et al.*, 1991). These pentapeptide sequences do not, however, appear to be sufficient to mediate fully the specific interactions with TonB (Brewer *et al.*, 1990; Hannavy *et al.*, 1990). When bound to the receptor protein, TonB is believed to induce conformational changes in the receptor that allow the ferric-siderophore to enter the periplasmic space. Recent work on FepA has led to the interesting suggestion that all of these outer-membrane receptors may be 'gated porins' (Rutz *et al.*, 1992). FepA is a 723-amino-acid protein that can be considered to have three distinct domains: (i) a region of the molecule exposed on its surface that binds ferric enterobactin, (ii) a β-barrel domain located in the membrane bilayer that may act as a non-specific membrane channel and (iii) a 'TonB box', which can interact with TonB and is the part of the molecule located within the periplasmic space. When the cell-surface ligand-binding peptides are deleted, mutant FepA proteins are generated that are incapable of high-affinity enterobactin uptake. Instead, surprisingly they form non-specific passive channels in the outer membrane that act independently of TonB and allow enterobactin to pass through into the periplasmic space (Rutz *et al.*, 1992). It is proposed that in normal FepA protein the channel would be closed at the cell surface by loops of hydrophilic peptides that selectively bind enterobactin. Once activated by TonB, the 'gate' would be opened by conformational alterations in FepA that allow ferric enterobactin to pass into the channel and through into the periplasm. Such a mechanism preserves the permeability of the outer membrane, but operates in response to the interaction of ferric-siderophore with FepA and of FepA with the TonB protein.

The extensive sequence homology among the TonB-dependent

receptors of *E. coli* suggests that the other receptors may transport their siderophores by this 'gated' porin mechanism, with the TonB protein acting as a kind of 'molecular gatekeeper'. Once in the periplasm the various siderophores would bind to the other components of the transport system located in the periplasm and periplasmic membrane, and the ferric-siderophore, or iron, would then be translocated across the cytoplasmic membrane into the cell by another energy-dependent process.

Much of the work on high-affinity iron transport in *E. coli* has been carried out with avirulent laboratory strains, such as *E. coli* K-12. From the point of view of infection, however, it is important to understand what happens in pathogenic strains and, since surface components play such an important part in host–bacteria interactions, the iron-regulated proteins of pathogenic *E. coli* are clearly of particular interest. Pathogenic strains of *E. coli* produce the same new proteins as *E. coli* K-12, when growing in the presence of iron-binding proteins *in vitro* (Griffiths *et al.*, 1983, 1985a,b), but the relative abundance of these proteins expressed in different pathogenic strains of *E. coli* varies considerably under the same iron-restricted growth conditions. As we have seen, some *E. coli* strains produce iron-regulated receptor proteins in their outer membrane, which are not seen in *E. coli* K-12. These include IutA, the ColV plasmid-encoded 74-kDa aerobactin receptor of pathogenic *E. coli* that cause extra-intestinal infections, and the 76-kDa aerobactin receptor protein of enteroinvasive strains of *E. coli* (EIEC) (Griffiths *et al.*, 1985b). Interestingly, upon sodium dodecyl sulphate polyacrylamide gel electrophoresis (SDS-PAGE), EIEC exhibit an iron-regulated outer-membrane profile that is identical to that seen with laboratory-constructed *E. coli* K-12–*Shigella flexneri* hybrids under the same growth conditions (Griffiths *et al.*, 1985b). During iron restriction, the *S. flexneri* parent strain used in these constructions also produces a 76-kDa protein that is believed to be its aerobactin receptor. Analysis of more than 70 strains of *E. coli* from various human and animal infections has shown considerable differences between the SDS-PAGE patterns of iron-regulated outer-membrane proteins from the various strains (Chart *et al.*, 1988). Three distinct and characteristic outer-membrane protein profiles could be identified (Fig. 12.5), but not all isolates produced patterns that matched exactly one of these. Only isolates from human extra-intestinal infections gave rise to the patterns seen in lanes 2 and 3 (Figure 12.5).

Strains of *E. coli* isolated from cases of human enteric diseases, or

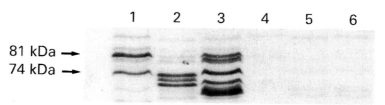

Fig. 12.5. Representatives of three characteristic SDS-PAGE profiles distinguished amongst the iron-regulated outer-membrane proteins of *Escherichia coli* isolates (lanes 1–3); only the relevant portion of the gel is shown. The SDS-PAGE profiles of the outer-membrane proteins from the same organisms grown under iron-replete conditions are shown in lanes 4–6. Lanes 1 and 4, *E. coli* 025:H⁻ (enterotoxigenic strain); lanes 2 and 5, *E. coli* O1:K1 (from human urinary tract infection): lanes 3 and 6, *E. coli* 018:K1 (from meningitis and septicaemia in human newborn). Each lane carried 25 μg protein (from Chart *et al.*, 1988; reproduced by permission of the Society for General Microbiology).

from animal septicaemia or enteric diseases, produced the pattern seen in Figure 12.5 lane 1. Human EIEC exhibited a profile similar to that of the other human enteric strains, except that they produced the additional 76-kDa protein, the aerobactin receptor. These differences between strains are missed when the SDS-PAGE profiles of the outer-membrane proteins of the iron-replete organisms are examined (Figure 12.5, lanes 4–6). Caution should, however, be exercised when interpreting data relating to the nature of the iron-regulated proteins produced by various strains, if these are obtained with chemical iron-chelating agents. This is particularly the case when results obtained from studies on bacterial iron uptake *in vitro* are extrapolated to the events that may be taking place in the host during infection. In the laboratory, iron-regulated proteins are induced by growing *E. coli* in the presence of iron-binding proteins or, more frequently, by adding to the growth medium chelators such as αα'-dipyridyl, ethylenediamine-di-(*o*-hydroxyphenylacetic acid) (EDDA), or desferrioxamine mesylate (Desferal, CIBA-GEIGY). Although chemical chelators are convenient to use, it should be noted that the protein patterns obtained may not always be the same as those obtained with naturally occurring iron-binding proteins (Chart *et al.*, 1986). The results obtained with bacteria grown in media that contain transferrins probably most closely resemble conditions *in vivo*. It has been shown that some of the iron-regulated receptors are expressed *in vivo* during infection (Griffiths *et al.*, 1983). Indeed, the iron-regulated outer-membrane proteins of *E. coli* O111, recovered without subculture from the peritoneal cavities of infected guinea-pigs, are major components of the outer-membrane and are present in amounts equal to, or even greater than, the so-called major outer-membrane proteins that have apparent molecular weights in the range 30–42 kDa. Unlike *E. coli* O111, which shows the same pattern of iron-regulated outer-membrane proteins when grown *in vivo* and *in vitro* in the presence of ovotransferrin, *E. coli* O18:K1, a pathogenic strain that carries a ColV plasmid, produces not only the iron-regulated proteins seen *in vitro* but also a new protein during growth *in vivo* (Griffiths *et al.*, 1985a). The latter is not associated with the presence of the ColV plasmid. Differences in the pattern of the major outer-membrane proteins of *E. coli* O18 have also been noted in cells grown *in vivo* and these probably reflect other environmental changes, such as osmotic changes, experienced by the bacteria (Griffiths, 1991). *E. coli* and other pathogens isolated directly from human clinical material have also been shown to express iron-regulated proteins. This undoubtedly shows that these pathogens were growing under conditions of iron restriction during natural infection of the human host (Brown *et al.*, 1984; Lam *et al.*, 1984; Shand *et al.*, 1985).

Antibodies that react with some of the iron-regulated receptor proteins of *E. coli* and other pathogens have also been detected in human and animal sera, again clearly showing that these proteins are expressed by pathogens growing *in vivo* (Griffiths *et al.*, 1985a; Shand *et al.*, 1985; Fernandez-Beros *et al.*, 1989; Todhunter *et al.*, 1991). It is not clear whether these antibodies play any part in protecting the host against infection, possibly by interfering with siderophore-mediated iron uptake. As part of an investigation into the possible protective role of anti-receptor antibodies, Chart & Griffiths (1985, and unpublished data) examined the antigenic homology of FepA in different strains of *E. coli* with polyclonal and monoclonal antibodies. The results showed that the molecular weight and some of the antigenic properties of the enterobactin receptor are highly conserved. It is perhaps not surprising that antibodies raised against purified and denatured FepA fail to react with the protein *in situ* on the surface of the *E. coli* strain tested, and have no effect on bacterial multiplication. However, Coulton (1982) was able to raise antibodies to the FhuA protein of *E. coli* that partially inhibit ferrichrome-mediated iron transport and adsorption of phage T5 to the Fhu receptor. Similarly, polyclonal antibodies against the ColV plasmid-encoded IutA receptor inhibit the binding of aerobactin to membranes that contain the Iut A protein and to *E. coli* K-12 that expresses IutA (Roberts *et al.*, 1989). However, even if antibodies recognise the native receptor, they may not always be able to interact with the bacterial cell surface. In some cases, the lipopolysaccharide probably interferes with the antibody–antigen interaction by masking the receptor proteins, just as the lipopolysaccharide can interfere with the interaction between cloacin DF13 and its receptor IutA (Derbyshire *et al.*, 1989). Thus, polyclonal antibodies against the IutA protein, which can react with the receptor in *E. coli* K-12, fail to inhibit the binding of aerobactin to clinical isolates of *E. coli* that express IutA (Roberts *et al.*, 1989). Nevertheless, Bolin & Jensen (1987) have reported that turkeys passively immunised with antibodies against the iron-regulated outer-membrane proteins of *E. coli* O78:K80:H9 were protected against experimental *E. coli* septicaemia, but the actual mechanisms responsible for this protection have never clearly been shown to be due to antibodies against iron-regulated receptors.

Use of haem iron

In addition to obtaining iron from iron-binding protein, *E. coli* can, under certain circumstances, obtain sufficient iron from cell-free haemoglobin or haem for multiplication *in vivo*. It has long been known that haem and haemoglobin can greatly enhance the susceptibility of animals and humans to *E. coli* infections (Davis & Yull, 1964; Bornside *et al.*, 1968; Bullen *et al.*, 1968, 1991), and that it is the iron component of these molecules that is the important factor (Lee *et al.*, 1979). Though much is known about mechanisms of siderophore-mediated iron uptake in *E. coli*, it is surprising that little is known about the mechanisms by which this organism obtains iron from haem or haemoglobin. More is known about such systems in other organisms, in which several haem-binding proteins have been found (Hanson *et al.*, 1992; Lee, 1992; Bramanti & Holt, 1993). It has recently been shown that the iron in haemoglobin is used in preference to that in ovotransferrin when both are present at the same time. The uptake of ovotransferrin-bound iron took place only after haemoglobin-derived iron had been exhausted (Law *et al.*, 1992). This confirms the general belief that haem iron is more readily available than that bound to iron-binding proteins (Griffiths, 1987b). Law *et al.* (1992) also found that growth rate was related to the concentration of haemoglobin and that it was much higher than that of the same strain growing in the same medium in the absence of haemoglobin. During haemoglobin-stimulated growth of *E. coli*, the enterobactin-mediated iron-uptake system was expressed and it was suggested that this system may be involved in the transport into the cell of iron derived from haemoglobin, but how this occurs is unclear (Law *et al.*, 1992).

Under normal circumstances only a trace of free haem is found in serum and it is bound to haemopexin or serum albumin (Hershko, 1975; Smith, 1990). Similarly, the small amount of haemoglobin that may appear in serum during red blood cell breakdown is bound to hap-toglobin (Hershko, 1975; Eaton *et al.*, 1982). Interestingly, the con-centration of haptoglobin increases dramatically in the serum of patients with acute or chronic infections (Owen *et al.*, 1964; Chiancone *et al.*, 1968). If pathogens like *E. coli* are to use this source of iron, sufficient free haemoglobin or haem must be present in the circulation to over-whelm the appropriate binding protein, otherwise the pathogens must acquire it directly from protein complexes. It has been reported that *E. coli* is unable to use, as a source of iron, haemoglobin bound to haptoglobin, which suggests that haptoglobin might be used to treat potentially fatal haemoglobin-promoted infections (Eaton *et al.*, 1982). However, the strains of *E. coli* studied by these workers appear not to have been well characterised, and it is unclear whether other strains of *E. coli*, possibly those associated with septicaemia, may be able to do so. It is also quite clear that certain other pathogens, such as *Vibrio vulnificus*, can use haemoglobin in the haemoglobin–haptoglobin com-plex (Helms *et al.*, 1984). Similarly, *Haemophilus influenzae* can use the haem–haemopexin complex, and an iron-regulated haemopexin recep-tor has been identified in this organism (Wong *et al.*, 1994).

It has been suggested that haemolysin-induced haemolysis *in vivo* is a way of increasing the level of cell-free haem or haemoglobin and, coincidentally, the available iron pool (Linggood & Ingram, 1982). Haemolysins are well-known virulence determinants of *E. coli* (see Chapter 11) and the association between haemolytic *E. coli* and disease has long been recognised (Dudgeon *et al.*, 1921). In particular, strains of *E. coli* that cause extra-intestinal infections produce haemolysins (Opal *et al.*, 1990), and these appear to be derepressed under iron-restricted growth conditions (Lebek & Grünig, 1985; Grünig *et al.*, 1987). Haemolysin production by *V. cholerae*, *V. parahaemolyticus* and *Serratia marcescens* is also iron-regulated (Poole & Braun, 1988; Stoebner & Payne, 1988; Dai *et al.*, 1992). Linggood & Ingram (1982) found that the transfer of a Hly plasmid to a non-haemolytic strain of *E. coli* increased its virulence for mice. Injection of non-toxic amounts of iron, haemoglobin, α-haemolysin or phenylhydrazine, which causes haemolysis, simulated the effect of the Hly plasmid by stimulating bacterial growth. An iron-sequestering system that depends on haemolysin-induced liberation of haemoglobin from erythrocytes may be expected to be important only for the growth of bacteria in blood, and their ability to make haemolysins would have little effect on bacterial growth on mucosal surfaces, as in the bowel, and this, indeed, appears to be the case (Smith & Linggood, 1971). Why haemolysin-producing strains of *E. coli* should be associated with human pyelonephritis is unclear. A connection between haemolysin production and the ability of *E. coli* to produce pyelonephritis in mice and rats after intravenous injection has been demonstrated experimentally. This suggests that the ability to multiply in the bloodstream may be an important factor that permits the initiation of infection by this route (Fried *et al.*, 1971; Van den Bosch *et al.*, 1979, 1981). Waalwijk *et al.* (1983) have shown that the α-haemolysin itself enhances the pathogenicity of *E. coli* in the mouse haematogenous pyelonephritis model, and that this enhanced virulence is due to the erythrocyte lysis, which liberates haemoglobin that acts as a ready iron source for the organisms. When a Tn5-induced non-haemolytic mutant strain and the haemolytic parent were injected simultaneously into mice, both strains multiplied. The fact that both organisms multiplied in the kidney suggests that the α-haemolysin produced by the haemolytic strain acted as a growth factor *in vivo* for the non-haemolytic mutant. The virulence of the mutant *E. coli* was similarly enhanced by injection of α-haemolysin, haemoglobin or iron salts. Haemolysins do not only lyse erythrocytes, but also other mammalian cells, which undoubtedly contributes to their role in pathogenesis.

Iron as a regulatory signal

A significant development in the understanding of microbial pathogenicity has been the recognition that the restricted availability of iron in tissue fluids presents not only *E. coli* but also other pathogens with the difficulty of acquiring sufficient of the metal for multiplication *in vivo*. This iron limitation constitutes a major environmental signal that acts alone, or in conjunction with other controls, to regulate the expression of a number of virulence and metabolic genes (Griffiths, 1987b; Mekalanos, 1992). Analysis of pathogens grown under specific environmental conditions, such as iron restriction, is now leading to a clearer picture of the characteristics associated with virulence. This is because some of the crucial determinants are either not produced or are produced only at very low levels by organisms grown in rich broth media and, thus, have been missed by investigators. Similarly, other bacterial components may be down-regulated *in vivo*. Such information is crucial for understanding microbial pathogenicity and has important consequences for vaccine design (Griffiths, 1991). The co-ordinated response of *E. coli* to low levels of iron includes the expression of high-affinity iron-acquisition systems and the synthesis of a number of factors that are apparently not directly related to iron metabolism. These include the phage-encoded Shiga-like toxin type 1 (SLT 1) (Calderwood & Mekalanos, 1987; see also Chapter 10), a recently discovered entero-toxin from EIEC (Fasano *et al.*, 1990; see also Chapter 16), superoxide dismutase (Niederhoffer *et al.*, 1990; Fee, 1991) and the haemolytic activity encoded by some Hly plasmids (Grünig *et al.*, 1987). Production of Shiga toxin (Dubos & Geiger, 1946; Van Heyningen & Gladstone, 1953) and a number of other important toxins, including diphtheria toxin (Pappenheimer, 1977) and *Pseudomonas* exotoxin A (Bjorn *et al.*, 1978), is similarly iron-regulated.

Considerable progress has now been made in understanding the molecular mechanisms by which iron co-ordinately regulates the expression of a number of unlinked genes in *E. coli*. Most of the genes involved in siderophore biosynthesis and transport are negatively regulated at the transcriptional level by a 17-kDa repressor protein, Fur, which uses ferrous (Fe^{2+}) iron as the co-repressor (Bagg & Neilands, 1987a,b; O'Halloran, 1993). Fur is the product of the regulatory gene *fur* that is located at about 15.5 minutes on the *E. coli* chromosome. Mutations in *fur* are constitutively de-repressed for iron assimilation (Hantke, 1981), including the uptake of uncomplexed Fe^{2+} (Hantke, 1987a). Other *E. coli* genes under Fur control include the phage-encoded *slt* genes for SLT 1, the superoxide dismutase genes, *sodA* and *sodB*, the *tonB* gene, the haemolytic activity encoded by some Hly plasmids, and *fur* itself (Grünig *et al.*, 1987; de Lorenzo *et al.*, 1988b; Niederhoffer *et al.*, 1990; Postle, 1990b; Fee, 1991; Stojiljkovic *et al.*, 1994). Binding sites for the active Fe^{2+}-Fur repressor protein, the so-called 'iron box', have been identified in the promoters of many of these iron-regulated genes, including *fur* (Bagg & Neilands, 1987a,b; Calderwood & Mekalanos, 1987; Grünig *et al.*, 1987; Elkins & Earhart, 1989; Griggs & Konisky, 1989; Niederhoffer *et al.*, 1990; Postle, 1990b). The DNA sequences of the iron boxes consist of a highly A- and T-rich palindrome, and deletions that disrupt the palindrome structure make the promoter unresponsive to regulation by iron. It has also been shown that the presence of a consensus 'iron-box' sequence, 5'-GATAATGATAAT-CATTATC, is sufficient to allow Fur-mediated iron regulation of a gene (Calderwood & Mekalanos, 1988). The general mode of action of Fur is shown schematically in Figure 12.6. When iron supply is plentiful, this involves the binding of the Fur protein–Fe^{2+} complex to the operator, with the Fur protein binding as a dimer. This blocks transcription of relevant mRNA species and iron-related functions are not expressed. As the intrabacterial iron concentration falls during iron restriction, less Fe^{2+} is available for binding to Fur. Since Fur in its metal-free state binds poorly to the 'iron-box', or not at all, this leads to derepression of iron-regulated operons and to the synthesis of iron-related functions. In addition, at least two other *E. coli* genes appear to be positively regulated either directly or indirectly by Fur (Hantke, 1987b; Niederhoffer *et al.*, 1990). In contrast to the fairly simple on–off model of regulation by iron and Fur just described, control of the *fur* gene itself is more complicated. It is not only negatively autoregulated by Fur and Fe^{2+}, but also positively regulated through the cAMP–CAP system (catabolite activator protein) (de Lorenzo *et al.*, 1988b). It has been suggested that this type of regulation establishes a link between the modulation of iron metabolism and the metabolic status of the cell (de Lorenzo *et al.*, 1988b). A role for cAMP–CAP control, operating in conjunction with Fur, has also been found in the *cir* gene (Griggs *et al.*, 1990). Fur regulation of the citrate-mediated iron-transport system in *E. coli* is also complicated because it involves induction by Fe^{3+}-dicitrate, though citrate does not enter the cell (Hussein *et al.*, 1981; Zimmerman *et al.*, 1984). In this case regulation is believed to involve, in addition to Fur, two other regulatory proteins, FecR and FecI, which are responsible, respectively, for monitoring Fe^{3+}-dicitrate levels in the periplasm and for gene induction (Van Hove *et al.*, 1990).

In addition to Fur-controlled regulation, a global response to iron restriction has been found at the level of transfer RNA (tRNA) modification (Griffiths, 1987b; Persson, 1993). Growth of *E. coli* in the presence of an iron-binding protein results in the generation of specifically altered tRNA molecules that elute earlier during chromatography than do the same tRNAs from iron-replete cells (Griffiths & Humphreys, 1978; Buck & Griffiths, 1981, 1982). The same iron-related modification of tRNA occurs in *E. coli* growing *in vivo* during infection (Griffiths *et al.*, 1978). Indeed, it was this discovery that first provided positive proof that bacteria growing *in vivo* during infection were doing

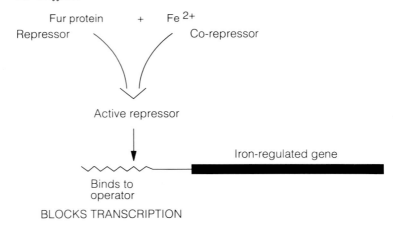

Fig. 12.6. Schematic representation of Fur-mediated iron regulation of gene expression in *Escherichia coli*, Fur, ferric uptake regulation.

so under iron-restricted conditions. These altered tRNAs lack the methyl-thio (ms^2) moiety of the 2-methylthio-N^6-(Δ^2-isopentenyl)-adenosine (ms^2i^6A) adjacent to the 3' end of the anticodon (A37) of the tRNAs from iron-replete *E. coli* (Buck & Griffiths, 1982). Such altered tRNAs, including the tRNAs for phenylalanine, tyrosine, tryptophan and serine, recognise codons with a 5'-uridine (UXY codons). The change in structure for the tRNA for phenylalanine is shown in Figure 12.7.

Similar tRNA changes have been observed in *Salmonella typhimurium*, *Klebsiella pneumoniae* and *Pseudomonas aeruginosa* (McLennan *et al.*, 1981; Buck & Ames, 1984). Originally, it was thought that the alteration of tRNAs was associated with inhibition of bacterial growth, because they were found in pathogenic *E. coli* inhibited by human milk, bovine colostrum or serum, in which bacteriostasis is induced by the combined action of antibody and iron-binding proteins (Griffiths, 1972; Griffiths & Humphreys, 1977,1978), but not all strains of *E. coli* were inhibited by these body fluids. This was believed to be due to the absence of the appropriate antibodies. Since the altered tRNA population was also found in pathogenic *E. coli* that grew well in human milk, bovine colostrum or in synthetic media containing iron-binding protein, it was proposed that these alterations were connected not with the growth inhibition, but with the adaptation of *E. coli* to an iron-restricted environment (Griffiths & Humphreys, 1978). A regulatory role that possibly controls aspects of bacterial metabolism essential for pathogenicity has been suggested for the changes in the tRNAs.

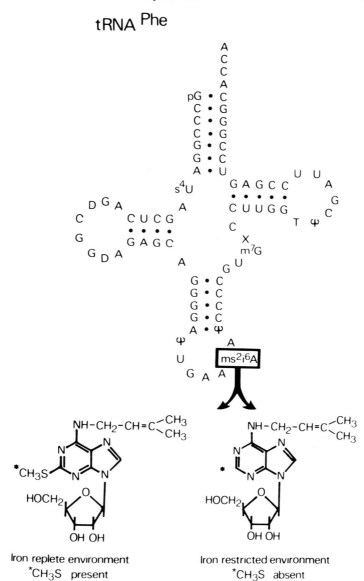

Fig. 12.7. Effect of iron on the post-transcriptional modification of phenylalanine tRNA. [ms²i⁶A, 2-methylthio-N^6– (Δ^2-isopentenyl)-adenosine] (from Griffiths, 1981; reproduced by permission of Raven Press, New York).

Subsequent work has shown that under-modification of these tRNAs induces pleiotropic effects on bacterial physiology. In some instances these effects are on the translational efficiency of the tRNAs, in others they alter the effect of the context in which the codons occur, and in yet others the mechanisms are unknown (Buck & Griffiths, 1981, 1982; Bouadloun *et al.*, 1986; Ericson & Björk, 1986; Petrullo & Elseviers, 1986; Blum, 1988; Persson, 1993). For example, failure to methylthiolate tRNA by iron restriction significantly decreases the translational efficiencies of the tRNAs affected. These, in turn, by attenuation mechanisms, lead to increased synthesis of aromatic amino-acids and possibly enterobactin, as well as to increased transport of aromatic amino-acids into the cell. All of these processes are interrelated through the aromatic biosynthetic pathway (Buck & Griffiths, 1981, 1982; Buck & Ames, 1984). It is believed that such regulatory features are involved in adapting *E. coli* for growth in iron-restricted environments (Buck & Griffiths, 1982; Griffiths, 1987b).

Enterobactin is synthesised from chorismic acid by way of a branch of the aromatic amino-acid biosynthetic pathway (Figure 12.3). Derepression of the enterobactin system during iron restriction necessitates adjustments to the whole aromatic pathway to ensure production of essential aromatic compounds, such as *p*-aminobenzoate, and aromatic amino-acids, if these are required. The ability to regulate the expression of various operons in this pathway through the level of charging of the tRNA (classical attenuation; Yanofsky, 1981) and by iron-related post-transcriptional tRNA modification can provide the bacterial cell with considerable regulatory flexibility that may be important for growth under conditions of iron restriction. There is also evidence that under-modification of the adenosine (A37) located next to the anticodon of certain tRNAs leads to increased frequency of spontaneous mutations when the cell has to adapt to environmental stress (Connolly & Winkler, 1989, 1991).

High-affinity siderophore-mediated iron-uptake systems and virulence

Developments during the past few years have significantly increased our understanding of the wide-ranging effects of the iron-restricted environment of the host on invading pathogens such as *E. coli*. Nevertheless, some aspects remain unclear. In only isolated instances has it been shown with certainty that a siderophore-mediated iron-uptake system is essential for virulence. For example, highly virulent strains of *Vibrio anguillarum*, which are responsible for a devastating septicaemic disease of fish, carry a plasmid that encodes a siderophore-dependent iron-transport system, which allows the organism to grow under iron-restricted conditions. On loss of the plasmid, *V. anguillarum* loses its ability to grow under such conditions and its virulence (Crosa, 1989). In the case of *E. coli*, the contribution to virulence of the siderophores, especially enterobactin, is less clear. Although ability to produce and use aerobactin is thought to play an important part in the virulence of invasive *E. coli* strains, it is not clear why acquisition of the ability to make this second siderophore confers a selective advantage on bacteria already able to make enterobactin, but a number of hypotheses has been proposed (Griffiths, 1987b; de Lorenzo & Martinez, 1988; Crosa, 1989; Wooldridge & Williams, 1993). In terms of kinetics, hydroxamate-based iron chelators, such as aerobactin, appear to be inferior to catecholate-type siderophores in their ability to remove iron from transferrin (Carrano & Raymond, 1979). However, the presence of other factors in body fluids may influence the overall effectiveness of different siderophores *in vivo*. Care is, therefore, necessary when extrapolating data from experiments *in vitro* to the situation in host tissues during infection. Pollack *et al.* (1976) and Konopka *et al.* (1982) have shown that the kinetic disadvantage of hydroxamate-mediated removal of iron from transferrin can be partially overcome by adding other anions to the system. Another important difference between the mode of action of these two chelators is that aerobactin is recycled while enterobactin is used only once to transport iron into the cell (Raymond & Carrano, 1979; Braun *et al.*, 1984). Moreover, serum albumin has been reported to bind enterobactin, but not aerobactin, so decreasing its effective concentration in serum (Konopka & Neilands, 1984). In addition, anti-enterobactin antibodies (Moore *et al.*, 1980; Moore & Earhart, 1981) and anti-O-polysaccharide antibodies that interfere with enterobactin secretion (Fitzgerald & Rogers, 1980) have been detected in sera. All of these mechanisms, as well as the relatively low solubility in water (Pollack & Neilands, 1970) and chemical instability of enterobactin (Neilands, 1981) may well restrict the overall effectiveness of enterobactin-mediated iron-uptake systems in serum and favour aerobactin-mediated iron transport. The growth of *E. coli* strains that rely entirely on enterobactin for their iron supply may then be expected to be restricted and such organisms would be at a disadvantage when compared with aerobactin producers. The fact that higher dose levels of aerobactin-negative (ColV⁻) *E. coli* O18:K1:H7 grew as well in host tissues as the aerobactin-positive ColV$^+$ strain suggests that enterobactin-mediated iron uptake can function *in vivo*, but that aerobactin iron-uptake systems may be more important at low infective doses (Smith & Huggins, 1980). Roberts *et al.* (1989) have shown, using a mouse peritonitis model, that the aerobactin-mediated iron-uptake system of plasmid ColV-K30, genetically isolated by molecular cloning from other plasmid determinants, is sufficient to restore to full virulence a clinical *E. coli* strain whose aerobactin-positive ColV plasmid had been lost. It is not known, however, whether enterobactin and aerobactin are both required for full virulence. So far, well-characterised Ent$^-$Aero$^+$ strains of *E. coli* have not been reported amongst clinical isolates from septicaemic disease, but most strains of *Shigella flexneri* produce only aerobactin. The failure of *Sh. flexneri* to produce enterobactin is due to a defect in the expression of *ent* genes and not to their absence (Schmitt & Payne, 1988; Payne, 1989). The loss by mutation of the ability to synthesise enterobactin inhibits the ability of *Salmonella typhimurium* to grow in human serum and also markedly reduces its virulence for mice, suggesting that enterobactin production is important for virulence (Yancey *et al.*, 1979). Subsequently, however, Benjamin *et al.* (1985) found that although enterobactin-negative mutants of *S. typhimurium* fail to multiply in normal mouse serum, inability to make enterobactin does not alter its virulence for several inbred strains of mice. Since *S. typhimurium* is an intracellular pathogen, it is suggested that failure of the *ent* mutation to affect virulence is due to the lack of a growth requirement for enterobactin once the pathogen has entered the cell. *Shigella flexneri* is also an intracellular pathogen, and it has been shown that its ability to synthesise aerobactin does not affect intracellular multiplication, but it appears to provide a selective advantage for extracellular growth (Nassif *et al.*, 1987). Payne (1989) suggested that siderophores may be called into play when *Shigella* multiply in the extracellular compartments of host tissues and they may also be important for the survival of the pathogen in the environment outside the host. More recently, Brock *et al.* (1991) have presented evidence that suggests that enterobactin and aerobactin fulfil somewhat different functions in that they may acquire iron *in vivo* from different sources; enterobactin by scavenging predominantly transferrin-bound iron and aerobactin obtaining iron preferentially from cells. Interest has also been aroused by the additional contribution that siderophores may make to the pathogenesis of infection by suppressing host immune responses (Autenrieth *et al.*, 1991) and by promoting tissue damage and inflammation at sites of infection, through siderophore-induced free radical formation (Coffman *et al.*, 1990). Depending on their biochemical properties, siderophores behave differently in such systems and this may have different clinical consequences.

Conclusions

Though considerable advances have been made in understanding the molecular basis of iron-related virulence processes, less progress has been made in assessing the contribution to host defences of the bacteriostatic effects of the combined action of iron-binding proteins and antibodies that appear to function by interfering with enterobactin production and iron acquisition (Fitzgerald & Rogers, 1980; Brock *et al.*, 1983; Rogers, 1983; Griffiths & Bullen, 1987). There is evidence that the combined action of secretory IgA and lactoferrin in the bowel contribute to the protective effect of human milk against neonatal enteritis due to *E. coli* (Bullen *et al.*, 1972; Griffiths & Bullen, 1987). A similar function has been attributed to the IgG and lactoferrin present in bovine colostrum. The activities of other milk components are also likely to play a part in the well-known protective effect of breast milk against enteric infections in infants (Griffiths & Bullen, 1987), including the bactericidal activity of apolactoferrin (Bellamy *et al.*, 1992), which is unrelated to bacterial iron metabolism. However, the bactericidal activity of plasma, which does seem to involve transferrin and bacterial iron metabolism, has not been explained satisfactorily (Griffiths & Bullen, 1987; Bullen *et al.*, 1992).

Similarly, little progress has been made in understanding the consequences for clinical infections of increased availability of iron, and this continues to be a controversial topic (Hershko *et al.*, 1988; Bullen *et al.*, 1991). It would be expected that the abnormal presence of freely available iron *in vivo* would increase the rate of bacterial multiplication and to tip the balance in favour of the pathogen. For example, certain strains of *E. coli* have a doubling time of about 35 minutes in the presence of an iron-binding protein, but this is reduced to approximately 25 minutes when iron is freely available in the medium (Griffiths & Humphreys, 1978). Even a modest reduction in the rate of bacterial growth can make a significant difference to the size of the bacterial population over a matter of hours, and this may be crucial to the outcome of an infection. Bullen *et al.* (1991) cited clinical examples to support the importance of increased iron availability in determining infection, whereas Hershko *et al.*

(1988) remained sceptical and quoted alternative, sometimes rather ill-defined, explanations of the same data. In reality, the factors that determine the outcome of infections are numerous and complex, and it is not surprising that it is often difficult to establish their relative contributions in clinical settings.

There is no doubt that the availability of iron can, in some circumstances, be crucial to the clinical outcome of infection. Freely available haem or haemoglobin clearly promote infection and the catastrophic effects of the combination of cell-free haemoglobin and *E. coli* in the peritoneal cavity in humans has long been known (Kluger & Bullen, 1987). Proposals to use cross-linked haemoglobins as erythrocytes substitutes in transfusion medicine should, therefore, be evaluated very carefully, particularly because pyridoxalated polymerised haemoglobin has been shown to promote fulminating *E. coli* sepsis in mice. Indeed, the results suggest that cross-linked haemoglobin may be more of a problem than the native molecule, because it has been designed for a longer half-life in the circulation and will, therefore, be available to potential pathogens for far longer (Griffiths *et al.*, 1995). Any advantages of these products over whole blood may be outweighed, therefore, by the promotion of bacterial proliferation *in vivo* and a resulting increase in the susceptibility of recipients to infection. Further research is clearly necessary into the effect of changes in host iron metabolism and transferrin saturation levels on the susceptibility of compromised individuals to infection by *E. coli* and other pathogens.

References

Ainscough, E. W., Brodie, A. M., Plowman, J. E., Bloor, S. J., Loehr, J. S. & Loehr, T. M. (1980). Studies on human lactoferrin by electron paramagnetic resonance, fluorescence and resonance Raman spectroscopy. *Biochemistry*, **19**, 4072–9.

Armstrong, S. K., Pettis, G. S., Forrester, L. J. & McIntosh, M. A. (1989). The *Escherichia coli* enterobactin biosynthesis gene, *ent* D: nucleotide sequence and membrane localization of its protein product. *Molecular Microbiology*, **3**, 757–66.

Autenrieth, I., Hantke, K. & Heesemann, J. (1991). Immunosuppression of the host and delivery of iron to the pathogen: a possible dual role of siderophores in the pathogenesis of microbial infections? *Medical Microbiology and Immunology*, **180**, 135–41.

Bagg, A. & Neilands, J. B. (1987a). Molecular mechanism of regulation of siderophore-mediated iron assimilation. *Microbiological Reviews*, **51**, 509–18.

Bagg, A. & Neilands, J. B. (1987b). Ferric uptake regulation protein acts as a repressor, employing iron (II) as a co-factor to bind the operator of an iron transport operon in *Escherichia coli*. *Biochemistry*, **26**, 5471–7.

Bellamy, W., Takase, M., Yamauchi, K., Wakabayashi, H., Kawase, K. & Tomita, M. (1992). Identification of the bactericidal domain of lactoferrin. *Biochimica et Biophysica Acta*, **1121**, 130–6.

Benjamin, W. H. Jr., Turnbough, C. L. Jr., Posey, B. S. & Briles, D. E. (1985). The ability of *Salmonella typhimurium* to produce the siderophore enterobactin is not a virulence factor in mouse typhoid. *Infection and Immunity*, **50**, 392–7.

Bindereif, A., Braun, V. & Hantke, K. (1982). The cloacin receptor of Col V-bearing *Escherichia coli* is part of the Fe^{3+}-aerobactin transport system. *Journal of Bacteriology*, **150**, 1472–5.

Bjorn, M. J., Iglewski, B. H., Ives, S. K., Sadoff, J. C. & Vasil, M. L. (1978). Effect of iron on yields of exotoxin A in cultures of *Pseudomonas aeruginosa* PA-103. *Infection and Immunity*, **19**, 785–91.

Blum, P. H. (1988). Reduced *leu* operon expression in a *mia A* mutant of *Salmonella typhimurium*. *Journal of Bacteriology*, **170**, 5125–33.

Bolin, C. A. & Jensen, A. E. (1987). Passive immunization with antibodies against iron-regulated outer membrane proteins protects turkeys from *Escherichia coli* septicaemia. *Infection and Immunity*, **55**, 1239–42.

Bornside, G. H., Bouis, P. J. & Cohn, I. (1968). Haemoglobin and *Escherichia coli*, a lethal intraperitoneal combination. *Journal of Bacteriology*, **95**, 1567–71.

Bouadloun, F., Srichaiyo, T., Isaksson, L. A. & Björk, G. R. (1986). Influence of modification next to the anticodon in tRNA on codon context sensitivity of translational suppression and accuracy. *Journal of Bacteriology*, **166**, 1022–7.

Bramanti, T. E. & Holt, S. C. (1993). Hemin uptake in *Porphyromonas gingivalis*: Omp 26 is a Hemin-binding surface protein. *Journal of Bacteriology*, **175**, 7413–20.

Braun, V., Brazel-Faisst, C. & Schneider, R. (1984). Growth stimulation of *Escherichia coli* in serum by iron(III)-aerobactin: recycling of aerobactin. *FEMS Microbiology Letters*, **21**, 99–103.

Braun, V., Günter, K. & Hantke, K. (1991). Transport of iron across the outer membrane. *Biology of Metals*, **4**, 14–22.

Brewer, S., Tolley, M., Trayer, I. P., Barr, G. C., Dorman, C. J., Hannavy, K., Higgins, C. F., Evans, J. S., Levin, B. A. & Wormald, M. R. (1990). Structure and function of X-Pro dipeptide repeats in the Ton B proteins of *Salmonella typhimurium* and *Escherichia coli*. *Journal Molecular Biology*, **216**, 883–95.

Brickman, T. J. & McIntosh, M. A. (1992). Overexpression and purification of ferric enterobactin esterase from *Escherichia coli*: demonstration of enzymatic hydrolysis of enterobactin and its iron complex. *Journal Biological Chemistry*, **267**, 12350–5.

Brock, J. H., Pickering, M. G., McDowall, M. C. & Deacon, A. G. (1983). Role of antibody and enterobactin in controlling growth of *Escherichia coli* in human milk and acquisition of lactoferrin- and transferrin-bound iron by *Escherichia coli*. *Infection and Immunity*, **40**, 453–9.

Brock, J. H., Williams, P. H., Licéaga, J. & Woodridge, K. G. (1991). Relative availability of transferrin-bound iron and cell-derived iron to aerobactin-producing and enterochelin-producing strains of *Escherichia coli* and to other microorganisms. *Infection and Immunity*, **59**, 3185–90.

Brown, M. R. W., Anwar, H. & Lambert, P.A. (1984). Evidence that mucoid *Pseudomonas aeruginosa* in the cystic fibrosis lung grows under iron-restricted conditions. *FEMS Microbiology Letters*, **21**, 113–17.

Buck, M. & Ames, B.N. (1984). A modified nucleotide in tRNA as a possible regulator of anaerobiosis: synthesis of *cis*-2-methylthio-ribosylzeatin in the tRNA of *Salmonella*. *Cell*, **36**, 523–31.

Buck, M. & Griffiths, E. (1981). Regulation of aromatic amino acid transport by tRNA: role of 2-methylthio-N^6-(Δ^2-isopentenyl) adenosine. *Nucleic Acids Research*, **9**, 401–14.

Buck, M. & Griffiths, E. (1982). Iron-mediated methylthiolation of tRNA as a regulator of operon expression in *Escherichia coli*. *Nucleic Acids Research*, **10**, 2609–24.

Bullen, J. J. & Griffiths, E. (1987) In *Iron and Infection: Molecular, Physiological and Clinical Aspects*, eds. J. J. Bullen & E. Griffiths. Chichester: John Wiley.

Bullen, J. J., Leigh, L. C. & Rogers, H. J. (1968). The effect of iron compounds on the virulence of *Escherichia coli* for guinea pigs. *Immunology*, **15**, 581–8.

Bullen, J. J., Rogers, H. J. & Leigh, L. (1972). Iron-binding proteins in milk and resistance to *Escherichia coli* infections in infants. *British Medical Journal*, **1**, 69–75.

Bullen, J. J., Spalding, P. B., Ward, C. G. & Rogers, H. J. (1992). The role of Eh, pH and iron in the bactericial power of human plasma. *FEMS Microbiology Letters*, **94**, 47–52.

Bullen, J. J., Ward, C. G. & Rogers, H. J. (1991). The critical role of iron in some clinical infections. *European Journal Clinical Microbiology and Infectious Diseases*, **10**, 613–17.

Byrd, T. F. & Horwitz, M. A. (1989). Interferon gamma-activated human monocytes down-regulate transferrin receptors and inhibit the intracellular multiplication of *Legionella pneumophila* by limiting the availability of iron. *Journal Clinical Investigation*, **83**, 1457–65.

Calderwood, S. B. & Mekalanos, J. J. (1987). Iron regulation of Shiga-like toxin expression in *Escherichia coli* is mediated by the *fur* locus. *Journal of Bacteriology*, **169**, 4759–64.

Calderwood, S. B. & Mekalanos, J. J. (1988). Confirmation of the Fur operator site by insertion of a synthetic oligonucleotide into an operon fusion plasmid. *Journal of Bacteriology*, **170**, 1015–17.

Carmel, G., Hellstren, D., Henning, D. & Coulton, J.W. (1990). Insertion mutagenesis of the gene encoding the ferrichrome-iron receptor of *Escherichia coli* K12. *Journal of Bacteriology*, **172**, 1861–9.

Carrano, C. J. & Raymond, K. N. (1979). Ferric iron sequestering agents: 2. Kinetics and mechanisms of iron removal from transferrin by enterochelin and synthetic tricatechols. *Journal of the American Chemical Society*, **101**, 5401–4.

Chart, H., Buck, M., Stevenson, P. & Griffiths, E. (1986). Iron regulated outer membrane proteins of *Escherichia coli* : variations in expression due to the chelator used to restrict the availability of iron. *Journal of General Microbiology*, **132**, 1373–8.

Chart, H. & Griffiths, E. (1985). Antigenic and molecular homology of the ferric-enterobactin receptor protein of *Escherichia coli*. *Journal of General Microbiology*, **131**, 1503–9.

Chart, H., Stevenson, P. & Griffiths, E. (1988). Iron-regulated outer-membrane proteins of *Escherichia coli* strains associated with enteric or extraintestinal diseases of man and animals. *Journal of General Microbiology*, **134**, 1549–59.

Chenault, S. S. & Earhart, C. F. (1991). Organisation of genes encoding membrane proteins of the *Escherichia coli* ferric enterobactin permease. *Molecular Microbiology*, **5**, 1405–13.

Chiancone, E., Alfsen, A., Ioppalo, C., Vecchini, P., Finazzi-Agro, A., Wyman, J. & Antonini, E. (1968). Studies on the reaction of haptoglobin and haemoglobin and haemoglobin chains I: stoichiometry and affinity. *Journal of Molecular Biology*, **34**, 347–56.

Coffman, T. J., Cox, C. D., Edeker, B. L. & Britigan, B. E. (1990). Possible role of bacterial siderophores in inflammation: iron bound to the *Pseudomonas* siderophore pyochelin can function as a hydroxyl radical catalyst. *Journal of Clinical Investigation*, **86**, 1030–7.

Connolly, D. M. & Winkler, M. E. (1989). Genetic and physiological relationships among the *mia* A gene, 2-methylthio-N^6-(Δ^2-isopentenyl)-adenosine tRNA modification and spontaneous mutagenesis in *Escherichia coli* K12. *Journal of Bacteriology*, **171**, 3233–46.

Connolly, D. M. & Winkler, M. E. (1991). Structure of *Escherichia coli* K12 *mia* A and characterization of the mutator phenotype caused by *mia* A insertion mutations. *Journal of Bacteriology*, **173**, 1711–21.

Cooper, S. R., McArdle, J. V. & Raymond, K. N. (1978). Siderophore electrochemistry: relation to intracellular release mechanism. *Proceedings of the National Academy of Sciences, USA*, **75**, 3551–4.

Coulton, J. W. (1982). The ferrichrome-iron receptor of *Escherichia coli* K12: antigenicity of the Fhu A protein. *Biochimica et Biophysica Acta*, **717**, 154–62.

Coulton, J. W., Mason, P. & Allatt, D. D. (1987) *fhu* C and *fhu* D genes for iron (III)-ferrichrome transport into *Escherichia coli* K12. *Journal of Bacteriology*, **169**, 3844–9.

Coulton, J. W., Mason, P. & DuBow, M. S. (1983). Molecular cloning of the ferrichrome-iron receptor of *Escherichia coli* K12. *Journal of Bacteriology*, **156**, 1315–21.

Crichton, R. R. & Ward, R. J. (1992). Structure and molecular biology of iron binding proteins and the regulation of 'free' iron pools. In *Iron and Human Disease*, ed. R.B. Lauffer, pp. 23–75. Boca Raton, FL: CRC Press.

Crosa, J. H. (1987). Bacterial iron metabolism, plasmids and other virulence factors. In *Iron and Infection: Molecular, Physiological and Clinical Aspects*, eds. J. J. Bullen & E. Griffiths, pp 139–170, Chichester: John Wiley.

Crosa, J. H. (1989). Genetics and molecular biology of siderophore-mediated iron transport in bacteria. *Microbiology Reviews*, **53**, 517–30.

Curtis, N. A. C., Eisenstadt, R. L., East, S. J., Cornford, R. J., Walker, L. A. & White, A. J. (1988). Iron-regulated outer membrane proteins of *Escherichia coli* K12 and mechanism of action of catechol substituted cephalosporins. *Antimicrobial Agents and Chemotherapy*, **32**, 1879–86.

Dai, J. H., Lee, Y. S. & Wong, H. C. (1992). Effects of iron limitation on production of a siderophore, outer membrane proteins, and hemolysin and on hydrophobicity, cell adherence, and lethality for mice of *Vibrio parahemolyticus*. *Infection and Immunity*, **60**, 2952–6.

Davis, J. H. & Yull, A. B. (1964). A toxic factor in abdominal injury II. The role of the red cell component. *Journal of Trauma*, **4**, 84–7.

De Lorenzo, V., Herrero, M. & Neilands, J. B. (1988a). IS1-mediated mobility of the aerobactin system of p Col V-K30 in *Escherichia coli*. *Molecular and General Genetics*, **213**, 487–90.

De Lorenzo, V., Herrero, M., Giovannini, F. & Neilands, J. B. (1988b). Fur (ferric uptake regulation) protein and CAP (catabolite activator protein) modulate transcription of *fur* gene in *Escherichia coli*. *European Journal of Biochemistry*, **173**, 537–46.

De Lorenzo, V. & Martinez, J. L. (1988). Aerobactin production as a virulence factor: a re-evaluation. *European Journal of Clinical Microbiology and Infectious Diseases*, **7**, 621–9.

Derbyshire, P., Baldwin, T., Stevenson, P., Griffiths, E., Roberts, M., Williams, P., Hall, T. L. & Formal, S. B. (1989). Expression in *Escherichia coli* K12 of the 76000-dalton iron-regulated outer membrane protein of *Shigella flexneri* confers sensitivity to Cloacin DF13 in the absence of *Shigella* O antigen. *Infection and Immunity*, **57**, 2794–8.

Dubos, R. J. & Geiger, J. W. (1946). Preparations and properties of shiga toxin and toxoid. *Journal of Experimental Medicine*, **84**, 143–56.

Dudgeon, L. S., Wordley, E. & Bawtree, F. (1921). On bacillus coli infections of the urinary tract, especially in relation to haemolytic organisms. *Journal of Hygiene, Cambridge*, **20**, 137–64.

Earhart, C. F. (1987). Ferri-enterobactin transport in *Escherichia coli*. In *Iron Transport in Microbes, Plants and Animals*, eds. G. Winkelmann, D. van der Helm & J. B. Neilands, pp. 67–84, Weinheim: VCH Publishers.

Eaton, J. W., Brandt, P., Mahoney, J. R. & Lee, J. T. (1982). Haptoglobin: a natural bacteriostat. *Science*, **215**, 691–3.

Elkins, M. F. & Earhart, C. F. (1989) Nucleotide sequence and regulation of the *Escherichia coli* gene for ferrienterobactin transport protein Fep B. *Journal of Bacteriology*, **171**, 5443–51.

Elwell, L. P. & Shipley, P. L. (1980). Plasmid-mediated factors associated with virulence of bacteria to animals. *Annual Review of Microbiology*, **34**, 465–96.

Ericson, J. U. & Björk, G.R. (1986). Pleiotropic effects induced by modification deficiency next to the anticodon of tRNA from *Salmonella typhimurium* LT2. *Journal of Bacteriology*, **166**, 1013–21.

Fasano, A., Kay, B. A., Russell, R. G., Maneval D. R. Jr. & Levine, M. M. (1990). Enterotoxin and cytotoxin production by enteroinvasive *Escherichia coli*. *Infection and Immunity*, **58**, 3717–23.

Fee, J. A. (1991). Regulation of *sod* genes in *Escherichia coli*: relevance to superoxide dismutase function. *Molecular Microbiology*, **5**, 2599–610.

Fernandez-Beros, M. E., Gonzalez, C., McIntosh, M. A. & Cabello, F. C. (1989). Immune response to the iron-deprivation-induced proteins of *Salmonella typhi* in typhoid fever. *Infection and Immunity*, **57**, 1271–5.

Fitzgerald, S. P. & Rogers, H. J. (1980). Bacteriostatic effect of serum: role of antibody to lipopolysaccharide. *Infection and Immunity*, **27**, 302–8.

Fleming, T. P., Nahlik, M. S., Neilands, J. B., & McIntosh, M. A. (1985). Physical and genetic characterization of cloned enterobactin genomic sequences from *Escherichia coli*. *Gene*, **34**, 47–54.

Fried, F. A., Vermuelen, C. W., Ginsburg, M. J. & Cone, C. M. (1971). Etiology of pyelonephritis: further evidence associating the production of experimental pyelonephritis and haemolysin in *Escherichia coli*. *Journal of Urology*, **103**, 718–21.

Frost, G. & Rosenberg, H. (1973). The inducible citrate-dependent iron transport system in *Escherichia coli* K12. *Biochimica et Biophysica Acta*, **330**, 90–101.

Gadó, I., Milch, H., Czirók, E. & Herpay, M. (1989). The frequency of aerobactin production and its effect on the pathogenicity of human *Escherichia coli* strains. *Acta Microbiologica Hungarica*, **36**, 51–60.

Gibson, F. & Magrath, D. I. (1969). The isolation and characterization of a hydroxamic acid (aerobactin) formed by *Aerobacter aerogenes* 62–1. *Biochimica et Biophysica Acta*, **192**, 175–84.

Gonzalo, M. P., Martinez, J. L., Baguero, F., Gómez-Lus, R. & Pérez-Diaz, J. C. (1988). Aerobactin production linked to transferable antibiotic resistance in *Escherichia coli* strains isolated from sewage. *FEMS Microbiology Letters*, **50**, 57–9.

Greenwood, K. T. & Luke, R. K. J. (1976). Studies on the enzymatic synthesis of enterochelin in *Escherichia coli* K12: four polypeptides involved in the conversion of 2,3-dihydroxybenzoate to enterochelin. *Biochimica et Biophysica Acta*, **454**, 285–97.

Greenwood, K. T. & Luke, R. K. J. (1978). Enzymic hydrolysis of enterochelin and its iron complex in *Escherichia coli* K12. *Biochimica et Biophysica Acta*, **525**, 209–18.

Grewal, K. K., Warner, P. J. & Williams, P. H. (1982). An inducible outer membrane protein involved in aerobactin mediated iron transport by Col V strains of *Escherichia coli*. *FEBS Letters*, **140**, 27–30.

Griffiths, E. (1972). Abnormal phenylalanyl-tRNA found in serum inhibited *Escherichia coli* strain O111. *FEBS Letters*, **25**, 159–64.

Griffiths, E. (1983). Adaptation and multiplication of bacteria in host tissues. *Philosophical Transactions of the Royal Society (London) B*, **303**, 85–96.

Griffiths, E. (1987a). Iron in biological systems. In *Iron and Infection: Molecular Physiological and Clinical Aspects*, eds. J. J. Bullen & E. Griffiths, pp. 1–25, Chichester: John Wiley.

Griffiths, E. (1987b). The iron-uptake systems of pathogenic bacteria. In *Iron and Infection: Molecular, Physiological and Clinical Aspects*, eds. J. J. Bullen & E. Griffiths, pp. 69–137, Chichester: John Wiley.

Griffiths, E. (1991). Environmental regulation of bacterial virulence– implications for vaccine design and production. *Trends in Biotechnology*, **9**, 309–15.

Griffiths, E. & Bullen, J. J. (1987). Iron-binding proteins and host defence. In *Iron and Infection: Molecular, Physiological and Clinical Aspects*, eds. J. J. Bullen & E. Griffiths, pp. 171–209, Chichester: John Wiley.

Griffiths, E., Cortes, A., Gilbert, N., Stevenson, P., MacDonald, S. & Pepper, D. (1995). Haemoglobin-based blood substitutes and sepsis. *Lancet*, **345**, 158–60.

Griffiths, E. & Humphreys, J. (1977). Bacteriostatic effect of human and bovine colostrum on *Escherichia coli*: the importance of bicarbonate. *Infection and Immunity*, **15**, 396–401.

Griffiths, E. & Humphreys, J. (1978). Alterations in tRNAs containing 2-methylthio-N^6-(Δ^2-isopentenyl)-adenosine during growth of enteropathogenic *Escherichia coli* in the presence of iron-binding proteins. *European Journal of Biochemistry*, **82**, 503–13.

Griffiths, E. & Humphreys, J. (1980). Isolation of enterochelin from the peri-toneal washings of guinea-pigs lethally infected with *Escherichia coli*. *Infection and Immunity*, **28**, 286–9.

Griffiths, E., Humphreys, J., Leach, A. & Scanlon, L. (1978). Alterations in the tRNAs of *Escherichia coli* recovered from lethally infected animals. *Infection and Immunity*, **22**, 312–17.

Griffiths, E., Rogers, H. J. & Bullen, J. J. (1980). Iron, plasmids and infection. *Nature*, **284**, 508–9.

Griffiths, E., Stevenson, P., Hale, T. L. & Formal, S. B. (1985b). The synthesis of aerobactin and a 76000 dalton iron-regulated outer membrane protein by *Escherichia coli* K12 – *Shigella* hybrids and by enteroinvasive strains of *Escherichia coli*. *Infection and Immunity*, **49**, 67–71.

Griffiths, E., Stevenson, P. & Joyce, P. (1983). Pathogenic *Escherichia coli* express new outer membrane proteins when growing *in vivo*. *FEMS Microbiology Letters*, **16**, 95–9.

Griffiths, E., Stevenson, P., Thorpe, R. & Chart, H. (1985a). Naturally occurring antibodies in human sera that react with the iron-regulated outer membrane proteins of *Escherichia coli*. *Infection and Immunity*, **47**, 808–13.

Griggs, D. W., Kafka, K., Nau, C. D. & Konisky, J. (1990). Activation of expression of the *Escherichia coli cir* gene by an iron-independent regulatory mechanism involving cyclic AMP–cyclic AMP receptor protein complex. *Journal of Bacteriology*, **172**, 3529–33.

Griggs, D. W. & Konisky, J. (1989). Mechanism for iron-regulated trans-cription of the *Escherichia coli cir* gene: metal-dependent binding of Fur protein to the promoters. *Journal of Bacteriology*, **171**, 1048–54.

Grünig, H. M., Rutschi, D., Schoch, C. & Lebek, G. (1987). The chromo-somal *fur* gene regulates the extracellular haemolytic activity encoded by certain Hly plasmids. *Zentralblatt für Bakteriologie und Hygiene A*, **266**, 231–8.

Hancock, R. E. W., Hantke, K. & Braun, V. (1976). Iron transport in *Escherichia coli* K12: involvement of the colicin B receptor and of a citrate-inducible protein. *Journal of Bacteriology*, **127**, 1370–5.

Hannavy, K., Barr, G. C., Dorman, C. J., Adamson, J., Mazengera, L. M., Gallagher, M. P., Evans, J. S., Levin, B. A., Trayer, I. P. & Higgins, C. F. (1990). Ton B protein of *Salmonella typhimurium*: a model for signal transduction between membranes. *Journal of Molecular Biology*, **216**, 897–910.

Hanson, M. S., Slaughter, C. & Hansen, E. J. (1992). The *hbp* A gene of *Haemophilus influenzae* type b encodes a heme-binding lipoprotein con-served among heme-dependent *Haemophilus* species. *Infection and Immunity*, **60**, 2257–66.

Hantke, K. (1981). Regulation of ferric ion transport in *E. coli*. Isolation of a constitutive mutant. *Molecular and General Genetics*, **182**, 288–92.

Hantke, K. (1983). Identification of an iron uptake system specific for coprogen and rhodotorulic acid in *Escherichia coli* K12. *Molecular and General Genetics*, **191**, 301–6.

Hantke, K. (1987a). Ferrous iron transport mutants in *Escherichia coli* K12. *FEMS Microbiology Letters*, **44**, 53–7.

Hantke, K. (1987b). Selection procedure for deregulated iron transport mutants (fur) in *Escherichia coli* K12: *fur* not only affects iron metabolism. *Molecular and General Genetics*, **210**, 135–9.

Hantke, K. (1990). Dihydroxybenzoylserine–a siderophore for *E. coli*. *FEMS Microbiology Letters*, **67**, 5–8.

Hantke, K. & Zimmermann, L. (1981). The importance of the *exb* B gene for vitamin B_{12} and ferric iron transport. *FEMS Microbiology Letters*, **12**, 31–5.

Harris, W. R., Carrano, C. J. & Raymond, K. N. (1979a). Spectrophotometric determination of the proton dependent stability constant of ferric enterochelin. *Journal of the American Chemical Society*, **101**, 2213–14.

Harris, W. R., Carrano, C. J. & Raymond, K. N. (1979b). Co-ordination chemistry of microbial iron transport compounds: 16: Isolation, characterization and formation constants of ferric aerobactin. *Journal of the American Chemical Society*, **101**, 2722–7.

Harris, W. R., Carrano, C. J., Cooper, S. R., Sofen, S. R., Avdeef, A. E., McArdle, J. V. & Raymond K. N. (1979c). Co-ordination chemistry of microbial iron transport compounds. 19: Stability constants and electrochemical behaviour of ferric enterobactin and model complexes. *Journal of the American Chemical Society*, **101**, 6097–104.

Hartmann, A. & Braun, V. (1980). Iron transport in *Escherichia coli*: uptake and modification of ferrichrome. *Journal of Bacteriology*, **143**, 246–55.

Helms, S. D., Oliver, J. D. & Travis, J. C. (1984). Role of heme compounds and haptoglobin in *Vibrio vulnificus* pathogenicity. *Infection and Immunity*, **45**, 345–9.

Hershko, C. (1975). The fate of circulating haemoglobin. *British Journal of Haematology*, **29**, 199–204.

Hershko, C., Peto, T. E. A. & Weatherall, D. J. (1988). Iron and Infection. *British Medical Journal*, **296**, 660–4.

Hider, R. C., Silver, J., Neilands, J. B., Morrison, I. E. G. & Rees, L. V. C. (1979). Identification of iron (II)–enterobactin and its possible role in *Escherichia coli* iron transport. *FEBS Letters*, **102**, 325–8.

Hollifield, W. C. Jr. & Neilands, J. B. (1978). Ferric enterobactin transport system of *Escherichia coli* K12: extraction, assay and specificity of the outer membrane receptor. *Biochemistry*, **17**, 1922–8.

Hussain, S., Hantke, K. & Braun, V. (1981). Citrate-dependent iron transport system in *Escherichia coli* K12. *European Journal of Biochemistry*, **117**, 431–7.

Jacobson, S. H., Tullus, K., Wretlind, B. & Brauner, A. (1988). Aerobactin-mediated uptake of iron by strains of *Escherichia coli* causing pyelonephritis and bacteraemia. *Journal of Infection*, **16**, 147–52.

Kluger, M. J. & Bullen, J. J. (1987). Clinical and physiological aspects. In *Iron and Infection: Molecular, Physiological and Clinical Aspects*, eds. J. J. Bullen & E. Griffiths, pp. 243–82, Chichester: John Wiley.

Konijn, A. M. & Hershko, C. (1989). The anaemia of inflammation and chronic disease. In *Iron in Immunity, Cancer and Inflammation*, eds. M. de Sousa & J. H. Brock, pp. 111–43, Chichester: John Wiley.

Konopka, K., Bindereif, A. & Neilands, J. B. (1982). Aerobactin-mediated utilization of transferrin iron. *Biochemistry*, **21**, 6503–8.

Konopka, K. & Neilands, J. B. (1984). Effect of serum albumin on siderophore-mediated utilization of transferrin iron. *Biochemistry*, **23**, 2122–7.

Köster, W. (1991). Iron (III) hydroxamate transport across the cytoplasmic membrane of *Escherichia coli*. *Biology of Metals*, **4**, 23–32.

Köster, W. & Böhm, B. (1992). Point mutations in two conserved glycine residues within the integral membrane protein Fhu B affect iron (III) hydroxamate transport. *Molecular and General Genetics*, **232**, 399–407.

Köster, W. & Braun, V. (1989). Iron-hydroxamate transport into *Escherichia coli* K12: localization of Fhu D in the periplasm and of Fhu B in the cytoplasmic membrane. *Molecular and General Genetics*, **217**, 233–9.

Köster, W. & Braun, V. (1990a). Iron (III) hydroxamate transport in *Escherichia coli*: substrate binding to the periplasmic Fhu D protein. *Journal Biological Chemistry*, **265**, 21407–10.

Köster, W. & Braun, V. (1990b). Iron (III)-hydroxamate transport of *Escherichia coli*: restoration of iron supply by coexpression of the N- and C-terminal halves of the cytoplasmic membrane protein Fhu B cloned on separate plasmids. *Molecular and General Genetics*, **223**, 379–84.

Lafont, J. P., Dho, M., D'Hanteville, H. M., Bree, A. & Sansonetti, P. J. (1987). Presence and expression of aerobactin genes in virulent avian strains of *Escherichia coli*. *Infection and Immunity*, **55**, 193–7.

Lam, C., Turnowsky, F., Schwarzinger, E. & Neruda, W. (1984). Bacteria recovered without subculture from infected human urines expressed iron regulated outer membrane proteins. *FEMS Microbiology Letters*, **24**, 255–9.

Langman, L., Young, I. G., Frost, G., Rosenberg, H. & Gibson, F. (1972). Enterochelin system of iron transport in *Escherichia coli*: mutations affecting ferric-enterochelin esterase. *Journal of Bacteriology*, **112**, 1142–9.

Law, D., Wilkie, K. M., Freeman, R. & Gould, F. K. (1992). The iron uptake mechanisms of enteropathogenic *Escherichia coli*: the use of haem and haemoglobin during growth in an iron-limited environment. *Journal of Medical Microbiology*, **37**, 15–21.

Lawlor, K. M., Daskaleros, P. A., Robinson, R. E. & Payne, S. M. (1987). Virulence of iron-transport mutants of *Shigella flexneri* and utilization of host iron compounds. *Infection and Immunity*, **55**, 594–9.

Lawlor, K. M. & Payne, S. M. (1984). Aerobactin genes in *Shigella* spp. *Journal of Bacteriology*, **160**, 266–72.

Lebek, G. and Grünig, H. M. (1985). Relation between the hemolytic property and iron metabolism in *Escherichia coli*. *Infection and Immunity*, **50**, 23–30.

Lee, B. C. (1992). Isolation of haemin-binding proteins of *Neisseria gonorrhoeae*. *Journal of Medical Microbiology*, **36**, 121–7.

Lee, J. T., Arenholz, D. A., Nelson, R. D. & Simmonds, R. L. (1979). Mechanism of the adjuvant effect of haemoglobin in experimental peritonitis V. The significance of the co-ordinated iron component. *Surgery*, **86**, 41–7.

Leong, J. & Neilands, J. B. (1976). Mechanisms of siderophore iron transport in enteric bacteria. *Journal of Bacteriology*, **126**, 823–30.

Linggood, M. A. & Ingram, P. L. (1982). The role of alpha haemolysin in the virulence of *Escherichia coli* for mice. *Journal of Medical Microbiology*, **15**, 23–30.

Liu, J., Duncan, K. & Walsh, C. T. (1989). Nucleotide sequence of a cluster of *Escherichia coli* biosynthesis genes: identification of *ent* A and purification of its product 2,3-dihydro-2,3-dihydroxybenzoate dehydrogenase. *Journal of Bacteriology*, **171**, 791–8.

Liu, J., Quinn, N., Berchtold, G. A. & Walsh, C. T. (1990). Overexpression, purification and characterization of isochorismate synthetase (Ent C), the first enzyme in the biosynthesis of enterobactin from chorismate. *Biochemistry*, **29**, 1417–25.

Marolda, C. L., Valvano, M. A., Lawlor, K. M., Payne, S. M. & Crosa, J. H. (1987). Flanking and internal regions of chromosomal genes mediating aerobactin iron uptake systems in enteroinvasive *Escherichia coli* and *Shigella flexneri*. *Journal of General Microbiology*, **133**, 2269–78.

Martinez, J. L., Delgado-Iribarren, A. & Baquero, F. (1990). Mechanisms of iron acquisition and bacterial virulence. *FEMS Microbiology Reviews* **75**, 45–56.

McClelland, D. B. L. & van Furth, R. (1976). Antimicrobial factors in the exudates of skin windows in human subjects. *Clinical and Experimental Immunology*, **25**, 442–8.

McDougall, S. & Neilands, J. B. (1984). Plasmid- and chromosome-coded aerobactin synthesis in enteric bacteria: insertion sequences flank operon in plasmid-mediated systems. *Journal of Bacteriology*, **159**, 300–5.

McLennan, B. D., Buck, M., Humphreys, J. & Griffiths, E. (1981). Iron related modification of bacterial tRNA. *Nucleic Acids Research*, **9**, 2629–40.

Mekalanos, J. J. (1992). Environmental signals controlling expression of virulence determinants in bacteria. *Journal of Bacteriology*, **174**, 1–7.

Moore, D. G. & Earhart, C. F. (1981). Specific inhibition of *Escherichia coli* ferrienterochelin uptake by a normal human serum immunoglobulin. *Infection and Immunity*, **31**, 631–5.

Moore, D. G., Yancey, R. J., Lankford, C. E. & Earhart, C. F. (1980). Bacteriostatic enterochelin-specific immunoglobulin from normal human serum. *Infection and Immunity*, **27**, 418–23.

Nahlik, M. S., Brickman, T. J., Ozenberg, B. A. & McIntosh, M. A. (1989). Nucleotide sequence and transcriptional organization of the *Escherichia coli* enterobactin biosynthesis cistrons *ent* B and *ent* A. *Journal of Bacteriology*, **171**, 784–90.

Nassif, X., Mazert, M. C., Mournier, J. & Sansonetti, P. J. (1987). Evaluation with *iuc*: TN10 mutant of the role of aerobactin production in the virulence of *Shigella flexneri*. *Infection and Immunity*, **55**, 1963–9.

Neilands, J. B. (1981). Microbial iron compounds. *Annual Review of Biochemistry*, **50**, 715–31.

Neilands, J. B. (1982). Microbial envelope proteins related to iron. *Annual Review of Microbiology*, **36**, 285–309.

Neilands, J. B. (1990). Molecular biology and regulation of iron acquisition by *Escherichia coli* K12. In *The Bacteria* vol. 11, eds. B. H. Iglewski & V. L. Clark, pp. 205–23. New York: Academic Press.

Neilands, J. B. (1991). Mechanism and regulation of synthesis of aerobactin in *Escherichia coli* K12 (p Col V-K30). *Canadian Journal of Microbiology*, **38**, 728–33.

Nelson, M., Carrano, C. J. & Szaniszlo, P. J. (1992). Identification of the ferrioxamine B receptor, Fox B, in *Escherichia coli* K12. *Biometals*, **5**, 37–46.

Niederhoffer, E. C., Naranjo, C. M., Bradley, K. L. & Fee, J. A. (1990). Control of *Escherichia coli* superoxide dismutase (*sod* A and *sod* B) genes by the ferric uptake regulation (*fur*) locus. *Journal of Bacteriology*, **172**, 1930–8.

Nikaido, H. (1979). Non specific transport through the outer membrane. In *Bacterial Outer Membranes: Biogenesis and Functions*, ed. M. Inoue, pp. 361–407, New York: John Wiley.

O'Brien, I. G. & Gibson, F. (1970). The structure of enterochelin and related 2,3-dihydroxy-N-benzoylserine conjugates from *Escherichia coli*. *Biochimica et Biophysica Acta*, **215**, 393–402.

O'Halloran, T. V. (1993). Transition metals in control of gene expression. *Science*, **261**, 715–25.

Opal, S. M., Cross, A. S., Gemski, P. & Lyhte, L. W. (1990). Aerobactin and α-hemolysin as virulence determinants in *Escherichia coli* isolated from human blood, urine and stool. *Journal of Infectious Diseases*, **161**, 794–6.

Owen, J. A., Smith, R., Padaya, R. & Martin, J. (1964). Serum haptoglobin in disease. *Clinical Science*, **26**, 1–6.

Ozenberger, B. A., Brickman, T. J. & McIntosh, M. A. (1989). Nucleotide sequence of the *Escherichia coli* isochorismate synthetase gene *ent* C and evolutionary relationship of isochorismate synthetase and other chorismate-utilizing enzymes. *Journal of Bacteriology*, **171**, 775–83.

Ozenberger, B. A., Nahlik, M. S. & McIntosh, M. A. (1987). Genetic organization of multiple *fep* genes encoding ferric enterobactin transport functions in *Escherichia coli*. *Journal of Bacteriology*, **169**, 3638–46.

Pappenheimer, A.M. Jr. (1977). Diphtheria toxin. *Annual Review of Biochemistry*, **46**, 69–94.

Payne, S. M. (1989). Iron and virulence in *Shigella*. *Molecular Microbiology*, **3**, 1301–6.

Payne, S. M., Niesel, D. W., Peixotto, S. S. & Lawlor, K. M. (1983). Expression of hydroxamate and phenolate siderophores by *Shigella flexneri*. *Journal of Bacteriology*, **155**, 949–55.

Perez-Casal, J. F. & Crosa, J. H. (1984). Aerobactin iron uptake sequences in plasmid Col V-K30 are flanked by inverted IS1-like elements and replication regions. *Journal of Bacteriology*, **160**, 256–65.

Persson, B. C. (1993). Modification of tRNA as a regulatory device. *Molecular Microbiology*, **8**, 1011–16.

Petrullo, L. A. & Elseviers, D. (1986). Effect of a 2-methylthio-N[6]-isopentyladenosine deficiency on peptidyl-tRNA release in *Escherichia coli*. *Journal of Bacteriology*, **165**, 608–11.

Pollack, J. R. & Neilands, J. B. (1970). Enterobactin, an iron transport compound from *Salmonella typhimurium*. *Biochemical and Biophysical Research Communications*, **38**, 989–92.

Pollack, S., Aisen, P., Lasky, F. D. & Vanderhoff, G. (1976). Chelate mediated transfer of iron from transferrin to desferrioxime. *British Journal of Haematology*, **34**, 231–5.

Poole, K. & Braun, V. (1988). Iron regulation of *Serratia marcescens* hemolysin gene expression. *Infection and Immunity*, **56**, 2967–71.

Postle, K. (1990a). Ton B and the Gram-negative dilemma. *Molecular Microbiology*, **4**, 2019–25.

Postle, K. (1990b). Aerobic regulation of the *Escherichia coli ton* B gene by changes in iron availability and the *fur* locus. *Journal of Bacteriology*, **172**, 2287–93.

Postle, K. & Skare, J. T. (1988). *Escherichia coli* Ton B protein is exported from the cytoplasm without proteolytic cleavage of its amino terminus. *Journal of Biological Chemistry*, **262**, 11000–7.

Pressler, U., Staudenmaier, H., Zimmermann, L. & Braun, V. (1988). Genetics of the iron dicitrate transport system in *Escherichia coli*. *Journal of Bacteriology*, **170**, 2716–24.

Rabsch, R. & Reissbrodt, W. (1988). Further differentiation of Entero-bacteriaceae by means of siderophore pattern analysis. *Zentralblatt für Bakteriologie und Hygiene A*, **268**, 306–17.

Raymond, K. N. & Carrano, C. J. (1979). Co-ordination chemistry of microbial iron transport. *Accounts of Chemical Research*, **12**, 183–90.

Reid, R. T., Live, D. H., Faulkner, D. J. & Butler, A. (1993). A siderophore from a marine bacterium with an exceptional ferric ion affinity constant. *Nature*, **366**, 455–8.

Roberts, M., Partha Sarathy, S., Lam-Po-Tang, M. K. L. & Williams, P. H. (1986). The aerobactin iron uptake system in enteropathogenic *Escherichia coli*: evidence for an extinct transposon. *FEMS Microbiology Letters*, **37**, 215–19.

Roberts, M., Wooldridge, K. G., Garine, H., Kuswandi, S. I. & Williams, P. H. (1989). Inhibition of biological activities of the aerobactin receptor protein in rough strains of *Escherichia coli* by polyclonal antiserum raised against native protein. *Journal of General Microbiology*, **135**, 2387–98.

Rogers, H. J. (1973). Iron-binding catechols and virulence in *Escherichia coli*. *Infection and Immunity*, **7**, 445–56.

Rogers, H. J. (1983). Role of iron chelators, antibodies and iron-binding proteins in infection. In *Microbiology 1983*, ed. D. Slessinger, pp. 334–37, Washington DC: American Society for Microbiology.

Rogers, H. J., Synge, C., Kimber, B. & Bayley, P. M. (1977). Production of enterochelin by *Escherichia coli* O111. *Biochimica et Biophysica Acta*, **497**, 548–57.

Rosenberg, H. & Young, I. G. (1974). Iron transport in the enteric bacteria, In *Microbial Iron Metabolism*, ed. J. B. Neilands, pp. 67–82, New York: Academic Press.

Rusnak, F., Faraci, W. S. & Walsh, C. T. (1989). Subcloning, expression and purification of the enterobactin biosynthetic enzyme 2,3-dihydroxy-benzoate–AMP ligase: demonstration of enzyme-bound (2,3-dihydroxy-benzoyl) adenylate product. *Biochemistry*, **28**, 6827–35.

Rusnak, F., Liu, J., Quinn, N., Berchtold, G. A. & Walsh, C. T. (1990). Sub-cloning of the enterobactin biosynthetic gene *ent* B: expression, puri-fication, characterization and substrate specificity of isochorismatase. *Biochemistry*, **29**, 1425–35.

Rutz, J. M., Liu, J., Lyons, J. A., Goranson, J., Armstrong, S. K., McIntosh, M. A., Feix, J. B. & Klebba, P. E. (1992). Formation of a gated channel by a ligand-specific transport protein in the bacterial outer membrane. *Science*, **258**, 471–5.

Schmitt, M. P. & Payne, S. M. (1988). Genetics and regulation of enterobactin genes in *Shigella flexneri*. *Journal of Bacteriology*, **170**, 5579–87.

Shand, G. H., Anwar, H., Kadurugamuwa, J., Brown, M. R. W., Silverman, S. H. & Melling, J. (1985). *In vivo* evidence that bacteria in urinary tract infection grow under iron-restricted conditions. *Infection and Immunity*, **48**, 35–9.

Shea, C. M. & McIntosh, M. A. (1991). Nucleotide sequence and genetic organization of the ferric enterobactin transport system: homology to other periplasmic binding protein-dependent systems in *Escherichia coli*. *Molecular Microbiology*, **5**, 1415–28.

Skare, J. T., Ahmer, B. M. M., Seachord, C. L., Darveau, R. P. & Postle, K. (1993). Energy transduction between membranes: Ton B, a cytoplasmic membrane protein, can be chemically cross-linked *in vivo* to outer membrane receptor Fep A. *Journal of Biological Chemistry*, **268**, 16302–8.

Smith, A. (1990). Transport of tetrapyrroles: mechanisms and biological and regulatory consequences. In *Biosynthesis and Metabolism of Heme and Chlorophyll*, ed. H. A. Dailey, pp. 435–89, New York: McGraw Hill.

Smith, H. W. & Huggins, M. B. (1980). The association of the O18K1 and H7 antigens and the Col V plasmid of a strain of *Escherichia coli* with its virulence and immunogenicity. *Journal of General Microbiology*, **121**, 387–400.

Smith, H. W. & Linggood, M. A. (1971). Observations on the pathogenic properties of the K88, Hly and Ent plasmids of *Escherichia coli* with particular reference to porcine diarrhoea. *Journal of Medical Microbiology*, **4**, 467–85.

Smith, H. W., Parsell, Z. & Green, P. (1978). Thermosensitive H1 plasmids determining citrate utilization. *Journal of General Microbiology*, **109**, 305–11.

Stoebner, J. A. & Payne, S. M. (1988). Iron-regulated hemolysin production and utilization of heme and hemoglobin by *Vibrio cholerae*. *Infection and Immunity*, **56**, 2891–5.

Stojiljkovic, I., Bäumler, A. J. & Hantke, K. (1994). Fur Regulon in Gram-negative bacteria: identification and characterization of new iron-regulated *Escherichia coli* genes by a Fur titration assay. *Journal of Molecular Biology*, **236**, 531–45.

Tidmarsh, G. F. & Rosenberg, L. T. (1981). Acquisition of iron from transferrin by *Salmonella paratyphi* B. *Current Microbiology*, **6**, 217–20.

Todhunter, D. A., Smith K. L. & Hogan, J. S. (1991). Antibodies to iron-regulated outer membrane proteins of coliform bacteria isolated from bovine intramammary infections. *Veterinary Immunology and Immunopathology*, **28**, 107–15.

Valvano, M. A. & Crosa, J. H. (1984). Aerobactin iron transport genes commonly encoded by certain Col V plasmids occur in the chromosome of a human invasive strain of *Escherichia coli* K1. *Infection and Immunity*, **46**, 159–67.

Valvano, M. A., Silver, R. P. & Crosa, J. H. (1986). Occurrence of chromosome–or plasmid-mediated aerobactin iron transport systems and hemolysin production among clonal groups of human invasive strains of *Escherichia coli* K1. *Infection and Immunity*, **52**, 192–9.

Van den Bosch, J. F., de Graaf, F. & MacLaren, D. M. (1979). Virulence of *Escherichia coli* in experimental hematogenous pyelonephritis in mice. *Infection and Immunity*, **25**, 68–74.

Van den Bosch, J. F., Postma, P., de Graaf, F. & MacLaren, D. M. (1981). Haemolysis by urinary *Escherichia coli* and virulence in mice. *Journal of Medical Microbiology*, **14**, 321–31.

Van Heyningen, W. E. & Gladstone, G. P. (1953). The neurotoxin of *Shigella shigae* 3. The effect of iron on production of the toxin. *British Journal of Experimental Pathology*, **34**, 221–9.

Van Hove, B., Staudenmaier, H. & Braun, V. (1990). Novel two-component transmembrane transcription control: regulation of iron dicitrate transport in *Escherichia coli* K12. *Journal of Bacteriology*, **172**, 6749–58.

Waalwijk, C., MacLaren, D. M. & de Graaf, J. (1983). *In vivo* function of hemolysin in the nephropathogenicity of *Escherichia coli*. *Infection and Immunity*, **42**, 245–9.

Wagegg, W. & Braun, V. (1981). Ferric citrate transport in *Escherichia coli* requires outer membrane receptor protein Fec A. *Journal of Bacteriology*, **145**, 156–63.

Watanabe, N. A., Nagasu, T., Katsu, K. & Kitoh, K. (1987). E-0702, a new cephalosporin, is incorporated into *Escherichia coli* cells via the *ton* B-dependent iron transport system. *Antimicrobial Agents and Chemotherapy*, **31**, 497–504.

Waters, V. L. & Crosa, J. H. (1986). DNA environment of the aerobactin iron uptake system genes in prototypic Col V plasmids. *Journal of Bacteriology*, **167**, 647–54.

Weinberg, E. D. (1989). Cellular regulation of iron assimilation. *Quarterly Review of Biology*, **64**, 261–90.

Williams, P. & Griffiths, E. (1992). Bacterial transferrin receptors – structure, function and contribution to virulence. *Medical Microbiology and Immunology*, **181**, 301–22.

Williams, P. H. (1979). Novel iron uptake system specified by Col V plasmids: an important component in the virulence of invasive strains of *Escherichia coli*. *Infection and Immunity*, **26**, 925–32.

Williams, P. H. & Warner, P. J. (1980). Col V-plasmid-mediated, Colicin V-independent iron uptake system of invasive strains of *Escherichia coli*. *Infection and Immunity*, **29**, 411–16.

Wong, J. C. Y., Holland, J., Parsons, T., Smith, A. & Williams, P. (1994). Identification and characterization of an iron-regulated hemopexin receptor in *Haemophilus influenzae* type b. *Infection and Immunity*, **62**, 48–59.

Woodrow, G. C., Langman, L., Young, I. G. & Gibson, F. (1978). Mutations affecting the citrate-dependent iron uptake systems in *Escherichia coli*. *Journal of Bacteriology*, **133**, 1524–6.

Wooldridge, K. G. & Williams, P. H. (1993). Iron uptake mechanisms of pathogenic bacteria. *FEMS Microbiology Reviews*, **12**, 325–48.

Yancey, R. J., Breeding, S. A. L. & Lankford, C. E. (1979). Enterochelin (enterobactin): virulence factor for *Salmonella typhimurium*. *Infection and Immunity*, **24**, 174–80.

Yanofsky, C. (1981). Attenuation in the control of expression of bacterial operons. *Nature*, **289**, 751–8.

Young, I. G., Langman, L., Luke, R. K. J. & Gibson, F. (1971). Biosynthesis of the iron transport compound enterochelin: mutants of *Escherichia coli* unable to synthesize 2,3-dihydroxy-benzoate. *Journal of Bacteriology*, **106**, 51–7.

Zimmermann, L., Hantke, K. & Braun, V. (1984). Exogenous induction of the iron dicitrate transport system of *Escherichia coli* K12. *Journal of Bacteriology*, **159**, 271–7.

13

Co-ordinate regulation of virulence gene expression in *Escherichia coli*

C. J. DORMAN and N. NÍ BHRIAIN

The interaction between a bacterium and its host during infection imposes many environmental stresses on the micro-organism to which it must adapt if it is to survive. Since *Escherichia coli* is clearly very successful at such adaptations, it must possess mechanisms that enable it to interpret its surroundings and to mount an appropriate and co-ordinated response. Most of the information available about environmental adaptation by *E. coli* comes from research with *E. coli* K12, which is a non-pathogen. Nevertheless, the insights gained from studies with this organism are highly relevant to pathogenic forms of this species.

Environmental sensing and response

Escherichia coli appears to sense its surroundings to be composed of a series of 'physical' signals, such as temperature and osmotic pressure, and 'chemical' signals, such as the presence or absence of iron and carbon sources. Changes in these signals call for specific responses, which usually require changes in gene expression. This implies a link between the environmental sensing systems and the bacterial genome. Intensive research in recent years has uncovered the mechanisms by which some of these sensing and response links operate. In the case of a response to a chemical change, such as the presence or absence of a particular ligand, the bacterium frequently employs a specific DNA-binding protein that binds the same ligand. Ligand binding alters the ability of the protein to bind to DNA, and this can result in either activation or repression of transcription. Such proteins recognise and bind to specific DNA sequences and can, in this way, regulate transcription of all genes that possess the same DNA sequence in their promoter regions. Such a group of co-regulated genes is called a *regulon* and expression of its members is

373

co-ordinately controlled in response to the presence or absence of the cognate ligand.

When a physical change to the environment takes place, such as an alteration in osmolarity, another form of sensing and response may be employed. In this case the change in the physical parameter is detected by the periplasmic domain of a sensor protein located in the bacterial inner membrane. This protein is a kinase and in response to the signal it undergoes autophosphorylation. The phosphate group is then transferred to a DNA-binding protein located in the cytoplasm. Transcription of certain genes will depend on whether or not the DNA-binding protein is phosphorylated. In this case, the environmental signal does not directly alter the DNA-binding activity of the regulatory protein. Rather, it acts through an intermediate sensor protein, the kinase. This type of sensing and response system is referred to as a 'two-component' system. Once again, the genes of the response system possess characteristic binding sites for the regulatory protein close to their promoters making all the co-regulated genes members of a regulon.

Sensing and response systems for chemical or physical signals cannot be broken down into neat groups simply on the basis of mechanism. For example, in many virulence systems of enteric bacteria, response to temperature changes (a physical stimulus) involves gene activation by a DNA-binding protein that has no kinase partner. Conversely, response to nitrogen starvation (a chemical response) involves a 'two-component' protein kinase/DNA-binding-protein partnership. Furthermore, a particular stimulus can effect a response by more than one route and a particular gene or operon can be affected by more than one stimulus (see below). The sensing and response system of the cell is therefore complex, but this is not surprising because the environment is also complex. This complexity means that bacteria rarely encounter environmental signals one at a time. Instead, they face multiple challenges simultaneously and must respond to each appropriately if the organism is to survive. To meet this challenge successfully calls for co-ordination of the response systems.

Co-ordination of response systems

Bacteria appear to have solved the problem of co-ordinating their environmental response systems by employing multiple regulators in a hierarchical manner. Each system possesses its specific regulator, which may be shared with other genes or operons that contribute to the same response (Table 13.1). In addition, different response systems may be co-

Table 13.1. *Operons and regulators discussed in the text*

Operon	Product	Regulator	Regulator type
cfa/I	CFA/I adhesin	CfaD	AraC-like transcription factor
		H-NS	DNA curve binding protein
cfa/II	CS1 CS2 adhesin	Rns	AraC-like transcription factor
csgA	Curli adhesin	Crl	*Trans*-acting transcription factor
		H-NS	DNA curve binding protein
		RpoS	Stationary phase sigma factor
eae	Intimin	Per	AraC-like transcription factor
fan	K99 adhesin	FanA	Transcription regulator
		FanB	Transcription regulator
		Lrp	DNA-bending protein
fap	987P adhesin	FapR	AraC-like transcription factor
fim	Type-1 fimbriae	FimB	Site-specific recombinase
		FimE	Site-specific recombinase
		H-NS	DNA curve binding protein
		IHF	DNA-bending protein
		Lrp	DNA-bending protein
hly	α-haemolysin	*hlyR*	*Cis*-acting regulatory sequence
		Hha	Histone-like protein
		Transcription antitermination	Allows full-length *hlyCABD* transcription
ipa	Invasion protein	VirF	AraC-like transcription factor
		VirB	Transcription factor
		H-NS	DNA curve binding protein
		Topo I	Type-1 DNA topoisomerase
ompB	EnvZ/OmpR	IHF	DNA-bending protein
		cAMP–CRP	DNA-bending complex
ompC ompF	Porins	EnvZ	Histidine protein kinase
		OmpR	Transcription factor
		IHF	DNA-bending protein
		cAMP–CRP	DNA-bending complex (via *ompB*)
pap	Pap adhesin	PapB	Transcription regulator
		PapI	Transcription regulator
		H-NS	DNA curve binding protein
		Lrp	DNA-bending protein
		Dam	DNA methylase
		cAMP–CRP	DNA-bending complex
slt	Shiga-like toxin	Fur	Iron regulatory protein

Table 13.2. *Proteins of* Escherichia coli *discussed in the text that alter the topology of DNA*

Protein	Structure	Subunit molecular weight (kDa)	Function	Gene (map location in minutes)
Topo I	α	97	Type-I topoisomerase	*opA* (28)
Topo II (gyrase)	$\alpha_2\beta_2$	97 (α) 90 (β)	Type-2 topoisomerase	*gyrA* (α; 48.3) *gyrB* (β; 83.5)
Topo III	α	73.2	Type-1 topoisomerase	*topB* (38.7)
Topo IV	$\alpha_2\beta_2$	75 (α) 66.8 (β)	Type-2 topoisomerase	*parC* (α; 65.6) *parE* (β; 66)
Hha	?	8.6	Histone-like protein	*hha* (10.3)
H-NS	α_2	11.2	DNA curve binding	*hns* (27.5)
IHF	αβ	11.2 (α) 10.5(β)	DNA bending	*himA* (α; 37.5) *himD* (β; 20.3)
Lrp	α_2	18.8	DNA bending	*lrp* (19.6)

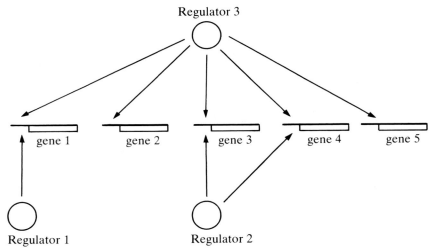

Fig. 13.1. Co-ordinated regulation of transcription. Five idealised and unlinked structural genes are shown. Gene 1 is controlled by regulator 1, which is specific to it. It is also controlled by the highly pleiotropic regulator 3, which also regulates genes 2, 3, 4 and 5. Regulator 2 affects only genes 3 and 4. The three notional regulators may be ranked according to the extent of their influence on structural gene transcription. Regulator 3 is the most pleiotropic, affecting transcription of all five structural genes; regulator 2 is of intermediate rank, affecting genes 3 and 4; regulator 1 is specific to gene 1 and so ranks below regulator 2. The regulators also network expression of the structural genes; potentially, each regulator may alter transcription in response to a different environmental stimulus.

regulated by proteins with much more wide-ranging effects on gene expression (Figure 13.1). These may affect the transcription of genes that contribute to unrelated functions, so as to allow their expression to be regulated by a network of control systems. Some pleiotropic regulators are structurally very distinct from the specific regulatory proteins. Many are concerned with the organisation of the nucleoprotein complex of the bacterial genome and have secondary roles as gene regulators (Table 13.2). These are very important proteins whose contributions to the co-ordination of gene expression, particularly virulence gene expression, have only recently come to be appreciated.

Classical regulators

Truly satisfactory classifications for gene regulators are difficult to establish because of the number of exceptions that inevitably arise whenever an attempt is made to determine rules for nomenclature. In the following sections of this chapter, regulators will be considered in two groups. Firstly, the system-specific regulators that alter transcription in response to particular signals, such as a change in iron levels, cAMP concentration, osmotic pressure, temperature or growth phase will be considered. The second group comprises transcription regulators that operate mainly by altering DNA topology. This division into two groups is not entirely satisfactory; it will be seen that some 'classical' regulators (such as cAMP-CRP, or cAMP catabolite repression protein) also alter DNA topology.

The system-specific regulators of the first group are generally proteins that bind to operator-like sequences associated with the transcription initiation sites of their subservient genes. Changes in the specific environmental parameter sensed by the protein will alter its conformation, resulting in a change in its ability to bind to DNA or to interact with other proteins on DNA.

The system-specific regulators can be subdivided into four subgroups: (i) proteins that alter transcription upon binding a specific small co-effector molecule, (ii) proteins related to the AraC DNA-binding protein of the arabinose utilisation operon, but which alter gene expression in response to changes in temperature rather than the presence of a carbohydrate co-effector molecule; (iii) proteins of the 'two-component' histidine protein kinase/response regulator family, in which the activity of the DNA-binding protein, or response regulator, is modulated by phospho-transfer from the kinase partner; and (iv) proteins that are alternative sigma factors, capable of reprogramming RNA polymerase and directing it to initiate transcription from 'non-standard' promoters in response to particular environmental signals.

Fur protein and iron regulation

The Fur (ferric uptake regulation) protein of *E. coli* is specifically concerned with the regulation of the iron starvation response. It is a 17-kDa DNA-binding protein that acts as a transcriptional repressor of the iron assimilation pathway genes (Hantke, 1981; 1987; Schäffer *et al.*, 1985; Hantke, 1987). The DNA-binding domain of Fur lies within the amino-terminus and its function is modulated by binding ferrous iron (Fe^{2+}) within a pocket at the carboxyl-terminus (Coy & Neilands, 1991; Saito & Williams, 1991). In the absence of Fe^{2+}, Fur dissociates from the DNA and transcription of iron assimilation genes is activated, so allowing *E. coli* to acquire iron from the environment. In the presence of iron the protein binds to its operator sequence, which is known as the 'iron box' and is located at the promoter of Fur-regulated genes (Calderwood & Mekalanos, 1987; De Lorenzo *et al.*, 1987). This results in repression of transcription (see Chapter 12).

Apart from its house-keeping functions concerned with iron metabolism, Fur plays a role in controlling transcription of virulence genes in *E. coli*. An example is the Fur-mediated repression of Shiga-like toxin (Slt) gene transcription in the presence of high levels of iron (Table 13.1). This two-subunit toxin is elaborated by *E. coli* strains that cause diseases such as haemorrhagic colitis and it is structurally closely related to the Shiga toxin of *Shigella dysenteriae* type 1. Two toxin genes *sltA* and *sltB* are involved, organised as an operon and carried by a bacteriophage (Calderwood *et al.*, 1987; Jackson *et al.*, 1987). The *sltAB* operon is under the control of Fur acting through an 'iron box' at the promoter. Transcription is triggered by iron starvation (Calderwood & Mekalanos, 1987). This is believed to be because expression of the toxin results in host tissue damage accompanied by release of nutrients, including iron.

The cAMP–CRP system

The cAMP catabolite repression protein (CRP) regulates gene expression in response to intracellular cAMP levels, which are themselves modulated by the nature of the carbon sources available to the organism (Magasanik & Neidhardt, 1987). When CRP binds cAMP, it becomes proficient at binding to specific sequences in DNA. These are associated with the promoters of CRP-regulated genes and the effect of cAMP–CRP binding is generally to activate transcription. This is achieved by making physical contacts with RNA polymerase to allow the latter to promote open complex formation at the promoter. Since CRP is a DNA-bending protein, its action on transcription also involves a change in DNA structure. This bending of the DNA helix is believed to assist in transcription activation. In some instances, cAMP–CRP acts as a transcriptional repressor, but such cases are rare (Botsford & Harman, 1992).

The classical examples of cAMP–CRP in the activation of transcription are the promoters of the *lac* operon and the *mal* regulon, which are concerned respectively with the uptake and utilisation of the carbon sources lactose and maltose. Much of the current understanding of how this protein controls transcription comes from studies of these systems and of the galactose utilisation operon, *gal* (Botsford & Harman, 1992). The contribution of cAMP–CRP to the control of bacterial virulence has recently come to be appreciated. For example, in uropathogenic strains of *E. coli,* it contributes to the regulation of the *pap* operon which codes for P-pili adhesins (Forsman *et al.* 1989; see below) (Table 13.1). Further evidence for its role in virulence comes from work with the enteric pathogen *Salmonella typhimurium.* In this case, mutations that inactivate cAMP–CRP expression render the organism avirulent in mice (Curtiss & Kelly, 1987).

Leucine-responsive regulatory protein

The leucine-responsive regulatory protein, Lrp, regulates the expression of a large number of genes in *E. coli* (Calvo & Matthews, 1994) (Table 13.2). Unlike histone-like protein (H-NS), which usually has a negative effect on transcription, Lrp represses some genes but activates others. In many cases, the action of Lrp on particular genes is modulated by leucine. The protein is a homodimer composed of 18.8-kDa subunits and is present in *E. coli* K12 at approximately 3000 molecules per cell (Willins *et al.*, 1991). It consists of three domains, an amino-terminal domain concerned with DNA binding via a helix-turn-helix motif, a central domain concerned with transcriptional regulation and a carboxyl-terminal domain that is required for interaction with leucine (Platko & Calvo, 1993). With the *E. coli ilvIH* promoter as a model system, Wang & Calvo (1993) showed that the binding of Lrp to DNA produces bends in the helix and that the resulting nucleoprotein structure probably contributes to the effects of Lrp on transcription.

The Lrp protein regulates transcription of the *pap* operon in uropathogenic *E. coli* (Fig. 13.5) (see Chapter 8). Transcription of this operon is under phase-variable control. This means that individual bacteria within the population either express (phase ON) or do not express (phase OFF) Pap fimbriae. Switching between these two states is controlled at the level of transcription by Dam methylation at two 5'-GATC-3' sites in the *papI–papB* intergenic region. These sites are called $GATC_{1028}$ and $GATC_{1130}$ from their locations in the regulatory region (Blyn *et al.*, 1990). Transcription of the *pap* genes is regulated in part by the differential protection of these sites from Dam methylation. In phase ON cells, $GATC_{1028}$ is unmethylated, while in phase OFF cells, $GATC_{1130}$ is unmethylated. Protection of $GATC_{1130}$ against methylation requires the Mbf (Methylation blocking factor) protein, while protection of $GATC_{1028}$ requires both Mbf and the *pap*-operon-encoded PapI regulatory protein (Braaten *et al.*, 1991). The Mbf protein is now known to be Lrp. Methylation of $GATC_{1028}$ inhibits binding of Lrp/PapI at this site and alters binding of Lrp at $GATC_{1130}$ (Braaten *et al.*, 1992). Thus, the regulatory mechanism is founded on the competition between Lrp/PapI and Dam methylase for binding near $GATC_{1028}$ and the methylation/non-methylation of this site, which regulates *pap* transcription (Nou *et al.*, 1993) (Figure 13.5). The *pap* operon is one of the Lrp-dependent operons that is not affected by leucine (Braaten *et al.*, 1992).

The *fan* operon of ETEC encodes the K-99 fimbriae that mediate attachment of ETEC to the small intestine of lambs, calves and piglets (De Graaf, 1988) (Table 13.1). Expression of the *fan* operon is regulated positively by Lrp. Mutations in *lrp* result in a 70-fold reduction in transcription of *fanC*, the pilus subunit gene (Braaten *et al.*, 1992). The expression of *fan* is leucine sensitive. Addition of L-leucine or L-alanine to the growth medium represses expression of K99-pili by 25- to 50-fold, an effect that is, at least in part, caused by a repression of *fan* transcription (Braaten *et al.*, 1992). The *fan* operon does not appear to undergo phase variation and no 5'-GATC-3' sequences are found within the *fan* regulatory region (Van der Woude *et al.*, 1992). This suggests that the mechanism by which Lrp regulates *fan* is different from that by which it controls *pap*.

Type-1 fimbriae are a third category of *E. coli* adhesive fimbriae whose expression is regulated by Lrp (Figure 13.5; Table 13.1). In this case, Lrp exerts its major effect on the site-specific recombination system that controls the orientation of the invertible promoter fragment. In *lrp* mutants, the rate of inversion of this fragment is reduced (Blomfield *et al.*, 1993).

AraC-like regulators

The arabinose utilisation systems of enteric bacteria, including *E. coli,* are regulated by the DNA-binding protein AraC (Schleif, 1987), which has two domains. The first, in the amino-terminal part of the protein, is concerned with binding arabinose and the second, in the carboxyl-terminal part of the protein, is concerned with binding to a specific DNA sequence that is found in a reiterated form in the regulatory region of the *ara* operon (Brunelle & Schleif, 1989). The ability of AraC to bind DNA is modulated by conformational changes that result from arabinose binding within the amino-terminal domain. This is analogous to the effect of Fe^{2+} on the DNA-binding ability of Fur. AraC is now recognised as a prototypic member of a family of DNA-binding proteins that share significant amino-acid sequence homology at their carboxyl-terminal domains (Gallegos *et al.*, 1993). Thus, it is probable that these molecules interact with DNA in a similar manner. The AraC family members can be divided into two classes; one consists of proteins that regulate gene expression in response to carbohydrate molecules, while the other are proteins that regulate virulence gene expression (Gallegos *et al.*, 1993) (Figure 13.2). Members of the latter class are usually encoded by plasmid-linked genes.

In *E. coli,* at least four virulence systems are regulated by AraC-like proteins at the transcriptional level. Firstly, enterotoxigenic *E. coli* (ETEC) strains synthesise plasmid-encoded fimbrial antigens, such as colonisation factor I (CFA/I) and colonisation factor II (CFA/II). CFA/II is composed of three distinct 'coli surface' (CS) antigens, CS1, CS2 and CS3. Transcription of the genes that code for CS1 and CS2 is positively regulated in response to temperature by the plasmid-encoded protein, Rns (Caron *et al.*, 1989) (Figure 13.2). This regulatory protein is a member of the AraC family. Expression of CFA/I is also regulated in response to temperature. Here, a plasmid-encoded AraC-like protein, CfaD, acts as a positive transcription regulator. CfaD and Rns are very closely related and can functionally substitute for one another (Savelkoul *et al.*, 1990) (Figure 13.2).

Secondly, enteroinvasive strains of *E. coli* (EIEC) possess a plasmid-encoded virulence gene regulon that is transcriptionally activated in response to temperature. This virulence system is closely related to that of the enteroinvasive pathogen, *Shigella flexneri* (Hale, 1991; see Chapter 16). The detail of thermal activation of the invasion genes has been worked out in *Sh. flexneri* and similar events are believed to occur in

```
E. coli AraC     196  DIASVAQHVCLSPSRLSHLFRQQLGISVLSWREDQRISQAKLLLSTRMPIATVGRNVGFDDQLYFSRVFKKCTGASPSEFRAGCEEKVNDVAVKLS

E. coli Rns      178  WTLGIIASAFNASEITIRKRLESENTNFNQILMQLRMSKAALLLENSYQISQISNMIGISSASYFIRIFNKHYGVTPKQFFTYFKGG

E. coli CfaD     178  WTLGIIADAFNVSEITIRKRLESENTNFNQILMQLRMSKAALLLENSYQISQISNMIGISSASYFIRVFNKHYGVTPKQFFTYFKGG

Sh. flexneri VirF 175  WRLSSISNNLNLSEIAVRKRLESEKLTFQQILLDIRMHHAAKLLLNSNSYINDVSRLLIGISSPSYFIRKFNEYGITPKKFVLYHKKF

E. coli EnvY     162  WNLRIVASSLCLSPSLLKKKLKNENTSYSQIVTECRMRYAVQMLLMDNKNITQVAQLCGYSSTSYFISVFKAFYGLTPLNYLAKQRQKVMW

E. coli FapR     168  WKLSDIAEEMHISEISVRKRLEQECLNFNQLILDVRLMKARHLLRHSEASVTDIAYRCGFSDSNHFSTLFRREFNWSPKKFEIGIKENLRCNR

Consensus             W L IA    SEI RKRLE E  F  QI    RM A LLL    I        G SS SYFIR F  YG TPK F   K
```

Fig. 13.2. An alignment of the amino-acid sequences of the carboxyl-terminal domains of those members of the AaC family of transcriptional regulators discussed in Chapter 13. Residues in the consenses sequence occur at that position in at least four of the six polypeptides shown. Alignments are based on those in Gallegos *et al.* (1993).

EIEC (Dagberg & Uhlin, 1992). A primary regulatory protein, VirF, activates transcription of the gene that codes for a secondary regulatory protein, VirB, in response to an increase in growth temperature. VirF is a member of the AraC family (Dorman, 1992) (Figure 13.2). The secondary regulator, VirB, is also a DNA-binding protein, which activates transcription of the structural genes that code for the virulence factors. VirF activates at least one structural gene (*virG*) directly, showing that the regulatory cascade in which VirF activates *virB* is not shared by all of the virulence genes on the plasmid (Adler *et al.*, 1989; Tobe *et al.*, 1991).

Thirdly, expression of the 987P fimbrial adhesin in ETEC is subject to complex regulation. This adhesin, which is required for attachment to the brush border cells of the pig intestine, is produced in association with heat-stable enterotoxin (ST_{pa}). The genes that code for the toxin are part of a transposon called Tn*1681*. When this mobile genetic element inserts near the 987P genes, it activates transcription of a fimbrial regulatory gene, *fapR*. The latter gene codes for an AraC-like protein (FapR), which activates transcription of the structural genes that code for 987P-fimbriae (Figure 13.2). This activation may also occur in response to environmental signals (Klaasen & De Graaf, 1990; Klaasen *et al.*, 1990).

Finally, the *eae* locus on the chromosome of enteropathogenic *E. coli* (EPEC) strains encodes a 94-kDa outer-membrane protein, intimin, that is required for the attachment and effacement phenotype associated with the pathogenicity of these organisms (see Chapter 14). It is also found on the chromosomes of enterohaemorrhagic *E. coli* (EHEC) strains (Donnenberg & Kaper, 1992). Intimin shows homology with the invasin proteins of *Yersinia enterocolitica* and *Y. pseudotuberculosis* that promote invasion by binding to integrin receptors on host epithelial cells (Isberg & Leong, 1990). Expression of intimin in EPEC is enhanced by the presence of a plasmid known as EAF (Jerse & Kaper, 1991). This harbours the *per* gene, which codes for a *trans*-acting regulatory protein, Per. This molecule displays homology with the AraC family members, particularly with protein EnvY, which is a thermoregulator of porin gene expression in *E. coli* K12 (Lundgrigan & Earhardt, 1984; Lundrigan *et al.*, 1989; Klaasen & De Graaf, 1990; Donnenberg & Kaper, 1992). (Figure 13.2). Presumably, Per activates gene expression in response to signals from the environment.

The EnvZ/OmpR histidine protein kinase/response regulator system

The *ompB* operon of *E. coli* codes for the regulatory proteins OmpR and EnvZ (Bachmann, 1990). Counterparts of this system occur in other enteric bacteria (see below). These are prototypic members of a class of bacterial regulators known as 'two-component systems'. Such systems are composed of a sensor partner, a histidine protein kinase, and a response regulator, which is often, but not always, a DNA-binding protein (Stock *et al.*, 1989). The sensor protein detects one or more specific environmental signals and transmits this signal, via the response regulator, to the response apparatus, usually the genome. The response regulator may, however, receive signals from kinases other than its dedicated partner. This phenomenon is known as 'cross-talk' and has

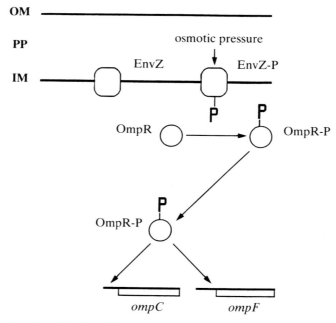

Fig. 13.3. The EnvZ/OmpR two-component regulatory system. Osmotic pressure in the periplasm results in autophosphorylation of the cytoplasmic domain of EnvZ. Phospho-transfer to OmpR activates this protein for DNA binding. Phospho–OmpR then induces transcription of either the *ompC* or the *ompF* porin genes, depending on the cytoplasmic concentration of phospho–OmpR (see the section on the EnvZ/OmpR system in the text). IM, inner membrane; OM, outer membrane; PP, periplasm.

been shown to occur in several of the best studied 'two-component' systems (Wanner, 1992).

EnvZ, a 50-kDa histidine protein kinase, is associated with the cytoplasmic membrane and possesses periplasmic and cytoplasmic domains. OmpR is a 27-kDa DNA-binding protein that regulates transcription of the genes that code for the OmpC and OmpF outer-membrane porin proteins (Stock *et al.*, 1989) (Figure 13.3). EnvZ is concerned primarily with sensing changes in the osmotic pressure of the periplasm. Increases in osmolarity induce autophosphorylation of EnvZ on His-243 within its cytoplasmic domain. Phospho-transfer to OmpR allows this protein to bind DNA (Figure 13.3). At high osmolarity, the level of phospho–OmpR in the cell is high, while at low osmolarity phospho-OmpR levels are low. The OmpC porin is expressed preferentially at high osmolarity. Its gene has low-affinity binding sites for phospho–OmpR in its promoter region. When this form of the OmpR protein is in low abundance, that is at low osmolarity, transcription of *ompC* is precluded. The OmpF porin is expressed preferentially at low osmolarity. The *ompF* gene possesses high-affinity sites for phospho–OmpR. These sites are organised so that, when occupied, the gene is activated and this happens at low osmolarity. The *ompF* gene also has alternative, low-affinity binding sites for phospho–OmpR. When these sites are also occupied, at high osmolarity, the gene is repressed. In this way, the cell expresses OmpF and OmpC porins in a reciprocal manner. Their regulation is fine-tuned by several other regulatory inputs (Stock *et al.*, 1989; Dorman & Ní Bhriain, 1992). Direct evidence that EnvZ/OmpR contributes to *E. coli* virulence is lacking, but it is required for virulence in other enteric bacteria, including *Sh. flexneri*. In the latter, mutations in *envZ* disrupt normal regulation of invasion gene expression (Bernardini *et al.*, 1990). It is, therefore, highly likely to have a similar role in EIEC. EnvZ/OmpR is also required for mouse virulence in *Salmonella typhimurium* (Dorman *et al.*, 1989). Here, the EnvZ/OmpR-dependent genes that code for OmpC and OmpF are involved, but additional and as yet unidentified EnvZ/OmpR-regulated genes also seem to be required for full mouse virulence (Chatfield *et al.*, 1991).

RpoS, an alternative sigma factor

Escherichia coli possesses several sigma factors that can displace the 'vegetative' sigma factor, RpoD, and redirect RNA polymerase to initiate transcription at non-standard promoters. Alternative sigma factors that activate transcription in response to heat shock (RpoH), nitrogen starvation (RpoN) and the onset of stationary phase (RpoS) have been described. RpoS is required for stationary phase expression of, among others, HPII catalase, which is encoded by *katE*, exonuclease III, which is encoded by *xthA* and plays an important part in the repair of oxidatively damaged DNA, and the morphogene *bolA* whose product contributes to the determination of the shape of *E. coli* cells in stationary phase (Demple *et al.*, 1986; Aldea *et al.*, 1989; Mulvey & Loewen, 1989; Bohannon *et al.*, 1991; Lange & Hengge-Aronis, 1991; Tanaka *et al.*, 1993). The RpoS sigma factor is required for virulence gene expression in enteric bacteria. In fibronectin- and lamin-binding strains of *E. coli*, it contributes to the positive control of curli adhesin gene expression (Olsén *et al.*, 1993) (Table 13.1; see below). Recently, awareness has developed that the stationary phase of growth is particularly relevant to studies aimed at understanding bacterial behaviour during infection. Presumably, this stressful physiological state includes many of the stimlui encountered by organisms when they interact with the host *in vivo*. The observation that RpoS makes a central contribution to stationary phase adaptation and is required for the expression of at least some virulence genes makes it possible to appreciate more fully the molecular events that occur during virulence gene activation.

Regulators of DNA topology

Recent research has highlighted the importance of non-classical regulators of transcription in the control of virulence genes. Many of these are proteins that affect the topology of bacterial DNA (Dorman & Ní Bhriain, 1993). These proteins can be divided into two groups, namely catalytic proteins, called topoisomerases, that alter the topology of DNA by breaking and rejoining the helix (Drlica, 1990) and architectural proteins that alter local DNA structure (Drlica & Rouvière-Yaniv, 1987) (Table 13.2). Both groups of proteins have been studied intensively in *E. coli* and are reviewed here briefly in terms of their contributions to the control of virulence gene expression.

DNA topoisomerases

Escherichia coli expresses at least four different topoisomerases. The first of these, DNA gyrase, can introduce negative supercoils into DNA by a double-stranded breakage and reunion mechanism. It changes the linking number of DNA in steps of two, and is therefore classified as a type-2 enzyme; it requires ATP for this reaction. The second, DNA topoisomerase I, is a type-1 enzyme that changes the linking number of DNA in steps of one. It acts on supercoiled DNA, relaxing it by a single-stranded break-swivel-reunion mechanism; it uses the free energy stored in the supercoiled molecule to drive the reaction. The third, topoisomerase III, is a type-1 enzyme with a decatenase activity and the fourth, topoisomerase IV, is a type-2 enzyme with a decatenase activity that is required for normal segregation of daughter chromosomes after replication (Table 13.2).

The global level of supercoiling in *E. coli* DNA is set by the opposing activities of DNA gyrase and DNA topoisomerase I. However, the value at which this is set can be affected by the external environment. Thus, changes in parameters such as osmotic stress, temperature, oxygen availability, glucose levels and others can result in adjustments in the global level of DNA supercoiling. This provides the bacterium with a mechanism for resetting the superhelical density of its DNA in response to fluctuations in environmental signals. Genes required to respond to these environmental changes may be expected to have promoters whose activites are modulated by changes in DNA supercoiling. In many cases, this appears to be the case (Dorman & Ní Bhriain, 1993). Since very many virulence genes are regulated by environmental signals, it has been suggested that these genes may also have supercoiling-sensitive promoters (Dorman, 1991). This has been shown to be so in *Sh. flexneri* and can also be expected to occur in EIEC. In *Sh. flexneri,* transcription of invasion genes is regulated by temperature and osmolarity, and normal expression of these genes requires functional DNA topoisomerase I and gyrase (Dorman *et al.*, 1990; Hale, 1991; Ní Bhriain & Dorman, 1993; Tobe *et al.*, 1993; Porter & Dorman, 1994). DNA topoisomerase I is also required for normal regulation of invasion gene expression in *S. typhimurium.* Furthermore, at least one of these invasion genes possesses an osmotically sensitive promoter (Galán & Curtiss, 1990). There is now an impressive body of evidence from studies of Gram-negative and Gram-positive bacteria to support the hypothesis that many bacterial virulence genes are sensitive to changes in DNA supercoiling (Dorman & Ní Bhriain, 1993).

Histone-like proteins

The role of genome architectural proteins in virulence gene regulation has also become well-established. These proteins act on DNA in different ways to alter its topology. Some wrap the DNA into structures approximating to eukaryotic chromatin, while others bend the DNA, altering its path and influencing long-range interactions that affect gene expression. Their low molecular weight and highly basic amino-acid composition has led to the classification of these proteins as 'histone-like'. Their cellular location has led to them being referred to as 'nucleoid-associated'. Despite their general role in genome organisation, these proteins are capable of making specific contributions to the control of the expression of particular genes.

H-NS

The H-NS protein is a 15.4-kDa polypeptide that forms an integral part of *E. coli* chromatin (Table 13.2). About 20,000 copies are present per cell and it binds preferentially to curved DNA (Higgins *et al.*, 1990; Yamada *et al.*, 1991; Owen-Hughes *et al.*, 1992; Ussery *et al.*, 1994). H-NS also regulates transcription, usually negatively (Ueguchi & Mizuno, 1993). In EIEC, and *Sh. flexneri*, it acts as a repressor of invasion gene expression (Dorman *et al.*, 1990; Dagberg & Uhlin, 1992; Hromockyj *et al.*, 1992) (Figure 13.4). In uropathogenic strains of *E. coli*, it represses expression of genes that code for Pap fimbrial adhesins (Göransson *et al.*, 1990) (Figure 13.5). It also regulates the rate of the site-specific recombination event that governs transcription of the type-1 fimbrial subunit gene in *E. coli* K12 (Higgins *et al.*, 1988; Kawula & Orndorff, 1991) (Figure 13.5). Expression of the thermally regulated CFA/I adhesin is also negatively regulated by H-NS in ETEC (Figure 13.4). In the absence of H-NS, the need for the positively acting CfaD transcription factor, an AraC-like protein, is partially removed. This has been interpreted as implying that the role of the CfaD protein *in vivo* is to overcome the normal barrier to transcription activation imposed by H-NS (Jordi *et al.*, 1992). A similar role has been proposed for the AraC-like VirF protein in thermal activation of the invasion genes of EIEC (Dagberg & Uhlin, 1992).

H-NS has been shown to contribute to the control of curli expression (Figure 13.4). These are thin, coiled fibres found on the surface of fibronectin- and laminin-binding strains of *E. coli* (Olsén *et al.*, 1989; see Chapter 2). The curlin subunit protein is encoded by the *csgA* gene,

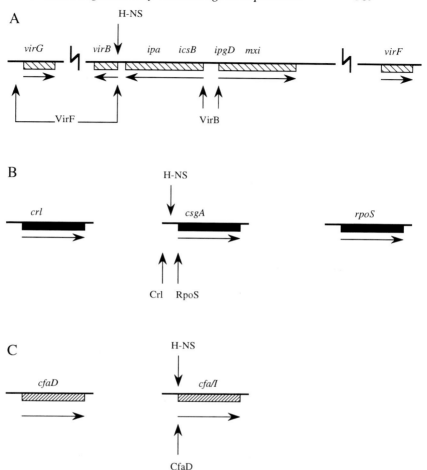

Fig. 13.4. Virulence gene regulatory systems in which histone-like protein (H-NS) plays an antagonistic role with a specific transcriptional activator. Downard-pointing vertical arrows: negative inputs; upward-pointing vertical arrows: positive inputs. (A) The invasion gene regulon of *Shigella flexneri* and enteroinvasive *Escherichia coli*. The primary regulator VirF activates *virG* and the secondary regulatory gene *virB* in response to increased temperature. VirB then activates the invasion genes (*icsBipa*) and the accessory virulence genes (*ipgDmxi*). H-NS represses transcription of *virB*. (B) Regulation of curli expression. Crl induces transcription of the *csgA* structural gene; the sigma factor RpoS is required for expression in stationary phase; H-NS regulates *csgA* transcription negatively. (C) The colonisation factor antigen I (CFA/I) system. The AraC-like protein CfaD activates transcription of the *cfa/I* structural gene; H-NS represses this gene.

which is transcriptionally activated by the *trans*-acting regulatory gene *crl* at 26°C but not at 37°C. The *crl* gene is not itself thermoregulated. In *E. coli* K12 strain HB101, the *crl* gene is absent and the *csgA* gene is cryptic. Transcriptional activation of *csgA* can be achieved by introducing *crl* (Arnqvist *et al.*, 1992) or by mutating the *hns* gene (Olsén *et al.*, 1993). This shows that H-NS regulates *csgA* negatively and suggests that curli expression may be affected by DNA topolgy. Additional indications that DNA topology may affect curli expression comes from the observations that curlin gene expression is regulated by osmolarity and by anaerobiosis (Provence & Curtiss, 1992), two environmental parameters that alter DNA topology in bacteria (see above).

Curli expression is also regulated positively by RpoS, which is the sigma factor required for stationary phase gene expression (Tanaka *et al.*, 1993) (Figure 13.4). This links their expression to other stationary-phase- and osmotic-stress-controlled genes (Hengge-Aronis, 1993; Olsén *et al.*, 1993). The function of RpoS appears to be to relieve H-NS-imposed transcriptional repression of *csgA* during the stationary growth phase (Olsén *et al.*, 1993). This antagonism is reminiscent of the proposed roles of AraC-like transcription factors, such as CfaD in *E. coli* and VirF in *Sh. flexneri* and EIEC, which relieve transcriptional repression of virulence factor genes imposed by H-NS (see above) (Figure 13.4).

Integration host factor

The integration host-factor (IHF) is a sequence-specific DNA-binding protein that interacts with the minor groove of DNA. It introduces bends of up to 140° into the helix and so dramatically alters the path of the DNA (Table 13.2). This heterodimeric protein was originally characterised as a host-encoded contributor to bacteriophage lambda integration and excision. More recently, its many roles in controlling *E. coli* gene expression have become appreciated (Friedman, 1988; Freundlich *et al.*, 1992). IHF is required for the site-specific recombination event that regulates expression of the type-1 fimbrial subunit gene (Dorman & Ní Bhriain, 1993) (Figure 13.5; Table 13.1). IHF also negatively regulates transcription of the *ompB* locus in *E. coli* (Tsui *et al.*, 1991), which was discussed above as a potential regulator of virulence gene expression in EIEC.

Hha

Hha is a 8.6-kDa polypeptide with histone-like properties that negatively regulates the expression of the genes that code for α-haemolysin expres-

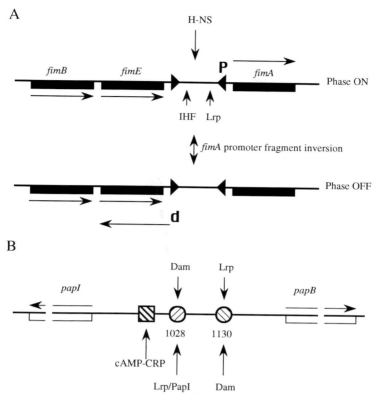

Fig. 13.5. Regulation of phase-variable adhesin gene expression by multiple regulators. Downward-pointing vertical arrows: negative inputs; upward-pointing vertical arrows: positive inputs (A) The type-1 fimbrial system. The site-specific recombinases are encoded by the *fimB* and *fimE* genes. The inverted repeats at which these proteins act are represented by the thick horizontal arrow heads between *fimE* and *fimA*. The *fimA* gene codes for the fimbrial subunit protein. The *fimA* promoter (P) is carried on the invertible seqeunce lying between the inverted repeats; inversion of this segment of DNA changes the orientation of the promoter with respect to *fimA*. In Phase ON, *fimA* is transcribed; in Phase OFF, *fimA* is silent. The rate of inversion is affected positively by leucine-responsive regulatory protein (Lrp) and integration host-factor (IHF) and negatively by histone-like protein (H-NS). (B) The segment of DNA between the divergently transcribed *papI* and *papB* regulatory genes of the Pap pilus operon is shown. The positions of two DNA adenine methylase (Dam) methylation sites (1028 and 1130) are indicated, together with a binding site for the cAMP–CRP (where CRP is catabolite repression protein) complex. The mechanism by which the interplay of these factors controls expression of Pap fimbriae is discussed in the text (see the section on Lrp). Note that the *papI* promoter is negatively regulated by H-NS (Göransson *et al.*, 1990).

sion in *E. coli* strains associated with extra-intestinal infections (Nieto *et al.*, 1991; see Chapter 11). The haemolysin operon is composed of four genes, *hlyCABD*. The *hlyA* gene codes for the toxin, which requires the *hlyC* gene product for activation. The products of *hlyBD* are required for toxin secretion. The operon is expressed as a major transcript (*hlyCA*) and a minor transcript (*hlyCABD*), both of which originate at a common promoter. Transcript length is thought to be a function of an anti-termination system that acts at a rho-independent terminator located between *hlyA* and *hlyB* (Koronakis *et al.*, 1988). Transcription of *hly* is also affected by a *cis*-acting sequence, *hlyR*, located upstream of *hlyC* (Vogel *et al.*, 1988). If this sequence is deleted, expression of haemolysin is poor. If the *hha* gene is then inactivated, high haemolysin expression is restored (Nieto *et al.*, 1991) (Table 13.1). The observations of *hlyR hha* were made with the plasmid-encoded *hly* operons typically found in strains isolated from infected animals. A sequence analogous to *hlyR* has also been found in the chromosomally encoded *hly* operon of strains isolated from infected human urinary tract (Cross *et al.*, 1990). Hha is closely related to the histone-like protein YmoA that regulates virulence gene expression negatively in *Yersinia enterocolitica* (Cornelis *et al.*, 1991; De la Cruz *et al.*, 1992). The mechanism by which Hha affects *hly* expression is currently unclear. Given its 'histone-like' properties, it would not be surprising if some modulation of DNA structure were involved.

Conclusions

This brief review of some of the mechanisms by which virulence gene expression is co-ordinated in *E. coli* illustrates a number of themes that are also emerging in studies of other bacterial pathogens. Firstly, virulence genes are rarely expressed constitutively. Rather, their expression has to be induced, usually by a stimulus from the external environment. Induction of gene expression generally involves a change in transcription. Post-transcriptional regulation also occurs in some systems but this aspect is beyond the scope of the present chapter. Secondly, there is no single mechanism by which environmental signals are transmitted to the genome. Physical and chemical signals exploit a variety of transmission pathways. Thirdly, transcriptional control is hierarchical. There are regulatory proteins that control a very small number of genes, or only a single gene, while others control very large numbers of genes. Individual genes or operons can be subject to control by more than one regulator, which means that they can belong simultaneously to more than one regulon. This networking of regulons increases the capacity of the bacterium to respond to a multifactorial environment. The fourth point is that determinants of bacterial genome structure can themselves contribute to the control of expression of particular genes, including virulence genes. This can involve crude changes in the global level of DNA supercoiling that result from environmental insults, such as osmotic stress, temperature change, carbon source depletion, or more localised changes in DNA topology, such as local variations in supercoiling due to the activities of neighbouring genes, DNA looping caused by DNA-binding proteins, DNA bending due to the action of proteins or the inherent properties of specific DNA sequences, and the conversion of transcriptionally proficient DNA into silent DNA by formation of higher-order nucleoprotein structures that approximate to eukaryotic chromatin.

Examples of these control systems have been considered in the preceding pages. The Pap and type-1 pilus adhesin systems serve to illustrate how particular genes can be integrated into many regulons with diverse membership, making them subject to multiple regulators. Thus, expression of the *pap* pilus operon of *E. coli* is governed in a number of ways. These are its own specific Pap regulatory proteins (PapB and PapI), the histone-like protein H-NS that represses *pap* transcription and links its expression to all other H-NS-controlled systems, such as the porin genes *ompC* and *ompF,* the type-1 fimbriae, the invasion genes in EIEC, curli, etc. (reviewed in Dorman & Ní Bhriain, 1993); the cAMP–CRP system, which is a DNA-bending protein and links *pap* expression to the *lac* operon, the *ompB* operon and scores of other genes; (reviewed in Botsford & Harman, 1992); the Lrp protein is also a DNA-bending protein and links *pap* expression to type-1 fimbriae, *ompC* and *ompF* expression and at least 15 other systems (reviewed in Calvo & Matthews, 1994). Type-1 fimbriae are controlled by H-NS and Lrp, in common with Pap fimbriae, but, unlike Pap, not by cAMP–CRP. They are, however, controlled by IHF, in common with *ompC* and *ompF*, and many more genes (reviewed in Freundlich *et al.*, 1992). In this way, they allow the cell to respond in different degrees to a complex external environment and provide the means for the cell subtly or dramatically to vary its transcription profile as the need arises. Measures aimed at preventing or treating bacterial infection may be made more effective if these regulatory features are taken into account.

Acknowledgements

C. J. Dorman acknowledges support from the Royal Society (London), the Medical Research Council (UK), the Engineering and Physical Sciences Research Council (UK), the Wellcome Trust (UK), Forbairt (Irish Republic) and the University of Dublin.

References

Adler, B., Sasakawa, C., Tobe, T., Makino, S., Komatsu, K. & Yoshikawa, M. (1989). A dual transcriptional activation system for the 230 kb plasmid genes coding for virulence-associated antigens of *Shigella flexneri*. *Molecular Microbiology*, **3**, 627–35.

Aldea, M., Garrido, T., Hernández-Chico, C., Vincente, M. & Kushner, S. R. (1989). Induction of a growth-phase-dependent promoter triggers transcription of *bolA*, an *Escherichia coli* morphogene. *EMBO Journal*, **8**, 3923–31.

Arnqvist, A., Olsén, A., Pfeifer, J., Russell, D. G. & Normark, S. (1992). The Crl protein activates cryptic genes for curli formation and fibronectin binding in *Escherichia coli*. *Molecular Microbiology*, **6**, 2443–52.

Bachmann, B. J. (1990). Linkage map of *Escherichia coli* K-12, edition 8. *Microbiological Reviews*, **54**, 130–97.

Bernardini, M. L., Fontaine, A. & Sansonetti, P. J. (1990). The two-component regulatory system OmpR-EnvZ controls the virulence of *Shigella flexneri*. *Journal of Bacteriology*, **172**, 6274–81.

Blomfield, I. C., Calie, P. J., Eberhardt, K. J., McClain, M. S. & Eisenstein, B. I. (1993). Lrp stimulates phase variation of type 1 fimbriation in *Escherichia coli* K-12. *Journal of Bacteriology*, **175**, 27–36.

Blyn, L. B., Braaten, B. A. & Low, D. A. (1990). Regulation of *pap* pilin phase variation by a mechanism involving differential Dam methylation states. *EMBO Journal*, **9**, 4045–54.

Bohannon, D. E., Connell, N., Keener, J., Tormo, A., Espinosa-Urgel, M., Zambrano, M. M. & Kolter, R. (1991). Stationary phase-inducible 'gear-box' promoters: differential effects of *katF* mutations and role of s[70]. *Journal of Bacteriology*, **173**, 4482–92.

Botsford, J. L. & Harman, J. G. (1992). Cyclic AMP in prokaryotes. *Microbiological Reviews*, **56**, 100–22.

Braaten, B. A., Blyn, L. B., Skinner, B. S. & Low, D. A. (1991). Evidence for a methylation-blocking factor (*mbf*) locus involved in *pap* pilus expression and phase variation in *Escherichia coli*. *Journal of Bacteriology*, **173**, 1789–800.

Braaten, B. A., Platko, J. V., Van der Woude, M. W., Simons, B. H., de Graaf, F. K., Calvo, J. M. & Low, D. A. (1992). Leucine-responsive regulatory protein controls the expression of both *pap* and *fan* pili operons in *Escherichia coli*. *Proceedings of the National Academy of Sciences, USA*, **89**, 4250–4.

Brunelle, A. & Schleif, R. (1989). Determining residue-base interactions between AraC protein and *araI* DNA. *Journal of Molecular Biology*, **209**, 607–22.

Calderwood, S. B., Auclair, F., Donohue-Rolfe, A., Keusch, G. T. & Mekalanos, J. J. (1987). Nucleotide sequence of the shiga-like toxin genes of *Escherichia coli*. *Proceedings of the National Academy of Sciences, USA*, **84**, 4364–8.

Calderwood, S. B. & Mekalanos, J. J. (1987). Iron regulation of shiga-like toxin expression in *Escherichia coli* is mediated by the *fur* locus. *Journal of Bacteriology*, **169**, 4759–64.

Calvo, J. M. & Matthews, R. G. (1994). The leucine-responsive regulatory protein, a global regulator of metabolism in *Escherichia coli*. *Microbiological Reviews*, **58**, 466–90.

Caron, J., Coffield, L. M. & Scott, J. R. 1989. A plasmid-encoded regulatory gene, *rns*, required for expression of CS1 and CS2 adhesins of enterotoxigenic *Escherichia coli*. *Proceedings of the National Academy of Sciences, USA*, **86**, 963–7.

Chatfield, S. N., Dorman, C. J., Hayward, C. & Dougan, G. (1991). Role of *ompR*-dependent genes in *Salmonella typhimurium* virulence: mutants defective in both OmpC and OmpF are attenuated *in vivo*. *Infection and Immunity*, **59**, 449–52.

Cornelis, G. R, Sluiters, C., Delor, I., Geib, D., Kaniga, K., Lambert de Rouvroit, C., Sory, M.-P., Vanooteghem, J.-C. & Michiels, T. (1991). *ymoA*, a *Yersinia enterocolitica* chromosomal gene modulating the expression of virulence functions. *Molecular Microbiology*, **5**, 1023–34.

Coy, M. & Neilands, J. B. (1991). Structural dynamics and functional domains of the Fur protein. *Biochemistry*, **30**, 8201–10.

Cross, M. A., Koronakis, V., Stanley, P. L. D. & Hughes, C. (1990). HlyB-dependent secretion of haemolysin by uropathogenic *Escherichia coli* requires conserved sequences flanking the chromosomal *hly* determinant. *Journal of Bacteriology*, **172**, 1217–24.

Curtiss, R. III & Kelly, S. M. (1987). *Salmonella typhimurium* deletion mutants lacking adenylate cyclase and cyclic AMP receptor protein are avirulent and immunogenic. *Infection and Immunity*, **55**, 3035–43.

Dagberg, B. & Uhlin, B. E. (1992). Regulation of virulence-associated plasmid genes in enteroinvasive *Escherichia coli*. *Journal of Bacteriology*, **174**, 7606–12.

De la Cruz, F., Carmona, M. & Juárez, A. (1992). The Hha protein from *Escherichia coli* is highly homologous to the YmoA protein from *Yersinia enterocolitica*. *Molecular Microbiology*, **6**, 3451–4.

De Lorenzo, V., Wee, S., Herrero, M. & Neilands, J. B. (1987). Operator sequences of the aerobactin operon of plasmid ColV-K30 binding the ferric uptake regulation (*fur*) repressor. *Journal of Bacteriology*, **169**, 2624–30.

Demple, B., Johnsonon, A. & Fung, D. (1986). Exonuclease III and endonuclease IV remove 3′ blocks from DNA synthesis in H_2O_2-damaged *Escherichia coli*. *Proceedings of the National Academy of Sciences, USA*, **83**, 7731–5.

Donnenberg, M. S. & Kaper, J. B. (1992). Enteropathogenic *Escherichia coli*. *Infection and Immunity*, **60**, 3953–61.

Dorman, C. J. (1991). DNA supercoiling and environmental regulation of gene expression in pathogenic bacteria. *Infection and Immunity*, **59**, 745–9.

Dorman, C. J. (1992). The VirF protein from *Shigella flexneri* is a member of the AraC transcription factor superfamily and is highly homologous to

Rns, a positive regulator of virulence genes in enterotoxigenic *Escherichia coli. Molecular Microbiology*, **6**, 1575.

Dorman, C. J., Chatfield, S., Higgins, C. F., Hayward, C. & Dougan, G. (1989). Characterization of porin and *ompR* mutants of a virulent strain of *Salmonella typhimurium: ompR* mutants are attenuated *in vivo. Infection and Immunity*, **57**, 2136–40.

Dorman, C. J. & Ní Bhriain, N. (1992). Global regulation of gene expression during environmental adaptation: implications for bacterial pathogens. In *Molecular Biology of Bacterial Infection,* eds. C. E. Hormaeche, C. W. Penn & C. J. Smyth, pp. 193–230. Cambridge: Cambridge University Press.

Dorman, C. J. & Ní Bhriain, N. (1993). DNA topology and bacterial virulence gene regulation. *Trends in Microbiology*, **1**, 92–9.

Dorman, C. J., Ní Bhriain, N. & Higgins, C. F. (1990). DNA supercoiling and environmental regulation of virulence gene expression in *Shigella flexneri. Nature*, **344**, 789–92.

Drlica, K. (1990). Bacterial topoisomerases and the control of DNA super-coiling. *Trends in Genetics*, **6**, 433–7.

Drlica, K. & Rouvière-Yaniv, J. (1987). Histone-like proteins of bacteria. *Microbiological Reviews*, **51**, 301–19.

Forsman, K., Göransson, M. & Uhlin, B. E. (1989). Autoregulation and multiple DNA interactions by a transcriptional regulatory protein in *E. coli* pili biosynthesis. *EMBO Journal*, **8**, 1271–7.

Freundlich, M., Ramani, N., Mathew, E., Sirko, A. & Tsui, P. (1992). The role of integration host factor in gene expression in *Escherichia coli. Molecular Microbiology*, **6**, 2557–63.

Friedman, D. I. (1988). Integration host factor: a protein for all reasons. *Cell*, **55**, 545–54.

Galán, J. E. & Curtiss, R. III. (1990). Expression of *Salmonella typhimurium* genes required for invasion is regulated by changes in DNA supercoiling. *Infection and Immunity*, **58**, 1879–85.

Gallegos, M.-T., Michán, C. & Ramos, J. L. (1993). The XylS/AraC family of regulators. *Nucleic Acids Research*, **21**, 807–10.

Göransson, M., Sonden, B., Nilsson, P., Dagberg, B., Forsman, K. Emanuelsson, K., & Uhlin, B. E. (1990). Transcriptional silencing and thermoregulation of gene expression in *Escherichia coli. Nature*, **344**, 682–5.

de Graaf, F. K. (1988). Fimbrial structures of enterotoxigenic *E. coli. Antonie Van Leeuwenhoek*, **54**, 395–404.

Hale, T. L. (1991). Genetic basis of virulence in *Shigella* species. *Micro-biological Reviews*, **55**, 206–24.

Hantke, K. (1981). Regulation of ferric ion transport in *E. coli*. Isolation of a constitutive mutant. *Molecular and General Genetics*, **182**, 288–92.

Hantke, K. (1987). Ferrous iron transport mutants in *Escherichia coli* K-12. *FEMS Microbiology Letters*, **44**, 53–7.

Hengge-Aronis, R. (1993) Survival of hunger and stress: the role of *rpoS* in early stationary phase gene expression. *Cell*, **72**, 165–8.

Higgins, C. F., Dorman, C. J., Stirling, D. A., Waddell, L., Booth, I. R., May, G. & Bremer, E. (1988). A physiological role for DNA supercoiling in the osmotic regulation of gene expression in *S. typhimurium* and *E. coli. Cell*, **52**, 569–84.

Higgins, C. F., Hinton, J. C. D., Hulton, C. S. J., Owen-Hughes, T., Pavitt, G. D. & Seirafi, A. (1990). Protein H1: a role for chromatin structure in the regulation of bacterial gene expression and virulence? *Molecular Microbiology*, **4**, 2007–12.

Hromockyj, A. E., Tucker, S. C. & Maurelli, A. T. (1992). Temperature regulation of *Shigella* virulence: identification of the repressor gene *virR*, an analogue of H-NS, and partial complementation by tyrosyl transfer RNA (tRNA$_{Tyr}$). *Molecular Microbiology*, **6**, 2113–24.

Isberg, R. R. & Leong, J. M. (1990). Multiple b1 chain integrins are receptors for invasin, a protein that promotes bacterial penetration into mammalian cells. *Cell*, **60**, 861–71.

Jackson, M. P., Newland, J. W., Holmes, R. K. & O'Brien, A. D. (1987). Nucleotide sequence analysis of the structural genes for shiga-like toxin I encoded by bacteriophage 933J from *Escherichia coli. Microbial Pathogenesis*, **2**, 147–53.

Jerse, A. E. & Kaper, J. B. (1991). The *eae* gene of enteropathogenic *Escherichia coli* encodes a 94-kilodalton membrane protein, the expression of which is influenced by the EAF plasmid. *Infection and Immunity*, **59**, 4302–9.

Jordi, B. J. A. M., Dagberg, B., De Haan, L. A. M., Hamers, A. M., Van der Zeijst, B. A. M., Gaastra, W. & Uhlin, B. (1992). The positive regulator CfaD overcomes the repression mediated by histone-like protein H-NS (H1) in the Cfa/I fimbrial operon of *Escherichia coli. EMBO Journal*, **11**, 2627–32.

Kawula, T. H. & Orndorff, P. E. (1991). Rapid site-specific DNA inversion in *Escherichia coli* mutants lacking the histone-like protein H-NS. *Journal of Bacteriology*, **173**, 4116–23.

Klaasen, P. & de Graaf, F. K. (1990). Characterization of FapR, a positive regulator of expression of the 987P operon in enterotoxigenic *Escherichia coli. Molecular Microbiology*, **4**, 1779–83.

Klaasen, P., Woodward, M. J., van Zijderveld, F. G. & de Graaf, F. K. (1990). The 987P gene cluster in enterotoxigenic *Escherichia coli* contains a ST$_{pa}$ transposon that activates 987P expression. *Infection and Immunity*, **58**, 801–7.

Koronakis, V., Cross, M. & Hughes, C. (1988). Expression of the *E. coli* hemolysin secretion gene *hlyB* involves transcript anti-termination within the *hly* operon. *Nucleic Acids Research*, **16**, 4789–800.

Lange, R. & Hengge-Aronis, R. (1991). Growth phase-regulated expression of *bolA* and morphology of stationary-phase *Escherichia coli* cells are controlled by the novel sigma factor σ^s. *Journal of Bacteriology*, **173**, 4474–81.

Lundrigan, M. D. & Earhardt, C. F. (1984). Gene *envY* of *Escherichia coli* K-12 affects thermo-regulation of major porin expression. *Journal of Bacteriology*, **157**, 262–8.

Lundrigan, M. D., Friedrich, M. J. & Kadner, R. J. (1989). Nucleotide sequence of the *Escherichia coli* porin thermoregulatory gene *envY. Nucleic Acids Research*, **17**, 800.

Magasanik, B. & Neidhardt, F. C. (1987). Regulation of carbon and nitrogen utilisation. In Escherichia coli *and* Salmonella typhimurium: *Cellular and Molecular Biology*, eds. F. C. Neidhardt, J. L. Ingraham, K. B. Low, B. Magasanik, M. Schaechter & H. E. Umbarger, pp. 1318–25. Washington DC: American Society for Microbiology.

Mulvey, M. R. & Loewen, P. C. (1989). Nucleotide sequence of *katF* of *Escherichia coli* suggests KatF is a novel σ transcription factor. *Nucleic Acids Research*, **17**, 9979–91.

Ní Bhriain, N. & Dorman, C. J. (1993). Isolation and characterisation of a *topA* mutant of *Shigella flexneri*. *Molecular Microbiology*, **7**, 351–8.

Nieto, J. M., Carmona, M., Bolland, S., Jubete, Y., De la Cruz, F. & Juárez, A. (1991). The *hha* gene modulates haemolysin expression in *Escherichia coli*. *Molecular Microbiology*, **5**, 1285–93.

Nou, X., Skinner, B., Braaten, B., Blyn, L., Hirsch, D. & Low, D. (1993). Regulation of pyelonephritis-associated pili phase-variation in *Escherichia coli*: binding of the PapI and the Lrp regulatory proteins is controlled by DNA methylation. *Molecular Microbiology*, **7**, 545–53.

Olsén, A, Arnqvist, A., Sukupolvi, S. & Normark, S. (1993). The RpoS sigma factor relieves H-NS-mediated repression of *csgA*, the subunit gene of fibronectin-binding curli in *Escherichia coli*. *Molecular Microbiology*, **7**, 523–36.

Olsén, A., Jonsson, A. & Normark, S. (1989). Fibronectin binding mediated by a novel class of surface organelles on *Escherichia coli*. *Nature*, **338**, 652–5.

Owen-Hughes, T. A., Pavitt, G. A., Santos, D. S., Sidebotham, J. M., Hulton, C. S., Hinton, J. C. D. & Higgins, C. F. (1992). The chromatin-associated protein H-NS interacts with curved DNA to influence DNA topology and gene expression. *Cell*, **71**, 255–65.

Platko, J. V. & Calvo, J. M. (1993). Mutations affecting the ability of *Escherichia coli* Lrp to bind DNA, activate transcription, or respond to leucine. *Journal of Bacteriology*, **175**, 1110–7.

Porter, M. E. & Dorman, C. J. (1994). A role for H-NS in the thermo-osmotic regulation of virulence gene expression in *Shigella flexneri*. *Journal of Bacteriology*, **176**, 4187–91.

Provence, D. L. & Curtiss, R. III. (1992). Role of *crl* in avian pathogenic *Escherichia coli*: a knockout mutation of *crl* does not affect haemag-glutination activity, fibronectin binding or curli production. *Infection and Immunity*, **60**, 4460–7.

Saito, T. & Williams, R. P. J. (1991). The binding of the ferric uptake regulation protein to a DNA fragment. *European Journal of Biochemistry*, **197**, 43–7.

Savelkoul, P. H. M., Willshaw, G. A., McConnell, M. M., Smith, H. R., Hamers, A. M., van der Zeijst, B. A. M., & Gaastra, W. (1990). Expression of Cfa/I fimbriae is positively regulated. *Microbial Pathogenesis*, **8**, 91–9.

Schäffer, S., Hantke, K. & Braun, V. (1985). Nucleotide sequence of the iron regulatory gene *fur*. *Molecular and General Genetics*, **200**, 110–13.

Schleif, R. (1987). The L-arabinose operon. In Escherichia coli *and* Salmonella typhimurium. *Cellular and Molecular Biology*, eds. F. C. Neidhardt, J. L. Ingraham, K. B. Low, B. Magasanik, M. Schaechter & H. E. Umbarger, pp. 1473–81. Washington DC: American Society for Microbiology.

Stock, J. B., Ninfa, A. J. & Stock, A. M. (1989). Protein phosphorylation and regulation of adaptive responses in bacteria. *Microbiological Reviews*, **53**, 450–90.

Tanaka, K., Takayanagi, Y., Fujita, N., Ishihama, A. & Takahashi, H. (1993). Heterogeneity of the principal σ factor in *Escherichia coli*: the *rpoS* gene product, σ^{38}, is a second principal σ factor of RNA polymerase in stationary-phase *Escherichia coli*. *Proceedings of the National Academy of Sciences, USA*, **90**, 3511–15.

Tobe, T., Nagai, S., Okada, N., Adler, B., Yoshikawa, M. & Sasakawa, C.

(1991). Temperature-regulated expression of invasion genes in *Shigella flexneri* is controlled through the transcriptional activation of the *virB* gene on the large plasmid. *Molecular Microbiology*, **5**, 887–93.

Tobe, T., Yoshikawa, M., Mizuno, T. & Sasakawa, C. (1993). Transcriptional control of the invasion regulatory gene *virB* of *Shigella flexneri*: activation by VirF and repression by H-NS. *Journal of Bacteriology*, **175**, 6142–9.

Tsui, P., Huang, L. & Freundlich, M. (1991). Integration host factor binds specifically to multiple sites in the *ompB* promoter of *Escherichia coli* and inhibits transcription. *Journal of Bacteriology*, **173**, 5800–7.

Ueguchi, C. & Mizuno, T. (1993). The *Escherichia coli* nucleoid protein HN-S functions directly as a transcriptional repressor. *EMBO Journal*, **12**, 1039–46.

Ussery, D. W., Hinton, J. C. D., Jordi, B. J. A. M., Granum, P. E., Seirafi, A., Stephen, R. J., Tupper, A. E., Berridge, G., Sidebotham, J. M. & Huggins, C. F. (1994). The chromatin-associated protein H-NS. *Biochemie*, **76**, 968–80.

Van der Woude, M. W., Braaten, B. A. & Low, D. A. (1992). Evidence for global regulatory control of pilus expression in *Escherichia coli* by Lrp and DNA methylation: model building based on analysis of *pap*. *Molecular Microbiology*, **6**, 2429–35.

Vogel, M., Hess, J., Then, I., Juárez, A. & Goebel, W. (1988). Characterization of a sequence (*hlyR*) which enhances synthesis and secretion of hemolysin in *Escherichia coli*. *Molecular and General Genetics*, **212**, 76–84.

Wang, Q. & Calvo, J. M. (1993). Lrp, a major regulatory protein in *Escherichia coli*, bends DNA and can organize the assembly of a higher-order nucleoprotein structure. *EMBO Journal*, **12**, 2495–501.

Wanner, B. L. (1992). Is cross regulation by phosphorylation of two-component response regulator proteins important in bacteria? *Journal of Bacteriology*, **174**, 2053–8.

Willins, D. A., Ryan, C. W., Platko, J. V. & Calvo, J. M. (1991). Characterization of Lrp, an *Escherichia coli* regulatory protein that mediates a global response to leucine. *Journal of Biological Chemistry*, **266**, 10768–74.

Yamada, H., Yoshida, T., Tanaka, K.-I., Sasakawa, C. & Mizuno, T. (1991). Molecular analysis of the *Escherichia coli hns* gene encoding a DNA-binding protein, which preferentially recognises curved DNA sequences. *Molecular and General Genetics*, **230**, 332–6.

Part three

Mechanisms of disease

14

Enteropathogenic *Escherichia coli*

P. H. WILLIAMS, T. J. BALDWIN and
S. KNUTTON

The identification of *Escherichia coli* as the causative agent of summer diarrhoea was at first hampered by the fact that the organism is also a component of the normal intestinal flora. Standard bacteriological examination showed little or no difference between patients with gastroenteritis and healthy individuals. Only when antibodies were raised against an *E. coli* strain isolated from a child with severe protracted diarrhoea, who later died, was it possible to distinguish between strains associated with disease and those that were part of the normal intestinal flora (Bray, 1945). It then became apparent that the vast majority of outbreaks of summer diarrhoea among infants were associated with infection by antigenically similar populations of *E. coli*, while isolates from healthy adults, children and animals did not react with the antiserum. The development of a defined serotyping system for *E. coli* by Kauffman (1947) allowed a systematic categorisation of isolates based on their serological characteristics. Study of Bray's strains showed that they belonged to serogroup O55, while later analysis of stored samples of faeces indicated that strains of serogroup O111 were similarly associated with hospital outbreaks of infantile diarrhoea. The virulence of *E. coli* strains of serogroups O55 and O111 was subsequently confirmed in healthy adult volunteers (Ferguson & June, 1952).

The term 'enteropathogenic', to describe *E. coli* strains incriminated in infantile diarrhoea, was coined by Neter *et al.* (1955). By 1957 a total of 13 enteropathogenic O-serogroups had been recognised, O18ab, O18ac, O26, O44, O55, O86, O111, O114, O119, O125, O126, O127 and O128 and serogroups O142 and O158 were added later. In the case of some of these, such as O55, which is rarely isolated from healthy individuals, O-serotyping alone is sufficient to indicate the presence of a potential enteropathogen. It soon became clear, however, that different serotypes within other incriminated serogroups were not equally pathogenic, and that the ability to cause diarrhoea in infants was associated only with particular O:H-serotypes (Ewing *et al.*, 1963). Thus, O86:H34 is the only serotype in the O86-serogroup implicated in diarrhoeal disease; other H-types of the group are commonly found in the intestinal flora of healthy individuals but they are non-pathogenic. Traditionally, enteropathogenic *E. coli* (EPEC) have been defined on the basis of these classical O:H-serotypes (Robins-Browne, 1987) but as the understanding of EPEC pathogenicity improves, it is becoming clear that EPEC strains will be better described in terms of specific virulence characteristics.

Interest in the pathogenicity of *E. coli* involved in enteric disease increased dramatically in the early 1970s. Strains, designated enterotoxigenic *E. coli* (ETEC), were shown to produce cholera-like or other enterotoxins, while other strains, designated enteroinvasive *E. coli* (EIEC), were like *Shigella* and invaded the intestinal mucosa to cause an inflammatory dysentery-like disease. It had long been known that *E. coli* were also associated with urinary tract and other extra-intestinal infections. The word 'enteropathogenic' was, therefore, used for a heterogeneous group of organisms that did not produce recognisable toxins and did not invade intestinal cells. Some workers considered that EPEC isolates were simply ETEC that had, during storage, lost the plasmids that had encoded toxin production. The controversy was resolved when it was shown that EPEC strains, which did not produce enterotoxins and were not invasive, were still able cause diarrhoea in adult volunteers (Levine *et al.*, 1978). In this way EPEC were confirmed as a class of diarrhoea-producing strains of *E. coli* distinct from ETEC and EIEC. They were still, however, identified by what they did *not* do, and by the fact that they belonged to particular O:H-serotypes.

The pathology of enteropathogenic *Escherichia coli* infection

The first ultrastructural examination of EPEC-infected bowel tissue was carried out on piglets infected with *E. coli* O55:H7. This revealed a series of characteristic changes in the absorptive cells of the small bowel, including lengthening and loss of microvilli at sites of bacterial adherence, invagination and apparent thickening of the plasma membrane and increased electron density in the adjacent cytoplasm (Staley *et al.*, 1969). These observations were subsequently confirmed with the use of a variety of animal models of EPEC infection. The term 'attaching and effacing' (AE) was introduced to describe these characteristic

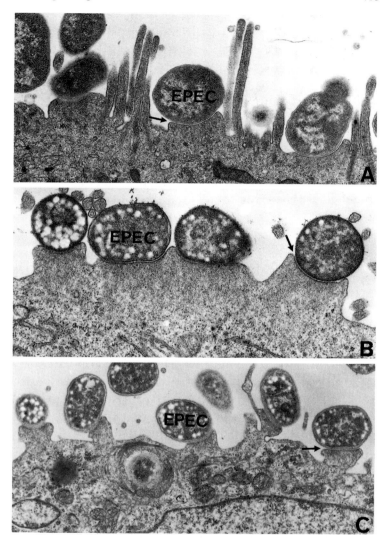

Fig. 14.1. Electron micrograph of EPEC-infected (EPEC, enteropathogenic *Escherichia coli*) human small intestinal mucosa showing the
characteristic attaching and effacing (AE) lesion with localised destruction of microvilli, intimate attachment of bacteria (arrows) and a dense
plaque of filaments beneath adherent bacteria (A). Identical lesions are
seen in cultured human intestinal (Caco-2) cells (B) and human
epithelial (HEp-2) cells (C). A, B × 22,000; C × 15,000. (Reprinted
with permission of the American Society for Microbiology.)

morphological changes and the *E. coli* strains that cause them, because of the intimate bacterial attachment and localised effacement of brush border microvilli (Moon *et al.*, 1983).

Ultrastructural studies of biopsy material from children with EPEC infections confirmed the formation of AE lesions in human disease (Ulshen & Rollo, 1980; Rothbaum *et al.*, 1982). In severe infections there is almost complete destruction of the absorptive surface of the jejunum and ileum, with extensive villus atrophy and thinning of the mucosal lining, wherever bacterial colonisation is particularly heavy. Changes in cell organelles indicative of intracellular damage are also seen in heavily colonised enterocytes; such changes are thought to precede the eventual death and loss of cells from the villous surface. Crypt cells show distinctive cytoplasmic vacuolation and loss of the normal basal location of the nucleus. Regions of the lamina propria in the ileum and the colon show evidence of cellular infiltration by lymphocytes, plasma cells and eosinophils, but with a virtual absence of polymorphs. A significant increase in permeability of EPEC-infected epithelium, probably indicative of the disruption of cellular tight junctions, has been shown with cultured intestinal cells that differentiate to form polarised, microvillated monolayers (Collington *et al.*, 1993).

Biopsies of small intestine infected *in vitro* with known diarrhoea-producing EPEC strains show AE lesions identical with those seen in patients (Knutton *et al.*, 1987a) (Figure 14.1A). These include intimate bacterial attachment, loss of microvilli and cupping of the plasma membrane around bacteria to form a pedestal-like structure. Extensive vesiculation of the microvillous membrane and accumulation of cytoskeletal elements in a dense plaque beneath intimately adherent bacteria were newly observed features of lesion formation and crucial to progress in the understanding of the pathogenesis of EPEC.

Adherence of enteropathogenic *Escherichia coli*

The lack of obvious virulence characteristics in EPEC isolates (Law, 1988) prompted the detailed investigation of their adherence properties. Early studies with clinical isolates focused on their adhesion to cultured epithelial cells, such as HEp-2 and HeLa cells. Cravioto *et al.* (1979) showed that 80 per cent of classical EPEC strains attach to these cells in a mannose-resistant manner, as compared with only 19 per cent of non-pathogenic strains. Later, two characteristic patterns of EPEC attachment were observed, namely localised adherence (LA) in which bacteria adhere in discrete microcolonies (Figure 14.2B) and diffuse adherence (DA) in which bacteria adhere uniformly over the cell surface (Scaletsky *et al.*, 1984). EPEC strains that displayed LA also produce AE lesions in cultured epithelial cells morphologically identical to those seen in infected intestinal epithelial cells. Bacteria attach intimately to the apical cell surface, frequently on pedestal-like structures with dense plaques of cytoskeletal filaments beneath attached bacteria (Knutton *et al.*, 1987b) (Figure 14.1B, C). Strains with the DA adherence phenotype do not possess the AE property and are now generally grouped together as diffusely adherent *E. coli* (DAEC). In the absence of direct evidence from volunteer studies for the induction of disease, the role of DAEC in infantile diarrhoea remains uncertain.

During AE lesion formation, EPEC disrupt the brush border cytoskeleton and cytoskeletal elements accumulate beneath adherent bacteria. Since actin is the major component of the brush border cytoskeleton, it seemed likely that the filamentous plaque formed beneath adherent EPEC, in intestinal epithelial cells and in cultured cells, was composed predominantly of actin. This was confirmed by staining filamentous actin with fluorescein-isothiocyanate-(FITC-) conjugated phalloidin, a toxin that binds specifically to polymerised actin. Intense spots of fluorescence are seen at sites that correspond exactly to the position of each bacterium (Figure 14.2A,D). Such a pattern of actin accumulation is caused only by AE bacteria and so fluorescence actin staining (FAS) is a highly specific test for the identification of bacteria that have AE activity (Knutton *et al.*, 1989). Other cytoskeletal proteins, including myosin, α-actinin, talin and ezrin also co-localise with actin at sites of EPEC attachment (Finlay *et al.*, 1992; Manjarrez-Hernandez *et al.*, 1992).

In tissue culture cell adhesion assays, EPEC display LA and AE activity. The LA phenotype is associated with a high-molecular-weight (55–70 MDa) EPEC adherence factor (EAF) plasmid that is found in most classical EPEC strains (Baldini *et al.*, 1983). A 1-kb DNA fragment, the EAF probe, from an uncharacterised region of the 60-MDa EAF plasmid pMAR2 of EPEC strain E2348 (O127:H6) hybridises with DNA from virtually all LA strains and has been used extensively in epidemiological studies (Levine *et al.*, 1988). For AE lesion formation there is not, however, an absolute requirement for the EAF plasmid, the genetic determinants for which are located on the bacterial chromosome (Knutton *et al.*, 1987b). Thus, a plasmid-cured derivative of E2348, although only very weakly adherent, retained AE activity, as assessed by the FAS assay (Figure 14.2C, D) (Knutton *et al.*, 1989) and by electron

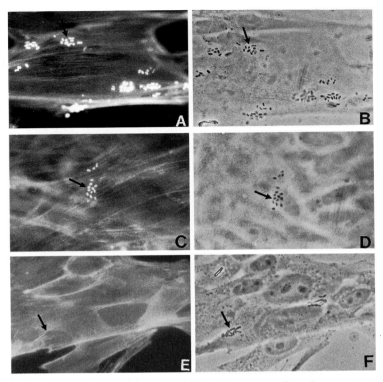

Fig. 14.2. Actin fluorescence (A,C,E) and corresponding phase contrast (B,D,F) micrographs showing cultured cells infected with enteropathogenic *Escherichia coli* (EPEC) strain E2348 (A,B), with E2348 cured of its EPEC adherence factor (EAF) plasmid (C,D), and with EAF plasmid transformant of a laboratory strain of *E. coli* (E,F). Positive fluorescence actin staining (FAS) tests are seen with the wild-type EPEC and with the plasmid-cured derivative, but not with the plasmid transformant (arrows). ×500. (Reprinted with permission of the American Society for Microbiology.)

microscopy (Knutton *et al.*, 1987a). On the other hand, a laboratory strain of *E. coli*, into which pMAR2 had been introduced by transformation, showed clear LA but was FAS-negative (Figure 14.2E,F) and did not exhibit intimate attachment (Knutton *et al.*, 1987b).

EAF plasmids are, nevertheless, important in EPEC pathogenesis. Plasmid-cured E2348 is a poor coloniser of the intestine and is significantly less pathogenic in volunteers than the parent E2348 strain (Levine *et al.*, 1985). The important function of the EAF plasmid is to encode an adhesin responsible for tissue culture cell adherence, the role of which *in vivo* is probably to promote the initial attachment of EPEC to brush borders. The identity of the plasmid-encoded adhesin has, however, remained elusive.

Enteropathogenic *E. coli* produce several types of fimbriae that may function as adhesins, including rod-like structures, fine fibrillae and rope-like bundles of thin filaments termed bundle-forming pili (BFP) (Girón *et al.*, 1993). The latter are a member of the type-IV group of fimbriae that includes those of *Vibrio cholerae, Pseudomonas aeruginosa, Neisseria gonorrhoeae* and *Bacteroides nodosus* (Donnenberg *et al.*, 1992). Rod-like and fibrillar EPEC fimbriae show homology with fimbriae of uropathogenic *E. coli* and DAEC (Girón *et al.*, 1993). Expression of BFP (Figure 14.3), which bind bacteria together to give autoaggregation (Figure 14.3, inset), is associated with the presence of the EAF plasmid and localised adherence to HEp-2 cells (Girón *et al.*, 1993). However, autoaggregation of bacteria should not be confused with localised adherence, because EPEC that lack EAF plasmids and BFP expression, and therefore do not autoaggregate, still display a localised pattern of adherence to HEp-2 cells (Figure 14.2D) (Knutton *et al.*, 1991). While there is no direct evidence that BFP are an adhesin that promotes cell attachment, antiserum against BFP reduces the ability of EPEC to adhere (Girón *et al.*, 1991). The role in attachment of other fimbrial types produced by EPEC has still to be assessed.

Fluorescence actin staining provides a simple diagnostic assay for the AE lesion and has allowed the characterisation of the genes involved in AE activity. Jerse *et al.* (1990) used transposon Tn*phoA* insertion mutate, which is specific for genes that specify exported proteins, to mutagenise a plasmid-cured derivative of EPEC strain E2348, and then screened for loss of fluorescence in the FAS assay. One FAS-negative mutant was unable to adhere intimately to epithelial cells, and an oligonucleotide probe derived from the nucleotide sequence adjacent to the inserted transposon was then used to select a hybridising clone from a cosmid gene bank. The chromosomal gene interrupted by Tn*phoA* was designated *eae* (for <u>E</u>. *coli* <u>a</u>ttaching and <u>e</u>ffacing). Its role in EPEC pathogenesis was confirmed in volunteers, who received either the wild-type E2348 strain or an isogenic mutant in which the *eae* gene had been deleted. The 11 volunteers who received E2348 developed diarrhoea, while only four of the 11 who received the deletion mutant did so (Donnenberg & Kaper, 1992). The development of disease in some of the latter group is indicative of the existence of other, as yet undefined, determinants of EPEC-associated diarrhoea.

The cloned *eae* gene, later designated *eaeA*, has been sequenced and a

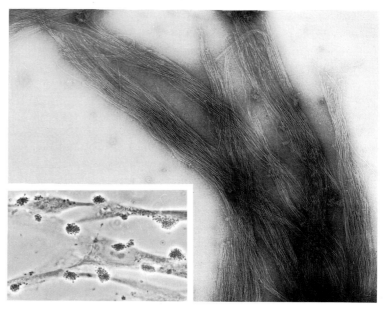

Fig. 14.3. Electron micrograph of bundle-forming pili (BFP) showing long, rope-like bundles of laterally aggregated filaments. Entero-pathogenic (EPEC) *Escherichia coli* producing BFP adhere to cultured cells in small localised aggregates (inset). ×1000,000; inset ×400.

gene probe (*eaeA* probe), that consists of an internal 1-kb fragment of the *eaeA* gene, is highly sensitive and specific for the detection EPEC strains (Jerse *et al.*, 1990). The product of the *eae* gene is a 94-kDa outer-membrane protein, named intimin because of its suggested role as the intimate adhesin in the adherence of EPEC to epithelial cells (Jerse & Kaper, 1991; Donnenberg & Kaper, 1992). This is supported by the observation that an *eaeA* deletion mutant attaches to epithelial cells but does not show intimate adhesion or give a positive FAS test (Donnenberg & Kaper, 1991). Adhesion causes some degree of actin condensation, however, since the mutant produces what has been termed a 'shadow' phenotype in the FAS assay (Donnenberg *et al.*, 1990). Reintroduction of the cloned *eaeA* gene on a plasmid into the deletion mutant restores a positive FAS reaction and AE activity (Donnenberg & Kaper, 1991). Thus, intimin is necessary, but not by itself sufficient, to produce full AE activity. Expression of *eaeA* has been shown to be affected by genes of the EAF plasmid (Jerse & Kaper, 1991), which may explain the weak adherence properties and low levels of virulence of plasmid-cured strains (Levine *et al.*, 1985). A second gene necessary for intimate attachment of

EPEC to epithelial cells is located immediately downstream of *eaeA* (Donnenberg *et al.*, 1993). This gene, termed *eaeB*, is involved in signal transduction in target cells (Foubister *et al.*, 1994).

All the known determinants of the AE phenotype have now been localised to a 35-kb region of the chromosome called the locus of enterocyte effacement (LEE), which is conserved in all pathogens that produce the AE lesion (McDaniel *et al.*, 1995). In addition to *eaeA* and *eaeB*, LEE contains genes similar to those that encode a specialised secretion pathway for virulence factors in animal and plant pathogens (Van Gijsegem *et al.*, 1993). A mutation of one of these genes, *sepA* (for secretion of EPEC proteins), eliminates the ability of EPEC to induce AE lesions and to secrete a number of proteins.

Host signalling in infection with enteropathogenic *Escherichia coli*

During the course of the formation of the AE lesion, EPEC induce the destruction of microvilli by cytoskeletal breakdown and membrane vesiculation, and cytoskeletal elements accumulate beneath intimately adherent bacteria. Since EPEC remain predominantly extracellular during the infection process, such gross cytoskeletal reorganisation must involve membrane signal transduction in the infected cells; there is no evidence for elevation in the levels of cyclic nucleotides (cAMP, cGMP) in EPEC-infected cells. However, treatment of brush border cells with calcium-mobilising hormones or calcium ionophores *in vitro* has effects that are, at least superficially, strikingly similar to the morphological changes seen during EPEC infection, namely breakdown of the actin core of the microvilli, effacement of the brush border and extensive membrane vesiculation (Goligorsky *et al.*, 1986). This observation led Baldwin *et al.* (1991) to investigate the possible role of calcium in EPEC pathogenicity. They showed that infection of cultured HEp-2 cell monolayers with EPEC results in significantly elevated intracellular free calcium concentrations ($[Ca^{2+}]_i$), as measured by enhanced calcium-dependent fluorescence of the indicator dye Quin-2.[1] Free calcium levels in uninfected monolayers are typically in the range 40–75 nM; within an hour of infection with EPEC, concentrations have doubled and after about four hours, when cells in the monolayer are just beginning to die, overall calcium concentrations are in excess of 300 nM. The source of the additional free

1 Quin-2 is 2-({2-[bis(carboxymethyl)amino]-5-methylphenoxy}-methyl)-6-methoxy-8-bis (carboxymethyl) aminoquinoline.

cytosolic calcium is from within the cell itself; chelation or removal of calcium from the external medium does not affect the ability of EPEC to raise $[Ca^{2+}]_i$. The effect is not uniform throughout the monolayer or, indeed, throughout a particular infected cell in the monolayer. Use of the calcium indicator dyes Fura-2,[2] with a computer imaging technique, and Fluo-3,[3] which emits in the visible range of the spectrum, clearly shows that increases in calcium concentration in infected Hep-2 and Caco-2 cells are confined specifically to the vicinity of adherent EPEC microcolonies and levels in these regions of the cell are probably greater than 1 μM.

In intestinal epithelial cells, increased $[Ca^{2+}]_i$ activates actin de-polymerisation and inhibits bundling of actin by the calcium-dependent microvillus protein villin. This causes loss of cytoskeletal integrity by the breakdown of actin in the microvillus core (Bretscher & Weber, 1979, 1980). The cytoskeleton of non-intestinal cell types, such as HEp-2, contains the related calcium-dependent actin-severing protein gelsolin (Pontremoli *et al.*, 1986). The classical pathway of calcium mobilisation from intracellular stores involves initial binding of agonists to host cell receptors and subsequent activation of the effector protein phos-pholipase C, via GTP-binding proteins. The enzyme mediates cleavage of the membrane phospholipid phosphatidylinositol bisphosphate to yield two second messenger molecules, inositol 1,4,5-trisphosphate [Ins $(1,4,5)P_3$) and diacylglycerol. The former is hydrophilic; it enters the cytoplasm and acts on endoplasmic reticulum membrane receptors to mediate efflux of calcium. Increased inositol phosphate fluxes have recently been detected directly in EPEC-infected cells (Foubister *et al.*, 1994). Diacylglycerol is hydrophobic and remains in the membrane, where it acts as a membrane receptor for the calcium-phospholipid-dependent protein kinase C (PKC).

Second messengers generally exert their effects by direct or indirect activation of specific protein kinases. It is possible, therefore, to deter-mine pathological changes due to abnormal signal transduction by identi-fying alterations in the phosphorylation states of various cellular proteins in response to bacterial infection. Adherence of EPEC to cultured HEp-2 and Caco-2 cells stimulates a pattern of protein phosphorylation similar to that induced by agents, such as phorbol ester, that stimulate PKC (Baldwin *et al.*, 1990). The most prominent phosphoproteins induced in

2 Fura-2 is 1-[2-(5-carboxyoxazol-2-yl)-6-aminobenzoylfluran-5-oxyl]-2-2'-amino-5'-methylphenoxy)-ethane-*N*, *N*, *N'*, *N'*-tetra-acetic acid.
3 Fluro-3 is 1-[2-amino-5-(2, 7-dichloro-6-hydroxy-3-oxy-9-xanthenyl)-phenoxy]-2-[2-amino-5-methylphenoxy]ethane-*N*, *N*, *N'*, *N'*-tetra-acetic acid.

response to EPEC infection and phorbol ester treatment are a group of acidic species of approximately 20–21 kDa, identified as myosin light chain (MLC), on the basis of their reaction with antibodies raised against the denatured phosphorylated form of this protein (Manjarrez-Hernandez *et al.*, 1991, 1992). After stimulation by phorbol ester, phosphorylated MLC dissociates from the cytoskeletal actomyosin complex into a free cytosolic soluble form. A similar effect is observed with treatments of less than an hour with EPEC, but when infection is continued for up to four hours, an increasing proportion of the phosphorylated MLC is observed in a complexed form in the cytoskeleton. Immunofluorescence microscopy with anti-myosin antibodies clearly shows co-localisation of myosin with lesion-forming adherent bacteria on the surface of cultured cells after infection for longer periods (Figure 14.4A, B). Phosphoamino-acid analysis indicates differences in the phosphorylation patterns of MLC in the two conditions. After exposure to phorbol ester and short-lasting EPEC infections, serine residues are phosphorylated, indicating the activity of PKC. Longer-lasting EPEC infection results in threonine residue phosphorylation, which is suggestive of the activation of the specific enzyme MLC kinase, perhaps as part of a kinase cascade. Myosin light chain is also phosphorylated in biopsy samples of EPEC-infected human small intestine (Manjarrez-Hernandez *et al.*, 1992).

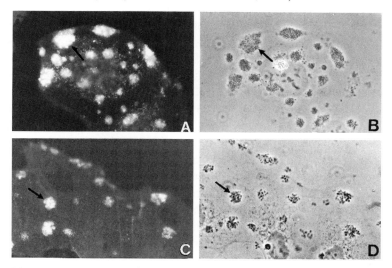

Fig. 14.4. Fluorescence (A, C) and corresponding phase-contrast (B, D) micrographs showing co-localisation of adherent bacteria with cytoskeletal myosin (A, B) and tyrosine phosphorylated protein(s) (C, D). ×500.

Among the other major proteins phosphorylated in response to EPEC infection, one of approximately 29 kDa (Baldwin *et al.*, 1990; Manjarrez-Hernandez *et al.*, 1991) has not yet been identified. In addition, infection with EPEC and other bacteria leads to the phosphorylation of HeLa cell 100- and 130-kDa proteins, which have been identified by immunoprecipitation as vinculin and α-actinin (Riley *et al.*, 1992).

It is interesting that some of these phosphoproteins, most notably MLC and the 29-kDa species, are also observed when cells are treated with epidermal growth factor (EGF) (Manjarrez-Hernandez *et al.*, 1991), the receptor of which is a tyrosine kinase; activation of tyrosine kinases is known to be an important early event in numerous signalling pathways. Some receptors, such as that for EGF, have intrinsic tyrosine kinase activity , while for others, such as integrins, a tyrosine kinase associates with the receptor once the agonist has bound. The activity of tyrosine kinases during EPEC infection has been confirmed by the use of antibodies against tyrosine phosphate; immunofluorescence microscopy shows a cross-reactive protein in infected cells that co-localises with adherent bacteria (Figure 14.4C, D), while Western blot analysis shows a major tyrosine phosphoprotein of approximately 90 kDa (Rosenshine *et al.*, 1992). Unlike EPEC *eaeA* deletion mutants, *eaeB* deletion mutants are defective in signalling and are unable to induce such tyrosine phosphorylation (Foubister *et al.*, 1994).

Actin accretion at sites of bacterial attachment

In addition to gross cytoskeletal changes, AE lesion formation is characterised by substantial deposition of filamentous actin beneath sites of bacterial attachment, detection of which is the basis of the FAS test. However, the concentration of actin as an electron-dense pad within AE lesions is far higher than would be likely to arise solely by accumulation of actin debris from cytoskeletal breakdown. This suggests significant *de novo* actin polymerisation during lesion development. This process is, however, independent of the small G-proteins Rac and Rho that, respectively, normally regulate localised actin polymerisation in membrane ruffles and stress fibres. Actin accretion within the pedestal is calcium-dependent (Baldwin *et al.*, 1993). Thus, loading cells with a calcium-buffering compound before EPEC infection considerably reduces actin polymerisation, as does treatment with a calmodulin inhibitor. Sodium dantrolene, a drug that modifies normal calcium mobilisation from intracellular stores, and so prevents the elevation of $[Ca^{2+}]_i$ in infected cultured cells, also significantly inhibits normal AE lesion formation. As we have seen above (p. 412), gelsolin and villin associate with and cleave F-actin non-proteolytically between G-actin monomers at high $[Ca^{2+}]_i$ (Matsudaira & Janmey, 1988). They remain associated with the ends of cleaved fragments, forming a cap that prevents elongation of filaments by further addition of actin monomers. As locally high calcium levels disperse, however, by diffusion or by active mobilisation of calcium into storage, binding of the cap to the phospholipid phosphatidylinositol 4,5-bisphosphate in the membrane results in dissociation of gelsolin or villin from the filament ends. This then allows an explosive burst of actin polymerisation at nucleation sites created by dissociation of gelsolin or villin. Thus, the presence of high concentrations of F-actin at sites of EPEC attachment may be explained by the changing activities of actin-severing proteins in response to changes in calcium concentrations within infected cells. Such a mechanism does not, however, explain the highly localised nature of the filamentous plaque or the co-localisation of other cytoskeletal elements.

Actin accretion does not occur in cells infected with an *eaeA* deletion mutant. This suggests that actin accretion during infection with wild-type EPEC may relate to aggregation of intimin-specific receptors at the surface of infected cells. One possibility is the integrin family of trans-membrane proteins (Schwartz, 1992), which normally function in cell morphology and tissue integrity. Indeed, intimin shows some homology with the protein invasin, of *Yersinia* spp. (Isberg & Leong, 1990), which is known to bind integrins. Moreover, integrins provide transmembrane links between the extracellular matrix and cytoskeletal actin via proteins, such as talin, α-actinin, vinculin and ezrin, some of which also co-localise with actin in the AE lesion. There is, however, currently no evidence for the presence of integrins on the apical surface of intestinal cell, and so their role, if any, in the pathogenesis of EPEC remains unclear. It is worthy of note, however, that EPEC adherence and lesion formation can be inhibited by factors that resemble the carbohydrate moiety of integrins (Cravioto *et al.*, 1991).

A unifying model of enteropathogenic *Escherichia coli* infection

Infection with EPEC is a complex and multifaceted process. In the infected host it is manifested as severe and persistent secretory diarrhoea, in which the intestinal mucosa undergoes gross morphological damage and individual enterocytes die as the result of disruption of the signalling mechanisms that normally control ion transport. Initial non-intimate

EPEC / Host Cell Interaction

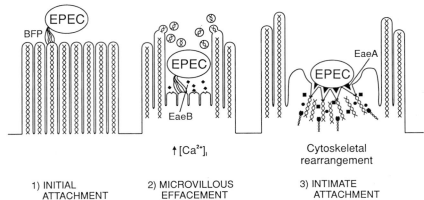

Fig. 14.5. The mechanism of attaching and effacing (AE) lesion formation by enteropathogenic *Escherichia coli* (EPEC). Stage 1. Non-
intimate bacterial attachment to the enterocyte brush border, most
probably mediated by a fimbrial adhesin, possibly bundle-forming pili
(BFP). Stage 2. Secretion of the EaeB protein (◆) stimulates localised
elevation of the intracellular free calcium concentration ($[Ca^{2+}]_i$), which,
in turn, stimulates the breakdown of actin (∞∞∞) by villin in the
microvillous core. Effacement of the brush border results from extensive
loss of microvilli by membrane vesiculation. Stage 3. Expression of the
EaeA protein intimin (▼) at the bacterial surface promotes intimate
adherence to the apical cell membrane. As high local calcium concentrations dissipate, polymerised actin (∞∞∞) forms a dense fibrous pad at
the point of bacterial attachment. Myosin light chain phosphorylated by
myosin light chain kinase (∞∞●) complexes with newly polymerised
actin, distorting the enterocyte membrane and forming the basis of the
pedestal lesion. Various other cytoskeletal proteins (●), including talin,
ezrin and α-actinin, and at least one tyrosine phosphoprotein (■), the
identity of which is as yet unknown, are also present in the pedestal.

binding of bacteria to brush border microvilli is mediated by plasmid-
encoded fimbrial structures. The subsequent process of lesion formation
can be considered in three stages (Figure 14.5).

Stage one is initial non-intimate adherence of bacteria to the microvilli
of the intestinal brush border. The nature of the plasmid-encoded
adhesin and its receptor in the brush border remain unclear, but bundle-
forming pili are candidate adhesins for EPEC that have EAF plasmids.

Stage two results in localised stimulation of host cell signal transduction
pathways that lead to significant elevation of $[Ca^{2+}]_i$. This in turn
promotes the actin-severing function of villin in the microvillous core and
results in extensive vesiculation of the microvillous membrane and

complete effacement of the microvilli. Secretion of a number of EPEC proteins, including the *eaeB* gene product, which is known to be involved in signalling, provides an explanation of how EPEC may stimulate host cell signal transduction while non-intimately attached to the cell surface (Haigh *et al.*, 1995). The overall effect of the second stage is a dramatic reduction in the absorptive capacity of the brush border.

In stage three, bacteria attach intimately to the apical membrane of the damaged enterocyte by means of the surface protein intimin. The nature of the receptor is not known, but the effect of intimin binding is an explosive burst of actin polymerisation in the apical cytoplasm that results in gross localised distortion of the membrane into a pedestal structure at the point of bacterial contact. In addition, several proteins undergo phosphorylation by a number of protein kinases in infected cells. Some are cytoskeletal components, which, as phosphoproteins, associate with polymerised actin in the pedestal. Others may be ion transport proteins, in which case phosphorylation may initiate a secretory response, particularly in the early stages of infection. Prolonged stimulation of signalling pathways will eventually result in the death of infected cells, and will undoubtedly contribute significantly to the persistence of EPEC disease.

References

Baldini, M. M., Kaper, J. B., Levine, M. M., Candy, D. C. & Moon, H. W. (1983). Plasmid-mediated adhesion in enteropathogenic *Escherichia coli*. *Journal of Pediatric Gastroenterology and Nutrition*, **2**, 534–8.

Baldwin, T. J., Brooks, S. F., Knutton, S., Manjarrez-Hernandez, A., Aitken, A. & Williams, P. H. (1990). Protein phosphorylation by protein kinase C in HEp-2 cells infected with enteropathogenic *Escherichia coli*. *Infection and Immunity*, **58**, 761–5.

Baldwin, T. J., Lee-Delauney, M. B., Knutton, S. & Williams, P. H. (1993). Calcium-calmodulin dependence of actin accretion and lethality in cultured HEp-2 cells infected with enteropathogenic *Escherichia coli*. *Infection and Immunity*, **61**, 760–3.

Baldwin T. J., Ward, W., Aitken, A., Knutton, S. & Williams, P. H. (1991). Elevation of intracellular free calcium levels in HEp-2 cells infected with enteropathogenic *Escherichia coli*. *Infection and Immunity*, **59**, 1599–604.

Bray, J. (1945). Isolation of antigenically homogeneous strains of *Bact. coli Neapolitanum* from summer diarrhoea of infants. *Journal of Pathology and Bacteriology*, **57**, 239–47.

Bretscher, A. & Weber, K. (1979). Villin: the major microfilament-associated protein of the intestinal microvillus. *Proceedings of the National Academy of Sciences, USA*, **76**, 2321–5.

Bretscher, A. & Weber, K. (1980). Villin is a major protein of the microvillus cytoskeleton which binds both G and F actin in a calcium-dependent manner. *Cell*, **20**, 839–47.

Collington, G. K., Shaw, R. K., Knutton, S. & Booth, I. W. (1993). Pathophysiology of enteropathogenic *Escherichia coli* diarrhoea: new insights using Caco-2 cells. *Zeitschrift für Gastroenterologie*, **31**, 567.

Cravioto, A., Gross, R. J., Scotland, S. M. & Rowe, B. (1979). An adhesive factor found in strains of *Escherichia coli* belonging to the traditional infantile enteropathogenic serogroups. *Current Microbiology*, **3**, 95–9.

Cravioto, A., Tello, A., Villafán, H., Ruiz, J., Del Vedovo, S. & Neeser, J.-R. (1991). Inhibition of localized adhesion of enteropathogenic *Escherichia coli* to HEp-2 cells by immunoglobulin and oligosaccharide fractions of human colostrum and breast milk. *Journal of Infectious Diseases*, **163**, 1247–55.

Donnenberg, M. S., Calderwood, S. B., Donohue-Rolfe, A., Keusch, G. T. & Kaper, J. B. (1990). Construction and analysis of Tn*phoA* mutants of enteropathogenic *Escherichia coli* unable to invade HEp-2 cells. *Infection and Immunity*, **58**, 1565–71.

Donnenberg, M. S., Girón, J. A., Nataro, J. P. & Kaper, J. B. (1992). A plasmid-encoded type IV fimbrial gene of enteropathogenic *Escherichia coli* associated with localized adherence. *Molecular Microbiology*, **6**, 3427–37.

Donnenberg, M. S. & Kaper, J. B. (1991). Construction of an *eae* deletion mutant of enteropathogenic *Escherichia coli* by using a positive-selection suicide vector. *Infection and Immunity*, **59**, 4310–17.

Donnenberg, M. S. & Kaper, J. B. (1992). Enteropathogenic *Escherichia coli*. *Infection and Immunity*, **60**, 3953–61.

Donnenberg, M. S., Yu, J. & Kaper, J. B. (1993). A second chromosomal gene necessary for intimate attachment of enteropathogenic *Escherichia coli* to epithelial cells. *Journal of Bacteriology*, **175**, 4670–80.

Ewing, W. H., Davis, B. R. & Montague, T. S. (1963). Studies on the occurrence of *Escherichia coli* serotypes associated with diarrhoeal disease. Atlanta, GA: US Department of Health, Education and Welfare, Public Health Service, Communicable Disease Center, 1963.

Ferguson, W. W. & June, R. C. (1952). Experiments on feeding adult volunteers with *Escherichia coli* 111, B$_4$, a coliform organism associated with infant diarrhoea. *American Journal of Hygiene*, **55**, 155–69.

Finlay, B. B., Rosenshine, I., Donnenberg, M. S. & Kaper, J. B. (1992). Cytoskeletal composition of attaching and effacing lesions associated with enteropathogenic *Escherichia coli* adherence to HeLa cells. *Infection and Immunity*, **60**, 2541–3.

Foubister, V., Rosenshine, I., Donnenberg, M. S. & Finlay, B. B. (1994a). The *eaeB* gene of enteropathogenic *Escherichia coli* is necessary for signal transduction in epithelial cells. *Infection and Immunity*, **62**, 3038–40.

Foubister, V., Rosenshine, I. & Finlay, B. B. (1994b). A diarrheal pathogen, enteropathogenic *Escherichia coli* (EPEC), triggers a flux of inositol phosphates in infected epithelial cells. *Journal of Experimental Medicine*, **179**, 993–8.

Girón, J. A., Donnenberg, M. S., Martin, W. C., Jarvis, K. G. & Kaper, J. B. (1993a). Distribution of the bundle forming pilus structural gene (*bfpA*) among enteropathogenic *Escherichia coli*. *Journal of Infectious Diseases*, **168**, 1037–41.

Girón, J. A., Ho, S. Y. & Schoolnik, G. K. (1991). An inducible bundle-forming pilus of enteropathogenic *Escherichia coli*. *Science*, **254**, 710–13.

Girón, J. A., Ho, S. Y. & Schoolnik, G. K. (1993b). Characterization of fimbriae produced by enteropathogenic *Escherichia coli*. *Journal of Bacteriology*, **175**, 7391–403.

Goligorsky, M. S., Menton, D. N. & Hruska, K. A. (1986). Parathyroid hormone-induced changes of the brush border topography and cytoskeleton in cultured renal proximal tubular cells. *Journal of Membrane Biology*, **92**, 151–62.

Haigh, R., Baldwin, T., Knutton, S. & Williams, P. H. (1995). Carbon dioxide regulated secretion of the EaeB protein of enteropathogenic *Escherichia coli*. *FEMS Microbiology Letters*, **129**, 63–8.

Isberg R. R. & Leong, J. M. (1990). Multiple b_1 chain integrins are receptors for invasin, a protein that promotes bacterial penetration into mammalian cells. *Cell*, **60**, 861–71.

Jerse, A. E. & Kaper, J. B. (1991). The *eae* gene of enteropathogenic *Escherichia coli* encodes a 94-kilodalton membrane protein, the expression of which is influenced by the EAF plasmid. *Infection and Immunity*, **59**, 4302–9.

Jerse, A. E., Yu, J., Tall, B. D. & Kaper, J. B. (1990). A genetic locus of enteropathogenic *Escherichia coli* necessary for the production of attaching and effacing lesions on tissue culture cells. *Proceedings of the National Academy of Sciences, USA*, **87**, 7839–43.

Kauffman, F. (1947). The serology of the coli group. *Journal of Immunology*, **57**, 71–100.

Knutton, S., Baldini, M. M., Kaper, J. B. & McNeish, A. S. (1987b). Role of plasmid-encoded adherence factors in adhesion of enteropathogenic *Escherichia coli* to HEp-2 cells. *Infection and Immunity*, **55**, 78–85.

Knutton, S., Baldwin, T., Williams, P. H. & McNeish, A. S. (1989). Actin accumulation at sites of bacterial adhesion to tissue culture cells: basis of a new diagnostic test for enteropathogenic and enterohemorrhagic *Escherichia coli*. *Infection and Immunity*, **57**, 1290–8.

Knutton, S., Lloyd, D. R. & McNeish, A. S. (1987a). Adhesion of enteropathogenic *Escherichia coli* to human intestinal enterocytes and cultured human intestinal mucosa. *Infection and Immunity*, **55**, 69–77.

Knutton, S., Phillips, A. D., Smith, H. R., Gross, R. J., Shaw, R., Watson, P. & Price, E. (1991). Screening of enteropathogenic *Escherichia coli* in infants with diarrhoea by fluorescent-actin staining test. *Infection and Immunity*, **59**, 365–71.

Law, D. (1988). Virulence factors of enteropathogenic *Escherichia coli*. *Journal of Medical Microbiology*, **26**, 1–10.

Levine, M. M., Bergquist, E. J., Nalin, D. R., Waterman, D. H., Hornick, R. B., Young, C. R., Sotman, S. & Rowe, B. (1978). *Escherichia coli* strains that cause diarrhoea but do not produce heat-labile or heat-stable enterotoxins and are non-invasive. *Lancet*, **i**, 1119–22.

Levine, M. M., Nataro, J. P., Karch, H., Baldini, M. M., Kaper, J. B., Black, R. E., Clements, M. L. & O'Brien, A. D. (1985). The diarrheal response of humans to some classic serotypes of enteropathogenic *Escherichia coli* is dependent on a plasmid encoding an enteroadhesiveness factor. *Journal of Infectious Diseases*, **152**, 550–9.

Levine, M. M., Prado, V., Robins-Browne, R., Lior, H., Kaper, J. B., Moseley, S. L., Gicquelais, K., Nataro, J. P., Vial, P. & Tall, B. (1988). Use of DNA probes and HEp-2 cell adherence assay to detect diarrheagenic *Escherichia coli*. *Journal of Infectious Diseases*, **158**, 224–8.

Manjarrez-Hernandez, H. A., Amess, B., Sellers, L., Baldwin, T. J.,

Knutton, S., and Williams, P. H. & Aitken, A. (1991). Purification of a 20 kDa phosphoprotein from epithelial cells and identification as a myosin light chain. *FEBS Letters*, **292**, 121–7.

Manjarrez-Hernandez, H. A., Baldwin T. J., Aitken, A., Knutton, S. & Williams, P. H. (1992). Intestinal epithelial cell protein phosphorylation in enteropathogenic *Escherichia coli* diarrhoea. *Lancet*, **339**, 521–3.

Matsudaira, P. & Janmey, P. (1988). Pieces in the actin-severing protein puzzle. *Cell*, **54**, 139–40.

McDaniel, T. K., Jarvis, K. G., Donnenberg, M. S. & Kaper, J. B. (1995). A genetic locus of enterocyte effacement conserved among diverse enterobacterial pathogens. *Proceedings of the National Academy of Sciences, USA*, **92**, 1664–8.

Moon, H. W., Whipp, S. C., Argenzio, R. A., Levine, M. M. & Gianella, R. A. (1983). Attaching and effacing activities of rabbit and human enteropathogenic *Escherichia coli* in pig and rabbit intestines. *Infection and Immunity*, **41**, 1340–51.

Neter, E., Westphal, O., Lederitz, O., Gino, R. M. & Gorzynski, E. A. (1955). Demonstration of antibodies against enteropathogenic *Escherichia coli* in sera of children of various ages. *Pediatrics*, **16**, 801–8.

Pontremoli, S., Melloni, E., Michetti, M., Sacco, O., Salamino, F., Sparatore, B. & Horecker, B. L. (1986). Biochemical responses in activated human neutrophils mediated by protein kinase C and a Ca^{2+}-requiring proteinase. *Journal of Biological Chemistry*, **261**, 8309–13.

Riley, L., Russell, B., Agarwal, S., Arruda, S. & Ho, J. (1992). Phosphorylation of cytoskeletal proteins by enteropathogenic *Escherichia coli*. *Abstracts of the 92nd General Meeting, American Society for Microbiology*, Abstract B-180. p. 56, Washington DC: American Society for Microbiology,

Robins-Browne, R. M. (1987). Traditional enteropathogenic *Escherichia coli* of infantile diarrhea. *Reviews of Infectious Diseases*, **9**, 28–53.

Rosenshine, I., Donnenberg, M. S., Kaper, J. B. & Finlay, B. B. (1992). Signal transduction between enteropathogemic *Escherichia coli* (EPEC) and epithelial cells: EPEC induces tyrosine phosphorylation of host cell proteins to initiate cytoskeletal rearrangements and bacterial uptake. *EMBO Journal*, **11**, 3551–60.

Rothbaum, R., McAdams, A. J., Gianella, R. & Partin, J. C. (1982). A clinicopathological study of enterocyte-adherent *Escherichia coli*: a cause of protracted diarrhea in infants. *Gastroenterology*, **83**, 441–54.

Scaletsky, I. C. A., Silva, M. L. M. & Trabulsi, L. R. (1984). Distinctive patterns of adherence of enteropathogenic *Escherichia coli* to HeLa cells. *Infection and Immunity*, **45**, 534–6.

Schwartz, M. A. (1992). Transmembrane signalling by integrins. *Trends in Cell Biology*, **2**, 304–8.

Staley, T. E., Jones, E. W. & Corley, L. D. (1969). Attachment and penetration of *Escherichia coli* into intestinal epithelium of the ileum in newborn pigs. *American Journal of Pathology*, **56**, 371–92.

Ulshen, M. H. & Rollo, J. L. (1980). Pathogenesis of *Escherichia coli* gastroenteritis in man – another mechanism. *New England Journal of Medicine*, **302**, 99–101.

Van Gijsegem, F., Genin, F. & Boucher, C. (1993). Conservation of secretion pathways for pathogenicity determinants of plant and animal bacteria. *Trends in Microbiology*, **1**, 175–80.

15

Vero-cytotoxin-producing *Escherichia coli*

G. A. WILLSHAW, S. M. SCOTLAND and
B. ROWE

Vero-cytotoxin- (VT-) producing *Escherichia coli* (VTEC) were first identified in 1977 (see Chapter 10). Their clinical importance was recognised in 1982 when VT-producing strains of *E. coli* O157:H7 (O157 VTEC) were isolated in the United States of America from the stools of patients during outbreaks of haemorrhagic colitis associated with the consumption of ground beef (Riley *et al.*, 1983). Since then O157 VTEC have been identified in many outbreaks and in sporadic cases of bloody diarrhoea in North America and Great Britain, and a close association has been established between VTEC and haemolytic uraemic syndrome (HUS) (Karmali, 1989). Although O157 strains are the most important in human disease, many serogroups of *E. coli* produce VT. In humans VTEC may be associated with clinical symptoms that range from mild non-bloody diarrhoea to severe manifestations, such as HUS (see Chapter 1). VTEC also cause disease in animals (Chapter 2). In this chapter the term VTEC is used to describe strains of *E. coli* defined by their ability to produce VT, including isolates from humans, animals and food. VTEC are sometimes termed enterohaemorrhagic *E. coli* (EHEC), but this designation is more appropriate for a subset of strains such as O26 and O157 that may be associated with bloody diarrhoea.

Strains of O157 VTEC have the H-antigen 7 or are non-motile. They have been identified in clinical laboratories by their failure to ferment D-sorbitol in 24 hours. Sorbitol fermenting O157 VTEC have, however, been identified in cases of HUS in Germany (Gunzer *et al.*, 1992). Isolation of O157 VTEC has been improved by the use of selective media combined with enrichment by immunomagnetic separation with beads coated with O157 antibody (Chapman *et al.*, 1994). For epidemiological purposes, O157 VTEC can be distinguished by phage typing (Ahmed *et al.*, 1987; Frost *et al.*, 1993), which can be combined with typing of the

VT genes to give added discrimination (Thomas *et al.*, 1993b; Chapter 10). Other methods, such as plasmid profile analysis, pulsed-field gel electrophoresis and multilocus enzyme electrophoresis, may further differentiate O157 VTEC and can be applied to VTEC of other serogroups (Scotland *et al.*, 1987; Böhm & Karch, 1992; Whittam *et al.*, 1993). Restriction fragment length polymorphism analysis of genomic DNA probed with phage λ (Paros *et al.*, 1993) or the DNA of a VT-encoding phage (Willshaw *et al.*, 1994b) have also been used to differentiate O157 VTEC strains. VTEC strains other than O157 do not have biochemical markers that assist in their identification and these strains must be tested for VT production or the presence of VT genes. Such tests are not usually carried out in clinical laboratories and the incidence of non-O157 VTEC is, therefore, likely to be underestimated.

Early studies of infection by VTEC and the properties of these strains have been reviewed by Karmali (1989). The epidemiology of VTEC has been extensively discussed (Griffin & Tauxe, 1991) and recent work on the properties and genetic control of VT are discussed elsewhere (Chapter 10). In this chapter the distribution of VTEC of different serogroups in human, animal and food sources will be reviewed. Recently there has been considerable interest in the factors that may contribute to the virulence of VTEC. These properties will be discussed and compared in VTEC strains of O157 and other serogroups.

Occurrence and distribution

VTEC from human infections

Stools from patients with diarrhoea, bloody diarrhoea and HUS have been examined for VTEC to assess the relative importance of O157 and other serogroups. Several surveys in North America and the United Kingdom identified O157 VTEC in 0.1 per cent to 2.7 per cent of non-selected diarrhoeal stools (Griffin & Tauxe, 1991; Griffin *et al.*, 1993; Maher & Stanley, 1992; Salmon & Smith, 1994). Non-O157 VTEC have been sought in few studies. In Canada, 0.7 per cent of more than 5000 stools contained VTEC other than O157, compared with 2.5 per cent that contained O157 VTEC (Pai *et al.*, 1988). A survey in Germany showed that 6.6 per cent of 668 diarrhoeal stools contained non-O157 VTEC belonging to 20 O-serogroups, but only 2.7 per cent of the specimens contained O157 VTEC (Gunzer *et al.*, 1992). Further work is necessary to determine the possible geographical variation in the relative contribution of VTEC serogroups to diarrhoea. Outside North America and Europe the importance of VTEC in diarrhoea has been less fully investigated. VTEC infections are more common at northern latitudes, and in less developed regions VTEC have not been recognised as a significant cause of infectious diarrhoea.

Examination of stools from cases of haemorrhagic colitis has established O157 VTEC as a major cause of the disease. In North America and the United Kingdom, these organisms have been isolated from 15 per cent to more than 70 per cent of bloody stools (Griffin & Tauxe, 1991). Strains of VTEC belonging to other serogroups are less likely to be associated with bloody stools. Thus, Pai *et al.* (1988) reported that 97 per cent of patients with diarrhoea and O157 VTEC had bloody stools, compared with 42 per cent of those infected with non-O157 strains, predominantly those of serotype O26:H11.

Strains of O157 VTEC have caused numerous outbreaks of bloody diarrhoea in North America and the United Kingdom. Some examples, together with the proven or likely vehicle of infection are given in Table 15.1. Outbreaks have often been recognised by the appearance of a cluster of HUS cases and have frequently been in 'institutional' settings, including hospitals, schools and day care centres, in which person-to-person spread has occurred. Community outbreaks have often been associated with restaurants. Strains of VTEC of serogroups other than O157 have been rarely recognised as causes of outbreaks of diarrhoea or bloody diarrhoea. One outbreak in Japan was associated with an O145:H− strain, but the patients did not appear to have bloody diarrhoea (Itoh *et al.*, 1985). Other Japanese outbreaks have involved O111:H− and O-untypable: H19 VTEC strains (Kudoh *et al.*, 1994). The small number of reported outbreaks is not due to lack of exposure, because non-O157 VTEC have commonly been isolated from food (see 'VTEC from non-human sources').

Since the early observations made by Karmali *et al.* (1983), many prospective and retrospective studies in North America, the United Kingdom and other parts of Europe have shown that O157 VTEC are more commonly isolated from the stools of patients with HUS than are VTEC of other O-serogroups. Isolation rates of O157 VTEC have ranged from 19 per cent to more than 60 per cent; less than ten per cent of specimens contain other VTEC (data summarised from Griffin & Tauxe, 1991). Two recent investigations of HUS in Germany have resulted in the isolation of VTEC from 32 per cent (Gunzer *et al.*, 1992) and 16 per cent (Bitzan *et al.*, 1993) of patients, and in both studies O157 VTEC were

Table 15.1. *Examples of various types of outbreaks of haemorrhagic colitis and the vehicle or likely vehicle of infection*

Year	Location	Cases	Fatalities	Vehicle	Reference
North America					
1982	Michigan and Oregon, USA (Fast food restaurants)	26		Beefburgers	Riley *et al.* (1983)
1985	Canada (Nursing home)	73 (12 HUS[a])	17	? Sandwich	Carter *et al.* (1987)
1989	Missouri, USA (Community)	243 (2 HUS)	4	? Water	Swerdlow *et al.* (1992)
1992/3	Western United States (Fast food restaurants)	477 (30 HUS)	3	Beefburgers	Bell *et al.* (1994)
Great Britain					
1985	East Anglia (Community)	49	1	? Vegetables	Morgan *et al.* (1988)
1987	Birmingham (Christening party)	26 (1 HUS)		? Turkey roll	Salmon *et al.* (1989)
1991	Preston (Fast food restaurant)	23 (3 HUS)		Beefburgers	Thomas *et al.* (1993a)
1992	Stockport (Hospital)	12	4	Cross infection	Thomas *et al.* (1993a)
1993	Sheffield (Dairy farm)	6 (3 HUS)		Raw milk	Chapman *et al.* (1993b)
1993	Gwent (Community)	7 (1 HUS)		Beefburgers	Willshaw *et al.* (1994b)

[a] Haemolytic-uraemic syndrome.

predominant. Surveillance of HUS in Britain has shown VTEC infection in 33 per cent of cases and 72 per cent of these were O157 VTEC (Scotland *et al.*, 1988; Kleanthous *et al.*, 1990). Reports from Italy (Caprioli *et al.*, 1994) and Australia (Cameron *et al.*, 1995) have described community outbreaks of HUS associated with VTEC strains of serogroup O111. The latter outbreak was linked to consumption of fermented salami-like products. The differences in the relative contribution of O157 and other VTEC to HUS are difficult to evaluate because the size of studies and the methods used to identify VTEC strains have varied. Since VTEC strains including O157 are usually shed in the faeces for only a short period, a critical factor appears to be the time of specimen collection (Milford *et al.*, 1990; Tarr *et al.*, 1990).

A few studies of HUS have been carried out in Argentina, Chile and Uruguay, where it is an important paediatric problem. In a small study of Chilean children with HUS, Cordévez *et al.* (1992) reported the isolation of VTEC, including O157, from 30 per cent of patients, but in an Argentinean study they were rarely isolated (Lopez *et al.*, 1989), though in the latter there was evidence of VTEC infection in most children with HUS and in about 30 per cent of those with uncomplicated diarrhoea. The contribution of VTEC to HUS in different geographical regions requires further study, because other organisms, particularly *Shigella dysenteriae*, are also associated with this disease (Karmali, 1989).

Although VTEC of many different serogroups have been isolated from human infections, serogroups other than O157 have not emerged as a major cause of diarrhoeal illness. The second most commonly reported serotype is O26:H11, which can be associated with haemorrhagic colitis, followed by strains of serotypes O103:H2 and O113:H21 and some H-types of serogroups O111 and O128. An increasing number of serogroups have been associated with HUS (Karmali, 1989; Bockemühl *et al.*, 1992; Willshaw *et al.*, 1992) and to establish the contribution of such strains to the disease, simpler tests for non-O157 VTEC would be valuable.

Examination of VTEC for the type of VT they produce has shown that, in Canada, O157 strains that produce both VT1 and VT2 predominate (Rowe *et al.*, 1993). Only about a quarter of strains from the United Kingdom are of this type; almost all the remainder produce only VT2, and VT1-producers are very rare (Thomas *et al.*, 1993a). Some evidence suggests that O157 VTEC that produce VT2 alone are more likely to be associated with the development of HUS than are strains that produce VT1 and VT2 or VT1 alone (Ostroff *et al.*, 1989). Among non-O157

VTEC, the VT types encountered are closely serotype related (Bockemühl *et al.*, 1992; Willshaw *et al.*, 1992), for example VTEC of serogroup O26 are associated with VT1 production.

Some evidence suggests that resistance to antimicrobial agents is becoming more prevalent in O157 VTEC strains. Between 1984 and 1987, all the 56 isolates examined in Washington State were antibiotic sensitive, while, between 1989 and 1991, 13 of 176 strains were resistant to streptomycin, sulphonamides and tetracyclines (Kim *et al.*, 1994). Similarly, in England and Wales the proportion of O157 VTEC resistant to at least one antimicrobial agent increased from ten per cent in 1992 to 20 per cent in 1994 (Thomas *et al.*, 1996). The most common pattern of resistance was the same as that observed in the United States of America, and was strongly associated with strains of phage type 2. Debate continues about the effectiveness of antimicrobial treatment for infections due to O157 VTEC (Karmali, 1989). The increasing resistance of this organism may complicate future treatment trials (Kim *et al.*, 1994).

VTEC from non-human sources

Diseased and healthy cattle have been investigated as a source of VTEC. Strains of O-serogroups O5, O26 and O111 can cause severe bloody diarrhoea in calves (Hall *et al.*, 1985; Sherwood *et al.*, 1985; Mainil *et al.*, 1987; Wieler *et al.*, 1992) and O157 VTEC have been isolated from calves with diarrhoea (Ørskov *et al.*, 1977; Synge & Hopkins, 1992), but their association with disease was not established. A longitudinal study in Sri Lanka showed that VTEC strains, but not O157, formed part of the intestinal flora of healthy calves and that they were associated with diarrhoea only in animals younger than ten weeks (Tokhi *et al.*, 1993).

Healthy cattle may harbour strains of VTEC but their presence does not usually result in disease. They have been isolated from between ten and 17 per cent of healthy cattle with the higher incidence among younger animals; a wide diversity of serotypes has been identified without an overwhelming prevalence of any particular VT type (Montenegro *et al.*, 1990; Willshaw *et al.*, 1993a). In most studies, a proportion of the VTEC belonged to O-serogroups or O:H-serotypes associated with human disease. Others were of types never, so far, isolated from humans, and their status as potential human pathogens is unknown. Carriage rates of O157 VTEC of less than one per cent have been reported for healthy adult cattle (Chapman *et al.*, 1989; Montenegro *et al.*, 1990), while among animals possibly epidemiologically linked to human disease, O157 VTEC were isolated from 2.8 per cent of heifers and calves and 0.15 per cent of adult cows (Wells *et al.*, 1991). In Great Britain, 3.6 per cent of cattle that passed through an abattoir, possibly linked to a cluster of human infections, carried O157 VTEC (Chapman *et al.*, 1992, 1993a).

Surveys for VTEC in beef from processing plants and retailers in North America, the United Kingdom and Thailand found that they can be recovered from between nine and 25 per cent of samples of beef and beef products, including sausages, beefburgers and ground beef (Read *et al.*, 1990; Suthienkul *et al.*, 1990; Smith *et al.*, 1991; Willshaw *et al.*, 1993b). Some of the large number of VTEC serogroups identified have also been found in cattle and from human disease, but VTEC of serogroups O26, O111 and O157 were not recovered. Other studies in North America have examined the prevalence of O157 VTEC. Doyle & Schoeni (1987) reported that the organism occurred in 3.7 per cent of retail ground beef specimens, including samples from a region with a high incidence of human infections. In a much larger study, however, O157 VTEC were found in only 0.12 per cent of raw beef samples and in 0.06 to 0.5 per cent of veal kidneys (Griffin & Tauxe, 1991).

In many instances, outbreaks of human infection have been epidemiologically linked to a food product of bovine origin, but a causative organism has rarely been isolated from a food item that was directly involved (see Table 15.1). In the United States of America, O157 VTEC were isolated from hamburger patties in the first documented outbreak of haemorrhagic colitis (Riley *et al.*, 1983; Wells *et al.*, 1983) and from a later and much larger outbreak (Bell *et al.*, 1994). The first isolation of O157 VTEC from a beefburger in Great Britain was associated with a small community outbreak (Willshaw *et al.*, 1994b). VTEC have also been isolated from unpasteurised milk. In one case, O157 VTEC were recovered from milk on a dairy farm possibly linked to a cluster of infections (Chapman *et al.*, 1993b) and, in another, identical strains of VT-producing O22:H8 were identified in faecal samples from a patient with HUS, and in milk from the patient's home and the supplying dairy (Bockemühl *et al.*, 1992). An outbreak of infection with O157 VTEC that involved more than 100 people in Scotland was associated with consumption of pasteurised milk; identical strains were isolated from patients and from dairy equipment leading from the pasteurisation apparatus (Upton & Coia, 1994).

Pigs are the only other well-documented animal source of VTEC strains (see Chapter 3). Early studies of *E. coli* of porcine origin showed that VT production was restricted to strains of O-serogroups 138, 139 and

141 (Dobrescu *et al.*, 1983). Smith *et al.* (1988) found that the majority of *E. coli* from post-weaning diarrhoea and oedema disease in weaned pigs were VT producers and belonged to the above serogroups. The strains produce a variant of VT2 toxin, termed VT2e (Marques *et al.*, 1987), that is identical with a heat-labile toxin known as 'oedema disease principle' by early workers. Some features of oedema disease have been seen in a proportion of HUS patients, who suffer neurological symptoms and peripheral oedema (Karmali *et al.*, 1985). However, VTEC of oedema disease serogroups have never been associated with human infection and appear to be highly adapted porcine pathogens. A strain of serogroup O101 that produced VT2e has been isolated from human infection (Pierard *et al.*, 1991). Such strains have been reported in healthy pigs at slaughter, which suggests a possible source of VTEC pathogenic for humans (Caprioli *et al.*, 1993). Many other VTEC serogroups have been reported in surveys of pork and pork products (Read *et al.*, 1990; Suthienkul *et al.*, 1990; Smith *et al.*, 1991), but in only one was isolation of O157 VTEC reported (Doyle & Schoeni, 1987).

In one of the few studies of VTEC carriage by other animals, Beutin *et al.* (1993) concluded that healthy domesticated animals were a reservoir of VTEC with pathogenic potential for humans. Species tested included sheep, goats and cattle, of which 66 per cent, 56 per cent and 21 per cent respectively harboured VTEC; these strains were also present, though at lower frequencies in pigs, cats and dogs. Almost 60 per cent of the serotypes encountered have been implicated as human pathogens, but they did not include O26, O111 or O157 strains. Several studies have indicated that chickens and chicken meat are not a significant source of VTEC (Doyle & Schoeni, 1987; Read *et al.*, 1990; Suthienkul *et al.*, 1990; Smith *et al.*, 1991; Beutin *et al.*, 1993). Water has rarely been reported as a vehicle for infection. A large water-borne outbreak in the United States was associated with a breakdown in a water supply, but the source of the O157 VTEC strain involved was not traced (Swerdlow *et al.*, 1992).

Virulence properties of VTEC

Production of VT

The association of VTEC with the distinct clinical syndromes of haemorrhagic colitis and HUS implies that VT is a major virulence factor in these diseases. The toxin can be detected in the faeces of patients and in intestinal contents during infection of animals (Pai *et al.*, 1986; Tzipori *et al.*, 1987; Karmali, 1989), and the effects of toxin administration to animals has been discussed in Chapter 10. The significance of VT production by whole bacteria has been investigated in experimental infections with strains that produce VT and variants that no longer produced toxin. The results showed that VT-negative variant strains still caused diarrhoea. Equally severe damage was caused to the intestinal mucosa of piglets by feeding either a wild-type O157 VTEC or a variant that had lost the ability to produce VT (Tzipori *et al.*, 1987). The damage included development of necrosis and oedema that might, to some extent, have been expected to be caused by toxic activity. Piglets may not, however, be an adequate model for the role of VT *in vivo* because neither VT1 nor VT2 produces fluid accumulation in a piglet jejunal loop test (Tzipori *et al.*, 1987). Francis *et al.* (1989) reported that the O157 VTEC strain 933 had effects on the central nervous system when administered to piglets, but such symptoms were absent when a derivative was used that produced VT1 but not VT2.

Virulence in animal infections

It is apparent from the observations described above that properties other than VT production may be essential for the full virulence of VTEC. Examination of human colonic material failed to show attachment of O157 VTEC (Kelly *et al.*, 1990) and the sites of VTEC colonisation in human disease are unknown. Natural and experimental VTEC infections of animals have, therefore, been important in demonstrating the adhesive properties of these strains.

Examination of calves during an outbreak of dysentery due to strain S102-9 (*E. coli* O5:H⁻ VT1⁺), showed a copious bloody diarrhoea, with severe reddening in the colon and petechial haemorrhages. Bacteria were seen closely attached to the surfaces of the colon and the microvilli were effaced, disorientated or shortened, so that bacteria often appeared to attach to characteristic cups or pedestals (Hall *et al.*, 1985). Similar lesions are caused by enteropathogenic *E. coli* (EPEC) in natural or experimental infections of humans, rabbits and piglets, and have been termed attaching and effacing (AE) lesions (Moon *et al.*, 1983) (see Chapter 14). Strain S102-9 was positive in the fluorescence actin staining (FAS, see section entitled '*In vitro* assays for adhesion'), which is considered to be a test for the ability to cause AE lesions *in vitro* (Hall *et al.*, 1990). Experimental infection of calves with strain S102-9 resulted in similar effects to those seen in the naturally occurring disease (Hall et al., 1985). VTEC of other serogroups isolated from calves with diarrhoea produced AE lesions, but the experimentally induced disease was often milder than the natural infection (Mainil et al., 1987).

No animal model adequately mimics the features of human VTEC infection. When animals are infected with VTEC from human disease, bloody diarrhoea or renal damage rarely occur, but some VTEC cause AE lesions in certain regions of the intestines of animals, and there is sometimes diarrhoea. Gnotobiotic piglets fed O157 VTEC develop non-bloody diarrhoea (Francis et al., 1986; Tzipori et al., 1986, 1987; Francis et al., 1989) with AE lesions predominantly in the caecum and necrosis of up to 80 per cent of the epithelial surface. Later, bacteria penetrate to deeper tissue layers but not beyond the submucosa and there is ulceration and colonic oedema. Some animals show neurological symptoms with damage to brain tissue similar to that seen in pigs during natural oedema disease. VTEC of serogroups 4, 5, 45, 103, 111 and 145 isolated from human disease also cause diarrhoea and produce AE lesions in piglets, but with some strain-to-strain variation in the severity of the disease and a few animals develop neurological abnormalities (Tzipori et al., 1988; Hall et al., 1990).

The ability of VTEC to colonise has been studied in experimental infections in other animals. Strains of O-serogroups 26, 111, 113, 121, 145 and 157, isolated from human infections, colonise the caecum, colon and distal ileum of young and weaned rabbits (Potter et al., 1985; Pai et al., 1986; Sherman et al., 1988). Such infections result in AE lesions and non-bloody diarrhoea. Day-old chicks fed an O157 VTEC strain became colonised and, although the birds appeared healthy, there was some damage to the caecum (Beery et al., 1985). A mouse model for intestinal colonisation by VTEC has been obtained by suppression of the normal intestinal flora with streptomycin (Wadolkowski et al., 1990a). In this model a wild-type O157 VTEC strain and a variant that lacked a 60-MDa plasmid colonised the caecum and proximal colon but, the animals remained healthy. Mice died when fed a derivative of the variant strain obtained by mouse passage and there was severe renal cortical tubular necrosis, but little glomerular damage that is a usual feature of human HUS (Wadolkowski et al., 1990b).

In vitro *assays for adhesion*

Epithelial tissue has been used to study attachment of VTEC strains. In one study, only one of five O157 VTEC adhered to human buccal epithelial cells or to isolated ileal enterocytes and colonocytes from histologically normal human surgical resection material (Durno *et al.*, 1989). The adherent strain expressed type-1 fimbriae and attachment was inhibited by D-mannose, its analogues and by treatment with α-mannosidase. Treatment of brush borders with sodium metaperiodate also inhibited attachment, and it was concluded that the receptor was a linked α-mannosyl-containing glycoprotein in the brush border membrane. However, most O157 VTEC do not express type-1 fimbriae, even after many subcultures in broth. There was considerable strain to strain variation in the adherence of O157 VTEC and non-O157 VTEC to cells derived from the distal ileum or colon of rabbits (Durno *et al.*, 1989; Ashkenazi *et al.*, 1992; Winsor *et al.*, 1992). Highest levels of attachment were generally given by fimbriate strains but some non-fimbriate strains also adhered well.

Strains of O157 VTEC do not give mannose-resistant haemagglutination of erythrocytes, a property often related to fimbriae associated with colonisation in diarrhoeagenic *E. coli*. In one study it was concluded that non-haemagglutinating fimbriae, distinct from type-1, were important in the attachment of O157 VTEC to INT407 cells (Karch *et al.*, 1987), but other workers have failed to confirm the involvement of fimbriae (Junkins & Doyle, 1989; Toth *et al.*, 1990). Fimbriae such as F107 may be important in the virulence of VTEC that cause porcine oedema disease (Imberechts *et al.*, 1993; see Chapter 3).

Outer-membrane constituents of HEp-2 cells have also been proposed as receptors for the adherence of O157 VTEC (Sherman & Soni, 1988; Sherman *et al.*, 1991). Pre-incubation with antiserum to a 94-kDa outer-membrane protein inhibited attachment and also reduced fluid accumulation when the bacteria were tested in a rabbit ileal loop.

Classical enteropathogenic strains of *E. coli* that cause AE lesions in animal models give a localised pattern of attachment (LA) to cells grown in tissue culture, including the HEp-2, HeLa, HEL and Caco-2 lines (Chapter 14). Filamentous actin concentrates beneath the attached bacteria and can be observed by the FAS test (Knutton *et al.*, 1989). These authors reported that two O157 VTEC strains gave a positive result for a FAS test carried out with HEp-2 and HEL cells. Many non-O157 VTEC from human infections also adhere to HEp-2 cells in a localised manner and are FAS positive (Willshaw *et al.*, 1992). Strains of O157 VTEC do not apparently adhere to the human colon carcinoma cell line Caco-2 that develops a defined brush border (Knutton *et al.*, 1989). We have, however, found that VTEC, including O157 strains, can attach to Caco-2 cells and give a positive FAS test (Scotland *et al.*, 1994; Nishikawa *et al.*, 1995).

Strains of O157 VTEC attach to T_{84} cells, another colon-derived cell line that gives polarised growth (Winsor *et al.*, 1992). One strain (O?:H21) adhered well to produce microcolonies at tight junctions. This cell line may be a good model of intestinal colonisation, since Tzipori *et al.* (1986) noted that VTEC proliferate and penetrate at intercellular junctions in the intestine of gnotobiotic piglets.

Genetic basis of adhesion

Role of plasmids

The enteropathogenic adherence factor (EAF) plasmid of some EPEC strains specifies a plasmid-encoded regulator (*per*) that is necessary for full expression of adherence (Chapter 14; Donnenberg & Kaper, 1992; Kaper, 1994). This plasmid also encodes bundle-forming pili involved in the localised adherence phenotype. VTEC strains do not hybridise with the EAF probe (Scotland *et al.*, 1990; Willshaw *et al.*, 1992) and it has been reported that enterohaemorrhagic *E. coli* of unspecified serotype do not possess genes for bundle-forming pili (Giron *et al.*, 1993). At present there is no evidence for a regulator homologous to *per* for the AE phenotype in O157 VTEC.

Almost all O157 VTEC carry a 55- to 60-MDa plasmid and its possible role in adhesion has been investigated. Piglets infected with a wild-type O157 VTEC, or with a variant strain that had lost this plasmid develop diarrhoea and AE lesions (Tzipori *et al.*, 1987). However, the importance of the plasmid, in attachment of O157 VTEC to cultured cells is unclear. According to Junkins & Doyle (1989), loss of the plasmid is associated with increased attachment, while Karch *et al.* (1987) observed decreased attachment. A probe (CVD419) derived from the plasmid of O157 VTEC (Levine *et al.*, 1987) hybridises with plasmids in about 60 per cent of VTEC of serogroups other than O26 and O157 (Willshaw *et al.*, 1992). A plasmid that hybridises with CVD419 is not necessary for formation of AE lesions during infection of piglets with VT1-producing O103:H2 strain S22-1 (Hall *et al.*, 1990), but plasmid loss resulted in decreased attachment to HEp-2 cells. Acquisition of the O157 VTEC plasmid by the non-adherent laboratory *E. coli* strains K-12 and HB101 has been reported to confer on them the ability to adhere without the association with AE lesion formation. Patterns of attachment other than LA have been described but there is poor agreement about the cell lines to which adhesion can occur (Sherman & Soni, 1988; Toth *et al.*, 1990).

Genetics of attaching and effacing activity

Jerse *et al.* (1990) showed, with an EPEC strain (E2348/69; O127:H6), that transposon-induced mutagenesis of the *eae* chromosomal locus results in failure to induce filamentous actin accumulation in HEp-2 cells or the attaching and effacing effect typical of EPEC infection. The *eae* gene alone was not sufficient to produce AE lesions, since K-12 strains that carry the cloned *eae* sequence were FAS-negative on HEp-2 cells (Jerse *et al.*, 1990). A 1-kb DNA probe derived from the *eae* gene detected homologous sequences in EPEC and VTEC of serotypes O157:H7 and O26:H11, but not in enterotoxigenic or enteroinvasive *E. coli*. The presence of genetically related sequences and the histo-pathological similarity of AE lesions induced by EPEC and VTEC strains have led to the cloning and characterisation of the *eae* gene homologue carried by O157 VTEC (Beebakhee *et al.*, 1992; Yu & Kaper, 1992).

Comparison of the *eae* sequences from EPEC and O157 VTEC strains has shown an overall homology of 86 per cent and 83 per cent respectively at the nucleotide and amino-acid levels. The first 2200 base pairs of the O157 *eae* gene are 97 per cent homologous to those of the EPEC gene, but the homology is only 59 per cent over the 800 base pairs at the carboxyl-terminus of the sequence. The central region is conserved, which accounts for the ability of the *eae* probe to detect some VTEC strains. The nucleotide sequences of the central one-third of the *eae* genes of EPEC and *E. coli* O157 are similar to the invasin gene of *Yersinia pseudotuberculosis* and *Yersinia enterocolitica* (Jerse *et al.*, 1990; Beebakhee *et al.*, 1992). The genes were most divergent at the carboxyl-terminus, the region said to be associated with binding to receptors on eukaryotic cells and with antigenic variation. Homologues of the *eae* gene have been identified in *Citrobacter freundii* biotype 4280 (Schauer & Falkow, 1993) and *Hafnia alvei* (Albert *et al.*, 1992). The carboxyl-terminus of these genes and those of EPEC and O157 VTEC have been expressed as fusion proteins that bind to HEp-2 cells, so confirming the role of this region of *eae* and *eae*-like genes in adhesion (Frankel *et al.*, 1994).

The product of the *eae* gene of EPEC, now renamed *eaeA*, is an outer membrane protein of molecular mass 94 kDa termed intimin. This has not, however, been shown to act as an adhesin. The product of the *eae* A gene from an O157 VTEC strain is expressed as a 97-kDa outer-membrane protein, intimin$_{O157}$, on the surface of wild-type strains and on *E. coli* K-12 that carry the cloned *eaeA* gene (Louie *et al.*, 1993), but the cloned sequence did not confer on *E. coli* K-12 the ability to cause AE lesions *in vitro*. Insertional inactivation of the *eaeA* gene of an O157 strain resulted in loss of FAS activity but did not affect adherence to HEp-2 cells. The importance of intimin$_{O157}$ *in vivo* was shown by the failure of an O157 VTEC strain that carries a mutant *eae* locus to attach intimately to the colonic epithelium of newborn piglets (Donnenberg *et al.*, 1993a). The *eae* sequences of EPEC and O157 VTEC complement each other *in vitro* (Louie *et al.*, 1993) and *in vivo* (Donnenberg *et al.*, 1993a), which indicates that the carboxyl-terminal sequence divergence of the two genes may not result in functional differences.

The importance of other chromosomal genes is indicated by the isolation of two mutant strains of O157 VTEC without insertions in *eaeA* that fail to produce AE lesions *in vitro* or *in vivo* (Dytoc *et al.*, 1993). The mutations could not be complemented by a cloned *eaeA* gene from an O157 strain and the functions of the inactivated genes are unknown. As we have seen above, a 94-kDa outer-membrane fraction from *E. coli* O157 blocks adhesion and AE lesion formation by O157 on cultured cells (Sherman *et al.*, 1991); this protein is not the product of the O157 *eaeA* gene (Dytoc *et al.*, 1993; Louie *et al.*, 1993).

Intimate adhesion of EPEC strain E2348/69 involves the protein product of the *eaeB* locus situated downstream of *eaeA* (Donnenberg *et al.*, 1993b). This protein, which appears to interact with epithelial cells to signal the cytoskeletal changes involved in AE lesion formation, is translocated from the bacterium by a secretory system encoded upstream of *eaeA*. Probes based on these EPEC regions hybridise with an O157:H7 strain, and it has been shown that *eaeA*, *eaeB* and associated genes are located on a 35-kb stretch of DNA in EPEC and O157:H7 (McDaniel *et al.*, 1995). This locus of enterocyte effacement is also present in *Hafnia alvei* and *Citrobacter freundii* 4280. Its site of insertion is the same as that of a length of DNA that carries the virulence genes of uropathogenic *E. coli* strains.

Distribution of eae sequences in VTEC

Results from several sources (see Table 15.2) illustrate the distribution of *eae* sequences in VTEC of human, animal and food origin. The strains were tested by hybridisation with the *eae* probe or by amplification of the conserved *eae* region in the polymerase chain reaction (PCR).

Carriage of *eae* sequences is serogroup related. Thus, whereas O26 and O157 VTEC have *eae* genes (Jerse *et al.*, 1990), only 18 of 48 VTEC of other serogroups are *eae*-positive (Willshaw *et al.*, 1992). The correlation between the presence of *eae* sequences, localised adherence to HEp-2 cells and a positive result in the FAS test is generally good. A few strains of serotypes O111ac:H− and O165:H25 are probe positive, but fail to give LA and cannot be examined in the FAS assay (Willshaw *et al.*, 1992). They may lack sequences involved in attachment, or the conditions necessary to observe maximal expression *in vitro* may not be fully known (Nishikawa *et al.*, 1995).

The *eae* gene is present in only certain H-antigen types in an O-serogroup. Thus, for example, serotype O128ab:H25 VTEC possess the *eae* sequence, while those with the H2-antigen do not. The latter include VTEC strains that adhere to HEp-2 cells in coiled chains rather than in a localised pattern (Willshaw *et al.*, 1992). With the exception of serotypes such as O111ac:H−, strains of the same serotype are usually uniform for the presence or absence of *eae* sequences, but in most cases only a very small number of strains has been examined. More hetero-geneity may become apparent, such as in the carriage of *eae* by strains of serotype O5:H− from humans, cattle, sheep and foods. These observa-tions may indicate that different clonal lines of VT-positive strains may be present within an O-serogroup.

Overall, many more serogroups of VTEC are *eae*-negative than are *eae*-positive (Table 15.2), and this property alone may not be a reliable indicator of pathogenic potential. Two strains of O91 VTEC from human infections have been found to be highly virulent in the mouse model, but they did not carry *eae* genes (Lindgren *et al.*, 1993). VTEC strains that are *eae*-negative have been isolated from sporadic cases of haemorrhagic colitis and HUS (Burnens *et al.*, 1992; Willshaw *et al.*, 1992; de Azavedo *et al.*, 1994). Variable patterns of adhesion to three different lines of cultured cells have been reported (de Azavedo *et al.*, 1994). None of the strains was FAS-positive and introduction of a cloned *eaeA* gene did not alter the phenotype. Screening by a PCR based on an EPEC sequence indicated that the strains also lacked the *eaeB* gene. VTEC that cause

Table 15.2. *Presence of eae gene sequence in VTEC strains from various sources*[a]

Source	VTEC strains	
	eae-positive	**eae-negative**
Human	O5:H−, O55:H7, O111ac:H−, O128ab:H25,H−, O157:H7,H−, O26:H11,H−, O103:H2,H−, O121:H19	O2:H6, O8:H14, O23:H7, O104:H2, O113:H21, O118:H12, O153:H25, O4:H5,H10, O18:H7, O55:H10, O105ac:H18, O114:H4, O128ab:H2, O163:H19, O6:H−, O22:H1, O91:H21,H−, O111ac:H−, O117:H4,H7, O145:H−, O168:H−
Bovine	O5:H−, O26:H11,H−, O80:H−, O111ac:H8,H11,H−, O145:H−, O19:H25, O49:H−, O136:H−	O1:H20, O8:H9, O29:H34, O46:H38, O86:H26, O113:H4, O126:H8, O149:H5, O156:H−, O172:H21,H−, O2:H7,H29, O22:H16, O40:H8, O55:H17, O88:H25, O115:H18, O136:H16,H−, O153:H12,H21,H25, O163:H19, O6:H34, O25:H5, O43:H2, O69:H−, O91:H−, O116:H−, O138:H−, O165:H8
Porcine	O103:H−, O130	O2, O120, O138:H4,H−, O65:H9, O121, O139:H1, O107, O130, O141:H4
Ovine	O6:H2, O26:H11	O5:H−, O168:H12, O6:H14, O113:21
Food	O111:H−, O157:H7	O5:H−, O8:H9,H19,H25,H30, O22:H8,H54, O91:H−, O114:H4, O128ab:H2, O163:H19, O6:H10, O60:H9, O100:H−, O115:H10, O146:H1,H8, O9a:H−, O79:H−, O113:H4,H21, O118:H12, O151:H12

[a] Results have been combined from the following sources: Jerse *et al.* (1990); Burnens *et al.* (1992); Gannon *et al.* (1992); Willshaw *et al.* (1992, 1993a, 1993b); de Azavedo *et al.* (1994); Beutin *et al.* (1994); Louie *et al.* (1994). Unpublished data from the Laboratory of Enteric Pathogens are also included.

oedema disease in pigs do not possess *eae* sequences (Gannon *et al.*, 1993). Strains isolated from food are usually *eae*-negative, but they may belong to the same serogroups as VTEC from human disease and cannot be excluded as potential pathogens for humans.

Sequence divergence at the carboxyl-terminus of *eaeA* gene homologues in O157 VTEC (Beebakhee *et al.*, 1992; Yu & Kaper, 1992) and other VTEC, such as O111 (Louie *et al.*, 1994), may form the basis of specific PCR or probe tests for these strains. Gannon *et al.* (1993) selected a primer pair that was relatively specific, in that it amplified DNA from all O157 VTEC tested but also from one VT-positive strain of serogroup O145 and from an EPEC strain of serogroup O55. A probe based on the carboxyl-terminal sequence of the O157 *eae* gene indicated highly homologous *eae* sequences in O157 and O145 VTEC and in O55:H7 stains of both EPEC and VTEC groups (Willshaw *et al.*, 1994a). DNA sequencing has indicated that the carboxyl-termini of the *eaeA* gene homologues in O157 VTEC and an O55:H7 EPEC strain were virtually identical (Louie *et al.*, 1994). These observations support the prediction, based on multi-locus enzyme electrophoresis, that O157 VTEC are most closely related to serotype O55:H7 strains, with which they probably share a common progenitor (Whittam *et al.*, 1993).

Production of enterohaemolysin

Several types of haemolysins have been described for different groups of pathogenic *E. coli* (Beutin, 1991; see also Chapter 11). The best studied is α-haemolysin, which belongs to a family of pore-forming cytolysins termed RTX toxins and is associated with strains that cause extra-intestinal infections. A phenotypically distinct enterohaemolysin (E-Hly) has been described in connection with many VTEC including most O157 strains (Beutin, 1991). This is detected as turbid zones around colonies grown overnight on agar containing washed erythrocytes of sheep, in contrast to the large clear zones produced, after a 3-h incubation, by α-haemolysin.

Production of E-Hly correlates with carriage of a plasmid that hybridises with the CVD419 sequence derived from the 60-MDa pO157 plasmid of O157 VTEC (Scotland *et al.*, 1990; Willshaw *et al.*, 1992). Loss of E-Hly production by a wild-type strain is often accompanied by loss of the plasmid, and a K-12 transconjugant with a CVD419-hybridising plasmid derived from strain H19(O26:H11) produces E-Hly (S. M. Scotland, unpublished).

The structural genes that encode production of E-Hly activity have been cloned from the pO157 plasmid of O157 VTEC strain EDL 933 (Schmidt *et al.*, 1994). Sequence analysis of a 5.4-kb cloned fragment has revealed two open reading frames that have about 60 per cent homology with the *hlyC* and *hlyA* genes of the α-haemolysin operon (Schmidt *et al.*, 1995). The genes appear to be organised in an operon-like structure similar to that of other RTX proteins. The predicted amino-acid sequence of the enterohaemolysin encoded by the O157 homologue of the *hlyA* gene is a protein of 107 kDa with structural characteristics common to the RTX cytolysins. The CVD419 probe sequence comprises most of the O157 *hlyA* gene and part of a putative *hlyB* gene.

Antibodies to O157 VTEC enterohaemolysin have been detected in serum samples from 19 of 20 patients with O157-associated HUS, but in only one control serum (Schmidt *et al.*, 1995). Although this enterohaemolysin appears to belong to the same class of cytolysin as α-haemolysin, its probable target cell specificity is different. This function is encoded at the amino-terminus of the molecule, in which there is a relatively low degree of homology between the two proteins (Schmidt *et al.*, 1995). The haemolysin activity of E-Hly may be of less importance than its effect on other cells. α-Haemolysin has been shown to release interleukin-1β from cultured cells (Bhakdi *et al.*, 1990). Since this increases the cytotoxicity of Shiga toxin for vascular epithelial cells, by stimulating production of globotriaosylceramide (Kaye *et al.*, 1993), it is possible that VT and enterohaemolysin act synergistically in infection with O157 VTEC.

Production of E-Hly by VT-negative strains has been reported for serogroups O26 and O114 (Scotland *et al.*, 1990; Beutin, 1991). Two genetically different types of enterohaemolysins, Ehly1 and Ehly2, are associated with temperate bacteriophages harboured by strains of O26:H− and O26:H11 that did not produce VT (Beutin *et al.*, 1993; Stroeher *et al.*, 1993). Sequences for the two haemolysins are present in some enterohaemolytic *E. coli* and in others that produce α-haemolysin. E-hly+ strains of O157, O111 and O116 were, however, among those that did not carry the sequences. DNA probes for Ehly1 and Ehly2 do not hybridise with the pO157 plasmid or cloned DNA derived from it (Schmidt *et al.*, 1994). More information is necessary before the importance of Ehly1 and Ehly2 in VTEC and their relationship to the E-Hly detected with the CVD419 probe can be assessed. Investigation of the role of E-Hly in the virulence of VTEC in experimental infection will be facilitated by the availability of cloned genes and derivatives of wild-type strains that do not produce E-Hly.

Conclusions

The importance of VTEC as a group of pathogenic *E. coli* has been established, but a more complete estimate of their incidence would be obtained by better surveillance. This is particularly necessary for non-O157 VTEC, and simpler tests are required for the identification of these organisms. Some evidence suggests that there is geographical variation in the significance of VTEC in infectious diarrhoea and HUS and in the relative contributions to these diseases of O157 and other serogroups of VTEC. Further research is necessary to extend these observations.

Persuasive evidence suggests that healthy cattle are a reservoir of O157 and other VTEC strains and that they can enter the food chain to provide a source of exposure for humans. A possible route of transmission of O157 VTEC may involve infections initially in calves that shed the organism into faecal slurry that may be used on grazing grass. This provides potential for infection of older animals from which the organism may contaminate milk or carcasses at slaughter. Possible sources of VTEC in healthy animals other than cattle and a wider range of foodstuffs require further investigation.

Many features of the virulence of VTEC strains remain poorly understood. Better animal models are needed to investigate the pathogenesis of HUS, and experiments to establish the importance of different types of VT are required. Little is as yet known about the mechanisms and genetic control of the initial attachment of VTEC *in vivo* and *in vitro*. Investigation of this subject should include O157 VTEC strains that are *eae*-probe-positive and the many strains that lack *eae* sequences. Such investigations should identify the properties that are most important for VTEC and O157 VTEC virulence and, in particular, they may result in more specific virulence-marker-derived tests for VTEC.

References

Ahmed, R., Bopp, C., Borczyk, A. & Kasatiya, S. (1987). Phage typing scheme for *Escherichia coli* O157:H7. *Journal of Infectious Diseases*, **155**, 806–9.

Albert, M. J., Faruque, S. M., Ansaruzzaman, M., Islam, M. M., Haider, K., Alam, K., Kabir, I. & Robins-Browne, R. (1992). Sharing of virulence associated properties at the phenotypic and genetic levels between entero-pathogenic *Escherichia coli* and *Hafnia alvei*. *Journal of Medical Microbiology*, **37**, 310–14.

Ashkenazi, S., La Rocco, M., Murray, B. E. & Cleary, T. G. (1992). The adherence of verocytotoxin-producing *Escherichia coli* to rabbit intestinal cells. *Journal of Medical Microbiology*, **37**, 304–9.

Beebakhee, G., Louie, M., De Azavedo, J. & Brunton, J. (1992). Cloning and nucleotide sequence of the *eae* gene homologue from enterohemorrhagic *Escherichia coli* serotype O157:H7. *FEMS Microbiology Letters*, **91**, 63–8.

Beery, J. T., Doyle, M. P. & Schoeni, J. L. (1985). Colonization of chicken cecae by *Escherichia coli* associated with hemorrhagic colitis. *Applied and Environmental Microbiology*, **49**, 310–15.

Bell, B. P., Goldoft, M., Griffin, P. M., Davis, M. A., Gordon, D. C., Tarr, P. I., Bartleson, C. A., Leuis, J. H., Barrett, T. J., Wells, J. G., Baron, R. & Kobayashi, J. (1994). A multi state outbreak of *Escherichia coli* O157:H7-associated bloody diarrhea and hemolytic uremic syndrome from hamburgers: the Washington experience. *Journal of the American Medical Association*, **272**, 1349–53.

Beutin, L., Geier, D., Steinrück, H., Zimmermann, S. & Scheutz, F. (1993). Prevalence and some properties of Verotoxin (Shiga-like toxin)-producing *Escherichia coli* in seven different species of healthy domestic animals. *Journal of Clinical Microbiology*, **31**, 2483–8.

Beutin, L. (1991). The different haemolysins of *Escherichia coli*. *Medical Microbiology and Immunology*, **180**, 167–82.

Beutin, L., Aleksic, S., Zimmermann, S. & Gleier, K. (1994). Virulence factors and phenotypic traits of Verotoxigenic strains of *Escherichia coli* from human patients in Germany. *Medical Microbiology and Immunology*, **183**, 13–21.

Beutin, L., Stroeher, U. H. & Manning, P. (1993). Isolation of enterohemolysin (Ehly2)-associated sequences encoded on temperate phages of *Escherichia coli*. *Gene* 132, 95–9.

Bhakdi, S., Muhly, M., Korom, S. & Schmidt, G. (1990). Effects of *Escherichia coli* hemolysin on human monocytes. Cytocidal action and stimulation of interleukin 1 release. *Journal of Clinical Investigation*, **85**, 1746–53.

Bitzan, M., Ludwig, K., Klemt, M., König, H., Büren, J. & Müller-Wiefel, D. E. (1993). The role of *Escherichia coli* O157 infections in the classical (enteropathic) haemolytic uraemic syndrome: results of a Central European, multicentre study. *Epidemiology and Infection*, **110**, 183–96.

Bockemühl, J., Aleksic, S. & Karch, H. (1992). Serological and biochemical properties of Shiga-like toxin (Verocytotoxin)-producing strains of *Escherichia coli*, other than O-group 157, from patients in Germany. *Zentralblatt für Bakteriologie A*, **276**, 189–95.

Böhm, H. & Karch, H. (1992). DNA fingerprinting of *Escherichia coli* O157:H7 strains by pulsed-field gel electrophoresis. *Journal of Clinical Microbiology*, **30**, 2169–72.

Burnens, A. P., Boss, P., Ørskov, F., Ørskov, I., Schoad, U. B., Müller, F., Heinzle, R. & Nicolet, J. (1992). Occurrence and phenotypic properties of Verotoxin producing *Escherichia coli* in sporadic cases of gastroenteritis. *European Journal of Clinical Microbiology and Infectious Diseases*, **11**, 631–4.

Cameron, S., Walker, C., Beers, M., Rose, N. & Anear, E. (1995). Enterohaemorrhagic *Escherichia coli* outbreak in South Australia associated with the consumption of mettwurst. *Communicable Disease Intelligence*, **19**, 70–1.

Caprioli, A., Luzzi, I., Rosmini, F., Resti, C., Edefonti, A., Perfumo, F., Farina, C., Goglio, A., Gianviti, A. & Rizzoni G. (1994). Community outbreak of hemolytic uremic syndrome associated with non-O157

Verocytotoxin-producing *Escherichia coli*. *Journal of Infectious Diseases*, **169**, 208–11.

Caprioli, A., Nigrelli, A., Gatti, R. & Lavanella, M. (1993). Isolation of Verotoxin-producing *Escherichia coli* from slaughtered pigs. *European Journal of Clinical Microbiology and Infectious Diseases*, **12**, 227–8.

Carter, A. O., Borczyk, A. A., Carlson, A. K., Harvey, B., Hockin, J. C., Karmali, M. A., Krishnan, C., Korn, M. D. & Lior, H. (1987). A severe outbreak of *Escherichia coli* O157:H7-associated hemorrhagic colitis in a nursing home. *New England Journal of Medicine*, **317**, 1496–9.

Chapman, P. A., Siddons, C. A., Wright, D. J., Norman, P., Fox, J. & Crick, E. (1992). Cattle as a source of verotoxigenic *Escherichia coli* O157. *Veterinary Record*, **131**, 323–4.

Chapman, P. A., Siddons, C. A., Wright, D. J., Norman, P., Fox, J. & Crick, E. (1993a). Cattle as a possible source of verocytotoxin-producing *Escherichia coli* O157 infections in man. *Epidemiology and Infection*, **111**, 439–47.

Chapman, P. A., Wright, D. J. & Higgins, R. (1993b). Untreated milk as a source of verotoxigenic *E. coli* O157. *Veterinary Record*, **133**, 171–2.

Chapman, P. A., Wright, D. J. & Norman, P. (1989). Verotoxin-producing *Escherichia coli* infections in Sheffield: cattle as a possible source. *Epidemiology and Infection*, **102**, 439–45.

Chapman, P. A., Wright, D. J. & Siddons, C. A. (1994). A comparison of immunomagnetic separation and direct culture for the isolation of *Escherichia coli* O157 from bovine faeces. *Journal of Medical Microbiology*, **40**, 424–7.

De Azavedo, J., McWhirter, E., Louie, M. & Brunton, J. (1994). *Eae*-negative Verotoxin-producing *Escherichia coli* associated with hemolytic uraemic syndrome and haemorrhagic colitis. In *Recent Advances in Verocytotoxin-producing* Escherichia coli *Infections*, eds. M. A. Karmali & A. G. Goglio pp. 265–8. Amsterdam: Elsevier.

Cordovéz, A., Prado, V., Maggi, L., Cordero, J., Martinez, J., Misraji, A., Rios, R., Soza, G., Ojeda, A. & Levine, M. M. (1992). Enterohemorrhagic *Escherichia coli* associated with hemolytic-uremic syndrome in Chilean children. *Journal of Clinical Microbiology*, **30**, 2153–7.

Dobrescu, L. (1983). New biological effect of edema disease principle *(Escherichia coli* – neurotoxin) and its use as an *in vitro* assay for this toxin. *American Journal of Veterinary Research*, **44**, 31–4.

Donnenberg, M. S. & Kaper, J. B. (1992). Enteropathogenic *Escherichia coli*. *Infection and Immunity*, **60**, 3953–61.

Donnenberg, M. S., Tzipori, S., McKee, M. L., O'Brien, A. D., Alroy, J. & Kaper, J. B. (1993a). The role of the *eae* gene of enterohemorrhagic *Escherichia coli* in intimate attachment *in vitro* and in a porcine model. *Journal of Clinical Investigation*, **92**, 1418–24.

Donnenberg, M. S., Yu, J. & Kaper, J. B. (1993b). A second chromosomal gene necessary for intimate attachment of enteropathogenic *Escherichia coli* to epithelial cells. *Journal of Bacteriology*, **175**, 4670–80.

Doyle, M. P. & Schoeni, J. L. (1987). Isolation of *Escherichia coli* O157:H7 from retail fresh meats and poultry. *Applied and Environmental Microbiology*, **53**, 2394–6.

Durno, C., Soni, R. & Sherman, P. (1989). Adherence of Vero cytotoxin-producing *Escherichia coli* serotype O157:H7 to isolated epithelial cells and brush border membranes *in vitro*: role of type 1 fimbriae (pili) as a bacterial adhesin expressed by strain CL-49. *Clinical and Investigative Medicine*, **12**, 194–200.

Dytoc, M., Soni, R., Cockerill, F. III. De Azavedo, J., Louie, M., Brunton, J. & Sherman, P. (1993). Multiple determinants of Verotoxin-producing *Escherichia coli* O157:H7 attachment-effacement. *Infection and Immunity*, **61**, 3382–91.

Francis, D. H., Collins, J. E. & Duimstra, J. R. (1986). Infection of gnotobiotic pigs with an *Escherichia coli* O157:H7 strain associated with an outbreak of hemorrhagic colitis. *Infection and Immunity*, **51**, 953–6.

Francis, D. H., Moxley, R. A. & Andraos, C. Y. (1989). Edema disease-like brain lesions in gnotobiotic piglets infected with *Escherichia coli* serotype O157:H7. *Infection and Immunity*, **57**, 1339–42.

Frankel, G., Candy, D. C. A., Everest, P. & Dougan, G. (1994). Characterization of the C-terminal dominions of intimin-like proteins of enteropathogenic and enterohaemorrhagic *Escherichia coli*, *Citrobacter freundii* and *Hafnia alvei*. *Infection and Immunity*, **62**, 1835–42.

Frost, J. A., Cheasty, T., Thomas, A. & Rowe, B. (1993). Phage typing of Vero cytotoxin-producing *Escherichia coli* O157 isolated in the United Kingdom: 1989–91. *Epidemiology and Infection*, **110**, 469–75.

Gannon, V. P. J., Rashed, M., King, R. K. & Golsteyn-Thomas, E. J. (1993). Detection and characterization of the *eae* gene of Shiga-like toxin-producing *Escherichia coli* using polymerase chain reaction. *Journal of Clinical Microbiology*, **31**, 1268–74.

Giron, J. A., Donnenberg, M. S., Martin, W. C., Jarvis, K. G. & Kaper, J. B. (1993). Distribution of the bundle-forming pilus structural gene (*bfp*A) among enteropathogenic *Escherichia coli*. *Journal of Infectious Diseases*, **168**, 1037–41.

Griffin, P. M. & Tauxe, R. V. (1991). The epidemiology of infections caused by *Escherichia coli* O157:H7, other enterohemorrhagic *E. coli* and the associated hemolytic uremic syndrome. *Epidemiologic Reviews*, **13**, 60–98.

Griffin, P. M., Ries, A. A. & Greene, K. D. (1993). *Escherichia coli* O157:H7 diarrhea in the US: a multi-center surveillance project. *Dairy, Food and Environmental Sanitation*, **13**, 598.

Gunzer, F., Böhm, H., Rüssmann, H., Bitzan, M., Aleksic, S. & Karch, H. (1992). Molecular detection of sorbitol-fermenting *Escherichia coli* O157 in patients with hemolytic-uremic syndrome. *Journal of Clinical Microbiology*, **30**, 1807–10.

Hall, G. A., Dorn, C. R., Chanter, N., Scotland, S. M., Smith, H. R. & Rowe, B. (1990). Attaching and effacing lesions *in vivo* and adhesion to tissue culture cells of Vero cytotoxin-producing *Escherichia coli* belonging to serogroups O5 and O103. *Journal of General Microbiology*, **136**, 779–86.

Hall, G. A., Reynolds, D. J., Chanter, N., Morgan, J. H., Parsons, K. R., Debney, T. G., Bland, A. P. & Bridger, J. C. (1985). Dysentery caused by *Escherichia coli* (S102–9) in calves: natural and experimental disease. *Veterinary Pathology*, **22**, 156–63.

Imberechts, H., de Greve, H., Hernalsteens, J.-P., Schlicker, C., Bouchet, H., Pohl, P., Charlier, G., Bertschinger, H. V., Wild, P., Vandekercthove, J., van Damme, J., van Montagu, M. & Lintermans, P. (1993). The role of adhesive F107 fimbriae and of SLT-IIv toxin in the pathogenesis of edema disease in pigs. *Zentralblatt für Bakteriologie A*, **278**, 445–50.

Itoh, T., Kai, A., Saito, K., Yanagawa, Y., Inaba, M., Takahashi, M., Takano, I., Matsushita, S., Kudoh, Y., Terayana, T., Ohashi, M., Karaki, K., Yamashita, H., Ikenque, S., Satoh, H., Seki, T., Katoh, K., Hirooka, Y., Yamada, M., Akiyana, H., Ohzeki, T., Ohshiba, Y., Yamanouchi, J., Tsuchikani, H., Tsunakawa, T. & Tazaki, T. (1985). Epidemiological and laboratory investigation on an outbreak of acute enteritis associated with cytotoxin-producing *Escherichia coli* O145:H-. *Annual Report of Tokyo Metropolitan Research Laboratory for Public Health*, **30**, 16–22.

Jerse, A. E., Yu, J., Tall, B. D. & Kaper, J. B. (1990). A genetic locus of enteropathogenic *Escherichia coli* necessary for production of attaching and effacing lesions, in tissue culture cells. *Proceedings of the National Academy of Sciences*, **87**, 7839–43.

Junkins, A. D. & Doyle, M. P. (1989). Comparison of adherence properties of *Escherichia coli* O157:H7 and a 60 megadalton plasmid-cured derivative. *Current Microbiology*, **19**, 21–7.

Kaper, J. B. (1994). Molecular genetics of attaching and effacing *E. coli*. In *Recent Advances in Verocytotoxin-producing* Escherichia coli *infections*, eds. M. A. Karmali & A. G. Goglio, pp. 223–31. Amsterdam: Elsevier Science.

Karch, H., Heesemann, J., Laufs, R., O'Brien, A. D., Tacket, C. O. & Levine, M. M. (1987). A plasmid of enterohemorrhagic *Escherichia coli* O157:H7 is required for expression of a new fimbrial antigen and for adhesion to epithelial cells. *Infection and Immunity*, **55**, 455–61.

Karmali, M. A. (1989). Infection by Verocytotoxin-producing *Escherichia coli*. *Clinical Microbiology Reviews*, **2**, 15–38.

Karmali, M. A., Petric, M., Lim, C., Fleming, P. C., Arbus, G. S. & Lior, H. (1985). The association between idiopathic hemolytic uremic syndrome and infection by Verotoxin-producing *Escherichia coli*. *Journal of Infectious Diseases*, **151**, 775–82.

Karmali, M. A., Steele, B. T., Petric, M. & Lim, C. (1983). Sporadic cases of haemolytic-uraemic syndrome associated with faecal cytotoxin and cytotoxin-producing *Escherichia coli* in stools. *Lancet*, **1**, 619–20.

Kaye, S. A., Louise, C. B., Boyd, B., Lingwood, C. A. & Obrig, T. G. (1993). Shiga toxin-associated hemolytic uremic syndrome: interleukin-1β enhancement of Shiga toxin cytotoxicity toward human vascular endothelial cells *in vitro*. *Infection and Immunity*, **61**, 3886–91.

Kelly, J., Oryshak, A., Wenetsek, M., Grabiec, J. & Handy, S. (1990). The colonic pathology of *Escherichia coli* O157:H7 infection. *American Journal of Surgical Pathology*, **14**, 87–92.

Kim, H. H., Samadpour, M., Grimm L., Clausen, C. R., Besser, T. E. Baylor, M., Kobayashi, J. M., Neill, M. A., Schoenknecht, F. D. & Tarr, P. I. (1994). Characteristics of antibiotic resistant *Escherichia coli* O157:H7 in Washington State, 1984–1991. *Journal of Infectious Diseases*, **170**, 1606–9.

Kleanthous, H., Smith, H. R., Scotland, S. M., Gross, R. J., Rowe, B., Taylor, C. M. & Milford, D. V. (1990). Haemolytic uraemic syndromes in the British Isles, 1985–8: association with Verocytotoxin producing *Escherichia coli*. Part 2: microbiological aspects. *Archives of Disease in Childhood*, **65**, 722–7.

Knutton, S., Baldwin, T., Williams, P. H. & McNeish, A. S. (1989). Actin accumulation at sites of bacterial adhesion to tissue culture cells: basis of a new diagnostic test for enteropathogenic and enterohemorrhagic *Escherichia coli. Infection and Immunity*, **57**, 1290–8.

Kudoh, Y., Kai, A., Obata, H., Kusonoki, J., Monma, C., Shingaka, M., Yanagawa, Y., Yamada, S., Matsushita, S., Itoh, T. & Ohta, K. (1994). Epidemiological surveys on Vero cytotoxin-producing *Escherichia coli* infections in Japan. In *Recent Advances in Vero Cytotoxin-Producing* Escherichia coli *infections*, eds. M. A. Karmali & A. G. Goglio, pp. 53–6. Amsterdam: Elsevier Science.

Levine, M. M., Xu, J. G., Kaper, J. B., Lior, H., Prado, V., Tall, B., Nataro, J., Karch, H. & Wachsmuth, K. (1987). A DNA probe to identify enterohemorrhagic *Escherichia coli* of O157:H7 and other serotypes that cause hemorrhagic colitis and hemolytic uremic syndrome. *Journal of Infectious Diseases*, **156**, 175–82.

Lindgren, S. W., Melton, A. R. & O'Brien, A. D. (1993). Virulence of enterohemorrhagic *Escherichia coli* O91:H21 clinical isolates in an orally infected mouse model. *Infection and Immunity*, **61**, 3832–42.

Lopez, E. L., Diaz, M., Grinstein, S., Devoto, S., Mendilaharzu, F., Murray, B. E., Ashkenazi, S., Rubeglio, E., Woloj, M., Vasquez, M., Turco, M., Pickering, L. K. & Cleary, T. G. (1989). Hemolytic uremic syndrome and diarrhea in Argentine children: the role of Shiga-like toxins. *Journal of Infectious Diseases*, **160**, 469–75.

Louie, M., De Azavedo, J., Clarke, R., Borczyk, A., Lior, H., Richter, M. & Brunton, J. (1994). Sequence heterogeneity of the *eae* gene and detection of verotoxin-producing *Escherichia coli* using serotype specific primers. *Epidemiology and Infection*, **112**, 449–61.

Louie, M., De Azavedo, J. C. S., Handelsman, M. Y. C., Clark, C. G., Ally, B., Dytoc, M., Sherman, P. & Brunton, J. (1993). Expression and characterization of the *eaeA* gene product of *Escherichia coli* serotype O157:H7. *Infection and Immunity*, **61**, 4085–92.

Maher, D. P. & Stanley, P. (1992). Verotoxin-producing *Escherichia coli* infection in hospitalised patients with acute gastro-enteritis. *Journal of Infection*, **24**, 220–1.

Mainil, J. G., Duchesne, C. J., Whipp, S. C., Marques, L. R. M., O'Brien, A. D., Casey, T. A. & Moon, H. W. (1987). Shiga-like toxin production and attaching effacing activity of *Escherichia coli* associated with calf diarrhea. *American Journal of Veterinary Research*, **48**, 743–8.

Marques, L. R. M., Peiris, J. S. M., Cryz, S. J. & O'Brien, A. D. (1987). *Escherichia coli* strains isolated from pigs with edema disease produce a variant of Shiga-like toxin II. *FEMS Microbiology Letters*, **44**, 33–8.

McDaniel, T. K., Jarvis, K. G., Donnenberg, M. S. & Kaper J. B. (1995). A genetic locus of enterocyte effacement conserved among diverse enterobacterial pathogens. *Proceedings of the National Academy of Sciences, USA*, **92**, 1664–8

Milford, D., Taylor, C. M., Guttridge, B., Hall, S. M., Rowe, B. & Kleanthous, H. (1990). Haemolytic uraemic syndromes in the British Isles, 1985–8: association with Verocytotoxin producing *Escherichia coli*. Part 1: clinical and epidemiological aspects. *Archives of Disease in Childhood*, **65**, 716–21.

Montenegro, M. A., Bülte, M., Trumpf, T., Aleksic, S., Reuter, G., Bulling, E. & Helmuth, R. (1990). Detection and characterization of faecal Verotoxin-producing *Escherichia coli* from healthy cattle. *Journal of Clinical Microbiology*, **28**, 1417–21.

Moon, H. W., Whipp, S. C., Argenzio, R. A., Levine, M. M. & Giannella, R. A. (1983). Attaching and effacing activities of rabbit and human enteropathogenic *Escherichia coli* in pig and rabbit intestines. *Infection and Immunity*, **41**, 1340–51.

Morgan, G. M., Newman, C., Palmer, S. R., Allen, J. B., Shepherd, W., Rampling, A., Warren, R. E., Gross, R. J., Scotland, S. M. & Smith, H. R. (1988). First recognized community outbreak of haemorrhagic colitis due to Verotoxin-producing *Escherichia coli* O157:H7 in the UK. *Epidemiology and Infection*, **101**, 83–91.

Nishikawa, Y., Scotland, S. M., Smith, H. R., Willshaw, G. A. & Rowe, B. (1995). Catabolite repression of the adhesion of Vero cytotoxin producing *Escherichia coli* of serogroups O157 and O111. *Microbial Pathogenesis*, **18**, 223–9.

Ørskov, F., Ørskov, I. & Villar, J. A. (1977). Cattle as reservoir of Verotoxin-producing *Escherichia coli* O157:H7. *Lancet*, **ii**, 276.

Ostroff, S. M., Tarr, P. I., Neill, M. A., Lewis, J. H., Hargrett-Bean, N. & Kobayashi, J. M. (1989). Toxin genotypes and plasmid profiles as determinants of systemic sequelae in *Escherichia coli* O157:H7 infections. *Journal of Infectious Diseases*, **160**, 994–8.

Pai, C. H., Ahmed, N., Lior, H., Johnson, W. M., Sims, H. V. & Woods, D. E. (1988). Epidemiology of sporadic diarrhea due to Verocytotoxin-producing *Escherichia coli*: a two year prospective study. *Journal of Infectious Diseases*, **157**, 1054–7.

Pai, C. H., Kelly, J. K. & Meyers, G. L. (1986). Experimental infection of infant rabbits with verotoxin-producing *Escherichia coli*. *Infection and Immunity*, **51**,16–23.

Paros, M., Tarr, P. I., Kim, H., Besser T. E. & Hancock, D. D. (1993). A comparison of human and bovine *Escherichia coli* O157:H7 isolates by toxin genotype, plasmid profile and bacteriophage λ-restriction fragment length polymorphism profile. *Journal of Infectious Diseases*, **193**, 1300–3.

Pierard, D., Huyghens, L., Lauwers, S. & Lior, H. (1991). Diarrhoea associated with *Escherichia coli* producing porcine oedema disease verotoxin. *Lancet*, **ii**, 762.

Potter, M. E., Kaufmann, A. F., Thomason, B. M., Blake, P. A. & Farmer, J. J. (1985). Diarrhea due to *Escherichia coli* O157:H7 in the infant rabbit. *Journal of Infectious Diseases*, **152**, 1341–3.

Read, S. C., Gyles, C. L., Clarke, R. C., Lior, H. & McEwen, S. (1990). Prevalence of Vero cytotoxigenic *Escherichia coli* in ground beef, pork and chicken in Southwestern Ontario. *Epidemiology and Infection*, **105**, 11–20.

Riley, L. W., Remis, R. S., Helgerson, S. D., McGee, H. B., Wells, J. G., Davis, B. R., Hebert, R. J., Olcott, E. S., Johnson, L. M., Hargrett, N. T., Blake, P. A. & Cohen, M. L. (1983). Hemorrhagic colitis associated with a rare *Escherichia coli* serotype. *New England Journal of Medicine*, **308**, 681–5.

Rowe, P. C., Orrbine, E., Lior, H., Wells, G. A., McLaine, P. N. and the CPKDRC co-investigators (1993). A prospective study of exposure to verotoxin-producing *Escherichia coli* among Canadian children with haemolytic uraemic syndrome. *Epidemiology and Infection*, **110**, 1–7.

Salmon, R. L., Farrell, I. D., Hutchinson, J. G. P., Coleman, D. J., Gross, R. J., Fry, N. K., Rowe, B. & Palmer, S. R. (1989). A christening party outbreak of haemorrhagic colitis and haemolytic uraemic syndrome associated with *Escherichia coli* O157:H7. *Epidemiology and Infection*, 103, 249–54.

Salmon, R. L. & Smith R. M. M. (1994). How common is *Escherichia coli* O157 and where is it coming from? Total population surveillance in Wales 1990–1993. In *Recent Advances in Vero cytotoxin-producing* Escherichia coli *infections*, eds. M. A. Karmali & A. G. Goglio, pp. 73–5. Amsterdam: Elsevier Science.

Schauer, D. B. & Falkow, S. (1993). Attaching and effacing locus of a *Citrobacter freundii* biotype that causes transmissible murine colonic hyperplasia. *Infection and Immunity*, 61, 2486–92.

Schmidt, H., Beutin, L. & Karch, H. (1995). Molecular analysis of the plasmid-encoded hemolysin of *Escherichia coli* O157:H7 strain EDL 933. *Infection and Immunity* 63, 1055–61.

Schmidt, H., Karch, H. & Beutin, L. (1994). The large-sized plasmids of enterohaemorrhagic *Escherichia coli* O157 strains encode hemolysins, which are presumably members of the *E. coli* α-hemolysin family. *FEMS Microbiology Letters*, 117, 189–96.

Scotland, S. M., Knutton, S., Said, B. & Rowe, B. (1994). Adherence to Caco-2 cells of Vero cytotoxin-producing strains of *Escherichia coli* belonging to serogroups other than O157. In *Recent Advances in Verocytoxin-producing* Escherichia coli *infections*, eds. M. A. Karmali, & A. G. Goglio, pp. 257–60. Amsterdam: Elsevier Science.

Scotland, S. M., Rowe, B., Smith, H. R., Willshaw, G. A. & Gross, R. J. (1988). Vero cytotoxin-producing strains of *Escherichia coli* from children with haemolytic uraemic syndrome and their detection by specific DNA probes. *Journal of Medical Microbiology*, 25, 237–43.

Scotland, S. M., Willshaw, G. A., Smith, H. R. & Rowe, B. (1987). Properties of strains of *Escherichia coli* belonging to serogroup O157 with special reference to production of Vero cytotoxins VT1 and VT2. *Epidemiology and Infection*, 99, 613–24.

Scotland, S. M., Willshaw, G. A., Smith, H. R. & Rowe, B. (1990). Properties of strains of *Escherichia coli* O26:H11 in relation to their enteropathogenic or enterohemorrhagic classification. *Journal of Infectious Diseases*, 162, 1069–74.

Sherman, P., Cockerill, F., Soni, R. & Brunton, J. (1991). Outer membranes are competitive inhibitors of *Escherichia coli* O157:H7 adherence to epithelial cells. *Infection and Immunity*, 59, 890–99.

Sherman, P. M. & Soni, R. (1988). Adherence of Vero cytotoxin-producing *Escherichia coli* serotype O157:H7 to human epithelial cells in tissue culture: role of outer membranes as bacterial adhesins. *Journal of Medical Microbiology*, 26, 11–17.

Sherman, P. M., Soni, R. & Karmali, M. (1988). Attaching and effacing adherence of Vero cytotoxin-producing *Escherichia coli* to rabbit intestinal epithelium *in vivo*. *Infection and Immunity*, 56, 756–61.

Sherwood, D., Snodgrass, D. R. & O'Brien, A. D. (1985). Shiga-like toxin production from *Escherichia coli* associated with calf diarrhoea. *Veterinary Record*, 116, 217–18.

Smith, H. R., Cheasty, T., Roberts, D., Thomas, A. & Rowe, B. (1991). Examination of retail chickens and sausages in Britain for Vero cytotoxin-producing *Escherichia coli*. *Applied and Environmental Microbiology*, 57, 2091–3.

Smith, H. R., Scotland, S. M., Willshaw, G. A., Wray, C., McLaren, I. M.,

Cheasty, T. & Rowe, B. (1988). Vero cytotoxin production and presence of VT genes in *Escherichia coli* strains of animal origin. *Journal of General Microbiology*, **134**, 829–34.

Stroeher, U. W., Bode, L., Beutin, L. & Manning, P. (1993). Characterization and sequence of a 33kDa enterohemoylsin (Ehly1)-associated protein in *Escherichia coli*. *Gene*, **132**, 89–94.

Suthienkul, O., Brown, J. E., Seriwatana, J., Tienthongdee, S., Sastravaha, S. & Echeverria, P. (1990). Shiga-like toxin-producing *Escherichia coli* in retail meats and cattle in Thailand. *Applied and Environmental Microbiology*, **56**, 1135–9.

Swerdlow, D. L., Woodruff, B. A., Brady, R. C., Griffin, P. M., Tippen, S., Donnell, H. O., Geldreich, E., Payne, B. J., Meyer, A., Wells, J. G., Greene, K. D., Bright, M., Bean, N. H. & Blake, P. A. (1992). A waterborne outbreak in Missouri of *Escherichia coli* O157:H7 associated with bloody diarrhea and death. *Annals of Internal Medicine*, **117**, 812–9.

Synge, B. A. & Hopkins, G. F. (1992). Verotoxigenic *Escherichia coli* O157 in Scottish calves. *Veterinary Record*, **130**, 583.

Tarr, P. I., Neill, M. A., Clausen, C. R., Watkins, S. L., Christie, D. L. & Hickman, R. O. (1990). *Escherichia coli* O157:H7 and the hemolytic uremic syndrome: importance of early cultures in establishing the etiology. *Journal of Infectious Diseases*, **162**, 553–6.

Thomas, A., Chart, H., Cheasty, T., Smith, H. R., Frost, J. A. & Rowe, B. (1993a). Vero cytotoxin-producing *Escherichia coli*, particularly serogroup O157, associated with human infections in the United Kingdom: 1989–91. *Epidemiology and Infection*, **110**, 591–600.

Thomas, A., Cheasty, T., Frost, J. A., Chart, H., Smith, H. R. & Rowe, B. (1996). Vero cytotoxin-producing *Escherichia coli*, particularly serogroup O157, associated with human infections in England and Wales: 1992–4. *Epidemiology and Infection*, **117**, 1–10.

Thomas, A., Smith, H. R. & Rowe, B. (1993b). Use of digoxigenin-labelled oligonucleotide DNA probes for VT2 and VT2 human variant genes to differentiate Vero cytotoxin-producing *Escherichia coli* strains of serogroup O157. *Journal of Clinical Microbiology*, **31**, 1700–3.

Tokhi, A. M., Peiris, J. S. M., Scotland, S. M., Willshaw, G. A., Smith, H. R. & Cheasty, T. (1993). A longitudinal study of Vero cytotoxin producing *Escherichia coli* in cattle calves in Sri Lanka. *Epidemiology and Infection*, **110**, 197–208.

Toth, I., Cohen, M. L., Rumschlag, H. S., Riley, L. W., White, E. H., Carr, J. H., Bond, W. W. & Wachsmuth, I. K. (1990). Influence of the 60-megadalton plasmid on adherence of *Escherichia coli* O157:H7 and genetic derivatives. *Infection and Immunity*, **58**, 1223–31.

Tzipori, S., Karch, H., Wachsmuth, I. K., Robins-Browne, R. M., O'Brien, A. D., Lior, H., Cohen, M. L., Smithers, J. & Levine, M. M. (1987). Role of a 60-megadalton plasmid and Shiga-like toxins in the pathogenesis of infection caused by enterohemorrhagic *Escherichia coli* O157:H7 in gnotobiotic piglets. *Infection and Immunity*, **55**, 3117–25.

Tzipori, S., Wachsmuth, I. K., Chapman, C., Birner, R., Brittingham, J., Jackson, C. & Hogg, J. (1986). The pathogenesis of hemorrhagic colitis caused by *Escherichia coli* O157:H7 in gnotobiotic piglets. *Journal of Infectious Diseases*, **154**, 712–16.

Tzipori, S., Wachsmuth, I. K., Smithers, J. & Jackson, C. (1988). Studies in gnotobiotic piglets on non-O157:H7 *Escherichia coli* serotypes isolated from patients with hemorrhagic colitis. *Gastroenterology,* **94**, 590–7.

Upton, P. & Coia, J. E. (1994). Outbreak of *Escherichia coli* O157 infection associated with pasteurised milk supply. *Lancet,* **344**, 1015.

Wadolkowski, E. A., Burris, J. A. & O'Brien, A. D. (1990a). Mouse model for colonization and disease caused by enterohemorrhagic *Escherichia coli* O157:H7. *Infection and Immunity,* **58**, 2438–45.

Wadolkowski, E. A., Sung, L. M., Burris, J. A., Samuel, J. E. & O'Brien, A. D. (1990b). Acute renal tubular necrosis and death of mice orally infected with *Escherichia coli* strains that produce Shiga-like toxin type II. *Infection and Immunity,* **58**, 3959–65.

Wells, J. G., Davis, B. R., Wachsmuth, I. K., Riley, L. W., Remis, R. S., Sokolow, R. & Morris, G. K. (1983). Laboratory investigation of hemorrhagic colitis outbreaks associated with a rare *Escherichia coli* serotype. *Journal of Clinical Microbiology,* **18**, 512–20.

Wells, J. G., Shipman, L. D., Greene, K. D., Sowers, E. G., Green, J. H., Cameron, D. N., Downes, F. P., Martin, M. L., Griffin, P. M., Ostroff, S. M., Potter, M. E., Tauxe, R. V. & Wachsmuth, I. K. (1991). Isolation of *Escherichia coli* serotype O157:H7 and other Shiga-like toxin-producing *E. coli* from dairy cattle. *Journal of Clinical Microbiology,* **29**, 985–9.

Whittam, T. S., Wolfe, M. L., Wachsmuth, I. K., Ørskov, F., Ørskov, I. & Wilson, R. A. (1993). Clonal relationships among *Escherichia coli* strains that cause hemorrhagic colitis and infantile diarrhea. *Infection and Immunity,* **61**, 1619–29.

Wieler, L. H., Bauerfeind, R. & Baljer, G. (1992). Characterization of Shiga-like toxin producing *Escherichia coli* (SLTEC) isolated from calves with and without diarrhea. *Zentralblatt für Bakteriologie A,* **276**, 243–53.

Willshaw, G. A., Scotland, S. M., Smith, H. R. & Rowe, B. (1992). Properties of Vero cytotoxin-producing *Escherichia coli* of human origin of O serogroups other than O157. *Journal of Infectious Diseases,* **166**, 797–802.

Willshaw, G. A., Cheasty, T., Jiggle, B., Rowe, B., Gibbons, D. & Hutchinson, D. N. (1993a). Vero cytotoxin-producing *Escherichia coli* in a herd of dairy cattle. *Veterinary Record,* **132**, 96.

Willshaw, G. A., Smith, H. R., Roberts, D., Thirlwell, J., Cheasty, T. & Rowe, B. (1993b). Examination of raw beef products for the presence of Vero cytotoxin producing *Escherichia coli,* particularly those of serogroup O157. *Journal of Applied Bacteriology,* **15**, 420–6.

Willshaw, G. A., Scotland, S. M., Smith, H. R., Cheasty, T., Thomas, A. & Rowe, B. (1994a). Hybridization of strains of *Escherichia coli* O157 with probes derived from the *eae*A gene of enteropathogenic *E. coli* and the *eae*A gene homolog from a Vero cytotoxin-producing strains of *E. coli* O157. *Journal of Clinical Microbiology,* **32**, 897–902.

Willshaw, G. A., Thirlwell, J., Jones, A. P., Parry, S., Salmon, R. L. & Hickey, M. (1994b). Vero cytotoxin-producing *Escherichia coli* O157 in beefburgers linked to an outbreak of diarrhoea, haemorrhagic colitis and haemolytic uraemic syndrome. *Letters in Applied Microbiology,* **18**, 304–7.

Winsor, D. K., Ashkenazi, S., Chiovetti, R. & Cleary, T. G. (1992). Adherence of enterohemorrhagic *Escherichia coli* strains to a human colonic epithelial cell line (T_{84}). *Infection and Immunity,* **60**, 1613–17.

Yu, J. & Kaper, J. B. (1992). Cloning and characterization of the *eae* gene of enterohaemorrhagic *Escherichia coli* O157:H7. *Molecular Microbiology,* **6**, 411–17.

16

Enteroinvasive *Escherichia coli*

T. L. HALE, P. ECHEVERRIA and J. P. NATARO

Enteroinvasive *Escherichia coli* (EIEC) are a small subset of *E. coli* biotypes that characteristically cause dysentery. In the late 1960s specific *E. coli* serotypes were clinically implicated as causative agents of enteritis or colitis (Sakazaki *et al.*, 1967). Volunteers challenged with isolates from patients with colitis-like symptoms developed bacillary dysentery (Du-Pont *et al.*, 1971). Most EIEC serogroups are closely related to *Shigella dysenteriae* or *Sh. boydii* serogroups (Cheasty & Rowe, 1983), and are *Shigella*-like in that they are non-motile, lactose negative and lysine decarboxylase negative (Toledo & Trabulsi, 1983). Other *Shigella*-like phenotypic characteristics of EIEC include the ability to invade HeLa cells (DuPont *et al.*, 1971) and to evoke keratoconjunctivitis in the guinea-pig eye (Sérény test) (Toledo & Trabulsi, 1983).

The epidemiology of enteroinvasive *Escherichia coli* infections

Epidemiological studies of EIEC infections are difficult to conduct, because the biochemical characteristics of the organisms are variable (Toledo & Trabulsi, 1983). While most strains are non-motile and lysine decarboxylase negative, EIEC may be either lactose-negative or lactose positive, and no single biochemical test is entirely specific. Moreover, not all isolates fall into the classical EIEC serogroups O28, O29, O112, O121, O124, O135, O136, O143, O144, O152, O164 and O167. Of the EIEC identified by non-serological methods in Thailand, ten per cent did not belong to these typical serogroups, and a new serogroup, O173, was identified (Ørskov *et al.*, 1991). DNA probes that specifically hybridise with genes carried on the EIEC virulence plasmid (Sethabutr *et al.*, 1985) have allowed epidemiological surveillance without the use of traditional

The views of the authors do not purport to reflect the position of the U.S. Department of the Army or the Department of Defense (para 4–3, AR 360–5).

serological or biochemical testing (Sethabutr *et al.*, 1993). The polymerase chain reaction (PCR) is an extremely sensitive detection technique for EIEC virulence genes (Echeverria *et al.*, 1992). Nevertheless,
these genetic screening techniques lack the necessary specificity to differentiate between *Shigella* and EIEC, and biochemical or serological
confirmation of the identity of probe- or primer-positive strains remains a
necessary component of epidemiological surveys (Echeverria *et al.*, 1991).

Though surveillance techniques for EIEC are limited, the essential
epidemiological characteristics of these infections have been described.
Outbreaks of EIEC are usually food-borne, but person-to-person transmission is possible in circumstances such as those in mental institutions
(Harris *et al.*, 1985). The first and largest identified epidemic of EIEC in
the United States of America affected 227 persons in 96 separate outbreaks. The organism belonged to serogroup O124 EIEC and the vehicle
of infection was imported French Camembert or Brie cheese (Tulloch
et al., 1973). Enteroinvasive *E. coli* have also been isolated from
passengers on an ocean cruise who developed diarrhoea after eating
potato salad (Snyder *et al.*, 1984) and a compilation of the incidence of

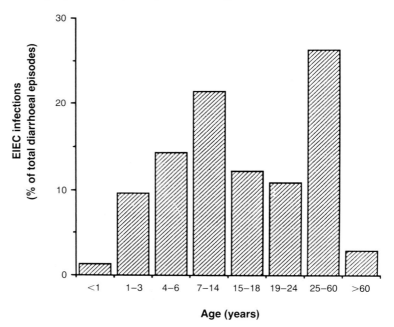

Fig. 16.1. The age distribution of *Escherichia coli* O124 infections in
Hungary, 1959–1962 (After Keyti, 1989). EIEC, enteroinvasive *Escherichia coli*.

EIEC O124 in Hungary during 1956–1966 showed that water-borne outbreaks were common (Keyti, 1989). The ability of these organisms to survive in water and to multiply in food (Keyti, 1989) apparently explains the pattern of sporadic outbreaks due to ingestion of sufficient quantities of contaminated substances. The incidence of EIEC in Hungary was evenly distributed across the age spectrum of three to 90 years (Figure 16.1). More recently EIEC was isolated in Thailand from approximately five per cent of hospital patients with diarrhoea (Echeverria *et al.*, 1991) and a similar proportion of travellers who developed diarrhoea while visiting Mexico or Nepal were infected with EIEC (Taylor *et al.*, 1988). The epidemiology of EIEC infections in children and adults in developing and developed countries has yet to be defined.

The clinical characteristics of enterinvasive *Escherichia coli* infection

Challenge of volunteers with O143 and O144 EIEC strains has provided graphic evidence of the virulence of these organisms (DuPont *et al.*, 1971). Within 24 hours of challenge (mean 11 hours), seven of 13 volunteers developed a febrile illness characterised by temperatures as high as 40°C, headache, myalgia, abdominal colic and profuse diarrhoea or dysentery. Although blood cultures were uniformly negative, two volunteers developed transient hypotension and severe systemic tox-aemia. Serious manifestations of colitis in five of the seven ill volunteers made treatment with intramuscular ampicillin necessary for three days. This resulted in rapid defervesence, firming of stools and bacteriological cure.

If EIEC colitis is presumed to be analogous to *Shigella* infections, it can be surmised that the dysentery elicited by both reflects inhibited colonic fluid absorption (Rout *et al.*, 1975) with the frequency of the small-volume stools determined by ileo–caecal flow. The presence of erythrocytes and sheets of neutrophils in the stool is almost diagnostic of enteroinvasive bacterial infection and reflects desquamation and ulceration of the colonic mucosa. The pathological changes produced by EIEC in ligated rabbit ileal loops consist of shigellosis-like colitis with mucosal disarray, necrosis, ulceration and intense acute inflammation. Examination, by immunofluorescence of ileal sections from guinea-pigs orally challenged with EIEC, shows extensive bacterial invasion of the epi-thelium (DuPont *et al.*, 1971).

Shigella and EIEC infections are frequently characterised by a prodrome of watery diarrhoea that precedes the onset of dysentery. Indeed, a majority of EIEC infections is characterised solely by watery diarrhoea (Tulloch *et al.*, 1973; Snyder *et al.*, 1984; Taylor *et al.*, 1988). In these cases, the clinical picture of EIEC infection is indistinguishable from that of enterotoxigenic *E. coli* (ETEC) infection. Net colonic water secretion has also been noted in patients suffering from extensive colitis (Butler *et al.*, 1986) and prostaglandins produced by the inflammatory response to bacterial invasion may contribute to the mucoid diarrhoea (Sharon *et al.*, 1978). The watery diarrhoea elicited by ETEC and *Shigella* infection may also be indicative of an enterotoxic syndrome.

Enterotoxins of enteroinvasive *Escherichia coli*

Evidence for enterotoxic activity in **Shigella** *species*

Active fluid secretion has been demonstrated by perfusion of the small intestine of monkeys after intragastric challenge with *Sh. flexneri* (Rout *et al.*, 1975), but dysentery without active fluid secretion was observed in animals inoculated intracaecally. This suggests that shigellae may produce enterotoxin(s) as the organisms pass through the small intestine, and enterotoxicity has been demonstrated *in vitro* with culture supernatants of several strains of *Sh. flexneri*. For example, intragastric administration of a partially purified *Sh. flexneri* 3a enterotoxin to suckling mice induces fluid secretion within 2.5 hours and this enterotoxin also elicits fluid accumulation in ligated rabbit ileal loops after four hours (Ketyi *et al.*, 1978a,b). In addition, EIEC K-12–*Sh. flexneri* hybrids induce fluid accumulation in rabbit ileal loops. This suggests that a *Sh. flexneri* chromosomal region linked to the Arg (90 minutes) and Mtl (81 minutes) markers confers a secretion-positive phenotype (Sansonetti *et al.*, 1983b).

Evidence for an enterotoxin in EIEC

The prominent watery diarrhoea of EIEC infections and the suggestive evidence for enterotoxic activity in *Shigella* spp. prompted a search for possible EIEC enterotoxins. Culture supernatants from nine EIEC strains induced significant increases in transepithelial electrical potential difference (PD) and short-circuit current (I_{sc}) when tested against rabbit ileum in Ussing chambers. Sterile culture supernatants from two of these stains produced moderate, but significant, fluid accumulation in ligated

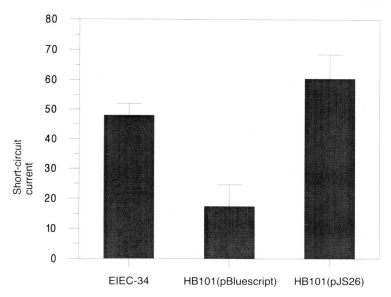

Fig. 16.2. Ussing chamber experiments with enteroinvasive *Escherichia coli* (EIEC) supernatants. Cultures were grown overnight at 37°C and the spent medium was filter-sterilised. Of each supernatant 200 μl was added to equilibrated Ussing chambers and changes in potential difference and in short-circuit current were determined. HB101(pJS26) is a 2.8-kb *Hind*III fragment cloned from EIEC-34 into pBluescript and expressed in *E. coli* HB101. Bars represent changes in short-circuit current as the mean of nine experiments; error bars represent the standard error of the mean.

rabbit ileal loops. As with the Shiga and Shiga-like cytotoxin/enterotoxins of *Sh. dysenteriae* type-1 and enterohaemorrhagic *E. coli*, expression of the extracellular enterotoxic activity of EIEC depends on iron-restricted growth conditions. The biological activity of EIEC culture supernatants was not, however, accompanied by tissue damage, either in Ussing chambers or in ileal loops. Although sterile supernatants of 35 EIEC strains were cytotoxic for Vero cell monolayers, this toxicity could not be neutralised with antitoxin raised against *E. coli* Shiga-like toxin (SLT), and homology with neither SLT-I nor SLT-II was found in the EIEC genome (Fasano *et al.*, 1990).

The enterotoxicity of the EIEC culture supernatant is relatively heat-stable and retains 75 per cent of its activity after boiling for 20 minutes. After high-pressure liquid chromatography, activity is present in a 68- to 80-kDa fraction of the supernatant. Cytotoxic activity is present below 30 kDa, which indicates that the enterotoxin, designated EIET for enteroinvasive enterotoxin, and cytotoxin are distinct (Fasano *et al.*, 1990). Antisera against the 30-100-kDa fraction of EIEC strain EI-34 supernatant neutralise the I_{sc} activity of EIET in Ussing chambers. In addition, sera obtained from volunteers after challenge with *Sh. flexneri* 2a neutralise the EIET activity of EI-34, which suggests that shigellae express a related toxin (J. P. Nataro, J. Seriwatana, J. G. Morris & A. Fasano, unpublished). Although EIET appears to be a cytotonic toxin, the physiological mechanism by which it alters fluid handling in the bowel remains unknown.

The genetics of EIET expression

A series of transposon Tn*phoA* gene fusions was generated in EIEC strain EI-34 in an attempt to clone the EIET locus (J. Nataro, J. Seriwatana, A. Fasano & J. G. Morris, unpublished). Alkaline-phosphatase-positive fusions were screened for enhanced expression when grown under conditions of iron restriction, and the iron-regulated fusions were then screened in Ussing chambers for decreased I_{sc} activity. DNA flanking Tn*phoA*- from EIET-negative strains was subcloned and used to probe a cosmid library of EI-34 DNA. In this way two cosmid clones, designated pJS34.1 and pJS34.5, that conferred the I_{sc} activity of EIET on a non-toxigenic *E. coli* recipient were identified. When these cosmids were subcloned into the pBluescript vector, a 2.8-kb *Hind*III fragment was identified that reproducibly causes the increases in I_{sc} that define EIET activity (Figure 16.2).

Determination of the DNA sequence of the 2.8-kb insert revealed two open reading frames (ORFs) that encode putative proteins, ORF1 (16.1 kDa) and ORF2 (63.1 kDa). Neither ORF contains a hydrophobic signal sequence at the 5'-end, but both display potential promoter sequences. The translated sequences of ORF1 and ORF2 did not reveal significant amino-acid similarity with any other known prokaryotic gene or protein. Both ORFs were separately subcloned for testing in Ussing chambers, and only ORF2 was found to give an increase in I_{sc}. An ORF2 DNA fragment probe was prepared from pJS26 and hybridised against a collection of EIEC and *Shigella* strains under high stringency. Homologous sequences were found in EIEC (75 per cent) and *Shigella* strains (80 per cent) that included members of all four *Shigella* species. None of 110 other enteric strains carried homologous sequences. The ORF2 gene appears to be identical to a plasmid-encoded *Shigella* enterotoxin, designated ShET2 to distinguish it from the previously described chromosomal *Shigella* enterotoxin designated ShET1 (Fasano *et al.*, 1995).

In order to estimate the effect of EIET on virulence, a deletion mutation of ORF2 was constructed and introduced by allelic exchange in place of the native gene in EIEC strain EI-34. Surprisingly, culture supernatants from this mutant gave decreased, but still significant, rises in I_{sc} in Ussing chamber experiments. This suggests that additional enterotoxin(s) are expressed by EIEC, and work is in progress to identify them. Further study of ORF2 deletion mutants in ligated rabbit ileal loops, in guinea-pigs and primates after intragastric challenge, and finally in challenged human volunteers will be necessary to establish the role of EIET in the virulence of EIEC and *Shigella* species. It should be possible to determine unambiguously the contribution of EIET by construction of an isogenic ORF2 mutant strain.

The genetic basis of invasion by enteroinvasive *Escherichia coli*

Evidence for plasmid-mediated virulence

Though enterotoxin(s) may contribute to EIEC virulence, the invasive phenotype is the defining characteristic of these pathogens. In seminal work, Sansonetti and his colleagues demonstrated that the invasive phenotype is associated with a 120-MDa (230-kb) plasmid of *Sh. sonnei* (Sansonetti *et al.*, 1981) and *Sh. flexneri* (Sansonetti *et al.*, 1982b). This suggested that a similar plasmid might carry genes that encode the invasive phenotype in '*Shigella*-like' strains of *E. coli* (Sansonetti *et al.*, 1982a). A survey of EIEC strains in the collections of the Institut Pasteur and the Walter Reed Army Institute of Research confirmed that a 120-MDa plasmid is present in all Sérény-positive cultures. Spontaneous plasmid loss in these EIEC strains correlated with a Sérény-negative phenotype, and virulence was restored by conjugal transfer of the pWR110 virulence plasmid of *Sh. flexneri* serotype 5. Although this showed that the *E. coli* and *Shigella* virulence plasmids are functionally interchangeable, *Eco*RI and *Bam*HI restriction analysis of the virulence plasmid of EIEC strain 4608-58 revealed a restriction profile significantly different from that of *Shigella* virulence plasmids. Nevertheless, Southern blot hybridisation with radiolabelled plasmid DNA from either EIEC or *Sh. flexneri* serotype 5 suggested extensive intergeneric homology (Sansonetti *et al.*, 1982a, 1983a, 1985; Hale *et al.*, 1983). From these studies it was surmised that *Shigella* and EIEC virulence plasmids are derived from a common ancestor, possibly a Gram-positive organism, to judge from their A+T content of 70 per cent, in comparison to 50 per cent for the *E. coli* chromosome (Baudry *et al.*, 1988; Adler *et al.*, 1989). Subsequent evolutionary divergence has apparently resulted in the loss or rearrangement of some restriction sites.

Nucleotide homology between EIEC and *Shigella* virulence plasmid genes is reflected in the similarity of the plasmid-encoded proteins detected by electrophoretic analysis of radiolabelled minicell constituents (Hale *et al.*, 1983) and by immunoblot analysis of whole-cell bacterial lysates probed with sera from convalescent rhesus monkeys that had been infected with *Sh. flexneri* serotype 2a. The latter experiments identified four immunodominant, plasmid-encoded proteins of 78 kDa, 62 kDa, 43 kDa, and 38 kDa that promote strong antibody responses after infection (Hale *et al.*, 1985). These products were subsequently designated 'invasion plasmid antigens' (IpaA, IpaB, IpaC and IpaD respectively) (Buysse *et al.*, 1987). Polyclonal and monoclonal antibodies elicited by *Shigella* Ipa proteins cross-react with proteins of similar molecular weight in Western blots and whole-cell enzyme-linked immunosorbent assay (ELISA), in which EIEC is the antigen (Hale *et al.*, 1985; Sansonetti *et al.*, 1985; Mills *et al.*, 1988).

Genetic mapping of the plasmid virulence loci in *Sh. flexneri* serotype 5 began with the identification of a 37-kb *Sau*3a fragment which, when cloned, restores to an avirulent strain that has lost the virulence plasmid the ability to invade HeLa cells *in vitro*. Clones of this fragment express the Ipa proteins, and Tn*5* insertions into three regions of the this fragment negate expression of the invasive phenotype (Maurelli *et al.*, 1985). *Eco*RI subclones of each of these three *Sh. flexneri* plasmid invasion regions hybridise with EIEC strains (Boileau *et al.*, 1984), and Tn*5* insertions in the same three areas of a 25-kb *Bam*HI fragment of the EIEC virulence plasmid also negate expression of the invasive phenotype (Small & Falkow, 1988). Five virulence-associated regions (Figure 16.3) were identified by more extensive Tn*5* mutagenesis of the *Sh. flexneri* serotype 2a virulence plasmid and hybridisation showed that these regions are also highly conserved in EIEC (Sasakawa *et al.*, 1988). Analysis of the products of ten non-invasive Tn*phoA* fusion mutants that map within a stretch of approximately 30 kb in the EIEC virulence plasmid suggests a transcriptional organisation that is identical to that found in *Sh. flexneri* serotype 2a (Hsia *et al.*, 1993).

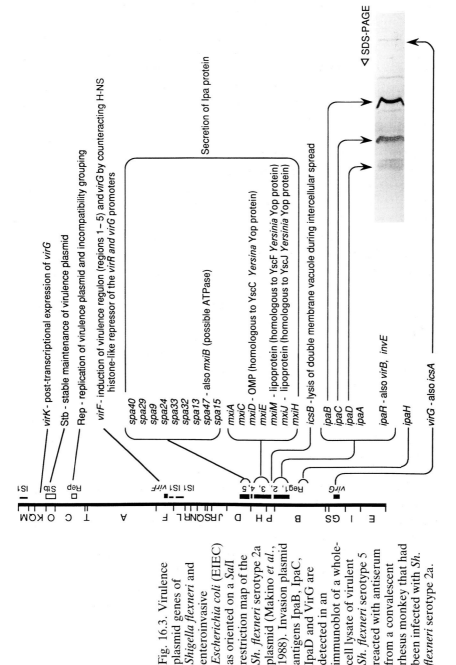

Fig. 16.3. Virulence plasmid genes of *Shigella flexneri* and enteroinvasive *Escherichia coli* (EIEC) as oriented on a *Sal*I restriction map of the *Sh. flexneri* serotype 2a plasmid (Makino *et al.*, 1988). Invasion plasmid antigens IpaB, IpaC, IpaD and VirG are detected in an immunoblot of a whole-cell lysate of virulent *Sh. flexneri* serotype 5 reacted with antiserum from a convalescent rhesus monkey that had been infected with *Sh. flexneri* serotype 2a.

virK - post-transcriptional expression of *virG*

Stb - stable maintenance of virulence plasmid

Rep - replication of virulence plasmid and incompatibility grouping

virF - induction of virulence regulon (regions 1 – 5) and *virG* by counteracting H-NS histone-like repressor of the *virR* and *virG* promoters

Secretion of Ipa protein

spa40
spa29
spa9
spa24
spa33
spa32
spa13
spa47 - also *mxiB* (possible ATPase)
spa15

mxiA
mxiC - OMP (homologous to YscC *Yersina* Yop protein)
mxiD
mxiE
mxiM - lipoprotein (homologous to YscF *Yersinia* Yop protein)
mxiJ - lipoprotein (homologous to YscJ *Yersinia* Yop protein)
mxiH

icsB - lysis of double membrane vacuole during intercellular spread

ipaB
ipaC
ipaD
ipaA

ipaR - also *virB, invE*

ipaH

virG - also *icsA*

◁ SDS-PAGE

Plasmid virulence genes

An annotated list of known virulence plasmid genes of *Sh. flexneri* is presented in Figure 16.3, and essential features of these genes are summarised below. The gene order is based on the *Sal*I restriction map of the *Sh. flexneri* serotype 2a virulence plasmid (Sawakawa *et al.*, 1986). The first gene, *virK*, is conserved in the large virulence plasmids of shigellae and EIEC. The VirK gene product plays an undefined role in the post-transcriptional expression of the *virG*(*icsA*) gene described below (Nakata *et al.*, 1992). The Rep region, which determines the plasmid incompatibility group, is homologous in EIEC and *Shigella* virulence plasmids. The EIEC virulence plasmid is, however, compatible with *Sh. flexneri* serotype 6, *Sh. boydii*, and *Sh. dysenteriae* but not with *Sh. flexneri* serotypes 1–5 or *Sh. sonnei* (Makino *et al.*, 1988). This suggests that there are at least two virulence plasmid incompatibility groups in enteroinvasive Enterobacteriaceae. The product of the *virF* gene is a *trans* activator of the *ipa*, *mxi*, *spa*, and *virG* loci (see below for further explanation). In EIEC, the VirF protein counteracts repression of *ipaR* and *icsA* by the H-NS histone-like protein that is encoded by *virR*, a chromosomal *drdX* allele (Dagberg & Uhlin, 1992).

The *spa* locus (surface presentation of Ipa antigen) consists of nine genes that correspond to invasion regions 4 and 5. This locus is necessary for the transport of Ipa proteins from the periplasm to the bacterial surface (Venkatesan *et al.*, 1992; Allaoui *et al.*, 1993; Sasakawa *et al.*, 1993). None of the *spa* ORFs contain typical signal sequences to suggest that they encode periplasmic or outer-membrane proteins. However, the second gene product in the *spa* operon (Spa47) has striking homology with the ATP-binding motif of protein-translocating ATPases from, for example, *Saccharomyces cerevisiae,* mammalian mitochondria, plant chloroplasts, and with certain ATP-binding, transport proteins of *Salmonella typhimurium* and *Bacillus subtilis* (Venkatesan *et al.*, 1992). Upstream of the *spa* operon, corresponding to invasion region 3 (Figure 16.3), lie six *mxi* genes (membrane expression of Ipa) that are also necessary for the export of Ipa proteins. Like the *spa* genes, *mxiA*, *mxiC* and *mixE* do not contain signal sequences, and the failure of alkaline-phosphatase-positive Tn*phoA* fusion mutants to map within any of these ORFs confirms that these genes do not encode periplasmic or outer membrane proteins (Allaoui *et al.*, 1993; Hsia *et al.*, 1993). In contrast, *mxiD, mxiM, mxiJ* and *mxiG* ORFs contain signal sequences, and Tn*phoA* fusions in these genes result in alkaline phosphatase-positive colonies (Allaoui *et al.*, 1992b, 1993; Hsia *et al.*, 1993). Four of the *mxi* genes have sequence homology with *Yersinia* genes, including the LcrD low-calcium response gene (*mxiA*) (Andrews & Maurelli, 1992), two Yop lipoproteins (*mxiJ* and *mxiH*) (Allaoui *et al.*, 1992b), and a putative Yop transport protein (*mxiD*) (Allaoui *et al.*, 1993). Although none of these findings can yet be integrated into a coherent model for the membrane transport of Ipa proteins, it is apparent that the *mxi–spa* loci encode components of a specialised system that has some of the characteristics of transport systems in other enteric bacteria.

Transcription in the virulence region diverges after the first gene in the *mxi* locus, *mxiH*, and proceeds in the opposite direction from *mxi–spa*. The next identified virulence gene is *icsB*, which corresponds to region 2 (Figure 16.3). The *icsB* gene product is necessary for the lysis of the inner leaflet of the double membrane that initially encloses shigellae as they spread to contiguous cells (Allaoui *et al.*, 1992a). This protein functions in concert with the *icsA*(*virG*) gene and *ipaB* in facilitating intercellular bacterial spread. Unlike mutants in *virF, virR* or the *spa* and *mxi* loci, *icsB* mutants can invade HeLa cells *in vitro*, but these mutants are avirulent in the Sérény test (Allaoui *et al.*, 1992a).

The *ipgC* gene (not shown) is located immediately upstream of the *ipaBCDA* operon, and this small ORF encodes a 17-kDa protein that serves as a molecular chaperon which prevents the premature association of IpaB and IpaC proteins in the bacterial cytoplasm (Menard *et al.*, 1994b). In the absence of this chaperon, IpaB is degraded before transport, and IpaC is destroyed as a bystander if it complexes with IpaB in the cytoplasm. The *ipgC* gene is in the same transcription unit as the *ipaBCDA* operon, and the next two genes to be transcribed, *ipaB* and *ipaC,* respectively encode 62-kDa and 45-kDa proteins. These form a complex during excretion into the extracellular milieu via the *mxi–spa* pathway. Release of the IpaBC complex is modulated by the 35-kDa *ipaD* gene product, and the release of this complex is triggered by contact with the plasma membrane of a mammalian cell (Menard *et al.*, 1994a).

The IpaBC complex is a key virulence determinant of *Sh. flexneri* and, by analogy, of other *Shigella* species and EIEC, but the exact biochemical role of any of the Ipa proteins in virulence remains to be defined. Insertion mutants in *ipaB, ipaC* and *ipaD* are non-invasive for HeLa cells, while insertions in *ipaA* still permit retention of the invasive phenotype (Baudry *et al.*, 1987). The virulence of mutants in *ipaCD* is restored in clones that express the complementary Ipa proteins (Sasakawa *et al.*, 1989). Like IpaB, IpaC contains a highly hydrophobic domain that may facilitate interactions with eukaryotic membranes (Baudry *et al.*, 1988; Venkatesan *et al.*, 1988). An *ipaB* gene replacement mutant, with programmed reinitiation of downstream *ipaCDA* transcription, is adherent but non-invasive in the HeLa cell model. This mutant is also unable to lyse endocytic vacuoles when ingested by cultured J774 macrophages (High *et al.*, 1992). Thus, in addition to being a major component of the invasion complex, IpaBC acts as a membrane-lysing toxin that enables bacteria to escape from endocytic vacuoles into the cytoplasmic compartment. The biochemical basis of these phenotypes is unknown, but it is thought that two highly hydrophobic domains in the *ipaB* ORF may facilitate the interaction of the protein product with eukaryotic membranes (High *et al.*, 1992).

Immediately downstream of the *ipaBCDA* operon is the *ipaR* gene, which is also designated *virB* or *invE* and positively regulates the *ipa*, *mxi* and *spa* virulence regulon (Buysse *et al.*, 1990). It has been postulated that the *ipaR* gene is subject to low temperature repression by the H-NS histone product of the chromosomal *virR* gene at temperatures below 35°C. The VirF plasmid gene product activates the virulence regulon at 37°C by counteracting histone repression of the *ipaR* gene (Dagberg & Uhlin, 1992). Tandem copies of an additional invasion plasmid antigen gene, designated *ipaH*, are located downstream of *ipaR* in *Shigella* spp. and EIEC (Venkatesan *et al.*, 1989; Sethabutr *et al.*, 1993). Like IpaBCDA, the 60-kDa IpaH protein product elicits serum antibody during *Shigella* infection, and the homology between the *ipaH* ORF and the YopM protein of *Yersinia pestis* suggests that this protein may contribute to the virulence of enteroinvasive pathogens by inhibiting platelet activation and fibrin clot formation in the immediate vicinity of colonic lesions (Hartman *et al.*, 1990).

Expression of *virG*, which is also designated *icsA* (to denote intercellular spread), is necessary for intercellular spread of *Shigella*, and a homologous region is present in the EIEC virulence plasmid (Makino *et al.*, 1986). Expression of *virG* is positively regulated by the VirF plasmid gene product (Adler *et al.*, 1989) and translation depends on the VirK gene product (Nakata *et al.*, 1992). The VirG or IcsA gene product is a 120-MDa outer-membrane protein that elicits an antibody response during infection. This protein is readily degraded by the chromosomal *E. coli* OmpT protease, previously identified as the KcpA⁻ phenotype, and it is a characteristic of EIEC and shigellae that the *ompT* gene has been deleted from the chromosome (Nakata *et al.*, 1993). In *Shigella*, and presumably in EIEC, the IcsA protein has a unipolar distribution that facilitates nucleation of actin microfilaments at the ends of daughter cells as the bacteria multiply in the cytoplasm of mammalian cells. It also has adenosine 5'-triphophatase (ATPase) activity that may play a role in actin polymerisation (Goldberg *et al.*, 1993).

Expression of the plasmid virulence operon is regulated by at least two chromosomal loci. The *virR* locus, which is linked to *galU* at 27 minutes on the *E. coli* chromosome, represses the *ipa, spa* and *mxi* loci at low temperature (Dagberg & Uhlin, 1992). In addition, the two-component osmolarity trans-membrane sensor system encoded by the *ompR–envZ* locus, located at 75 minutes, induces virulence operon expression in response to the high osmolarity in the bowel lumen (Bernardini *et al.*, 1990). Finally, a *Shigella* and EIEC chromosomal locus designated *vacB*, and linked to *purA* at 95 minutes, is necessary for expression at the post-transcriptional level of genes in the entire plasmid virulence operon (Tobe *et al.*, 1992).

The cellular and molecular basis of invasion by enteroinvasive *Escherichia coli*

The infectious dose of ETEC O143 and O144 is 1×10^8 colony-forming units (DuPont *et al.*, 1971) compared with the 1×10^2 colony forming units for *Sh. flexneri* (DuPont *et al.*, 1989). Nevertheless, Southern blot analysis and insertion mutagenesis have so far failed to identify virulence genes of *Shigella* species that do not have counterparts in EIEC strains. It may, therefore, be assumed that the basic pathogenetic mechanism of these enteroinvasive pathogens is similar. An insight into the initial stages of the invasion process has been gained from studies of *Sh. flexneri* strains injected into ligated rabbit ileal loops (Wassef *et al.*, 1989). These indicate that wild-type shigellae are preferentially taken up by the membranous M cells that overlie the lymphoid follicles. The organisms rapidly colonise the follicle-associated epithelial cells (FAE) by inter-cellular spread. This process depends on the plasmid-encoded invasive phenotype, since plasmid-negative strains do not colonise the FAE. Endoscopic examination of rhesus monkeys challenged with an avirulent *icsA* mutant of *Sh. flexneri* also suggests that the portal of infection in primates is the M cell that overlies lymphoid follicles in the colon (Sansonetti *et al.*, 1991).

A few hours after the uptake of virulent shigellae by M cells, the FAE ulcerate and the organisms spread to the villus epithelium. When either *Shigella* or EIEC are injected into rabbit ileal loops, this process is accompanied by acute inflammation in the lamina propria and by extensive migration of neutrophils through the epithelium into the lumen of the bowel (DuPont *et al.*, 1971). Recent experimental evidence suggests that invasion of epithelial cells is enhanced by neutrophil migration, which partially disrupts tight junctions and transiently exposes the basolateral surfaces of enterocytes to extracellular shigellae in the intestinal lumen. For example, inhibition of diapedesis, by injection of monoclonal antibody that neutralises neutrophil adhesion ligands (CD-31), protects ligated ileal loops from ulcerative lesions normally caused by *Sh. flexneri*. Neutrophil infiltration is elicited by cytokines, such as interleukin 1 (IL-1), that are elaborated by tissue macrophages that phagocytose shigellae in the lamina propria (Sansonetti, 1993; Zychlinsky, 1994). After phagocytosis by macrophages, the invasion plasmid antigen IpaB lyses the phagocytic vacuole (High *et al.*, 1992), and the shigellae induce apoptosis (programmed cell death) of the macrophage (Zychinsky *et al.*, 1992). Presumably EIEC, which also express the IpaB membrane-lysing toxin, induce a similar inflammatory cascade after transcytosis by M cells and phagocytosis by macrophages.

Experiments with cultured macrophages *in vitro* have revealed the role of IpaB in macrophage apoptosis, and five stages in the invasion and intercellular spread of these organisms have been recognised by the study of polarised colonic epithelial cells exposed to shigellae. As we have seen, bacterial endocytosis by these non-phagocytic cells is induced at the basolateral surface (Mounier *et al.*, 1992). This *first stage* of infection requires expression of virulence plasmid loci *ipa*, *mxi* and *spa*. In the *second stage* of infection the IpaBC complex causes lysis of the endocytic vacuole, and the shigellae multiply freely in the cytoplasm of the epithelial cell. In the *third stage* the organisms attach to the pre-formed actin microfilaments that constitute the perijunctional ring associated with the plasma membrane of polarised cells at the zonula adherens. The attached organisms spread within the cell in the plane of the zonula adherens by a unidirectional organelle-like movement (Vasselon *et al.*, 1992). The genetic and biochemical basis of this organelle-like intracellular bacterial movement is unknown. As the shigellae multiply, an occasional bacterium in the septation phase induces nucleation of F-actin at one or both of the cellular poles. This actin tail formation depends on the IcsA (or virG) protein (Goldberg *et al.*, 1993). During this *fourth stage* of infection, the actin-bundling protein, plastin, constricts the cylindrical actin tail just posterior to the bacterium, so inducing forward movement of the cell (Prevost *et al.*, 1992). The bacterium may have an impact on, and deform, the internal aspect of the plasma membrane resulting in a protrusion into the cytoplasm of the adjacent epithelial cell. In the *fifth and final stage* of infection, the interior membrane of this double membrane protrusion is lysed by the IcsB protein (Allaoui *et al.*, 1992a), and the external membrane is lysed by the IpaBC protein. As a result of this process, bacterial replication begins anew in the cytoplasm of the adjacent cell.

This pattern of bacterial invasion, multiplication, and intercellular spread *in vitro* gives *Sh. flexneri*, and presumably EIEC strains, the unique capacity to spread throughout the epithelial layer, while without further contact with the extracellular compartment. This intracellular life-style avoids host defence mechanisms, such as antibody, complement, neutrophils and natural killer cells. In addition, the intracytoplasmic milieu has ecological characteristics of an extreme environment with an absence of competition from other species and with access to unlimited pools of host cell nutrients (Moulder, 1974). Thus, the intracellular life-style presents a powerful selective advantage for enteroinvasive pathogens that allows them to escape the fully occupied ecological niche of the intestinal lumen and so to multiply in the intestinal epithelium.

References

Adler, B., Sasakawa, C., Tobe, T., Makino, S., Komatsu, K. & Yoshikawa, M. (1989). A dual transcriptional activation system for the 230 kb plasmid genes coding for virulence-associated antigens for *Shigella flexneri*. *Molecular Microbiology*, **3**, 627–35.

Allaoui, A., Mounier, J., Prevost, M.-C., Sansonetti, P. J. & Parsot, C. (1992a). *icsB*: a *Shigella flexneri* virulence gene necessary for the lysis of protrusions during intercellular spread. *Molecular Microbiology*, **6**, 1605–16.

Allaoui, A., Sansonetti, P. J. & Parsot, C. (1992b). MxiJ, a liopoprotein involved in secretion of *Shigella* Ipa invasions, is homologous to YscJ, a secretion factor of the *Yersinia* Yop proteins. *Journal of Bacteriology*, **174**, 7661–69.

Allaoui, A., Sansonetti, P. J. & Parsot, C. (1993). MxiD, an outer membrane protein necessary for the secretion of the *Shigella flexneri* Ipa invasions. *Molecular Microbiology*, **7**, 59–68.

Andrews, G. P. & Maurelli, A. T. (1992). *mxiA* of *Shigella flexneri* 2a which facilitates export of invasion plasmid antigens, encodes a homolog of the low-calcium response protein, LcrD of *Yersinia pestis*. *Infection and Immunity*, **60**, 3287–95.

Baudry, B., Kaczorek, K. & Sansonetti, P. J. (1988). Nucleotide sequence of the invasion plasmid antigen B and C genes (*ipa*B and *ipa*C) of *Shigella flexneri*. *Microbial Pathogenesis*, **4**, 345–57.

Baudry, B., Maurelli, A. T., Clerc, P., Sadoff, J. C. & Sansonetti, P. J. (1987). Localization of plasmid loci necessary for the entry of *Shigella flexneri* into HeLa cells, and characterization of one locus encoding four immunogenic polypeptides. *Journal of General Microbiology*, **133**, 3403–13.

Bernardini, M. L., Fontaine, A. & Sansonetti, P. J. (1990). The two-component regulatory system OmpR–EnvZ controls the virulence of *Shigella flexneri*. *Journal of Bacteriology*, **172**, 6274–81.

Boileau, C. R., d'Hauteville, H. & Sansonetti, P. J. (1984). DNA hybridization technique to detect *Shigella* species and enteroinvasive *Escherichia coli*. *Journal of Clinical Microbiology*, **20**, 959–61.

Butler, T., Speelman, P., Kabir, I. & Banwell, J. (1986). Colonic dysfunction during shigellosis. *Journal of Infectious Diseases*, **154**, 817–24.

Buysse, J. M., Stover, C. K., Oaks, E. V., Venkatesan, M. & Kopecko, D. J. (1987). Molecular cloning of invasion plasmid antigen (*ipa*) genes from *Shigella flexneri*: analysis of *ipa* gene products and genetic mapping. *Journal of Bacteriology*, **169**, 2561–69.

Buysse, J. M., Venkatesan, M., Mills, J. A. & Oaks, E. V. (1990). Molecular characterization of a *trans*-acting, postive effector (*ipaR*) of invasion plasmid antigen synthesis in *Shigella flexneri* serotype 5. *Microbial Pathogenesis*, **8**, 197–211.

Cheasty, T. & Rowe, B. (1983). Antigenic relationships between the enteroinvasive *Escherichia coli* O antigens O28ac, O112ac, O124, O136, O144, O152, and O164 and *Shigella* O antigens. *Journal of Clinical Microbiology*, **17**, 681–84.

Dagberg, B. & Uhlin, B. E. (1992). Regulation of virulence-associated plasmid genes in enteroinvasive *Escherichia coli*. *Journal of Bacteriology*, **174**, 7606–12.

DuPont, H. L., Formal, S. B., Hornick, R. B., Snyder, M. J., Libonati, J. P., Sheahan, D. G., LaBrec, E. H. & Kalas, J. P. (1971). Pathogenesis of *Escherichia coli* diarrhea. *New England Journal of Medicine*, **285**, 1–9.

DuPont, H. L., Levine, M. M., Hornick, R. B. & Formal, S. B. (1989). Inoculum size in shigellosis and implications for expected mode of transmission. *Journal of Infectious Diseases*, **159**, 1126–28.

Echeverria, P., Sethabutr, O. & Pitarangsi, C. (1991). Microbiology and diagnosis of infections with *Shigella* and enteroinvasive *Escherichia coli*. *Reviews of Infectious Diseases*, **13**, Supplement 4, S220–5.

Echeverria, P., Sethabutr, O., Serichatalergs, O., Lexomboon, U. & Tamura, K. (1992). *Shigella* and enteroinvasive *Escherichai coli* infections in households of children with dysentery in Bangkok. *Journal of Infectious Diseases*, **165**, 144–7.

Fasano, A., Kay, B. A., Russell, R. G., Maneval, D. R., Jr. & Levine, M. M. (1990). Enterotoxin and cytotoxin production by enteroinvasive *Eschercichi coli*. *Infection and Immunity*, **58**, 3717–23.

Fasano, A., Noriega, F. R., Maneval, D. R., Jr., Chanasogcram, S., Russell, R., Guandalini, S. & Levine, M. M. (1995). *Shigella* enterotoxin 1: an endotoxin of *Shigella flexneri* 2a active in rabbit small intestine *in vivo* and *in vitro*. *Journal of Clinical Investigation*, **95**, 2853–61.

Goldberg, M. B., Barzu, O., Parsot, C. & Sansonetti, P. J. (1993). Unipolar localization and ATPase activity of IcsA, a *Shigella flexneri* protein involved in intracellular movement. *Journal of Bacteriology*, **175**, 2189–96.

Hale, T. L., Oaks, E. V. & Formal, S. B. (1985). Identification and antigenic characterization of virulence-associated, plasmid-coded proteins of *Shigella* spp. and enteroinvasive *Escherchia coli*. *Infection and Immunity*, **50**, 620–9.

Hale, T. L., Sansonetti, P. J., Schad, P. A., Austin, S. & Formal, S. B. (1983). Characterization of virulence plasmids and plasmid-associated outer memberane proteins in *Shigella flexneri*, *Shigella sonnei*, and *Escherichia coli*. *Infection and Immunity*, **40**, 340–50.

Harris, J. R., Mariano, J., Wells, J. G., Payne, B. S., Donnell, H. D. & Cohen, M. L. (1985). Person to person transmission in an outbreak of enteroinvasive *Escherichia coli*. *American Journal of Epidemiology*, **122**, 245–52.

Hartman, A. B., Venkatesan, M., Oaks, E. V. & Buysse, J. M. (1990). Sequence and molecular characterization of a multicopy invasion plasmid antigen gene, *ipaH*, of *Shigella flexneri*. *Journal of Bacteriology*, **172**, 1905–15.

High, N., Mounier, J., Prevost, M. C. & Sansonetti, P. J. (1992). IpaB of *Shigella flexneri* causes entry into epithelial cells and escape from the phagocytic vacuole. *EMBO Journal*, **11**, 1991–9.

Hsia, R.-C., Small, P. L. & Bavoil, P. M. (1993). Characterization of virulence genes of enteroinvasive *Escherichia coli* by Tn*phoA* mutagenesis: identification of *invX*, a gene required for entry into HEp-2 cells. *Journal of Bacteriology*, **175**, 4817–23.

Keyti, I. (1989). Epidemiology of the enteroinvasive *Escherichia coli*. Observations in Hungary. *Journal of Hygeine, Epidemiology, Microbiology and Immunology*, **33**, 261–17.

Ketyi, I., Malovics, I., Vertenyi, A., Kontrohr, T. Pacsa, S. & Kuch, B. (1978a). Heat-stable enterotoxin produced by *Shigella flexneri*. *Acta Microbiological Academiae of Scientarum Hungarica*, **25**, 165–71.

Ketyi, I., Vertenyi, A., Malovics, I., Kontrohr, T. & Pacsa, S. (1978b). Unique features of heat-stable enterotoxin of *Shigella flexneri*. *Acta Microbiologica Academiae Scientarum Hungarica*, **25**, 219–27.

Makino, S., Sasakawa, C. Kamata, K., Kurata, T. & Yoshikawa, M. (1986). A genetic determinant required for continuous reinfection of adjacent cells on large plasmid in *S. flexneri* 2a. *Cell*, **46**, 551–5.

Makino, S., Sasakawa, C. & Yoshikawa, M. (1988). Genetic relatedness of the basic replicon of the virulence plasmid in shigellae and enteroinvasive *Escherichia coli*. *Microbial Pathogenesis*, **5**, 267–74.

Maurelli, A. T., Baudry, B., d'Hauteville, H., Hale, T. L. & Sansonetti, P. J. (1985). Cloning of plasmid DNA sequences involved in invasion of HeLa cells by *Shigella flexneri*. *Infection and Immunity*, **49**, 164–71.

Menard, R., Sansonetti, P. & Parsot, C. (1994a). The secretion of the *Shigella flexneri* Ipa invasins is activated by epithelial cells and controlled by IpaB and IpaD. *EMBO Journal*, **13**, 5293–302.

Menard, R., Sansonetti, P., Parsot, C. & Vasselon, T. (1994b). Extracellular association and cytoplasmic partitioning of the IpaB and IpaC invasions of *S. flexneri*. *Cell*, **79**, 515–25.

Mills, J. A., Buysse, J. M. & Oaks, E. V. (1988). *Shigella flexneri* invasion plasmid antigens B and C: epitope location and characterization with monoclonal antibodies. *Infection and Immunity*, **56**, 2933–41.

Moulder, J. W. (1974). Intracellular parasitism: life in an extreme environment. *Journal of Infectious Diseases*, **130**, 300–6.

Mounier, J., Vasselon, T., Hellio, R., Lesourd, M. & Sansonetti, P. J. (1992). *Shigella flexneri* enters human colonic Caco-2 epithelial cells though the basolateral pole. *Infection and Immunity*, **60**, 237–48.

Nakata, N., Sasakawa, C., Okada, N., Tobe, T., Fukuda, I., Suzuki, T., Komatsu, K. & Yoshikawa, M. (1992). Identification and characterization of *virK*, a virulence-associated large plasmid gene essential for intercellular spreading of *Shigella flexneri*. *Molecular Microbiology*, **6**, 2387–95.

Nakata, N., Tobe, T., Fukuda, I., Suzuki, T., Kamatsu, K., Yoshikawa, M. & Sasakawa, C. (1993). The absence of a surface protease, OmpT, Determines the intercellular spreading ability of *Shigella*: the relationship between the *ompT* and *kcpA* loci. *Molecular Microbiology*, **9**, 459–68.

Ørskov, I., Wachsmuth, I. K., Taylor, D. N., Echeverria, P., Rowe, B. & Sakazaki, R. (1991). Two new *Escherichia coli* O groups: O172 from Shiga-like toxin II producing strains (EHEC) and O173 from enteroinvasive *E. coli* (EIEC). *Acta Pathologica Microbiologica et Immunologica Scandanavica*, **99**, 30–2.

Perdomo, O. J. J., Cavaillon, J. M., Huerre, M., Ohayon, H., Gounon, P. & Sansonetti, P. J. (1994). Acute inflammation causes epithelial invasion and mucosal destruction in experimental shigellosis. *Journal of Experimental Medicine*, **180**, 1307–19.

Prevost, M. C., Lesourd, M., Arpin, M., Vernel, F., Mounier, J., Hellio, R. & Sansonetti, P. J. (1992). Unipolar reorganization of F-actin layer a bacterial division and bundling of actin filaments by plastin correlate with movement of *Shigella flexneri* within HeLa cells. *Infection and Immunity*, **60**, 4088–99.

Rout, W. R., Formal, S. B., Giannella, R. A. & Dammin, G. J. (1975). Pathophysiology of shigella diarrhea in the rhesus monkey: intestinal transport, morphological, and bacteriological studies. *Gastroenterology*, **68**, 270–8.

Sakazaki, R., Tamura, K. & Saito, M. (1967). Enteropathogenic *Escherichia coli* associated with diarrhea in children and adults. *Japanese Journal o Medical Science and Biology*, **20**, 387–99.

Sansonetti, P. J. (1993). Molecular and cellular mechanisms of cell invasion and killing by *Shigella flexneri*. In *Microbial Pathogenesis and Immune Response,* eds. E. W. Ades, S. A. Morse & R. F. Resdt, p. 20. Orlando, FL: The New York Acadamy of Sciences.

Sansonetti, P. J., Arondel, J., Fontaine, A., d'Hauteville, H. & Bernardini, M. L. (1991). *ompB* (osmo-regulation) and *icsA* (cell-to-cell spread) mutants of *Shigella flexneri*: vaccine candidates and probe to study the pathogenesis of shigellosis. *Vaccine*, **9**, 416–22.

Sansonetti, P. J., d'Hauteville, H., Ecobichon, C. & Pourcel, C. (1983a). Molecular comparison of virulence plasmids in *Shigella* and enteroinvasive *Escherichia coli*. *Annals de Microbiologie (Paris)*, **134A**, 295–318.

Sansonetti, P. J., Hale, T. L., Dammin, G. J., Kapfer, C., Collins, H. H. & Formal, S. B. (1983b). Alterations in the pathogenicity of *Escherichia coli* K-12 after transfer of plasmid and chromosomal genes from *Shigella flexneri*. *Infection and Immunity*, **39**, 1392–402.

Sansonetti, P. J., Hale, T. L., & Oaks, E. V. (1985). Genetics of virulence in enteroinvasive *Escherichia coli*. In *Microbiology–1985*, ed. D. Schlessinger, pp. 74–7. Washington DC: American Society for Microbiology.

Sansonetti, P. J., d'Hauteville, H., Formal, S. B. & Toucas, M. (1982a). Plasmid-mediated invasiveness of *"Shigella-*like" *Escherichia coli. Annals of Microbiology (Institue Pasteur)*, **132A**, 351–5.

Sansonetti, P. J., Kopecko, D. J. & Formal, S. B. (1981). *Shigella sonnei* plasmids: evidence that a large plasmid is necessary for virulence. *Infection and Immunity*, **34**, 75–83.

Sansonetti, P. J., Kopecko, D. J. & Formal, S. B. (1982b). Involvement of a plasmid in the invasive ablility of *Shigella flexneri. Infection and Immunity*, **35**, 852–60.

Sasakawa, C., Adler, B., Tobe, T., Okada, N., Nagai, S., Komatsu, K. & Yoshikawa, M. (1989). Functional organization and nucleotide sequence of virulence region-2 on the large virulence plasmid in *Shigella flexneri* 2a. *Molecular Microbiology*, **3**, 1191–201.

Sasakawa, C., Kamata, K., Sadai, T., Makino, S., Yamada, M., Okada, N. & Yoshikawa, M. (1988). Virulence-associated genetic regions comprising 31 kilobases of the 230-kilobase plamid in *Shigella flexneri* 2a. *Journal of Bacteriology*, **170**, 2480–4.

Sawakawa, C., Kamata, K., Sakai, T., Murayama, Y., Makino, S. & Yoshikawa, M. (1986). Molecular alteration of the 140-megadalton plasmid associated with loss of virulence and Congo red binding activty in *Shigella flexneri* 2a. *Infection and Immunity*, **51**, 470–5.

Sasakawa, C., Komatsu, K., Tobe, T., Suzuki, T. & Toshikawa, M. (1993). Eight genes in region 5 that form an operon are essential for invasion of epithelial cells by *Shigella flexneri* 2a. *Journal of Bacteriology*, **175**, 2334–46.

Sethabutr, O., Hanchalay, S., Echeverria, P., Taylor, D. N. & Leksomboon, U. (1985). A non-radioactive DNA probe to identify *Shigella* and enteroinvasive *Escherichia coli* in stools of children with diarrhea. *Lancet*, **2**, 1095–7.

Sethabutr, O., Venkatesan, M., Murphy, S., Eampokalap, B., Hoge, C. W. & Echeverria, P. (1993). Detection of *Shigella* and enteroinvasive *Echerichia coli* by amplification of the invasion plasmid antigen H DNA sequence in patients with dysentery. *Journal of Infectious Diseases*, **163**, 458–61.

Sharon, P., Ligumsky, M., Rachmilewitz, D. & Zor, U. (1978). Role of prostaglandins in ulcerative colitis. Enhanced production during active disease and inhibition by sulfasalazine. *Gastroenterology*, **75**, 638–40.

Small, P. L. & Falkow, S. (1988). Identification of regions on a 230-kilobase plasmid from enteroinvasive *Escherichia coli* that are required for entry into HEp-2; cells. *Infection and Immunity*, **56**, 225–9.

Snyder, J. D., Wells, J. G., Yashuk, J., Puhr, N. & Blake, P. A. (1984). Outbreak of invasive *Escherichia coli* gastroenteritis on a cruise ship. *American Journal of Tropical Medicine and Hygiene*, **32**, 281–4.

Taylor, D. N., Echeverria, P., Sethabutr, O., Pitarangsi, C., Leksomboon, U., Blacklow, N. R., Rowe, B., Gross, R. & Cross, J. (1988). Clinical and microbiologic features of *Shigella* and enteroinvasive *Escherichia coli* infections detected by DNA hybridization. *Journal of Clinical Microbiology*, **26**, 1362–6.

Tobe, T., Sasakawa, C., Okada, N., Honma, Y. & Yoshikawa, M. (1992). *vacB*, a novel chromosomal gene required for expression of virulence genes on the large plasmid of *Shigella flexneri. Journal of Bacteriology*, **174**, 6359–67.

Toledo, M. R. & Trabulsi, L. R. (1983). Correlation between biochemical and serological characteristics of *Escherichia coli* and results of the Séreny test. *Journal of Clinical Microbiology*, **17**, 419–21.

Tulloch, E. F., Ryan, K. J., Formal, S. B. & Franklin, F. A. (1973). Invasive enteropathogenic *Escherichia coli* dysentery: an outbreak of 28 adults. *Annals of Internal Medicine*, **79**, 13–17.

Vasselon, T., Mounier, J., Hellio, R. & Sansonetti, P. J. (1992). Movement along actin filaments on the perijunctional area and *de novo* polymerization of cellular actin are required for *Shigella flexneri* colonization of epithelial Caco-2 cell monolayers. *Infection and Immunity*, **60**, 1031–40.

Venkatesan, M. M., Buysse, J. M. & Kopecko, D. J. (1988). Characterization of invasion plasmid antien genes (*ipaBCD*) form *Shigella flexneri*. *Proceedings of the National Acadamy of Sciences, USA*, **85**, 9317–21.

Venkatesan, M. M., Buysse, J. M. & Kopecko, D. J. (1989). Use of *Shigella flexneri ipaC* and *ipaH* gene sequences for the general identification of *Shigella* spp. and enteroinvasive *Escherichia coli*. *Journal of Clinical Microbiology*, **27**, 2687–91.

Venkatesan, M. M., Buysse, J. M. & Oaks, E. V. (1992). Surface presentation of *Shigella flexneri* invasion plasmid antigens requires the products of the *spa* locus. *Journal of Bacteriology*, **174**, 1990–2001.

Wassef, J. S., Keren, D. F. & Mailloux, J. L. (1989). Role of M cells in initial antigen uptake and in ulcer formation in the rabbit intestinal loop model of shigellosis. *Infection and Immunity*, **57**, 858–63.

Zychlinsky, A., Fitting, C., Cavaillon, J.-M. & Sansonetti, P. J. (1994). Interleukin 1 is released by murine macrophages during apoptosis induced by *Shigella flexneri*. *Journal of Clinical Investigation*, **94**, 1328–32.

Zychinsky, A., Prevost, M. C. & Sansonetti, P. J. (1992). *Shigella flexneri* induces apoptosis in infected macrophages. *Nature*, **358**, 167–9.

17

Soft tissue infection and septicaemia

D. M. MACLAREN

Soft tissue infections

Skin and soft tissue infections

Skin and soft tissue infections are very common and are mainly due to pyogenic cocci. *L. coli* plays a very minor role in those infections and, in a series of 94 cases of cellulitis, Sigurdson & Gudmundsson (1989) isolated *E. coli* only once, from a perianal cellulitis. Maslow *et al.* (1993) found that only two of 170 episodes of *E. coli* septicaemia originated from a cellulitis. More extensive soft tissue infections, such as necrotising fasciitis have a sombre and life-threatening prognosis and are fortunately much less common. Various syndromes have been described on the basis of their presumed aetiology (clostridial versus non-clostridial) or on the basis of the structures involved. In this context, synergistic Gram-negative gangrene (Stone & Martin, 1972) is relevant, because its pathogenesis involves synergy between facultative anaerobes, such as *E. coli*, and members of the *Bacteroides* group. The onset is slower than that of necrotising fasciitis and gas formation is common. When the perineum is involved, the condition resembles classical Fournier's gangrene (Lewis, 1992).

Decubitus

Decubitus ulcers or pressure sores occur in patients who, for one reason or another, lie still in bed for long periods, so that the blood circulation in skin and subcutaneous tissues is impaired, which leads to their necrosis and ulceration. Sites at particular risk are the sacral areas, hips and heels, but pressure sores can also occur elsewhere. In view of the proximity of the perineal area to the most common sites of pressure sores, *E. coli* and *Bacillus fragilis* are often isolated. The matter of treatment is beyond the scope of this chapter, but, broadly speaking, the management of decubitus ulcers consists of measures to prevent continuous pressure on the area, removal of necrotic tissue and the local use of antiseptic ointments.

Infected decubitus ulcers can be the source of *E. coli* septicaemia. Indeed, Galpin *et al.* (1976) found decubitus ulcers to be a common source of *E. coli* sepsis, but this has not been the general experience. Thus, Maslow *et al.* (1993) found decubitus ulcers to be the source of *E. coli* septicaemia in only five out of 170 episodes. Nevertheless, infected decubitus ulcers are a potential source of Gram-negative septicaemia.

Wound infections

Contamination of wounds with *E. coli* may lead to wound infection. Such contamination may be endogenous, from the faecal flora, or exogenous, from water or soil. In Vietnam some 20 per cent of war wounds were contaminated with *E. coli* (Kovaric *et al.*, 1968). Surgical research has laid greater emphasis on the degree of contamination than on the nature of the contaminating flora (Edlich *et al.*, 1977). Retrospective analysis has shown that where the contaminating flora amounted to fewer than 10^5 bacteria per gram of tissue, 28 of 30 wounds healed after primary closure, but where the degree of contamination was greater, primary closure was unsuccessful because of the inevitability of infection (Robson *et al.*, 1968).

The number of bacteria cultured from wounds may reflect not merely the degree of contamination, but also the virulence of the infecting flora, since more virulent bacteria tend to grow more rapidly *in vivo* and they more successfully resist the defence systems of the host. Clearly, to assess the possibly enhanced growth of virulent bacteria, the time interval between injury and bacteriological sampling is important. In any event, the presence of anaerobic bacteria, even fewer than 10^5 bacteria per gram of tissue, may lead to infection (Tobin, 1984). This is attributable to the synergy between aerobic and anaerobic bacteria, which reduces the amount of inoculum required to initiate infection. On the other hand, endogenous contamination of wounds with *E. coli* reflects contamination with commensal flora in which both *E. coli* and anaerobes are present, such as the faecal, perineal, or vaginal flora. With this type of contamination, the synergy between the aerobic and anaerobic species reduces the amount of inoculum needed to initiate infection, thereby increasing the chances that it will occur. The role of anaerobes in wound infection is often underestimated (Polk, 1973; Willis, 1979), because in routine practice delays before culture reduce the likelihood that anaerobes are isolated. A survey of hospital infections in The Netherlands in 1987 showed that *E. coli* was the most common organism isolated (64 of 373 infections; Botman, personal communication), but Gram-negative anaerobes were not detected.

The 'diabetic foot'

The neuropathy and accelerated arteriosclerosis that may accompany diabetes mellitus mean that minor trauma in diabetic patients may go unheeded and lead firstly to the development of penetrating ulcers, and then to gangrene. Superficial cultures often yield a variety of microorganisms, including *Pseudomonas aeruginosa* and enterococci, whereas biopsies of deeper tissues yield *E. coli* or *Proteus* spp. together with Gram-negative anaerobes (Joseph, 1991). These cultures reveal the true pathogens, while more superficial cultures yield only contaminating bacteria (Sapico *et al.*, 1980).

Synergy between *Escherichia coli* and anaerobic bacteria

Clinical observations indicate that *E. coli* can cause soft tissue and wound infections (Conte, 1989), but make it apparent that the probability, the severity and the extent of the infection are greatly increased by the presence of anaerobic bacteria, especially of the *Bacteroides* group (Tobin, 1984). Infections of the biliary tract provide confirmatory evidence; in infections caused by aerobic bacteria alone, the prevalence of septicaemia was 34 per cent, whereas when *B. fragilis* was present, the prevalence rose to 45 per cent (Bourgault *et al.*, 1979), but the organisms that were responsible for the septicaemia were, with one exception, aerobes and particularly *E. coli*. Clearly, *B. fragilis* and *E. coli* together led to more extensive disease and a greater likelihood of septicaemia but *E. coli* was the invasive partner. An understanding of this bacterial synergy is vital to a full understanding of the pathogenesis of these infections (Table 17.1). A simple explanation may be that the more rapidly growing *E. coli* produces anaerobic conditions in which *B. fragilis* can flourish, but in reality the situation is more complex.

Table 17.1. *Possible mechanisms of synergy between* Escherichia coli *and* Bacteroides fragilis

---

Anaerobic conditions produced by *E. coli*
Haem-binding protein produced by *E. coli* and utilised by *B. fragilis*
Consumption of complement by *B. fragilis* and insufficient remaining for opsonisation of *E. coli*
Inhibitory substances that impair leucocyte function produced by *B. fragilis*, e.g. succinate

---

Interference with phagocytosis by anaerobic bacteria

A serendipitous observation was made by Ingham *et al.* (1977), namely that in specimens of pus, later shown to contain aerobes including *E. coli* and *B. fragilis*, the bacteria were predominantly extracellular. Treatment with metronidazole suppressed *B. fragilis*, and then the remaining bacteria were intracellular. The conclusion was drawn that the *B. fragilis* had somehow disturbed phagocytosis. This hypothesis was tested by a series of experiments *in vitro*, which confirmed that *B. fragilis* blocked the phagocytosis of *Proteus mirabilis* by human granulocytes. These findings were confirmed and extended by Namavar *et al.* (1983) in a study of other strains of *Bacteroides*. They concluded that strains of *Bacteroides* spp. excrete a low molecular weight heat-stable substance that disturbs granulocyte function. Rotstein *et al.* (1985) believed this substance to be succinate, a product of *B. fragilis* metabolism.

On the other hand, Vel *et al.* (1985, 1987) concluded that the inhibition of phagocytosis is cell-mediated and noted that it is found only if phagocytosis of the *E. coli* is complement-dependent. They believed that complement components are deposited on *B. fragilis* without leading to phagocytosis, and that after this preferential use of complement, an insufficient amount remained for the efficient opsonisation of the *E. coli*. They concluded that this is not a specific phenomenon, because other micro-organisms capable of depleting complement show a similar synergy with *E. coli*. Synergy between *B. fragilis* and *E. coli* was confirmed by means of a skin abscess model *in vivo*, in which *B. fragilis* leads to a local complement deficiency so that *E. coli* cannot be opsonised and cleared. This complement depletion did not fully explain the synergy *in vivo*, because *B. vulgatus* also depletes serum of complement *in vitro*, but synergy is not seen *in vivo*, presumably because *B. vulgatus* does not maintain itself long enough *in vivo* to be effective. The ability of

B. fragilis to grow in an iron-restricted environment, such as serum, which *B. vulgatus* cannot, would explain its greater prevalence in infection and seems an important factor in the complex interaction of anaerobes and *E. coli in vivo*.

Stimulation of growth of Bacteroides fragilis *by* Escherichia coli

The kinetics of bacterial growth in the peritoneum have been studied by Verweij *et al.* (1991) by use of a model of peritonitis that mimics the clinical situation (Dunn *et al.*, 1987). At an inoculum size at which *B. fragilis* was avirulent, *E. coli* led to small acute abscesses that healed, provided that the two organisms were given separately, but when they were inoculated together, larger persistent abscesses resulted. Kinetic studies showed that, within the first six hours, the number of *B. fragilis* declined while that of *E. coli* increased and, after six hours, *B. fragilis* began to multiply. Experiments *in vitro* confirmed that *E. coli* produces a substance, or substances, that stimulated the growth of *B. fragilis*. Preliminary experiments point to it being a haem-binding protein that *B. fragilis* can utilise to acquire iron for growth. Although bacteria can use siderophores produced by other bacteria, this is the first instance in which an iron-binding protein is shown to be used by another species. The suggested mechanism is shown in Figure 17.1 (Verweij, 1993). It would be interesting to know whether the growth of strains of *B. fragilis* that can acquire iron easily is stimulated by *E. coli*.

Clearly, the synergy between *B. fragilis* and *E. coli* is complex. It may depend, in part, on anaerobic conditions, or on the inhibition of phagocytosis by the production of succinate or by complement depletion by the anaerobe. A mechanism by which *E. coli* enables *B. fragilis* to acquire the iron necessary for growth may be the production of an iron-binding protein that *B. fragilis* can utilise. This may be particularly important, because a vaccine directed against this iron-binding protein might block its activity, but this possibility requires further study.

It may also be that strikingly different modes of synergy can show up in different models. For example, local complement deficiency may occur in small skin abscesses, but less readily in peritonitis. In any event, if the localised infection is not contained, it is *E. coli* that is usually able to invade and cause septicaemia (Weinstein *et al.*, 1974; Bourgault *et al.*, 1979).

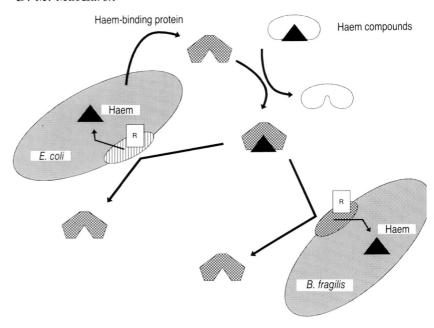

Fig. 17.1. Proposed mechanism by which *Bacteroides fragilis* utilises haem-binding protein produced by *Escherichia coli*.

Escherichia coli septicaemia

In the early years of this century *E. coli* was rarely responsible for septicaemia (Felty & Keefer, 1924), but its incidence in blood cultures has steadily increased since the 1930s (Finland *et al.*, 1959; Geerdes *et al.*, 1992). A dramatic increase in *E. coli* septicaemia in a London teaching hospital in the years 1966 to 1975 was observed by Williams *et al.* (1976) (Table 17.2). Circumstantial evidence points to the selective pressure of antibiotics as the factor responsible for this development (Finland, 1970). Advances in medicine have also affected the prevalence and pattern of septicaemia; seriously ill patients tend to survive longer and the administration of gastric acid inhibitors, for the prevention of stress ulceration, leads to colonisation of the stomach by facultative Gram-negative bacilli, such as *E. coli*. This is one source of pharyngeal colonisation by *E. coli*, a process promoted by the loss of epithelial fibronectin associated with serious illness. Thus, the risk of *E. coli* pneumonia is increased, a risk further amplified by endotracheal intubation for assisted respiration.

The prevalence of *E. coli* septicaemia appears to have reached a

Table 17.2. *Incidence of* Escherichia coli *septicaemia in a London Teaching Hospital, 1966–1975* (after Williams *et al.*, 1976)

Year	Cases of septicaemia per 10,000 admissions
1966–69	1.8
1970–71	3.3
1972	11.2
1973	11.4
1975	12.4

plateau (McGowan, 1985; Gransden *et al.*, 1990), and Gram-positive micro-organisms such as *Staphylococcus epidermidis* and enterococci are increasingly detected as the cause of septicaemia (Banerjee *et al.*, 1991; Donelly, 1993), perhaps as a consequence of selective bowel decontamination, which will be considered below (Bonten *et al.*, 1993), and the wider use of potent broad-spectrum cephalosporins with a predominantly Gram-negative spectrum of activity (Murray, 1990). Nevertheless, *E. coli* still remains the organism most commonly isolated in septicaemia (Geerdes *et al.*, 1992).

Escherichia coli septicaemia arises when the host is unable to contain this organism in its natural niche or at a site of localised infection. This failure of containment may be host-related, as in profound neutropenia, when intestinal *E. coli* may reach the local lymph nodes, grow there and then spread to the bloodstream. This possibility has led to the use of prophylactic antibiotics in so-called 'selective bowel decontamination', which aims to eliminate *E. coli* and other facultative Gram-negative bacteria, or to reduce them to levels that are unlikely to lead to septicaemia (Mulder *et al.*, 1979).

Failure of containment may also result from the presence of virulent strains of *E. coli* in localised infections. Much effort has been devoted to defining the responsible virulence factors.

Epidemiology

The incidence of Gram-negative septicaemia varies in different types of hospital. It is lowest in community hospitals and highest in tertiary referral hospitals (Bryan *et al.*, 1983). The urinary tract is the most

Table 17.3. *Possible virulence of*
Escherichia coli *factors in extra-intestinal infections*

O:K:H-serotype
Serum resistance
Haemolysin production
Aerobactin production
Fimbriae

common source (50–60 per cent); followed by the intestine (*c.* ten per cent), the biliary tract (*c.* ten per cent), wounds (*c.* four per cent), the respiratory tract (one to two per cent) and, rarely, soft tissue infections (Gransden *et al.*, 1990; Frasa *et al.*, 1993). In an appreciable number of cases (ten per cent) no focus is found, but it can be presumed that the intestinal tract is the most likely source.

Strains of *Escherichia coli* with enhanced virulence

Much attention has been devoted to the attributes that lead to enhanced virulence, because this knowledge is essential for planning preventive measures. From a biological point of view, *E. coli* has adapted to survival in the harshly competitive environment of the large intestine. It colonises the infant bowel soon after birth and then remains part of the commensal flora (see Chapter 3). Although always present, the composition of the *E. coli* flora varies and there are resident and transient strains (Simon & Gorbach, 1984). It should not be forgotten, however, that *E. coli* does not constitute more than a minute fraction of the intestinal flora. Should *E. coli* migrate to extra-intestinal tissue sites, it may not have to compete with a teeming commensal flora, but it will have to cope with other hostile factors such as the host immune system, cells with receptors different from those in the bowel, and alterations in the supply of nutrients. It is not surprising that only certain subsets of intestinal *E. coli* are able to survive in such a hostile environment (Brooks *et al.*, 1980). Comparison of faecal strains of *E. coli* and extra-intestinal strains, usually from urinary infection and septicaemia, have suggested that certain bacterial attributes enhance virulence and enable *E. coli* to widen its niche (Table 17.3). It will be convenient to consider these attributes and their relation to septicaemia individually, but it should not be forgotten that a strain may often possess one or more of these virulence properties and that they may well act in concert.

Serotypes

Determination of the O:K:H-serotype is a refined method for typing *E. coli*, because there are more than 170 O-antigens, about 100 K-antigens, and 56 H-antigens. Unfortunately, few laboratories possess all the necessary antisera, and most studies have relied on a limited range of antisera. This has certain inherent disadvantages, as will be considered below.

It was suggested by Sjöstedt (1946) that certain serotypes are more pathogenic than others. Later studies showed that a small number of antisera is sufficient to type the majority of *E. coli* isolated from urinary tract infection, which suggests that these strains may be nephropathogenic. Critics of this hypothesis pointed out that these O-antigens occurred quite commonly in faecal strains and that the same types occurred in *E. coli* septicaemia arising from infected foci other than the urinary tract (Kunin, 1978). Though this suggests that these O-serotypes were not especially uropathogenic, it is consistent with the notion of enhanced virulence. There is compelling evidence for the importance of K-antigens in invasive *E. coli* strains, but McCabe *et al.* (1978) was unable to find more K-antigens in strains isolated from septicaemia than in faecal strains. In neonatal sepsis and meningitis, where there is a pre-existing septicaemia, more than 75 per cent of strains possess the K1 antigen (Robbins, 1974).

In adult septicaemia K1-positive strains are more common than among faecal strains (Brauner *et al.*, 1987; Opal *et al.*, 1988). Nevertheless, virulence is multi-factorial and the cloning of K1-antigen in relatively avirulent strains does not significantly enhance their virulence (Silver *et al.*, 1981). The common occurrence in neonatal sepsis and meningitis of *E. coli* O7K1 and O18K1 strains, and the less common occurrence of O1:K1 in meningitis and the rarity of O18K1 strains in urinary tract infection are unexplained (Kusecek *et al.*, 1984).

It has implicitly been accepted that serotypes are clonal in origin (Achtman & Pluschke, 1986). Multi-locus isoenzyme analysis has shown that, in serotypes characterised by OK and H serology, genetic diversity is not great, but that strains that are not clonal may still be typed as having the same O- and K-antigens, and even the same serotypes need not be derived from the same clone. Thus, O1:K1 strains fell into three clones, two widely spread clones and a third less common clone (Ochman & Selander, 1984). One O1:K1 clone was involved in neonatal sepsis and meningitis, and the other was not. In future studies to relate subsets of

E. coli to particular disease entities, it will be necessary to type the strains fully or, preferably, to use genetic information to determine clonality. In any event, it is clear that certain K-antigens, such as K1, are associated with enhanced virulence and others, such as K100, are not.

K-antigens enhance virulence in a number of ways (see Chapter 4). They are not readily recognised as foreign in humans because of 'molecular mimicry', as a result they are poorly immunogenic and levels of natural anti-K opsonising antibodies are low. This is particularly true of the K1 antigen. Moreover, the negative charge of the capsule and its hydrophilic nature are essentially antiphagocytic, so that acidic capsular polysaccharide impairs phagocytosis. The degree of antiphagocytic activity is proportional to the amount of K-antigen present and capsular antigens reduce phagocytosis by interfering with complement deposition on the bacterium (Howard & Glynn, 1971). Capsular polysaccharides also increase the binding of the inhibitor β1H to C3b (Leying, 1990), thus preventing the normal activation of the complement cascade. In all these ways, therefore, the presence of an acidic polysaccharide capsule greatly assists *E. coli* to invade and to maintain itself in the bloodstream.

Serum resistance

Many facultative Gram-negative bacilli are rapidly killed in fresh normal serum by activation of the complement system, either by the classical pathway, when natural antibodies are present, or by the alternative pathway, when activation is by lipopolysaccharide (LPS) (Quie, 1981). Rough strains are exquisitely sensitive to complement-mediated killing, possibly because lipid A and core LPS activate complement very efficiently. Lipid A and core LPS may be shielded by oligosaccharide side chains in smooth LPS, so that complement activation occurs less readily (Goldman *et al.*, 1984). An alternative hypothesis is that complement activation by smooth LPS does takes place, but at some distance from its target because of the length of the polysaccharide side chains of LPS, which reduces the efficiency of the activated complement (Taylor, 1983). Such a mechanism would explain why serum resistance is proportional to the amount of polysaccharide present, the length of the side chain and the degree of substitution of core with the sugars of the smooth complete LPS (see Chapter 5).

Serum resistance is the outcome of the combined effects of LPS, capsule and certain membrane proteins (Montenegro *et al.*, 1985). As we have seen, the part that K-antigens play in serum resistance is debatable, with the notable exception of K1 antigen. Strains bearing K1 often possess only rough LPS, but are serum resistant, although less so than strains with a smooth O-phenotype (Vermeulen *et al.*, 1981). When K1 antigen is cloned into serum-sensitive avirulent strains, the serum resistance of the recipient increases (Silver *et al.*, 1981). Certain plasmids confer degrees of serum resistance. One of the best studied is the colicin virulence (ColV) plasmid that encodes the production of colicin V. It is, however, properties other than colicin V production that make the recipient more virulent, such as increased serum resistance, often, but not always, mediated by an iss (increased survival in serum) protein, impaired phagocytosis (Aguero & Cabello, 1983), increased fimbriation (Clancy & Savage, 1981) and aerobactin production (Bindereif & Neilands, 1985). ColV-positive strains are over-represented among *E. coli* isolates from pyelonephritis and they are common in septicaemia strains. Another membrane protein, traT, also confers serum resistance. Its importance in extra-intestinal *E. coli* infections may be deduced from its more frequent occurrence in invasive than in faecal isolates (Kanukollu *et al.*, 1985). However, it confers only moderate serum resistance and its importance has been debated.

Serum resistance is associated with certain O-serogroups of *E. coli*. In general, strains that belong to serogroups O2, O4, O6, O7, O18 and O75 are more serum resistant than those from other less common O-serogroups. McCabe *et al.* (1978) found that serogroups O2, O4, O6 and O16 were more common in septicaemia in infants and adults.

Serum resistance is undoubtedly a mark of invasive *E. coli*. Septicaemia strains are mostly resistant to serum-mediated killing. If killing by serum, mainly by alternative pathway complement activation, is the first line of host defence, serum-sensitive strains will find it very difficult to invade the bloodstream. However, when there is serious underlying disease and massive invasion of the blood stream, serum sensitive strains may succeed. In any event, not all septicaemia isolates of *E. coli* are serum-resistant. Other factors, such as overwhelming bacterial invasion, may account for the success of the minority of serum-sensitive strains in septicaemia.

Adhesins

Adherence is the first step in a complex process that results in bacterial colonisation and, under certain circumstances, in bacterial invasion. Factors that promote adherence may, therefore, justifiably be regarded as playing a vital role in the initiation of infection. Adherence by *E. coli* can be either sensitive or resistant to inhibition by mannose. The former is due to type-1 fimbriae (see Chapter 6) and the latter to P-fimbriae (see Chapter 8) or X-adhesins, a heterogeneous group that is shrinking as adhesins are characterised and named (Johnson, 1991; see also Chapter 18).

It is generally accepted that most *E. coli* strains can be induced to produce type-1 fimbriae but cultural conditions can greatly affect the result. Strains of *E. coli* responsible for septicaemia possess type-1 fimbriae more often than faecal strains (Opal *et al.*, 1988). This is difficult to explain in the light of the fact that type-1 fimbriae also promote adherence to leucocytes and often stimulate phagocytosis (Silverblatt *et al.*, 1979; Öhman *et al.*, 1982). *Proteus* in the fimbrial phase is less virulent than in the non-fimbrial phase, in a haematogenous experimental infection model. *Proteus* organisms, when fimbriated, cause an ascending infection of the urinary tract but, once in the kidney, they shed the fimbriae, presumably because they aid bacterial ascent, but are a disadvantage when the bacteria are confronted by phagocytic cells in the tissues (Silverblatt, 1974; Silverblatt & Ofek, 1978). It seems unlikely that *E. coli* would remain fimbriated in the bloodstream or that type-1 fimbriae play a role in septicaemia. While type-1 fimbriae stimulate phagocytosis, P-fimbriae reduce it, because they adhere poorly to human polymorphonuclear cells. Clearly, it would be interesting to know the state of fimbriation of *E. coli* in the bloodstream.

P-fimbriated *E. coli* can invade the normal urinary tract and cause serious pyelonephritis (Johnson *et al.*, 1987). Only where the resistance of the urinary tract is lowered as a consequence of anatomical or physiological abnormalities, can non-P-fimbriated *E. coli* cause pyelonephritis (Otto *et al.*, 1993). This has been suggested as a diagnostic screening test for occult urinary tract abnormalities (de Man *et al.*, 1989). Since the urinary tract is the most common source of septicaemia, one might expect P-fimbriated strains to be well represented in *E. coli* septicaemia and this is indeed the case (Brauner *et al.*, 1985, 1987). One study is exceptional in finding that P-fimbriated strains are over-represented in pyelonephritis, but uncommon in faecal and septicaemia strains (Opal *et al.*, 1982).

Since P-fimbriae are classically associated with uropathogenicity, P-fimbriation is more common where the urinary tract is the focus of infection than when it is not (Table 17.4). However, P-fimbriae appear to contribute to the ability of *E. coli* to maintain itself in the bloodstream,

Table 17.4. *Distribution of genes for adherence factors and haemolysin* production in Escherichia coli *from cases of septicaemia* (after Maslow, 1993)

Primary site of infection	No. of strains	Percentage positive strains			
		All adherence	P	S	Hly
Urinary tract	81	84	77	46	60
Gastro-intestinal tract	42	52	36	36	33
Respiratory tract	10	50	40	30	10
Other and unknown	37	48	29	21	12

P, P-fimbriae; S, S-fimbriae; Hly, Haemolysin.

Other – prostate, 3; cellulitis, 2; intravenous catheters, 2; paraspinal abscess, 1; decubitus ulcers, 5.

Table 17.5. *The relationship between the presence of adhesin-negative* Escherichia coli *in septicaemia and the immune status of patients* (after Maslow, 1993)

	Adhesin-positive	Adhesin-negative
Presence of local or general defects	71	34
Absense of local or general defects	22	1

presumably by virtue of their anti-phagocytic function. Adhesin-negative strains are virtually absent from patients without defects of their host defence (Table 17.5).

Of the non-P, mannose-resistant adhesins, S-adhesins are associated with septicaemia. The mechanism of this association is not clear. Their distribution in septicaemia parallels that of P-fimbriae, but they are less common.

Haemolysins

The suggestion that haemolysins contribute to virulence is due to Dudgeon *et al.* (1923), who observed the more frequent occurrence of haemolytic *E. coli* in urinary tract infection. In a haematogenous mouse model, the virulence of *E. coli* strains can be divided into three groups. Group I were avirulent and were rapidly cleared from the bloodstream, Group II were rapidly cleared from the blood and tissues, but grew in the

Table 17.6. *Properties of* Escherichia coli *according to the classification of van den Bosch* et al. (*1979*)

Virulence group	Percentage positive		
	K-antigen	Haemolysin	MRHA
I	84	16	14
II	76	57	24
III	84	45	17

MRHA, mannose-resistant haemagglutination.

kidney, while Group III multiplied rapidly in blood and tissues and caused early death (Van den Bosch *et al.*, 1979). Group II and III strains were more often haemolytic than those of Group I, which affords experimental evidence in favour of haemolysin as a virulence factor (Table 17.6).

Most research has centred on the α-haemolysin secreted by *E. coli*. Other haemolysins appear to be cell-bound and some may reflect the toxicity of metabolic products rather than true haemolysins. This account will be restricted to α-haemolysin, because the role in virulence played by cell-bound haemolysins has not been much studied (see Chapter 11). Transfer of a plasmid that codes for haemolysin does not render *E. coli* K-12 virulent, but insertion of a transposon to block haemolysin production reduces the nephropathogenicity of *E. coli* (Waalwijk & de Graaff, 1983). Moreover, although haemolysin was a decisive factor in uropathogenicity of Group II strains, it was of minor importance for the virulence of highly virulent Group III strains, and a non-haemolytic mutant of a Group III strain was almost as virulent as the parent (van den Bosch *et al.*, 1981)

Haemolysin production is often associated with other known virulence factors, such as P-fimbriae, serum resistance, common O-serogroups such as O4, O6, O18 and certain K-antigens.

Strains of *E. coli* isolated from septicaemia and pyelonephritis are more often haemolytic than faecal strains or strains isolated from cystitis, which suggests that haemolysin production promotes invasion by *E. coli*. Haemolysin may affect the course of *E. coli* septicaemia in several ways. Lysis of erythrocytes may provide a rich supply of iron-containing compounds and shortage of available iron is a problem that invasive *E. coli* must overcome (see Chapter 12). In addition, haemolysins are toxic to leucocytes (Gadeberg & Ørskov, 1984) and other tissue cells (Keane *et al.*, 1987), in this way contributing to inflammation, cell damage and evasion of phagocytosis. That α-haemolysin is produced *in vivo* is confirmed by the antibody response to haemolysin during infections by a haemolytic *E. coli* (Emody *et al.*, 1982).

Aerobactin

Although the human body has abundant stores of iron, this is almost entirely bound or deposited in body stores. There is, therefore, insufficient free iron for bacterial growth and pathogens require special mechanisms to scavenge bound iron (Otto *et al.*, 1992; and see Chapter 12). *Escherichia coli* accomplishes this by producing siderophores capable of extracting iron from iron complexes. Two siderophores are of particular interest, enterobactin, with an extremely high affinity for iron, and aerobactin, a hydroxamate with a lower affinity for iron, but which approaches that of human transferrin. Almost all *E. coli* strains produce enterobactin, but Miles & Khimji (1975) were unable to show any relationship between enterobactin production and virulence. Less than half of a small number of faecal strains produced aerobactin, but 75 per cent of septicaemia strains did so (Montgomerie *et al.*, 1984).

As we have noted in relation to soft tissue infection, *B. fragilis* also seems able to utilise a haem-binding protein produced by *E. coli* and this may be an important mechanism for obtaining iron in mixed infections. In an experimental model of peritonitis, this haem-binding protein of *E. coli* stimulated the growth of *B. fragilis*.

The gene for aerobactin production may be chromosomal or plasmid-borne, but in most clinical *E. coli* isolates it is chromosomal. The chromosomal aerobactin gene often occurs together with the determinants for haemolysin and P-fimbriae (Johnson *et al.*, 1988). Other workers were unable to find an association between aerobactin and haemolysin in urinary strains but they did not distinguish between strains with plasmid-borne and chromosomal aerobactin determinants (Ørskov *et al.*, 1988). The subset of *E. coli* strains with chromosomal aerobactin, haemolysin and P-fimbrial determinants are highly virulent, and cause invasive disease in immunocompetent hosts. Strains with plasmid-borne aerobactin did not show an association with haemolysin or P-fimbriae, but often had antimicrobial resistance genes, suggesting a possible way in which plasmid-borne aerobactin was selected. These strains were found only in infections in compromised hosts (Johnson *et al.*, 1988). These

Table 17.7. *The relationship between aerobactin production and the virulence of* Escherichia coli *in experimental ascending pyelonephritis in mice* (after Montgomerie *et al.*, 1984)

	Percentage of early death
Aerobactin-positive	35.4±12.0
Aerobactin-negative	11.4±3.4

$p = 0.02$.

observations may explain the conflicting reports in the literature on the association between aerobactin and other virulence factors, and in particular haemolysin.

In 1986 and 1987 there was an outbreak of *E. coli* O15 infections in England associated with septicaemia, meningitis and pneumonia. The strain of *E. coli* responsible carried a F1me plasmid that coded for aerobactin production and resistance to several antibiotics. This epidemic plasmid resembled *Salmonella* plasmids that also coded for aerobactin and antimicrobial resistance. Intergenus spread of the plasmid may have occurred under the selective pressure of antibiotics with the aerobactin gene endowing the recipient *E. coli* with the enhanced virulence (Phillips *et al.*, 1988).

In experimental infections, aerobactin-positive *E. coli* are more virulent than aerobactin-negative strains, the former being more lethal for mice (Table 17.7), and, in addition, aerobactin is less common in environmental *E. coli* strains than in septicaemia strains. It would seem that in the environment enterobactin plays a greater role in iron acquisition.

Miscellaneous virulence factors

No single biochemical test distinguishes faecal from septicaemia strains of *E. coli*, but certain biochemical profiles are more often associated with urosepsis (Brauner *et al.*, 1987). Carboxylesterase B exists as two variants, one moving rapidly on electrophoresis and the other more slowly. Invasive strains of *E. coli* possess the slowly migrating variant more commonly than environmental or faecal strains. It seems unlikely *a priori* that this contributes directly to the mechanism of invasion, but it may be linked to other properties that determine enhanced virulence and serve as markers of invasive strains (Goullet *et al.*, 1988).

Virulence factors as yet undetected

There is some evidence for as yet undetected virulence factors. Experimentally, an *E. coli* O18:K1 strain with the ColV plasmid was of reduced virulence if either of these properties was lost. Mutants of reduced virulence were found in which O18:K1 and the ColV plasmid were unchanged, suggesting that other factors are involved (Williams Smith & Huggins, 1980).

Septicaemia and shock due to *Escherichia coli*

The most serious complication of *E. coli* septicaemia is septic (endotoxic) shock, which is characterised by severe hypotension and progressive vital organ failure, including the lungs and kidneys. The mortality of established septic shock is between 50 and 75 per cent, even in the face of modern resuscitation methods and potent antibiotics (Cohen & Glauser, 1991).

In septic shock, a whole series of often interacting physiological mechanisms become activated and disordered, including the complement and coagulation cascades, and the cytokine regulatory system. Although a complex cascade of reactions has been described, it is generally accepted that endotoxin is the trigger, but there is some dissent from this hypothesis (Hurley, 1993) (see Chapter 5). The use of the term endotoxin is in some ways a misnomer, since endotoxin is not a toxin in the true sense of the word (Thomas, 1972), but is released by bacteria in the presence of serum. Cell-wall-active antibiotics may accelerate the release of endotoxin from *E. coli* and increased concentrations of plasma endotoxin have been detected in patients after antibiotic treatment, but there is no evidence that this is of any clinical significance (Hurley, 1993).

Endotoxin can activate complement, resulting in increased chemotaxis, increased leucocyte adherence and vasodilation. The 'sticky' leucocytes bind to each other and to vascular endothelium, resulting in the production and release of arachidonic acid derivatives, toxic oxygen radicals and lysosomal enzymes. In addition, endotoxin can activate Factor XII, to trigger the intrinsic coagulation pathway, and the extrinsic pathway via macrophages and endothelial cells. This leads to disseminated intravascular coagulation and consumption of clotting factors. LPS-activated Factor XII activates pre-kallikrein to kallikrein, which produces the potent hypotensive agent, bradykinin. Nitric oxide, also produced by vascular endothelium, is another powerful vasodilator and increases the hypotension. In this whole cascade of events, macrophages play an important role. Although the macrophage is beneficial in removing endotoxin from the circulation, it also produces cytokines such as interleukin-1, and tumour necrosis factor (TNF). The latter appears to be the central mediator of the pathophysiological response to LPS. LPS can bind directly to macrophages, but it can also bind to LPS-binding protein (LBP), an acute phase protein that forms a ligand with the macrophage. The LPS–LBP complex stimulates macrophages to produce cytokines, such as TNF, at lower concentrations than native LPS. From a biological view point, LBP assists the host by allowing earlier recognition of the presence of LPS.

There is little evidence to suggest that the endotoxin from one organism is more liable to give rise to shock than that from another. However, septicaemia due to serum-resistant strains more often leads to shock, probably because they can maintain themselves better in the bloodstream (McCabe *et al.*, 1978).

The evident shortcomings of antibiotics in the treatment of septic shock has led to other approaches. High doses of corticosteroids have been recommended to modulate the immunopathological response, but they have proved disappointing (Cohen & Glauser, 1991). Immunotherapy seems attractive, but a practical drawback is the great variety of *E. coli* serotypes. Lipid A and core polysaccharide are highly conserved regions of LPS, and antibodies directed against these might be expected to have a broad spectrum of activity. For practical reasons monoclonal antibodies against these regions of LPS seem ideal (see Chapter 5). Two such antibodies have been extensively tested. The first, E5, is a murine IgM monoclonal antibody that reacts with Lipid A, and the other, HA-IA, is a human monoclonal antibody active against the endotoxin core. In two large trials small subsets of patients seemed to benefit, but the patients who benefited could only be identified retrospectively (Cohen & Glauser, 1991), and this is rather disappointing. Moreover, after studying the reactions of several monoclonal antibodies with a range of endotoxins, it was concluded that the extent of cross-reactivity was less than had been predicted (B. J. Appelmelk, personal communication).

Another approach is to use monoclonal antibodies to block the effects of the cytokines that appear to be important in the pathogenesis of shock.

Monoclonal antibodies against TNF seem potentially useful and would have the advantage of also being effective in septic shock caused by Gram-positive bacteria (Cohen & Glauser, 1991). However, modulation of cytokines may well bring with it the disadvantage of impairing the host immune response. This is a challenging problem that is now being addressed (Dinarello *et al.*, 1993).

Acknowledgements

I should like to thank Dr. A. M. Simoons-Smit for her critical reading of the manuscript and helpful suggestions and Dr. B. Otto for discussing the 'shuttle protein' hypothesis illustrated in Figure 17.1. I am also very grateful to Mrs. R. Schoemaker who typed the manuscript with care and attention.

References

Achtman, M. & Pluschke, G. (1986). Clonal analysis of descent and virulence among selected *Escherichia coli*. *Annual Review of Microbiology*, **40**,185–210.

Aguero, M. E. & Cabello, F. C. (1983). Relative contribution of ColV plasmid and K1 antigen to the pathogenicity of *Escherichia coli*. *Infection and Immunity*, **40**, 359–68.

Banerjee, S. N., Emori, T. G., Culver, D. H., Gaynes, R. P., Jarvis, W. R., Horan, T., Edwards, J. R., Tolson, J., Henderson, T. & Martone, W. J. (1991). Secular trends in nosocomial primary bloodstream infections in the United States, 1980–1989. *American Journal of Medicine*, **91**, Supplement 3B, 86–9S.

Bindereif, A. & Neilands, J. B. (1985). Aerobactin genes in clinical isolates of *Escherichia coli*. *Journal of Bacteriology*, **161**, 727–35.

Bonten, M. J. M., van Tiel, F. H., van der Geest, S., Stobberingh, E. E. & Gaillard, C. A. (1993). *Enterococcus faecalis* pneumonia complicating topical antimicrobial prophylaxis. *New England Journal of Medicine*, **328**, 209–10.

Bourgault, A-M., England, D. M., Rosenblatt, J. E., Forgacs, P. & Bieger, R. C. (1979). Clinical characteristics of anaerobe bactibilia. *Archives of Internal Medicine*, **139**, 1347–9.

Brauner, A., Boeufgras, J.-M., Jacobson, S. H., Kaijser, B., Källenius, G., Svenson, S. B. & Wretlind, B. (1987) The use of biochemical markers, serotype and fimbriation in the detection of *Escherichia coli* clones. *Journal of General Microbiology*, **133**, 2825–34.

Brauner, A., Leissner, M., Wretlind, B., Julander, I., Svenson, S. B. & Källenius, G. (1985). Occurrence of P-fimbriated *Escherichia coli* in patients with bacteremia. *European Journal of Clinical Microbiology*, **4**, 566–9.

Brauner, A. & Østenson, C.-G. (1987) Bacteremia with P-fimbriated *Escherichia coli* in diabetic patients: correlation between proteinuria and non-P-fimbriated strains. *Diabetes Research*, **6**, 61–5.

Brooks, H. L., O'Grady, F., McSherry, M. A. & Cattell, W. R. (1980). Uropathogenic properties of *Escherichia coli* in recurrent urinary-tract infection. *Journal of Medical Microbiology*, **13**, 57–68.

Bryan, C. S., Reynolds, K. L. & Brenner, E. R. (1983). Analysis of 1,186 episodes of Gram-negative bacteremia in Non-University Hospitals: the effects of antimicrobial therapy. *Reviews of Infectious Diseases*, **5**, 629–38.

Clancy, J. & Savage, D. C. (1981). Another ColicinV phenomenon: *in vitro* adhesion of *Escherichia coli* to mouse intestinal epithelium. *Infection and Immunity*, **32**, 343–52.

Cohen, J. & Glauser, M. P. (1991). Septic shock: treatment. *Lancet*, **338**, 736–9.

Conte, J. E. (1989). Antibiotic prophylaxis: non-abdominal surgery. In *Current Clinical Topics in Infectious Diseases*, eds. J. S. Remington & M. N. Swartz, pp. 254–305. Cambridge, MA: Blackwell Scientific Publications.

De Man, P., Cläeson, I., Johanson, I.-M., Jodal, U. & Svanborg-Eden, C. (1989). Bacterial attachment as a predictor of renal abnormalities in boys with urinary tract infection. *Journal of Paediatrics*, **115**, 915–22.

Dinarello, C. A., Gelfand, J. A. & Wolff, S. M. (1993). Anticytokine strategies in the treatment of the systemic inflammatory response syndrome. *Journal of the American Medical Association*, **14**, 1829–35.

Donnelly, J. P. (1993). Selective decontamination of the digestive tract and its role in antimicrobial prophylaxis. *Journal of Antimicrobial Chemotherapy*, **31**, 813–29.

Dudgeon, L. S., Worldey, E. & Bawtree, F. (1923). On *Bacillus coli* infections of the urinary tract, especially in relation to haemolytic organisms. *Journal of Hygiene, Cambridge*, **21**, 168–98.

Dunn, D. L., Barke, R. A., Ewald, D. C. & Simmons, R. L. (1987). Macrophages and translymphatic absorption represent the first line of host defence of the peritoneal cavity. *Archives of Surgery*, **122**, 105–10.

Edlich, R. F., Rodeheaver, G. T., Thacker, J. G., Winn, H. R. & Edgerton, M. T. (1977). Management of soft tissue injury. *Clinics of Plastic Surgery*, **4**, 191–8.

Emody, L., Batai, I., Kerenyi, M., Szekely, J. & Polyak, L. (1982). Anti-*Escherichia coli* alpha-haemolysin in control and patient sera. *Lancet*, **ii**, 986.

Felty, A. R. & Keefer, C. S. (1924). Bacillus coli sepsis. *Journal of the American Medical Association*, **82**, 1430–3.

Finland, M. (1970). Changing ecology of bacterial infections as related to antibacterial therapy. *Journal of Infectious Diseases*, **122**, 419–31.

Finland, M., Johns, W. F. & Barnes, W. F. (1959). Occurrence of serious bacterial infections since introduction of antibacterial agents. *Journal of the American Medical Association*, **170**, 2188–97.

Frasa, H., Procee, J., Torensma, R., Verbruggen, A., Algra, A., Rozenberg-Arska, M., Kraaijeveld, K. & Verhoef J. (1993). *Escherichia coli* in bacteremia: O-acetylated K1 strains appear to be more virulent than non-O-acetylated K1 strains. *Journal of Clinical Microbiology*, **31**, 3174–8.

Gadeberg, O. V. & Ørskov, I. (1984). In vitro cytotoxic effect of an α-hemolytic *Escherichia coli* on human blood granulocytes. *Infection and Immunity*, **45**, 255–60.

Galpin, J. E., Chow, A. W. & Bayer, A. S. (1976). Sepsis associated with decubitus ulcers. *American Journal of Medicine*, **61**, 346–9.

Geerdes, H. F., Ziegler, D., Lode, H., Hund, M., Loehr, A., Fangmann, W. & Wagner, J. (1992). Septicemia in 980 patients at a University Hospital in Berlin: prospective studies during 4 selected years between 1979 and 1989. *Clinical Infectious Diseases*, **15**, 991–1002.

Goldman, R. C. K., Joiner, K. & Leive, L. (1984). Serum resistant mutants of *Escherichia coli* O111 contain increased lipopolysaccharide, lack an O-antigen-containing capsule and cover more of their lipid A core with O-antigen. *Journal of Bacteriology*, **159**, 877–82.

Gransden, W. R., Eykyn, S. J., Philips, I. & Rowe, B. (1990) Bacteremia due to *Escherichia coli*: a study of 861 episodes. *Reviews of Infectious Diseases*, **12**, 1008–18.

Goullet, P., Picard, B. & Sevali Garcia, J. (1986). Electrophoretic mobility of an esterase from *Escherichia coli* isolated from extraintestinal infections. *Journal of Infectious Diseases*, **154**, 727–8.

Howard, C. J. & Glynn, A. A. (1971). The virulence for mice of strains of *Escherichia coli* related to effects of K antigens on their resistance to phagocytosis and killing by complement. *Immunology*, **20**, 767–77.

Hurley, J. C. (1993). Reappraisal of the role of endotoxin in the sepsis syndrome. *Lancet*, **341**, 1133–5.

Ingham, H. R., Sisson, P. R., Tharagonnet, D., Selkon, J. B. & Codd, A. A. (1977). Inhibition of phagocytosis *in vitro* by obligate anaerobes. *Lancet*, **ii**, 1252–4.

Johnson, J. R. (1991). Virulence factors in *Escherichia coli* urinary tract infection. *Clinical Microbiology Reviews*, **4**, 80–128.

Johnson, J. R., Moseley, S. L., Roberts, P. L. & Stamm, W. E. (1988). Aerobactin and other virulence factor genes among strains of *Escherichia coli* causing urosepsis: association with patient characteristics. *Infection and Immunity*, **56**, 405–12.

Johnson, J. R., Roberts, P. L. & Stamm, W. E. (1987). P fimbriae and other virulence factors in *Escherichia coli* urosepsis: association with patients' characteristics. *Journal of Infectious Diseases*, **156**, 225–8.

Joseph, W. S. (1991). Treatment of lower extremity infections in diabetics. *Drugs*, **42**, 984–96.

Kanukollu, U., Bieler, S., Hull, S. & Hull, R. (1985). Contribution of the *tra*T gene to serum resistance among clinical isolates of enterobacteriaceae. *Journal of Medical Microbiology*, **19**, 61–7.

Keane, W. F., Welch, R., Gekker, G. & Peterson, K. (1987). Mechanism of *Escherichia coli* α-haemolysin-induced injury to isolated renal tubular cells. *American Journal of Pathology*, **126**, 350–7.

Kovaric, J. J., Matsumoto, T., Dobek, A. S. & Hamit, H. F. (1968). Bacterial flora of one hundred and twelve combat wounds. *Military Medicine*, **133**, 622–4.

Kunin, C. (1978). Microbiological aspects of urinary tract infection. In *Infections of the Urinary Tract*, eds. E. H. Kass & W. Brumfitt, pp. 37–43. Chicago: University of Chicago Press.

Kusecek, B., Wloch, H., Mercer, A., Vaisanen, C., Pluschke, G., Korhonen, T. & Achtman, M. (1984). Lipopolysaccharide capsule, and fimbriae as

490   D. M. MacLaren

virulence factors among O1, O7, O16, O18 or O75 and K1, K5, or K100 *Escherichia coli. Infection and Immunity*, **43**, 368–79.

Lewis, R. T. (1992). Necrotizing soft tissue infections. *Infectious Disease Clinics of North America*, **6**, 693–703.

Leying, H., Suerbaum, S., Kroll, H. P., Stahl, D. & Opferkuch, W. (1990). The capsular polysaccharide is a major determinant of serum resistance in K-1-positive blood culture isolates of *Escherichia coli. Infection and Immunity*, **58**, 222–7.

McCabe, W. R., Kaijser, B., Olling, S., Uwaydah, M. & Hanson, L. A. (1978). *Escherichia coli* in bacteremia: K and O antigens and serum sensitivity of strains from adults and neonates. *Journal of Infectious Diseases*, **138**, 33–41.

McGowan, J. E. (1985). Changing etiology of nosocomial bacteremia and fungemia and other hospital-acquired infections. *Reviews of Infectious Diseases*, **7**, Supplement 3, S357–70.

Maslow, J. N., Mulligan, M. E., Adams, K. S., Justis, J. C. & Arbeit, R. D. (1993). Bacterial adhesins and host factors: role in the development and outcome of *Escherichia coli* bacteremia. *Clinical Infectious Diseases*, **17**, 89–97.

Miles, A. A. & Khimji, P. L. (1975). Enterobacterial chelators of iron: their occurrence, detection and relation to pathogenicity. *Journal of Medical Microbiology*, **8**, 477–92.

Montenegro, M. A., Bitter-Suerman, D., Timmis, J. K., Aguero, M. E., Cabello, F. C., Sanyal, S. C. & Timmis, K. N. (1985). *tra*T gene sequences, serum resistance, and pathogenicity-related factors in clinical isolates of *Escherichia coli* and other Gram-negative bacteria. *Journal of General Microbiology*, **131**, 1511–27.

Montgomerie, J. Z., Bindereif, A., Neilands, J. B., Kalmanson, G. M. & Guze, L. B. (1984). Association of hydroxamate siderophore (aerobactin) with *Escherichia coli* isolated from patients with bacteremia. *Infection and Immunity*, **46**, 835–8.

Mulder, N. H., Nieweg, H. O., Sleijfer, D. T., de Vries-Hospers, H. G., van der Waaij, D., Fidler, V. & van Saene, H. K. F. (1979). Infection prevention in granulocytopenic patients by selective decontamination of the digestive tract. In *New Criteria for Antimicrobial Therapy*, eds. D. van der Waaij & J. Verhoef, pp. 113–16. Amsterdam: Excerpta Medica.

Murray, B. E. (1990). The life and times of the enterococcus. *Clinical Microbiology Reviews*, **3**, 46–65.

Namavar, F., Verweij-van Vught, A. M. J. J., Bal, M., van Steenbergen, T. J. M., de Graaff, J. & MacLaren, D. M. (1983). Effect of anaerobic bacteria on killing of *Proteus mirabilis* by human polymorphonuclear leucocytes. *Infection and Immunity*, **38**, 86–91.

Ochman, H. & Selander, R. K. (1984). Evidence for clonal population structure in *Escherichia coli. Proceedings of the National Academy of Sciences, USA*, **81**, 198–201.

Öhman, L., Hed, J. & Stendahl, O. (1982). Interaction between human polymorphonuclear leukocytes and two different strains of type 1 fimbriae-bearing *Escherichia coli. Journal of Infectious Diseases*, **146**, 751–7.

Opal, S. M., Cross, A., Gemski, P. & Lyhte, L. W. (1988). Survey of purported virulence factors of *Escherichia coli* isolated from blood, urine and stool. *European Journal of Clinical Microbiology and Infectious Diseases*, **7**, 425–7.

Ørskov, I. Svanborg-Eden, C., & Ørskov, F. (1988). Aerobactin production of serotyped *Escherichia coli* from urinary tract infections. *Medical Microbiology and Immunology*, **177**, 9–14.

Otto, B. R., Verweij-van Vught, A. M. J. J. & MacLaren, D. M. (1992). Transferrins and heme-compounds as iron sources for pathogenic bacteria. *Critical Reviews in Microbiology*, **18**, 217–33.

Otto, G., Sandberg, T., Marklund, B.-I., Ulleryd, P. & Svanborg, C. (1993). Virulence factors and pap genotype in *Escherichia coli* isolates from women with acute pyelonephritis, with or without bacteremia. *Clinical Infectious Diseases*, **17**, 448–56.

Philips, I., Eykyn, S., King, A., Gransden, W. R., Rowe, B., Frost, J. A. & Gross, R. (1988). Epidemic multiresistant *Escherichia coli* infection in West Lambeth Health District. *Lancet*, **ii**, 1038–41.

Polk, H. C. (1973). Postoperative wound infection: prediction of some responsible organisms. *The American Journal of Surgery*, **126**, 592–4.

Quie, P. G. (1981). Humoral factors in host defence against microbial invaders. *Scandinavian Journal of Infectious Diseases*, Supplement, **31**, 34–80.

Robbins, J. B., McCracken, G. H., Gotschlich, E. C., Ørskov, F., Ørskov, I. & Hanson, L. A. (1974). *Escherichia coli* K1 capsular polysaccharide associated with neonatal meningitis. *New England Journal of Medicine*, **22**, 73–80.

Robson, M. C., Lea, C. E., Dalton, J. B. & Heggers, J. P. (1968). Quantitative bacteriology and delayed wound closure. *Surgical Forum*, **19**, 501–10.

Rotstein, O. D., Pruett, T. L., Fiegel, V. D., Nelson, R. D. & Simmons, R. L. (1985) Succinic acid, a metabolic by-product of *Bacteroides* species, inhibits polymorphonuclear leukocyte function. *Infection and Immunity*, **48**, 402–8.

Sapico, F. L., Canawati, H. N., Witte, J. L., Montgomerie, J. Z., Wagner, F. W. & Bessman, A. N. (1980). Quantitative aerobic and anaerobic bacteriology of infected diabetic feet. *Journal of Clinical Microbiology*, **12**, 413–20.

Sigurdson, A. F. & Gudmundsson, S. (1989). The aetiology of bacterial cellulitis as determined by fine-needle biopsy. *Scandinavian Journal of Infectious Diseases*, Supplementum **21**, 537–42.

Silver, R. P., Finn, C. W., Vann, W. F., Aaronson, W., Schneerson, R., Kretschmer, P. J. & Garon, C. F. (1981). Molecular cloning of the K1 capsular polysaccharide genes of *E. coli*. *Nature*, **289**, 697–9.

Silverblatt, F. J. (1974). Host-parasite interaction in the rat renal pelvis. A possible role for pili in the pathogenesis of pyelonephritis. *Journal of Experimental Medicine*, **140**, 1696–1711.

Silverblatt, F. J., Dreyer, J. S. & Schauer, S. (1979). Effect of pili on susceptibility of *Escherichia coli* to phagocytosis. *Infection and Immunity*, 24, 218–23.

Silverblatt, F. J. & Ofek, I. (1978). Effects of pili on susceptibility of *Proteus mirabilis* to phagocytosis and on adherence to bladder cells. In *Infections of the Urinary Tract*, ed. E. H. Kass & W. Brumfitt, pp. 49–59. Chicago: University of Chicago Press.

Simon, G. L. & Gorbach, S. L. (1984). Intestinal flora in health and disease. *Gastroenterology*, **86**, 174–93.

Sjostedt, S. (1946). Pathogenicity of certain serological types of *E.coli*; their mouse toxicity, hemolytic power, capacity for skin necrosis and resistance to phagocytosis and bactericidal faculties of human blood. *Acta Pathologica Microbiologica Scandinavica*, **63**, 1–130.

Stone, H. H. & Martin, J. D. (1972). Synergistic necrotising cellulitis. *Annals of Surgery*, **175**, 702–11.

Taylor, P. W. (1983). Bactericidal and bacteriolytic activity of serum against Gram-negative bacteria. *Microbiological Reviews*, **47**, 46–83.

Thomas, L. (1972). Germs. *New England Journal of Medicine*, **287**, 553–5.

Tobin, G. R. (1984). Closure of contaminated wounds. *Surgical Clinics of North America*, **64**, 639–52.

Van den Bosch, J. F., de Graaff, J. & MacLaren, D. M. (1979). Virulence of *Escherichia coli* in experimental hematogenous pyelonephritis in mice. *Infection and Immunity*, **25**, 68–74.

Van den Bosch, J. F., Postma, P., de Graaf, J. & MacLaren, D. M. (1981). Haemolysis by urinary *Escherichia coli* and virulence in mice. *Journal of Medical Microbiology*, **14**, 321–31.

Vel, W. A. C., Namavar, F., Verweij-van Vught, A. M. J. J., Pubben, A. N. B. & MacLaren, D. M. (1985). Killing of *Escherichia coli* by human polymorphonuclear leucocytes in the presence of *Bacteroides fragilis*. *Journal of Clinical Pathology*, **38**, 86–91.

Vel, W. A. C., Namavar, F., Verweij-van Vught, A. M. J. J., Pubben, A. B. N. & MacLaren, D. M. (1987). Inhibition of the killing of *Escherichia coli* by human polymorphonuclear leucocytes in the presence of Bacteroides or Zymosan. In *Recent Advances in Anaerobic Bacteriology*, eds. S. P. Boriello & J. M. Hardie, pp. 289–91. Dordrecht: Martinus Nijhoff Publishers.

Vermeulen, C., Cross, A., Byrne, W. R. & Zollinger W. (1988). Quantitative relationship between capsular content and killing of K1-encapsulated *Escherichia coli*. *Infection and Immunity*, **56**, 2723–30.

Verweij, W. R. (1993). Mixed intra-abdominal infections and abscess formation in the rat: a study of cellular host reponse and bacterial ineractions. Thesis, Vrije Universiteit, Amsterdam.

Verweij, W. R., Namavar, F., Schouten, W. T. & MacLaren, D. M. (1991). Early events after intra-abdominal infection with *Bacteroides fragilis* and *Escherichia coli*. *Journal of Medical Microbiology*, **35**, 18–22.

Waalwijk, C. & de Graaff, J. (1983). Inactivation of hemolysin production in *Escherichia coli* by transposon insertion results in loss of virulence. *Antonie Van Leeuwenhoek*, **49**, 23–30.

Weinstein, W. M., Onderdonk, A. B., Bartlett, J. G. & Gorbach, S. L. (1974). Experimental intra-abdominal abscesses in rats: development of an experimental model. *Infection and Immunity*, **10**, 1250–5.

Williams, G. T., Houang, E. T., Shaw, E. J. & Tabaqchali, S. (1976). Bacteraemia in a London teaching hospital 1966–1975. *Lancet*, **ii**, 1291–3.

Williams Smith, H. & Huggins, M. B. (1980). The association of the O18, K1 and H7 antigens and the ColV plasmid of a strain of *Escherichia coli* with its virulence and immunogenicity. *Journal of General Microbiology*, **121**, 387–400.

Willis, A. T. (1979). Infections with obligate anaerobes. In *Recent Advances in Infection*, eds. D. Reeves & A. Geddes, pp. 205–21. Edinburgh: Churchill Livingstone.

18

Urinary tract infection

J. R. JOHNSON

Urinary tract infection (UTI) is the most common extra-intestinal infection due to *Escherichia coli*, and *E. coli* organism is the commonest cause of UTI. At some time during their lives, at least 12 per cent of men and 10 to 20 per cent of women experience an acute symptomatic UTI (Johnson & Stamm, 1989; Lipsky, 1989), and an even greater number develop asymptomatic (covert) bacteriuria. Each year in the United States of America more than 100,000 patients are admitted to hospital because of renal infection (Johnson & Stamm, 1989). During the past two decades there has been a great increase in knowledge about the virulence factors of uropathogenic *E. coli* (Harber *et al.*, 1985; Ørskov & Ørskov, 1985; Svanborg Eden & de Man, 1987; Eisenstein & Jones, 1988; Johnson, 1991a; Donnenberg & Welch, 1996). This chapter will summarise current knowledge about the role of *E. coli* virulence factors in the pathogenesis of UTI.

Adherence

Microbial attachment is a necessary first step in the colonisation of host mucosal surfaces, and often precedes invasive infections (Svanborg Eden, 1986; Reid & Sobel, 1987). The strains of *E. coli* that cause UTI typically adhere to human periurethral and uroepithelial cells (Svanborg Eden *et al.*, 1976, 1977, 1987a; Kallenius & Winberg, 1978; Kallenius *et al.*, 1980b) and agglutinate human erythrocytes in the presence of mannose, so-called mannose-resistant haemagglutination (MRHA) (Duguid *et al.*, 1979; Evans *et al.*, 1981; Green & Thomas, 1981). The close association between MRHA and adherence to uroepithelial cells (Kallenius & Mollby, 1979; Kallenius *et al.*, 1980b; Hughes *et al.*, 1983) was explained by the discovery that these two characteristics of urinary *E. coli*

Table 18.1. *The relationship between adherence to uroepithelial cells and mannose-resistant haemagglutination by* Escherichia coli *(after Brauner et al., 1990; Johnson, 1991a)*

	Per cent	
	Adherence to uroepithelial cells	Mannose-resistant haemagglutination
Pyelonephritis	70–100	50–83
Cystitis	50–60	17–52
Asymptomatic bacteriuria	22–36	11–19
Faecal *Escherichia coli*	10–36	2–29

are usually due to adhesive fimbriae (Svanborg Eden & Hanson, 1978b; Kallenius & Mollby, 1979; Korhonen *et al.*, 1980).

In animal models of UTI, strains that give MRHA are more virulent than strains that do not (Montgomerie, 1978; Van den Bosch *et al.*, 1980, 1982; Ketyi, 1981; Hughes *et al.*, 1983). Evidence that adherence is relevant *in vivo* in human UTI is provided by the presence of adhering bacteria on uroepithelial cells in the urine of infected patients (Ofek *et al.*, 1981; Ljungh & Wadstrom, 1983; Pere *et al.*, 1987). Adherence to uroepithelial cells is closely associated with the clinical category of UTI (Table 18.1). This suggests that these properties are related to ability to cause UTI, especially the more severe forms, and detailed characterisation of specific adhesins (Hacker, 1992) has shown that they contribute directly to urovirulence.

Mannose-resistant adhesins

The various mannose-resistant (MR) adhesins of uropathogenic *E. coli* are commonly divided into two groups, those that recognise P blood group antigens and related Gal(α1-4)Gal-containing structures, such as P-fimbriae and related adhesins, and other adhesins that have been termed 'X-adhesins' or 'X-fimbriae' (Johnson, 1991a) (Table 18.2). Now that the receptor specificity of many MR-adhesins, such as Dr, S, M, G (Table 18.2), has been identified, the designation 'X' has become potentially misleading. Precise nomenclature requires the use of receptor-specific designations, and a general term such as 'non-P MR-adhesins' seems appropriate when referring collectively to MR-adhesins other than those of the P-family.

P-fimbriae and related adhesins

Receptors

At first it seemed that the adherence of uropathogenic strains to human epithelial cells was due to their recognition, by way of adhesive fimbriae, of Gal(α1-4)Gal group (Gal–Gal) receptor epitopes present on host cells (Kallenius *et al.*, 1980a, 1981b; Korhonen *et al.*, 1980a; Leffler & Svanborg Eden, 1980, 1981; Korhonen *et al.*, 1982; Svenson *et al.*, 1983; Bock *et al.*, 1985). These strains and their purified fimbriae agglutinate erythrocytes and adhere to epithelial cells with surface antigens, such as the human P_1, P_2, and P^k phenotypes, which contain Gal–Gal, but they do not interact with cells that lack Gal–Gal-containing surface antigens, such as those from p̄ individuals (those who do not have any blood group antigens of the P class) (Table 18.3). Furthermore, this agglutination and/ or adherence is blocked by soluble Gal–Gal-containing substances. Finally, these strains bind immobilised glycolipids that contain, but not those that lack, the critical Gal–Gal moiety (Table 18.4). On the basis of this evidence, it was proposed that Gal–Gal is the minimal receptor for these adhesins, which were termed P-fimbriae to signify their interaction with P blood group antigens (Johnson, 1991a).

Wild-type strains of *E. coli* that recognise Gal–Gal differ in their precise binding specificity. Some adhere better to globoside than to globotriaosylceramide (Table 18.4), while the reverse is true of others (de Man *et al.*, 1987). Yet others bind preferentially to extended Gal–Gal-containing structures, such as Forssman antigen, human blood group A-antigen, or Stage-specific embryonic antigen 4 (SSEA-4, Table 18.4) (Lund *et al.*, 1988; Senior *et al.*, 1988; Karr *et al.*, 1989; Linstedt, 1989; Orino & Naiki, 1990). To accommodate this variety of receptor specificity and its corresponding genetic and structural diversity, it has been suggested that Gal–Gal-binding adhesins are termed 'G adhesins' and that three subclasses be distinguished (Strömberg *et al.*, 1990; Marklund *et al.*, 1992). In this scheme, Class I G-adhesins prefer Gal–Gal in the terminal position of a short oligosaccharide chain, as in the P^k-antigen (Table 418.). Class II G-adhesins, which are said to be characteristic of most human uropathogenic strains, prefer Gal–Gal in an internal position in a short oligosaccharide chain, as in globoside (Table 18.4). Finally, Class III G-adhesins prefer extended receptors, including the so-called 'F'-adhesins ('Forssman') (Orino & Naiki, 1990) and 'ONAP'-adhesins

Table 18.2. *Adhesins of uropathogenic* Escherichia coli

Adhesin type	Synonym(s)	Fimbriae present	Receptor	Role in UTI[a]
I. Mannose-resistant[b]				
A. P-related	Gal–Gal; G-adhesins; GS			
(classical) P	Gal–Gal; Pap; Class I+II G-adhesins	+	Gal(α1-4)Gal (P blood group antigens; Tables 18.3 & 18.4)	+++ (esp. pyelonephritis?)
F	Prs; Pap-2; ONAP; Class III G-adhesins	+	Extended structures containing Gal(α1-4)Gal (e.g. Forssman antigen, globo-A, SSEA-4, etc.; see Table 18.4)	++ (esp. cystitis)
B. non-P ('X') Dr-related				
Dr	O75-X	–	Dr blood group antigen (DAF)[c]; type IV collagen	++ (esp. cystitis)
AFA I, AFA III		–	Dr blood group antigen (DAF)[c]	++
S		+	Sialyl glycosides	+
M		–	M blood group antigen	?

	G	+	GlcNAc	?
	NFA-1 to NFA-6	−	N blood group antigen (NFA-3); M blood group antigen (NFA-4); others unknown	?
II.	Mannose-sensitive[d]			
	Type 1-fimbriae	+	Mannosides, +/− hydrophobic component	?
III.	Other[e]			
	F1C	+	N-acetyl-lactosamine, sialic acid	?

[a] UTI, urinary tract infection; scale is + to +++, in order of increasing importance in human UTI, based on human and animal model studies. ? – undefined.

[b] Mannose-resistant agglutination of human erythrocytes.

[c] Chloramphenicol and tyrosine analogues inhibit adherence mediated by the Dr hemagglutinin ('O75-X'), but not by AFA-I or AFA-III. DAF, decay accelerating factor.

[d] Mannose-sensitive agglutination of guinea-pig erythrocytes.

[e] Non-hemagglutinating; may be regarded non-P ('X') mannose-resistant adhesins.

Table 18.3. *P blood group antigens and phenotypes*[a]

P blood group phenotype	Antigens on erythrocytes[b]	Frequency in population
P_1	$P_1, P(P^k)$	75%
P_2	$P(P^k)$	25%
P_1^k	P_1, P^k	Very rare
P^k	None	Very rare

[a] See Fried & Wong , 1970; Fletcher *et al.*, 1979.
[b] Small amounts of P^k antigen are present on P_1 erythrocytes; P_2 erythrocytes contain smaller amounts.

('O-negative, A-positive', for agglutination of AP_1 but not OP_1 human erythrocytes) (Senior *et al.*, 1988).

Differential agglutination of Gal–Gal-coated latex beads, and rabbit, human and sheep erythrocytes has been proposed as a means to distinguish between these three classes of Gal–Gal adhesins (Marklund *et al.*, 1992) but the results have been conflicting (Karr *et al.*, 1990; Lindstedt *et al.*, 1989, 1991; Orino & Naiki, 1990; Strömberg *et al.*, 1990; Johanson *et al.*, 1992; Marklund *et al.*, 1992). Factors such as gene dose, bacterial concentration, assay temperature and the assay system, such as artificial versus natural membranes (Strömberg *et al.*, 1991), affect the observed phenotypes. It is desirable that the different binding specificities of pathogenic Gal–Gal-recognising strains should be clarified.

Gal–Gal-containing glycolipids are prominent in the kidney (Makita & Yamakawa, 1964; Martensson, 1966), the distribution of receptors for P-fimbriae in the urinary tract depends on the Gal–Gal-adhesin variant (Korhonen *et al.*, 1986b; Nowicki *et al*, 1986; Virkola *et al.*, 1988; Karr *et al.*, 1989) (Table 18.5). In general, blood group non-secretors have a greater receptor density for P-fimbriae on their uroepithelial cells than secretors (Lomberg *et al.*, 1986) and ABO blood group may also affect receptor density, particularly for class III Gal–Gal-adhesins (Lindstedt *et al.*, 1991). Colonisation of the human intestinal tract by P-fimbriated *E. coli* may be due to their attachment to a loosely adherent surface-associated substance on human colonic cells (Wold *et al.*, 1988). This may account for the greater frequency of P-fimbriae expression by resident colonic strains (19 per cent) than by transient colonisers (three per cent) (Wold *et al.*, 1992).

Table 18.4. *Gal(α1-4)Gal-containing glycolipids*[a]

Symbol[b]	P blood group antigen	Structure[b,c]
P₁	P₁	Galα1-4Galβ1-4GlcNAcβ1-3Galβ1-4Glcβ1-1cer
CTH	Pk	Galα1-4Galβ1-4Glcβ1-1cer
Globoside	P	GalNAcβ1-3Galα1-4Galβ1-4Glcβ1-1cer
Gal-globoside		Galβ1-3GalNAcβ1-3Galα1-4Galβ1-4Glcβ1-1cer
Forssman		GalNAcα1-3GalNAcβ1-3Galα1-4Galβ1-4Glcβ1-1cer
Para-Forssman		GalNAcβ1-3GalNAcβ1-3Galα1-4Galβ1-4Glcβ1-1cer
Globo-H		(Fucα1-2)Galβ1-3GalNAcβ1-3Galα1-4Galβ1-4Glcβ1-1cer
Globo-A		GalNAcα1-3(Fucα1-2)Galβ1-3GalNAcβ1-3Galα1-4Galβ1-4Glcβ1-1cer
SGG (SSEA-4)		NeuAcα2-3Galβ1-3GalNAcβ1-3Galα1-4Galβ1-4Glcβ1-1cer
DSGG		NeuAcα2-3(NeuAcα2-6)Galβ1-3GalNAcβ1-3Galα1-4Galβ1-4Glcβ1-1cer

[a] The Gal(α1-4)Gal moiety is underlined in each structure.

[b] CTH, ceramide trihexoside (globotriaosylceramide); globoside, globotetrasylceramide; Gal-globoside, galactosyl globoside; SGG, sialosyl Gal-globoside; SSEA-4, stage-specific embryonic antigen-4 (= Luke antigen); DSGG, disialosyl Gal-globoside.

[c] Glc, glucose; cer, ceramide; Gal, galactose; GalNAc, N-acetylgalactosamine; Fuc, fucose; NeuAc, neuraminic acid; GlcNAc, N-acetylglycosamine.

Table 18.5. *Distribution of receptors for* Escherichia coli *adhesins in the human urinary tract*

| | Receptors for[b] | | | | | | |
| | P-fimbriae (Gal–Gal adhesins) | | | Non-P mannose-resistant adhesins | | | |
Tissue site	Class I	Class II	Class III	Dr-adhesin	S-fimbriae	F1C-fimbriae	Type-1 fimbriae
Kidney							
Bowman's capsule	−	+++	+++	+++[c]	+++	−	−
Glomerulus	+++	+++	+++	−	+++	−	−
Proximal tubule	(+)	++	(+)	+++[c]	++	−	+++
Distal tubule	(+)	++	(+)	+++[c]	++	++	(+)
Collecting duct	−	+	+++	+++[c]	++	++	(+)
Vessel walls	?	+++[d]	?	−	+++[d]	+++[d]	+++
Renal pelvis epithelium	+++	?	+++	+	?	?	?
Bladder							
Epithelium	++	+	++	+	++	−	−
Vessel walls	?	+++[d]	?	−	+++[d]	+++[d]	++
Muscular layer	+++	+	+++	+	+	+	+++
Connective tissue	?	−	?	+++	++	−	−
Urine							
Epithelial cells[e]	+[e,f]	+[e]	+[e,f]	+[e]	+[e]	−	−

[a] From Korhonen et al., 1980; Ørskov et al., 1980; Korhonen et al., 1986a,b,c; Virkola, 1987, 1988; Nowicki et al., 1988; Karr et al., 1989; Linstedt et al., 1991; Johanson et al., 1992.
[b] Intensity of binding is indicated to − to +++; (+), weak and/or variable binding; ?, data unavailable.   [e] Only positive and negative are indicated.
[c] Endothelial cells.   [d] Basement membranes.
[f] Variable results reported. For class III adhesins, receptor density may depend on ABO phenotype and secretor status.

Association with other urovirulence factors

Determinants for P-fimbriae (*pap*) are characteristically present in strains that also produce haemolysin (Johnson *et al.*, 1988b; Arthur *et al.*, 1989b). In some strains, the *pap* gene cluster is genetically linked with determinants for other virulence factors, including haemolysin, P-fimbriae of other serological types, and other adhesins (Berger *et al.*, 1982; Low *et al.*, 1984; High *et al.*, 1988; Hull *et al.*, 1988; Arthur *et al.*, 1989a, 1990; Hacker *et al.*, 1990; Ott *et al.*, 1991). Such linked groups of virulence factor genes have been termed 'pathogenicity associated islands' (PAIs) (Swenson *et al.*, 1996), and they have been shown to undergo spontaneous deletion *in vitro* and *in vivo* (Hacker *et al.*, 1990).

Structural and antigenic considerations

Assembly of P-fimbriae is a complex, co-ordinated process (see Chapter 8). Though the overall genetic organisation of P-fimbriae from different strains is identical (van Die *et al.*, 1986), they are heterogeneous with respect to their subunit size and antigenic characteristics (Ørskov & Ørskov, 1983b; Hanley *et al.*, 1985; Pere *et al.*, 1986, 1988; Salit *et al.*, 1988b). The major fimbrial subunit, PapA, is antigenically dominant and responsible for the serological heterogeneity but, in spite of their serological differences, PapA from different P-fimbrial sero-variants have a high degree of amino-acid homology at the amino- and carboxyl-termini. However, the amino-acid sequence of the central parts of the molecule are highly variable. This may be accounted for by their exposed and hydrophilic nature, which is subject to maximum selective pressure by the host immune system while not essential for fimbrial function (O'Hanley *et al.*, 1983; Hanley *et al.*, 1985; Klemm, 1985; van Die *et al.*, 1987).

The serological heterogeneity of P-fimbriae poses a challenge for vaccine development. Sera, collected from patients after an episode of pyelonephritis, react with P-fimbriae from the patients' strain but they may not cross-react with other P-fimbriated strains, and they may not even block adherence with the homologous strain (de Ree & Van den Bosch, 1987; Salit *et al.*, 1988a). A peptide from the conserved amino-terminal region of PapA elicits cross-reactive antibodies against several P-fimbrial sero-variants and may represent a broadly cross-reactive immunogenic epitope for an anti-P-fimbrial vaccine (Schmidt *et al.*, 1988). An alternative approach may be to use as immunogens a 'cocktail' of P-fimbrial sero-variants to stimulate production of cross-reacting antibodies (Pecha *et al.*, 1989). An anti-adhesive monoclonal antibody that reacts with the PapG adhesin molecules of several serologically distinct P-fimbriae has been produced (Hoschützky *et al.*, 1989a). The inhibition of adherence by this monoclonal antibody may be due to binding to the conserved Gal–Gal recognition site of the adhesin molecules (Hoschützky *et al.*, 1989a). Thus, in spite their serological heterogeneity, several alternative strategies may allow stimulation of broadly active immunity against P-fimbriae.

Animal models

P-fimbriated *E. coli* elicit greater pyuria in mice after bladder inoculation than strains without P-fimbriae, and this inflammatory response is blocked by simultaneous administration of Gal–Gal. Aggregates of purified P-fimbriae and endotoxin behave like P-fimbriated bacteria, which suggests that P-fimbriae promote local inflammation by attaching a source of endotoxin to the urinary mucosa and possibly by stimulating local production of interleukin-6 (IL-6) (Linder *et al.*, 1988, 1990).

In mice, P-fimbriae are a major determinant of bacterial colonisation of the upper urinary tract but alone they are insufficient for renal invasion, which requires the presence of other factors, such as haemolysin (Hagberg *et al.*, 1983; O'Hanley *et al.*, 1985a, 1991; Domingue *et al.*, 1988). Administration of P-fimbrial receptor analogues with the bacterial inoculum protects mice from upper urinary tract colonisation with P-fimbriated organisms (Svanborg Eden *et al.*, 1982; Johnson & Berggren, 1994). Immunisation against P-fimbriae protects against renal infection by homologous P-fimbriated organisms (O'Hanley *et al.*, 1985a; Garg *et al.*, 1987; Schmidt *et al.*, 1988) and possibly also by heterologous strains (Pecha *et al.*, 1989).

In monkeys, P-fimbriated bacteria induce ureteritis and pyelonephritis (Kallenius *et al.*, 1983; Roberts *et al.*, 1984b, 1993), and simultaneous administration of Gal–Gal or inactivation of the *papG* adhesin gene protects against such infection (Svenson *et al.*, 1984; Roberts *et al.*, 1993). Pyelonephritis due to P-fimbriated strains can be prevented by vaccination with homologous P-fimbriae or with anti-Gal–Gal antibodies, which stimulate production of anti-idiotype antibodies and block adherence (Roberts *et al.*, 1984a; Kaack *et al.*, 1988, 1993).

Epidemiology

It has been firmly established that P-fimbriae are expressed *in vivo* during human UTI (Svenson *et al.*, 1982; Pere *et al.*, 1987; Kiselius *et al.*, 1989;

Table 18.6. *Association of virulence factor expression with clinical source of isolate[a]*

Virulence factor	Proportion (per cent) of strains that express virulence factors[b,c]				
	PN[b]	CY[b]	ABU[b]	UTI[b]	Faecal
P-fimbriae	1692/2491 (68)	691/2734 (25)	247/1169 (21)	2992/6904 (43)	166/1014 (16)
Type-1 fimbriae	304/508 (60)	489/693 (71)	316/541 (58)	1593/2491 (64)	365/608 (60)
Haemolysin	469/948 (49)	178/460 (39)	101/1473 (21)	1208/3486 (35)	359/3109 (12)
Aerobactin	501/690 (73)	239/484 (49)	72/188 (38)	1040/1774 (59)	179/423 (42)
K1 capsule	239/757 (32)	58/420 (14)	93/429 (22)	636/2927 (22)	818/3445 (24)
Serum resistance[d]	606/940 (64)	193/304 (63)	185/731 (25)	1181/2325 (51)	524/1013 (52)
Common O-groups[e]	329/464 (71)	216/339 (64)	139/365 (38)	783/1303 (60)	551/1432 (38)

[a] Based from Archambaud et al., 1988b; Conventi et al., 1989; Tomisawa et al., 1989; Blanco et al., 1990; Goullet & Picard, 1990; Opal et al., 1990; Österberg et al., 1990; Plos et al., 1990; Dalet et al., 1991; Johnson 1991a; Karkkainen et al., 1991; Majd et al., 1991; Rydberg & Helin, 1991; Benton et al., 1992; Jacobson et al., 1992; Schönian et al., 1992; Siitonen, 1992; Tambic et al., 1992; Tullus et al., 1992; Ikaheimo et al., 1993; Otto et al., 1993.

[b] PN, pyelonephritis or febrile UTI; CY, cystitis; ABU, asymptomatic bacteriuria; UTI, PN+CY+ABU plus any other UTI strains of unspecified clinical category.

[c] Differences in study design, populations, methods and definitions in different studies make it necessary to interpret total with caution.

[d] Serum resistance is variably defined; the table reflects designations used by various authors.

[e] From studies that recorded proportions of strains from eight common serogroups, including combinations of O1, O2, O4, O6, O7, O8, O16, O18, O25, O50, and O75.

Lichodziejewska *et al.*, 1989). The proportion of isolates that express P-fimbriae depends on the clinical setting and is greatest in pyelonephritis and UTI associated with fever. It is lower in cystitis and asymptomatic bacteriuria, and least among faecal *E. coli* strains (Table 18.6). The prevalence of P-fimbriation in UTI associated with septicaemia (urosepsis) can be as high as 71 per cent (Brauner *et al.*, 1985; Johnson *et al.*, 1987; Arthur *et al.*, 1990), which is similar to that in pyelonephritis (68 per cent; Table 18.6). Expression of P-fimbriae is much lower in septicaemia that results from other sources (28 per cent) (Brauner *et al.*, 1985). This suggests that P-fimbriae contribute to the ability of strains to cause UTI, especially its more severe forms.

The clinical significance of variant Gal–Gal-adhesins has been the subject of much speculation. The limited information available has been variously interpreted to suggest that Class III Gal–Gal adhesins are potentially uropathogenic (i) for dogs but not for humans (Strömberg *et al.*, 1990, 1991; Marklund *et al.*, 1992), (ii) for humans, but only those of the A$_1$ secretor phenotype, particularly for cystitis (Lindstedt *et al.*, 1991), (iii) for all Luke-positive individuals, that is most humans (Tippet *et al.*, 1986), and (iv) for pyelonephritis and cystitis (Karr *et al.*, 1990). The tests used in most clinical studies to establish the phenotype of P-fimbriae (Table 18.6), detect Class I and Class II Gal–Gal-adhesins, but might miss those of Class III. The data presented in Table 18.6 do not, therefore, reliably reflect the prevalence of Class III adhesins on human uropathogenic *E. coli*. The *prsG* adhesin gene, which encodes a Class III adhesin molecule, was found in only four per cent of pyelonephritis isolates, which suggests that they are not common in this condition (Otto *et al.*, 1993). These observations indicate that the ecological and pathogenic significance of variant Gal–Gal-adhesins are still incompletely understood.

The low prevalence of P-fimbriated strains in the faeces of healthy controls (16 per cent) contrasts with that in patients with pyelonephritis (Table 18.6). In some cases the P-fimbriated faecal strain is the same as the urinary isolate (Kallenius *et al.*, 1981a), which supports the hypothesis that UTI is an ascending infection (Stamm *et al.*, 1989). Nosocomially transmitted P-fimbriated *E. coli* have caused outbreaks of pyelonephritis in infants, with secondary transmission to household contacts (Tullus *et al.*, 1984, 1988).

In childhood UTI, strains of *E. coli* that are P-fimbriated cause more local and systemic inflammation than do non-P-fimbriated strains, even in the same clinical category (de Man *et al.*, 1988; Marild *et al.*, 1988). This is not so in women with pyelonephritis (Otto *et al.*, 1993). In asymptomatic bacteriuria during pregnancy, P-fimbriated but not non-P-fimbriated strains are associated with renal inflammation, as shown by a reduced renal concentrating capacity (Stenqkvist *et al.*, 1989). P-fimbriae stimulate production of IL-6 and IL-8 by human renal carcinoma cells *in vitro* (de Man *et al.*, 1990; Agace *et al.*, 1993) but, in experimental UTI in human volunteers, IL-6 production was the same with P-fimbriated and non-P-fimbriated strains (Hedges *et al.*, 1991). Thus, although P-fimbriae may help to localise infection to the kidney and stimulate an inflammatory response that gives rise to pain, fever, leucocytosis and renal dysfunction, the precise role of P-fimbriae in determining the site and clinical manifestations of UTI is still incompletely understood.

The compromised host

Anatomical and functional abnormalities of the urinary tract in children and adults are commonly associated with a decreased requirement for P-fimbriae in acute pyelonephritis (Table 18.7). A similar relationship has been observed in urosepsis due to *E. coli* (Brauner *et al.*, 1985; Johnson *et al.*, 1987; Karkkainen *et al.*, 1991; Maslow *et al.*, 1993; Otto *et al.*, 1993), in asymptomatic renal infection (Nicolle *et al.*, 1988), and in prostatitis and epididymitis (Dalet *et al.*, 1991). Furthermore, P-fimbriae are present in only ten per cent of *E. coli* that cause febrile UTI in hospital patients, most of whom had urinary catheters (Ikaheimo *et al.*, 1993). This suggests that urinary tract abnormalities or instrumentation, and serious illness may interfere with anatomical and functional defence mechanisms.

Recurrent UTI and renal scarring

The relationships between P blood group phenotype and secretor status, the uroepithelial cell receptor density for P-fimbriated organisms, and the development of recurrent UTI, renal scarring and renal dysfunction are complex and poorly understood. The vaginal, buccal, periurethral and uroepithelial cells of women predisposed to recurrent UTI have an increased binding capacity for uropathogenic bacteria (Fowler & Stamey, 1977; Kallenius & Winberg, 1978; Parsons *et al.*, 1979; Svanborg Eden & Jodal, 1979; Kallenius *et al.*, 1980b; Schaeffer *et al.*, 1981, 1982; Bruce *et al.*, 1983). Such individuals are also more likely than controls to be non-secretors of blood group substances (Kinane *et al.*, 1982; Sheinfeld *et al.*, 1989), possibly because the uroepithelial cells of non-secretors have an increased binding capacity for P-fimbriated organisms (Lomberg *et al.*,

Table 18.7. *Association between host compromise[a] and P-fimbriae in pyelonephritis*

Patient population	Proportion (per cent) of strains expressing P-fimbriae		Reference
	Non-compromised host	Compromised host	
Girls and boys	27/ 37 (73)	9/ 12 (75)	Arthur *et al.*, 1989b
Adults	112/126 (89)	22/110 (22)	Dalet *et al.*, 1991
Boys	52/ 63 (83)	19/ 33 (58)	De Lorenzo & Martinez, 1988
Adults	25/ 25 (100)	13/ 15 (87)	Dominigue *et al.*, 1985
Adults	17/ 21 (81)	5/ 17 (29)	Dowling *et al.*, 1987
Girls	25/ 31 (81)	15/ 17 (88)	Elo *et al.*, 1985
Girls	37/ 57 (65)	21/ 74 (28)	Lomberg *et al.*, 1983
Girls	75/105 (71)	28/ 78 (36)	Lomberg *et al.*, 1984
Girls	57/ 77 (74)	15/ 45 (33)	Lomberg *et al.*, 1989a
Women	53/ 67 (79)	14/ 25 (56)	Otto *et al.*, 1993
Girls and boys	8/ 8 (100)	2/ 4 (50)	Rydberg & Helin, 1991
Women	39/ 49 (80)	39/ 71 (55)	Sandberg *et al.*, 1988
Girls	12/ 14 (86)	2/ 3 (67)	Vaisanen *et al.*, 1981
Total[b]	374/487 (78)[b]	168/369 (46)[b]	

[a] Compromising conditions, as defined by various investigators, include anatomical urinary tract abnormalities, urinary tract instrumentation, medical illnesses, and pregnancy.
[b] Totals of results must be interpreted with caution because of differences in study design, populations, methods, and definitions in the various studies.

1986). The increased P-receptor density of uroepithelial cells from non-secretors may be due to their not being 'shielded' by the overhanging A, B, O, or Le[b] oligosaccharides that are present in secretors (Schoolnik, 1989). Moreover, uroepithelial cells from non-secretors express types of glycolipid (SGG, DSGG; see Table 18.4) that are absent from secretors and can serve as receptors for P-fimbriated *E. coli* (Stapleton *et al.*, 1992).

Though the P_1 phenotype is not associated with an increased uroepithelial cell receptor density for P-fimbriated organisms (Jacobson *et al.*, 1985; Lomberg *et al.*, 1986; Lomberg & Svanborg Eden, 1989b), it is associated with recurrent UTI and pyelonephritis in girls (Lomberg *et al.*, 1981, 1983, 1984; Leffler *et al.*, 1982) and possibly, but less clearly, in women (Mulholland *et al.*, 1984; Jacobson *et al.*, 1985; Lomberg & Svanborg Eden, 1989b; Sheinfeld *et al.*, 1989). The uroepithelial cells of adults with renal scarring, presumably due to infection, have an increased binding capacity for P-fimbriated bacteria, independent of their P blood group (Jacobson *et al.*, 1986a,b). Whether this contributes to the renal scarring by promoting renal infection is unclear, because in children renal scarring seems to result more commonly from infection with non-P-fimbriated than with P-fimbriated strains (de Man *et al.*, 1989; Lomberg *et al.*, 1989a).

Clinical application of tests for P-fimbriae

It has been suggested that testing for P-fimbriae may be useful for clinical purposes. For example, screening for faecal carriage of P-fimbriated *E. coli* in family contacts of patients with pyelonephritis, and treatment of asymptomatic carriers have been advocated as a means of preventing subsequent development of symptomatic UTI (Roberts, 1986). In children with cystitis treated for three days, treatment failure rate is high if the infecting organisms are P-fimbriated, but treatment is very successful if they are not. This led to the suggestion that the duration of treatment for cystitis in children could be determined by the presence of P-fimbriae on the causative organism (Tambic *et al.*, 1992). In boys, UTI due to a non-P-fimbriated *E. coli* predicts renal scarring (41 per cent against five per cent) and the presence of other urinary tract abnormalities (11 per cent against one per cent) (de Man *et al.*, 1989). Similarly, pyelonephritis or urosepsis due to non-P-fimbriated strains in adults suggests an underlying urological or medical condition. Testing for P-fimbriae has also has been proposed to identify pregnant woman with symptomatic bacteriuria who are at high risk of developing pyelonephritis (Stenqvist *et al.*, 1989).

Non-P MR-adhesins

As we have seen, most urinary strains exhibit MR adherence, as judged by Gal–Gal recognition, but some strains adhere without recognising Gal–Gal. These were termed 'X'-adhesins, i.e. of unknown specificity (Johnson, 1991a), but are now better termed non-P MR-adhesins and they are listed in Table 18.2 together with some of their characteristics. The proportion of clinical isolates that express such adhesins varies

Table 18.8. *The distribution of non-P mannose-resistant adhesins in various types of urinary tract infection (UTI). Data collected from the literature[a]*

	Per cent non-P MR adhesins
Pyelonephritis and febrile UTI	4–58
Cystitis	5–48
Asymptomatic bacteriuria	0–14

[a] Kallenius *et al.*, 1981a; Leffler & Svanborg Eden, 1981; Vaisanen *et al.*, 1981; Lomberg *et al.*, 1984; Vaisanen-Rhen *et al.*, 1984b; O'Hanley *et al.*, 1985b; Enerback *et al.*, 1987; Stenqvist *et al.*, 1987; Labigne-Roussel & Falkow, 1988; Nicolle *et al*, 1988; Sandberg *et al.*, 1988; Arthur *et al.*, 1989b; Plos *et al.*, 1990; Dalet *et al.*, 1991; Benton *et al.*, 1992; Ikäheimo *et al.*, 1993.

widely between studies, possibly because of differences in definitions, methods and patient populations (Table 18.8). This variability makes it unclear whether non-P MR-adhesins are more common among urinary than among faecal strains, but several surveys suggest that this is indeed the case (O'Hanley *et al.*, 1985b; Labigne-Roussel & Falkow, 1988; Arthur *et al.*, 1989b).

Dr and non-fimbrial adhesins

Most urinary isolates that express non-P MR-adhesins hybridise with DNA probes specific for non-fimbrial adhesins that recognise various portions of the Dr human blood group antigen (decay-accelerating factor, DAF) (Labigne-Roussel & Falkow, 1988; Nowicki *et al.*, 1988, 1990). The Dr family of adhesins includes the Dr haemagglutinin ('O75X adhesin') (Vaisanen-Rhen, 1984a; Nowicki *et al.*, 1988) and the non-fimbrial adhesins AFA-I and AFA-III (Labigne-Roussel & Falkow, 1988), which are genetically closely related (Nowicki *et al.*, 1990; Swanson *et al.*, 1991). These adhesins are physically distinct from traditional fimbrial *E. coli* adhesins, and appear on the cell surface as a fine mesh or coil (Vaisanen-Rhen, 1984a; Arthur *et al.*, 1989b).

Dr haemagglutinin binds to numerous sites in the urinary tract, including the renal interstitium and tubular basement membranes (Table 18.5). The latter may be due to recognition of the 7S domain of type-IV collagen (Westerlund *et al.*, 1989) but other evidence suggests that in human tissues the Dr antigen is the receptor for Dr-haemagglutinin (Kaul *et al.*, 1993).

Adhesins of the Dr family are more often associated with cystitis than are P-fimbriae. Dr-related sequences are present in 12 to 50 per cent of cystitis isolates, but in only two to 26 per cent of pyelonephritis isolates, six per cent of asymptomatic bacteriuria isolates, and 15 to 18 per cent of faecal isolates (Archambaud *et al.*, 1988a; Arthur *et al.*, 1989b; Nowicki *et al.*, 1989). The relative contribution of the several Dr variants is unknown, because adhesin-specific probes were not used in most of the epidemiological studies (Labigne-Roussel & Falkow, 1988; Arthur *et al.*, 1989b; Nowicki *et al.*, 1989).

S-fimbriae and F1C fimbriae

Closely related adhesins are expressed by some urinary *E. coli* strains (Ott *et al.*, 1986; Riegman *et al.*, 1990). S-fimbriae, so named because they bind specifically to sialosyl-oligosaccharide residues (Parkkinen *et al.*, 1983, 1989; Hanisch *et al.*, 1993), mediate non-P MRHA of human erythrocytes and are subject to phase variation (Nowicki *et al.*, 1985a,b). Multiple copies of the *sfa* operon are found in some uropathogenic strains (Zingler *et al.*, 1993). Binding sites for S-fimbriae are present throughout the urinary tract (Table 18.5). S-fimbriae recognise sialosyl-oligosaccharide chains on laminin in the extracellular matrix (Virkola *et al.*, 1993). They bind to and stimulate IL-6 production by renal epithelial cells (Kreft *et al.*, 1993) and contribute to virulence in animal models of infection, including UTI (Hacker *et al.*, 1986; Marre *et al.*, 1986). Epidemiological evidence suggests that S-fimbriae play a more prominent role in neonatal meningitis than in UTI (Ott *et al.*, 1986; Archambaud *et al.*, 1988b; Schönian *et al.*, 1992; Kunin *et al.*, 1993).

Strains that hybridise with a DNA probe for S-fimbriae but do not express these can sometimes be induced to express S-fimbriae by serial passage on agar (Schönian *et al.*, 1992). On the other hand, some strains cannot express S-fimbriae but are *sfa*-probe-positive because of the presence of determinants for F1C fimbriae, which share extensive homology with *sfa* determinants (Riegman *et al.*, 1990; Zingler *et al.*, 1993). F1C fimbriae do not mediate MRHA or adherence to uroepithelial cells, but they bind to buccal epithelial cells, renal tubular cells, and renal tissues (Table 18.5), and have a receptor specificity similar to that of S-fimbriae (Marre *et al.*, 1990). These fimbriae are expressed by approximately 20 per cent of uropathogenic strains (Pere *et al.*, 1987; Karkkainen *et al.*, 1991). Since these fimbriae are not present on organisms studied directly in the urine of infected patients, their significance in UTI is unclear (Pere *et al.*, 1987).

Other mannose-resistant adhesins

Individual representatives of a variety of other mannose-resistant adhesins have been described (see Table 18.2). These include so-called 'G-fimbriae', that recognise terminal *N*-acetylglucosamine (GlcNAc) moieties, a non-fimbrial adhesin with M blood group specificity, the so-called 'M-adhesin' (Vaisanen-Rhen *et al.*, 1983; Rhen *et al.*, 1986), and the non-fimbrial adhesins NFA-1 to NFA-6 (Goldhar *et al.*, 1987, 1991; Grünberg *et al.*, 1988; Hales *et al.*, 1988; Hoschützky *et al.*, 1989b; Kröncke *et al.*, 1990; Ahrens *et al.*, 1993). NFA-3 adhesin recognises glycophorin A^{NN}, the human blood group N-antigen (Grünberg *et al.*, 1988) and NFA-4 recognises glycophorin A^{MM}, the blood group M-antigen, but it is biochemically distinct from the former non-fimbrial 'M-adhesin' (Hoschützky *et al.*, 1989b). In view of their apparent rarity (Archambaud *et al.*, 1988b; Maslow *et al.*, 1993), these adhesins are of uncertain clinical relevance in the pathogenesis of UTI. They also present taxonomic challenges; for example, two biochemically distinct non-fimbrial adhesins which recognise the M blood group antigen, and both GlcNAc and Gal–Gal compete for the receptor designation 'G'.

Type-1 fimbriae

Receptors

With rare exceptions, mannose-sensitive adherence mediated by *E. coli* is due to type-1 fimbriae (Duguid & Old, 1980; Ofek *et al.*, 1982) (see Chapter 6). Since complex mannose-containing molecules are better inhibitors of binding than D-mannose or α-methylmannoside alone, the receptor for type 1-fimbriae is probably an extended structure (Firon *et al.*, 1984; Neeser *et al.*, 1986). The relevance of the paradoxical mannose-sensitive binding of type-1 fimbriae to a non-glycosylated region of fibronectin *in vivo* is unknown (Sokurenko *et al.*, 1992).

Receptors for type-1 fimbriae are present on human buccal (Ofek *et al.*, 1977), intestinal (Jann *et al.*, 1981; Neeser *et al.*, 1986; Wold *et al.*, 1988) and vaginal (Falkoski *et al.*, 1986) epithelial cells, which suggests a possible role for type-1 fimbriae in colonisation of the mouth, gut and vagina. The contradictory information about the role of type-1 fimbriae in adherence to uroepithelial cells may be due, in part, to the adherence of type-1 fimbriae to Tamm–Horsfall glycoprotein (uromucoid) (Duncan, 1988; Parkkinen *et al.*, 1988; Reinhart *et al.*, 1990). Since Tamm–Horsfall glycoprotein often coats uroepithelial cells, the cell-bound glycoprotein may promote the attachment of type-1 fimbriated organisms. Tamm–Horsfall glycoprotein in solution binds to type-1-fimbriated organisms and prevents their attachment to receptors on host cells and, *in vivo*, this may function as a natural defence mechanism by expelling type-1-fimbriated organisms in the urine (Ørskov *et al.*, 1980). Paradoxically, at low concentrations, even free Tamm–Horsfall glycoprotein promotes type-1-fimbrial adherence to uroepithelial cells (Dulawa *et al.*, 1988; Duncan, 1988; Sobota & Apicella, 1991). Type-1 fimbriae also bind to mannose-rich oligosaccharides present on immunoglobulin molecules, particularly IgA$_2$ (Wold *et al.*, 1990), which may provide a non-specific host defence against bacterial colonisation of the intestine and the urinary tract.

Though not observed by some investigators (Virkola *et al.*, 1988) (Table 18.5), binding of type-1-fimbriated bacteria to human bladder epithelium has been elegantly documented by scanning electron microscopy (Yamamoto *et al.*, 1990). These organisms bind to human ureteral epithelium (Fujita *et al.*, 1989) and to many mammalian renal cell lines (Salit & Gotschlich, 1977; Jann *et al.*, 1981; Korhonen *et al.*, 1981). Receptors for type-1 fimbriae are scantily distributed in the human kidney, as compared with those for P-fimbriae (Virkola, 1987) (Table 18.5).

Interaction with phagocytes

Much attention has recently been paid to interactions between type-1 fimbriae and human polymorphonuclear leucocytes (neutrophils) (Ofek *et al.*, 1992; see Chapter 19). Type-1 fimbriae mediate mannose-sensitive attachment to neutrophils and can stimulate phagocytosis in the absence of opsonins, a process termed 'non-opsonic lectinophagocytosis'. Depending on the hydrophobicity of the organism, attachment may or may not result in phagocytosis (Blumenstock & Jann, 1982; Öhman *et al.*, 1982). Several glycoprotein molecules have been proposed as neutrophil receptors for type-1 fimbriae, including the receptor for the third component of complement (CR3; the C$_3$bi receptor) (Rodriguez-Ortega *et al.*, 1987) and members of the carcinoembryonic antigen (CEA) family such as BGP-85 and NCA-55 (Leusch *et al.*, 1990, 1991; Sauter *et al.*, 1991).

Attachment of a type-1-fimbriated organism to neutrophils stimulates the release of their granular contents and generates a respiratory burst, perhaps by way of interactions with Fc receptors (Salmon *et al.*, 1987; Goetz, 1989). Bacteria that remain extracellular are killed by toxic products released from the stimulated neutrophil (Blumenstock & Jann, 1982; Öhman *et al.*, 1982) but, surprisingly, phagocytosed bacteria may escape killing (Goetz *et al.*, 1987). Whether the complex interactions between type-1 fimbriae and neutrophils promote or hinder the development of UTI remains unknown.

Animal models

Mice have receptors for type-1 fimbriae throughout their urogenital tract (O'Hanley *et al.*, 1985a) and type-1 fimbriae appear to be important in the colonisation of the mouse bladder (Hagberg *et al.*, 1983; Iwahi *et al.*, 1983; Keith *et al.*, 1986; Schaeffer *et al.*, 1987). Since fimbriated organisms adhere to the bladder wall, urine cultures may remain negative in spite of the presence of adherent organisms in the bladder (Hultgren *et al.*, 1985). In the absence of P-fimbriae, type-1 fimbriae contribute significantly to upper urinary tract colonisation (Hagberg *et al.*, 1983). In rats, the degree of chronic renal scarring that develops after intrarenal injection of *E. coli* is greatest with type-1-fimbriated strains (Topley *et al.*, 1989). Thus, type-1 fimbriae may play a role in bladder colonisation and possibly also in chronic inflammatory renal injury.

Administration of mannose or its analogues simultaneously with type-1-fimbriated organisms does not consistently protect mice from urinary tract colonisation by these organisms (Svanborg Eden *et al.*, 1982; Aronson *et al.*, 1987; Johnson & Berggren, 1994a). Antibodies against the adhesin or mannoside protect mice against subsequent bacterial challenge with type-1-fimbriated bacteria (Abraham *et al.*, 1985; Hultgren *et al.*, 1985; O'Hanley *et al.*, 1985a). Anti-fimbrial immunisation that blocks adherence protects rats from UTI (Silverblatt & Cohen, 1979; Silverblatt *et al.*, 1982).

Epidemiology

Direct examination of organisms in urine clearly shows that type-1 fimbriae are expressed during human UTI (Ljungh & Wadstrom, 1983; Pere *et al.*, 1987; Kiselius *et al.*, 1989; Lichodziejewska *et al.*, 1989). Phase variation can be observed *in vivo* in individual patients, and may be of pathogenic significance (Kiselius *et al.*, 1989). Direct comparison has shown that type-1 fimbriae are expressed by a similar proportion of urinary and faecal strains (Table 18.6) and various studies have suggested a specific association between type-1 fimbriae and pyelonephritis (Elo *et al.*, 1985), cystitis (Enerback *et al.*, 1987), pyelonephritis and cystitis (Brooks *et al.*, 1981; Hagberg *et al.*, 1981; Israele *et al.*, 1987), faecal strains (Arthur *et al.*, 1989b) and isolates from girls with UTI as opposed to boys with UTI (Westerlund *et al.*, 1988). These divergent findings may relate in part to the profound effect of cultural conditions on the expression of type-1 fimbriae and the use of different methods by the various investigators. A type-1 non-fimbriated strain was better able to colonise the bladder in human volunteers than was its isogenic type-1-fimbriated derivative (Andersson *et al.*, 1991). There is little evidence that production of type-1 fimbriae is less common in the setting of compromised hosts (Gander *et al.*, 1985; Johnson *et al.*, 1987; Arthur *et al.*, 1989b), and type-1 fimbriae may contribute to the persistence of *E. coli* in patients during long-term bladder catheterisation (Mobley *et al.*, 1987; Benton *et al.*, 1992).

Heamolysin

The cytolytic pore-forming toxin, α-haemolysin, of uropathogenic *E. coli* is a member of the RTX (repeat toxin) family of cytotoxins (Welch, 1991) (see Chapter 11). This haemolysin is toxic to a wide range of host cells, including neutrophils, monocytes, mast cells, basophils, lymphocytes, platelets and renal epithelial cells, in ways that contribute to inflamma-tion, tissue injury and impaired host defences. At low concentrations, α-haemolysin perturbs cellular functions and stimulates the release of mediators of inflammation, while at higher concentrations host cells are lysed (Bhakdi *et al.*, 1990; König *et al.*, 1990; Mobley *et al.*, 1990; Bhakdi & Martin, 1991; Johnson, 1991a; Jonas *et al.*, 1993). The cytolytic capacity of haemolytic strains is augmented by the presence of P-fimbriae (O'Hanley *et al.*, 1991), as is that of P-fimbriated strains by haemolysin production (Mobley *et al.*, 1990).

Haemolytic urinary strains of *E. coli* almost always also express MRHA or P-fimbriae (Green & Thomas, 1981; Hughes *et al.*, 1983; Johnson *et al.*, 1988b; Arthur *et al.*, 1989b). The *hly* gene sequences that determine haemolysin production are sometimes genetically linked with determinants for other virulence factors, including P-fimbriae and other adhesins (Low *et al.*, 1984; Hughes *et al.*, 1987; High *et al.*, 1988; Hacker *et al.*, 1990; Ott *et al.*, 1991) but the various genetic linkages in different strains indicate that they do not all carry the same block of virulence factor genes. Haemolysin production is especially common in strains of certain serogroups, such as O4, O6, O18, and possibly O75, and among

K2, K5, K12 and K13. It is uncommon in O1, O2, O7 and O9 strains (Evans *et al.*, 1981; Hughes *et al.*, 1982; Hacker *et al.*, 1983). The presence and absence of haemolysin production is also characteristic of certain O:K:H-serotypes (Ørskov *et al.*, 1988).

Animal models

Haemolytic strains are more lethal than non-haemolytic strains in a variety of animal infection models (Johnson, 1991a). Haemolysin appears to contribute to lethality by a direct toxic effect (Smith, 1963; Smith & Huggins, 1985) and by helping to provide iron for bacterial metabolism (Linggood & Ingram, 1982; Waalwijk *et al.*, 1983; Smith & Huggins, 1985; see Chapter 12). In models of ascending UTI, haemolysin production is associated with increased bladder colonisation and nephropathogenicity (Iwahi *et al.*, 1982; Ketyi *et al.*, 1983; Marre *et al.*, 1986; Domingue *et al.*, 1988). Cloned *hly* determinants introduced into non-haemolytic P-fimbriated strains converted these from non-invasive organisms that were merely able to colonise the kidney into renal-invasive pathogens, and anti-haemolysin immunity protects against this invasion but not against colonisation (O'Hanley *et al.*, 1991). Since HlyA, the structural haemolysin molecule, is, in broad terms, antigenically conserved in uropathogenic *E. coli* strains, an anti-haemolysin vaccine may have potential for human use (O'Hanley *et al.*, 1993).

Epidemiology

Since anti-haemolysin antibodies develop during UTI, it is likely that haemolysin is expressed *in vivo* (Emody *et al.*, 1982; Seetharama *et al.*, 1988). Haemolysin production is most common among strains from patients, and particularly children, with pyelonephritis (Brauner *et al.*, 1990). It is progressively less common in association with cystitis, asymptomatic bacteriuria and faecal strains (Table 18.5). Haemolysin production is also more common in UTI localised to the upper as opposed to the lower urinary tract (Brooks *et al.*, 1980, 1981). The association between haemolysin production and pyelonephritis persisted when other virulence factors were considered in a multivariate analysis (Tullus *et al.*, 1991). In children with UTI accompanied by fever, haemolysin production is as common when there is renal parenchymal involvement as when there is not (Jantausch *et al.*, 1992), and in women haemolysin production does not correlate with the development of septicaemia during acute pyelonephritis (Otto *et al.*, 1993). This suggests that while haemolysin may contribute to the development of clinical pyelonephritis and febrile

UTI, other factors determine renal parenchymal involvement and invasion of the bloodstream. Under conditions that compromise the host, haemolysin production in pyelonephritis is somewhat less common than when such conditions are absent (Johnson, 1991a; Benton *et al.*, 1992; Ikaheimo *et al.*, 1993; Otto *et al.*, 1993), which suggests that haemolysin helps to overcome host defences in individuals who are otherwise normal.

Aerobactin

The aerobactin system, which extracts iron from the host for bacterial metabolic processes, is the siderophore system of *E. coli* most clearly implicated in virulence. The genetic determinants of the aerobactin system may be chromosomal or plasmid-borne (Johnson, 1991a), and plasmids that carrying the aerobactin region sometimes also carry antimicrobial resistance genes (Colonna *et al.*, 1985, 1992; Delgado-Iribarren *et al.*, 1987; Johnson *et al.*, 1988b; Phillips *et al.*, 1988; Darja *et al.*, 1990). Strains with aerobactin plasmids are more common in the urosepsis of compromised than of uncompromised hosts (Johnson *et al.*, 1988b), possibly because compromised patients are subject to more exposure to antimicrobial agents. *Escherichia coli* may exchange large conjugative aerobactin-antimicrobial resistance plasmids with other genera, such as *Salmonella*, resulting in serious infections that are difficult to treat (Colonna *et al.*, 1985, 1992; Delgado-Iribarren *et al.*, 1987; Phillips *et al.*, 1988).

The association of aerobactin with P-fimbriae and haemolysin (Ørskov *et al.*, 1988; Jacobson *et al.*, 1990; Opal *et al.*, 1990; Tullus *et al.*, 1992) may depend on the plasmid as against the chromosomal location of the aerobactin system (Johnson *et al.*, 1988b). Direct genetic linkage between chromosomal *hly*, *pap* and aerobactin determinants has not been confirmed by DNA hybridisation (Ott *et al.*, 1991), but epidemiological evidence supports such an association (Johnson *et al.*, 1988b). Aerobactin production is more common in certain O:K:H-serotypes than in others (Ørskov *et al.*, 1988).

Animal models

Aerobactin production is associated with enhanced virulence in a variety of animal models (Williams, 1979; Williams & Warner, 1980; Lafont *et al.*, 1987; der Vartanian *et al.*, 1992). In ascending models of UTI, aerobactin-producing strains from patients with septicaemia are more virulent than strains that do not produce aerobactin (Montgomerie *et al.*,

1984). Even an incomplete aerobactin synthesis region appears to confer enhanced nephropathogenicity for mice, in addition to a growth advantage *in vitro* and enhanced cytotoxicity (Harjai *et al.*, 1993).

Attempts to protect animals against experimental infection with aerobactin-positive strains, by means of antibodies against the outer-membrane aerobactin receptor protein, have had mixed success. The reason may be that the receptor protein is inaccessible to antibody in the presence of intact wild-type lipopolysaccharide (Bolin *et al.*, 1987; Roberts *et al.*, 1989). Though aerobactin is non-immunogenic (Bindereif & Neilands, 1985), an anti-aerobactin monoclonal antibody that blocks the growth of aerobactin-positive bacteria in low-iron conditions can be produced if an aerobactin–protein conjugate is used as the immunogen (Le Roy *et al.*, 1992) but animal protection studies with this antibody have not been reported.

Epidemiology

The aerobactin system is more common in strains of *E. coli* isolated from patients with pyelonephritis and cystitis than in asymptomatic bacteriuria or faecal isolates (Table 18.5), which suggests that aerobactin contributes to urovirulence. However, when multivariate analysis was used to examine several virulence factors simultaneously, the association between aerobactin and pathogenicity documented by univariate analysis was no longer significant (Tullus *et al.*, 1991). There is little evidence that the aerobactin system is any less prevalent among strains from compromised as opposed to uncompromised hosts (Montogomerie *et al.*, 1984; Jacobson *et al.*, 1988; Johnson *et al.*, 1988b).

Capsular polysaccharide (K-antigen)

Capsular polysaccharides of *E. coli* are linear polymers of repeating carbohydrate subunits, with or without an amino-acid or lipid component, that coat the bacterial cell and protect it from host defence mechanisms (Ørskov, 1978; Jann & Jann, 1983; see Chapter 4). Most encapsulated uropathogenic strains express acidic, thermostable and highly anionic Group II capsules, in contrast to the Group I capsules of non-pathogenic strains (Jann & Jann, 1983).

The K1 capsule, a prototypic Group II capsular type, is antiphagocytic because of its negative charge and hydrophilicity (Jann & Jann, 1983; Harber *et al.*, 1986; Eisenstein & Jones, 1988; Silver *et al.*, 1988), and because it blocks activation of the alternative complement pathway, thereby reducing opsonisation (van Dijk *et al.*, 1979; Harber *et al.*, 1986). In some Group-II-encapsulated strains, serum resistance is due to the anti-complementary activity of the capsular polysaccharides (Verweij-van Vught *et al.*, 1983; Ørskov & Ørskov, 1985) and depends on the K-type (Opal *et al.*, 1982) and the amount of it that is present (Brooks *et al.*, 1980). However, capsular status is only one of several determinants of serum resistance, and often does not correlate with serum resistance in collections of clinical isolates (Bjorksten *et al.*, 1976; Taylor, 1976, 1983; McCabe *et al.*, 1978; Van Dijk *et al.*, 1978).

The K1, K5, and K12 capsules exhibit divergent associations with specific O-serogroups (Kaijser *et al.*, 1977b; Vaisanen-Rhen *et al.*, 1984b; Czirok *et al.*, 1986). Strains with K1 capsules commonly express MRHA (Evans *et al.*, 1981) and P-fimbriae (Vaisanen *et al.*, 1981; Siitonen, 1992) but not haemolysin (Hughes *et al.*, 1983; Czirok *et al.*, 1986), while K5 strains are commonly haemolytic (Hughes *et al.*, 1983).

Animal models

The presence and amount of capsular polysaccharide expressed by wild-type human urine isolates correlate with pathogenicity in mouse UTI models (Kalmanson *et al.*, 1975; Nicholson & Glynn, 1975; Ketyi *et al.*, 1983; Verweij-van Vught *et al.*, 1983; Domingue *et al.*, 1988) and non-encapsulated mutant strains are generally less virulent in mice than their encapsulated parents (Smith & Huggins, 1980; Verweij-van Vught *et al.*, 1983; Cross *et al.*, 1986). However, acquisition of capsule production by avirulent, non-encapsulated laboratory strains has little impact on their virulence (Silver *et al.*, 1981), which suggests that other factors present in wild-type strains are necessary for virulence.

Capsular polysaccharides are often poorly immunogenic (Kaijser & Olling, 1973b; Kaijser, 1981, 1983a; Hanson *et al.*, 1987; Salit *et al.*, 1988a), but immunogenicity is improved by using protein conjugate vaccines. Anti-capsular immunity protects mice, rats and rabbits against pyelonephritis due to the homologous strain or a strain that expresses a cross-reacting capsular polysaccharide (Robbins *et al.*, 1974; Kaijser & Ahlstedt, 1977a; Kaijser *et al.*, 1983b,c).

Epidemiology

A higher proportion of human urinary strains than faecal strains is encapsulated and typeable with standard anti-K sera (Vahlne, 1945; Kaijser *et al.*, 1977b). The common K types associated with UTI include K1, K2, K3, K5, K12, K13, K20 and K51 (Kaijser *et al.*, 1977b; Ørskov &

Ørskov, 1985; Svanborg Eden & de Man, 1987) and encapsulated urinary isolates produce more capsular substance compared to encapsulated faecal isolates (Glynn *et al.*, 1971; Kaijser, 1973a; Brooks *et al.*, 1980, 1981).

The most common capsular type overall, K1 (Ørskov, 1978), is more common in pyelonephritis than in other types of UTI or in the faecal flora (Table 18.6). In contrast, K1 strains are about equally common in asymptomatic bacteriuria and in faecal strains and may even be less common in cystitis (Table 18.6). The K1 isolates associated with more severe forms of UTI produce larger amounts of capsular substance (Kaijser, 1973a; Brooks *et al.*, 1981), which suggests that K1 contributes to the development of pyelonephritis but that it is not particularly important in the pathogenesis of other types of UTI.

Serum resistance

Bacterial resistance to killing by serum is the result of the individual or combined effects of capsular polysaccharide, O-polysaccharide side chains and surface proteins (Montenegro *et al.*, 1985; Timmis *et al.*, 1985). As we have seen, the evidence to support a major role for capsular polysaccharides in the serum resistance of clinical isolates is contradictory (Jann & Jann, 1983; Taylor, 1983; Ørskov & Ørskov, 1985; Eisenstein & Jones, 1988; Vermeulen *et al.*, 1988). O-polysaccharide is a component of smooth-type lipopolysaccharide and is associated with serum resistance (Lindberg *et al.*, 1975; Taylor, 1983; Goldman *et al.*, 1984; Ørskov & Ørskov, 1985; Timmis *et al.*, 1985). Serum-resistant strains, which have abundant O-polysaccharide, appear to activate complement to as great an extent as less well shielded serum-sensitive strains. This suggests that O-polysaccharide protects against complement-induced lysis by causing complement activation at a site distant from sensitive membrane target sites and not by preventing complement activation (Taylor, 1983; Goldman *et al.*, 1984). The *iss* and *traT* genes encode outer-membrane proteins that confer serum resistance by interfering with complement-mediated killing, perhaps by interfering with the membrane attack complex (Johnson, 1991a). Both these genes are present on ColV plasmids, and *traT* is also found on other F-like plasmids, sometimes accompanied by antimicrobial resistance genes (Moll *et al.*, 1980; Binns *et al.*, 1982; Nilius & Savage, 1984; Montenegro *et al.*, 1985; Timmis *et al.*, 1985; Fernandez-Beros *et al.*, 1990; Waters & Crosa, 1991). The outer-membrane protein OmpA confers serum resistance and enhanced virulence (Weiser & Gotschlich, 1991).

The serum resistance of the common serogroups O1, O2, O4, O6, O7, O18 and O75 is greater than that of uncommon O-serogroups, and it is lowest among rough O-polysaccharide-deficient strains (Olling *et al.*, 1973). Serum-resistant strains are usually more nephropathogenic in animal models compared to serum-sensitive strains (Montgomeri, 1978; Iwahi *et al.*, 1982; Marre *et al.*, 1986; Domingue *et al.*, 1988).

Epidemiology

The prevalence of serum resistance amongst pyelonephritis and cystitis isolates is similar and they are more commonly serum resistant than faecal and asymptomatic bacteriuria strains (Gower *et al.*, 1972; Brooks *et al.*, 1980) (Table 18.6). It seems, therefore, that serum resistance is important in the pathogenesis of symptomatic UTI, regardless of its severity. In conditions, other than pregnancy, in which the host may be compromised, the frequency of serum resistance among strains causing pyelonephritis is reduced (Lomberg *et al.*, 1984; Stenqvist *et al.*, 1987; Sandberg *et al.*, 1988; Lomberg *et al.*, 1989a).

Strains of *E. coli* that cause asymptomatic bacteriuria are less often serum resistant than faecal strains (Table 18.6) (Bjorksten & Kaijser, 1978), which suggests that serum-sensitive strains may have a selective advantage in bladder colonisation. Faecal strains that enter the bladder appear to adjust to the new environment by becoming more serum-sensitive with time (Lindberg *et al.*, 1975), possibly by a loss of O-polysaccharide side chains during prolonged bladder colonisation, as an adaptive response to the presence of urinary anti-O-antibodies.

Serotype and the 'clone concept'

Strains of *E. coli* that cause UTI can be distinguished from faecal strains by their O-polysaccharide antigens (Harber *et al.*, 1986). Although the same O-serogroups predominate among urinary and faecal strains (Turck *et al.*, 1962), certain of these O-serogroups are significantly more prevalent among urinary than among faecal strains (Johnson, 1991a), and among resident colonic strains than among transient faecal colonisers (Wold *et al.*, 1992). The O-serogroups most commonly associated with UTI are O1, O2, O4, O6, O7, O8, O16, O18, O25, O50 and O75 (Ørskov *et al.*, 1982).

Certain O-serogroups are clearly associated with the more severe forms of UTI, but there is little apparent difference between faecal isolates and those from asymptomatic bacteriuria (Table 18.6). Women colonised vaginally with O2, O4, O6 and O75 strains commonly go on to develop UTI, while those colonised with strains of other O-serogroups do not (Cooke & Ewins, 1975). The UTI-associated O-seroroups are less prevalent among patients with urinary tract abnormalities who develop pyelonephritis (Lomberg *et al.*, 1984). In mouse models, the UTI-associated O-serogroups are generally more urovirulent than other strains (Sjostedt, 1946; Van den Bosch *et al.*, 1979, 1982; Iwahi *et al.*, 1982). It appears, therefore, that specific O-polysaccharides identify strains with enhanced urovirulence.

As we have seen in relation to serum resistance, O-polysaccharides may contribute directly to virulence (see also Chapter 5). It is, however, likely that much of the virulence associated with certain O-serogroups is mediated by other virulence factors, such as P-fimbriae, MRHA, haemolysin and serum resistance, which are more common in UTI-associated O-serogroups. It should be noted that O-antigen alone is insufficient to define genetically distinct lineages of *E. coli* (Caugant *et al.*, 1985). Individual O-serogroups are heterogeneous with respect to virulence factor expression and other traits (Johnson, 1991a). The O:K:H-serotype affords finer resolution of genetic differences and similarities, and has traditionally been used to define distinct *E. coli* clones, a concept that is still useful in spite of evidence that genetic relationships in *E. coli* are more complex than was previously thought (Ørskov & Ørskov, 1983a). Examples of these genetic complexities are multiple outer-membrane protein groups, electrophoretic types and restriction fragment patterns, which may occur within individual O:K:H-serotypes, while other phenotypic properties are expressed consistently within, but not between, these subgroups (Kusecek *et al.*, 1984; Caugant *et al.*, 1985; Zingler *et al.*, 1990, 1992; Ott *et al.*, 1991).

These complexities notwithstanding, it is important to consider certain serotype-specific clinical associations. For example, there is no overlap in O:K:H-serotype between pyelonephritis and asymptomatic bacteriuria isolates (Stenqvist *et al.*, 1987). Although cystitis, pyelonephritis and asymptomatic bacteriuria isolates have serotypes in common, at least one serotype, O75:K100:H5, is unique to cystitis (Ørskov *et al.*, 1982). Furthermore, although no serotype is wholly unique to pyelonephritis, certain serotypes are regarded as distinctively pyelonephritogenic (Mabeck *et al.*, 1971; Ørskov et al., 1982; Vaisanen-Rhen *et al.*, 1984b). Thus, although the precise definition of genetically homogeneous clonal groups in *E. coli* is uncertain, certain groups of strains that share the same O-antigen or O:K:H-serotype are associated with UTI in general, and with specific UTI syndromes. The presence of other virulence factors in certain lineages probably accounts for most of these associations. The direct contribution to urovirulence of specific O- and possibly K- and H-antigens awaits clarification by the study of genetically manipulated strains.

Cytotoxic necrotising factor

Cytotoxic necrotising factor (CNF) is a toxic protein produced by many haemolytic strains of *E. coli*. It causes dermonecrosis in rabbits, is lethal for guinea-pigs and causes cell swelling and multinucleation in cell culture monolayers (Caprioli *et al.*, 1983, 1987, 1989; Blanco *et al.*, 1992a). Production of CNF is particularly common in serogroups O2, O6 and O75, but it is uncommon in others and rare in non-haemolytic strains (Blanco *et al.*, 1992a,b). The role of CNF in UTI has not, so far, been studied in animal models. In a univariate analysis, CNF production was a distinguishing feature between isolates from pyelonephritis and faecal isolates, but this could not be confirmed in a multivariate analysis (Brauner *et al.*, 1990). CNF is produced by 40 per cent of human urinary strains but not by faecal strains (Clay *et al.*, 1992). A more rigorous assessment of the contribution of CNF to urovirulence should be facilitated by the recent cloning of CNF determinants (Falbo *et al.*, 1992, 1993).

Carboxylesterase B

The B_2 variant of carboxylesterase B of human pathogenic, *E. coli* strains, including urinary isolates, is associated with the presence of haemolysin, P-fimbriae, UTI-associated O-serogroups and O:K:H serotypes, and the absence of antimicrobial resistance (Goullet & Picard, 1986, 1990; Johnson *et al.*, 1991b, 1994b). On the basis of this association of virulence factors, it is likely that the B_2 phenotype identifies an *E. coli* population with enhanced virulence, rather than itself contributing directly to virulence (Picard *et al.*, 1991).

Virulence factors in combination

The significance of virulence factors in UTI has usually been studied with one virulence factor at a time, but it is clear that uropathogenic strains commonly express several of these factors simultaneously. In some instances this is due to the presence of a block of genetically linked virulence determinants and in some strains diverse adhesin operons may be co-ordinately regulated (Hacker, 1992; see Chapter 13).

Animal models

The virulence of non-isogenic wild-type uroisolates in mouse models is not strictly determined by the number of virulence factors they express (Van den Bosch *et al.*, 1982; Domingue *et al.*, 1988). However, studies with genetically manipulated strains that carry a number of virulence factors suggest that each of these contributes to the net virulence of the organism, and that the outcome of infection depends on the particular combination of factors that is expressed (Smith & Huggins, 1980; Hagberg *et al.*, 1983; Ketyi *et al.*, 1983; Marre *et al.*, 1986; O'Hanley *et al.*, 1991). Further experiments with genetically modified strains will be necessary to clarify the interactions between the virulence factors that are most commonly present together in UTI isolates.

Epidemiology

Isolates of *E. coli* from cases of UTI express several virulence factors more commonly compared to faecal or periurethral isolates, and this correlates with the severity of the UTI (Brooks *et al.*, 1980, 1981; Hacker *et al.*, 1983; Lomberg *et al.*, 1984; Funfstuck *et al.*, 1986). In pyelonephritis and urosepsis most strains express multiple virulence factors, but in compromised hosts this is less likely to be the case (Lomberg *et al.*, 1984; Johnson *et al.*, 1988b; Tullus *et al.*, 1992). This suggests that these factors act additively or synergistically to overcome host defences, and that strains with several virulence factors are the most effective urinary pathogens in intact hosts.

Conclusions

Certain properties of *E. coli*, including P-fimbriae, haemolysin, aerobactin, serum resistance and the K1 capsule, are fairly well established as virulence factors in UTI. This is based on evidence from the evaluation of their mechanisms of action, from studies of animal models and from human epidemiological data. In the case of other traits, such as type-1 fimbriae and the UTI-associated O-antigens, the evidence for a direct pathogenetic role in UTI is less clear. Simultaneous expression of multiple virulence factors is clinically relevant and should be considered in future research. Conditions that compromise the host may allow virulence-factor-deficient organisms to cause serious UTI. The most meaningful insights into mechanisms of urovirulence will be gained when host factors, such as the nature of the clinical UTI, the anatomical site of the infection and the presence of underlying compromising features, are taken into account together with the properties of the strain of *E. coli* that has been isolated. This better understanding may make it possible to prevent human UTI by means of intervention directed specifically against the various virulence factors.

Acknowledgements

Jodi A. Aasmundrud helped to prepare the manuscript and Young Mee Chong helped to collect references. Grant Support: National Institutes of Health (DK-47504).

References

Abraham, S. N., Babu, J. P., Giampapa, C. P., Hasty, D. L., Simpson, W. A. & Beachey, E. H. (1985). Protection against *Escherichia coli*-induced urinary tract infections with hybridoma antibodies directed against type 1 fimbriae or complementary D-mannose receptors. *Infection and Immunity*, **48**, 625–8.

Agace, W., Hedges, S., Andersson, U., Andersson, J., Ceska, M. & Svanborg, C. (1993). Selective cytokine production by epithelial cells following exposure to *Escherichia coli*. *Infection and Immunity*, **61**, 602–9.

Ahrens, R., Ott, M., Ritter, A., Hoschützky, H., Bühler, T., Lottspeich, F., Boulnois, G. J., Jann, K. & Hacker, J. (1993). Genetic analysis of the gene cluster encoding nonfimbrial adhesin I from an *Escherichia coli* uropathogen. *Infection and Immunity*, **61**, 2505–12.

Andersson, P., Engberg, I., Lidin-Janson, G., Lincoln, K., Hull, R., Hull, S. & Svanborg, C. (1991). Persistence of *Escherichia coli* bacteriuria is not determined by bacterial adherence. *Infection and Immunity*, **59**, 2915–21.

Archambaud, M., Courcoux, P. & Labigne-Roussel, A. (1988a). Detection by molecular hybridization of *pap*, *afa*, and *sfa* adherence systems in *Escherichia coli* strains associated with urinary and enteral infections. *Annales de Microbiologie (Paris)*, **139**, 575–88.

Archambaud, M., Courcoux, P., Ouin, V., Chabanon, G. & Labigne-Roussel A. (1988b). Phenotypic and genotypic assays for the detection and identification of adhesins from pyelonephritic *Escherichia coli*. *Annales de Microbiologie (Paris)*, **139**, 557–73.

Aronson, M., Medalia, O., Schori, L., Mirelman, D., Sharon, N. & Ofek, I. (1987). Prevention of colonization of the urinary tract of mice with *Escherichia coli* by blocking adherence with methyl-α-D-mannopyranoside. *Journal of Infectious Diseases*, **139**, 329–32.

Arthur, M., Arbeit, R. D., Kim, C., Beltran, P., Crowe, H., Steinback, S., Campanelli, C., Wilson, R. A., Selander, R. K. & Goldstein, R. (1990). Restriction fragment length polymorphisms among uropathogenic

Escherichia coli isolates: *pap*-related sequences compared with *rrn* operons. *Infection and Immunity*, **58**, 471–9.

Arthur, M., Campanelli, C., Arbeit, R. D., Kim, C., Steinbach, S., Johnson, C. E., Rubin, R. H. & Goldstein, R. (1989a). Structure and copy number of gene clusters related to the *pap* P-adhesin operon of uropathogenic *Escherichia coli*. *Infection and Immunity*, **57**, 314–21.

Arthur, M., Johnson, C. E., Rubin, R. H., Arbeit, R. C., Campanelli, C., Kim, C., Steinbach, S., Agarwal, M., Wilkinson, R. & Goldstein, R. (1989b). Molecular epidemiology of adhesin and hemolysin virulence factors among uropathogenic *Escherichia coli*. *Infection and Immunity*, **57**, 303–13.

Benton, J., Chawla, J., Parry, S. & Stickler, D. (1992). Virulence factors in *Escherichia coli* from urinary tract infections in patients with spinal injuries. *Journal of Hospital Infection*, **22**, 117–27.

Berger, H., Hacker, J., Juarez, A., Hughes, C. & Goebel, W. (1982). Cloning of the chromosomal determinants encoding hemolysin production and mannose-resistant hemagglutination in *Escherichia coli*. *Journal of Bacteriology*, **152**, 1241–7.

Bhakdi, S. & Martin, E. (1991). Superoxide generation of human neutrophils induced by low doses of *Escherichia coli* hemolysin. *Infection and Immunity*, **59**, 2955–62.

Bhakdi, S., Muhly, M., Korom, S. & Schmidt, G. (1990). Effects of *Escherichia coli* hemolysin on human monocytes. *Journal of Clinical Investigation*, **85**, 1746–53.

Bindereif, A. & Neilands, J. B. (1985). Aerobactin genes in clinical isolates of *Escherichia coli*. *Journal of Bacteriology*, **161**, 727–35.

Binns, M. M., Mayden, J. & Levine, R. P. (1982). Further characterization of complement resistance conferred on *Escherichia coli* by the plasmid genes *ttraT* of R100 and *iss* of ColV, I-K94. *Infection and Immunity*, **35**, 654–9.

Bjorksten, B., Bortolussi, R., Gothefors, L. & Quie, P. G. (1976). Interaction of *E. coli* strains with human serum: lack of relationship to K1 antigen. *Journal of Pediatrics*, **89**, 892–7.

Bjorksten, B. & Kaijser, B. (1978). Interaction of human serum and neutrophils with *Escherichia coli* strains: differences between strains isolated from urine of patients with pyelonephritis or asymptomatic bacteriuria. *Infection and Immunity*, **22**, 308–11.

Blanco, J., Alonso, M. P., González, E. A., Blanco, M. & Garabal, J. I. (1990). Virulence factors of bacteraemic *Escherichia coli* with particular reference to production of cytotoxic necrotising factor (CNF) by P-fimbriate strains. *Journal of Medical Microbiology*, **31**, 175–83.

Blanco, J., Blanco, M., Alonso, M. P., Blanco, J. E., Garabal, J. I. & Gonzalez, E. A. (1992b). Serogroups of *Escherichia coli* strains producing cytotoxic necrotizing factors CNF1 and CNF2. *FEMS Microbiology Letters*, **96**, 155–60.

Blanco, J., Blanco, M., Alonso, M. P., Blanco, J. E., Gonzalez, E. A. & Garabal, J. I. (1992a). Characteristics of haemolytic *Escherichia coli* with particular reference to production of cytotoxic necrotizing factor type 1 (CNF1). *Research in Microbiology*, **143**, 869–78.

Blumenstock, E. & Jann, K. (1982). Adhesion of piliated *Escherichia coli* strains to phagocytes: differences between bacteria with mannose-sensitive pili and those with mannose-resistant pili. *Infection and Immunity*, **35**, 264–9.

Bock, K., Breimer, M. E., Brignole, A., Hannsson, G. C., Karlsson, K. A., Larson, G., Leffler, H., Samuelsson, B. E., Stromberg, N., Svanborg Eden, C. & Thurin, J. (1985). Specificity of binding of a strain of uropathogenic *Escherichia coli* to Galα1–4Gal-containing glycosphingolipids. *Journal of Biological Chemistry*, **260**, 8545–51.

Bolin, C. A. & Jensen, A. E. (1987). Passive immunization with antibodies against iron-regulated outer membrane proteins protects turkeys from *Escherichia coli* septicemia. *Infection and Immunity*, **55**, 1239–42.

Brauner, A., Katouli, M., Tullus, K. & Jacobson, S. H. (1990). Production of cytotoxic necrotizing factor, verocytotoxin and haemolysin by pyelonephritogenic *Escherichia coli*. *European Journal of Clinical Microbiology and Infectious Diseases*, **9**, 762–7.

Brauner, A., Leissner, M., Wretlind, B., Julander, I., Svenson, S. B. & Kallenius, G. (1985). Occurrence of P-fimbriated *Escherichia coli* in patients with bacteremia. *European Journal of Clinical Microbiology*, **4**, 566–9.

Brooks, H. J. L., Benseman, B. A. & Peck, J. (1981). Correlation between uropathogenic properties of *Escherichia coli* from urinary tract infections and the antibody-coated bacteria test and comparison with faecal strains. *Journal of Hygiene, Cambridge*, **87**, 53–61.

Brooks, H. J. L., O'Grady, F., McSherry, M. A. & Cattell, W. R. (1980). Uropathogenic properties of *Escherichia coli* in recurrent urinary-tract infection. *Journal of Medical Microbiology*, **13**, 57–68.

Bruce, A. W., Chan, R. C. Y., Pinkerton, D., Morales, A. & Chadwick, P. (1983). Adherence of Gram-negative uropathogens to human uroepithelial cells. *Journal of Urology*, **130**, 293–8.

Caprioli, A., Falbo, V., Roda, L. G., Ruggeri, F. M. & Zona, C. (1983). Partial purification and characterization of an *Escherichia coli* toxic factor that induces morphological cell alterations. *Infection and Immunity*, **39**, 1300–6.

Caprioli, A., Falbo, V., Ruggeri, F. M., Baldassarri, L., Bisicchia, R., Ippolito, G., Romoli, E. & Donelli, G. (1987). Cytotoxic necrotizing factor production by hemolytic strains of *Escherichia coli* causing extraintestinal infections. *Journal of Clinical Microbiology*, **25**, 146–9.

Caprioli, A., Falbo, V., Ruggeri, F. M., Minelli, F., Ørskov, I. & Donelli, G. (1989). Relationship between cytotoxic necrotizing factor production and serotype in hemolytic *Escherichia coli*. *Journal of Clinical Microbiology*, **27**, 758–61.

Caugant, D. A., Levin, B. R., Ørskov, I., Ørskov, F., Svanborg Eden, C. & Selander, R. K. (1985). Genetic diversity in relation to serotype in *Escherichia coli*. *Infection and Immunity*, **49**, 407–13.

Clay, C. G., Greeff, A. S., Crewe-Brown, H. H., de Villiers, B., Blanco, M., Gonzalez, E. A. & Blanco, J. (1992). Necrotizing *Escherichia coli* CNF+ from bacteraemia and urinary tract infections. In 92nd General Meeting, American Society for Microbiology, 26–30 May 1992, New Orleans. p. 56. Washington DC: American Society for Microbiology.

Colonna, B., Nicoletti, M., Visca, P., Casalino, M., Valenti, P. & Maimone, F. (1985). Composite IS*1* elements encoding hydroxamate-mediated iron uptake in FI*me* plasmids from epidemic *Salmonella* spp. *Journal of Bacteriology*, **162**, 307–16.

Colonna, B., Ranucci, L., Assunta Fradiani, P., Casalino, M., Calconi, A. & Nicoletti, M. (1992). Organization of aerobactin, hemolysin, and antibacterial resistance genes in lactose-negative *Escherichia coli* strains of serotype O4 isolated from children with diarrhea. *Infection and Immunity*, **60**, 5224–31.

Conventi, L., Errico, G., Mastroprimiano, S., D'Elia, R. & Busolo, F. (1989). Characterisation of *Escherichia coli* adhesins in patients with symptomatic urinary tract infections. *Genitourinary Medicine*, **65**, 183–6.

Cooke, E. M. & Ewins, S. P. (1975). Properties of strains of *Escherichia coli* isolated from a variety of sources. *Journal of Medical Microbiology*, **8**, 107–11.

Cross, A. S., Kim, K. S., Wright, D. C., Sadoff, J. C. & Gemski, P. (1986). Role of lipopolysaccharide and capsule in the serum resistance of bacteremic strains of *Escherichia coli*. *Journal of Infectious Diseases*, **154**, 497–503.

Czirok, E., Milch, H., Csiszar, K. & Csik, M. (1986). Virulence factors of *Escherichia coli*. *Acta Microbiologica Hungarica*, **33**, 69–83.

Dalet, F., Segovia, T. & Del Rio, G. (1991). Frequency and distribution of uropathogenic *Escherichia coli* adhesins: a clinical correlation over 2,000 cases. *European Urology*, **19**, 295–303.

Darja, Z. B., Modric, E. & Grabnar, M. (1990). Aerobactin uptake system, ColV production, and drug resistance encoded by a plasmid from an urinary tract infection *Escherichia coli* strain of human origin. *Canadian Journal of Microbiology*, **36**, 297–9.

De Lorenzo, V. & Martinez, J. L. (1988). Aerobactin production as a virulence factor: a reevaluation. *European Journal of Clinical Microbiology and Infectious Diseases*, **7**, 621–9.

De Man, P., Cedergren, B., Enerback, S., Larsson, A.C., Leffler, H., Lundell, A. L., Nilsson, B. & Svanborg Eden, C. (1987). Receptor-specific agglutination tests for detection of bacteria that bind globoseries glycolipids. *Journal of Clinical Microbiology*, **25**, 401–6.

De Man, P., Claeson, I., Johanson, I. M., Jodal, U. & Svanborg Eden, C. (1989). Bacterial attachment as a predictor of renal abnormalities in boys with urinary tract infection. *Journal of Pediatrics*, **115**, 915–22.

De Man, P., Jodal, U., Lincoln, K. & Svanborg Eden, C. (1988). Bacterial attachment and inflammation in the urinary tract. *Journal of Infectious Diseases*, **158**, 29–35.

De Man, P., Jodal, U., Van Kooten, C. & Svanborg, C. (1990). Bacterial adherence as a virulence factor in urinary tract infection. *Acta Pathologica Microbiologica et Immunologia Scandinavica*, **98**, 1053–60.

De Ree, J. M. & van den Bosch, J. F. (1987). Serological response to the P fimbriae of uropathogenic *Escherichia coli* in pyelonephritis. *Infection and Immunity*, **55**, 2204–7.

Delgado-Iribarren, A., Martinez-Suarez, J., Bazuero, F., Perez-Diaz, J. C. & Martinez, J. L. (1987). Aerobactin-producing multi-resistance plasmids. *Antimicrobial Agents and Chemotherapy*, **19**, 552–3.

Der Vartanian, M., Jaffeux, B., Contrepois, M., Chavarot, M., Girardeau, J-P., Bertin, Y. & Martin, C. (1992). Role of aerobactin in systemic spread of an opportunistic strain of *Escherichia coli* from the intestinal tract to gnotobiotic lambs. *Infection and Immunity*, **60**, 2800–7.

Domingue, G. J., Laucirica, R., Baglia, P., Covington, S., Robledo, J. A. & Li, S. C. (1988). Virulence of wild-type *Escherichia coli* uroisolates in experimental pyelonephritis. *Kidney International*, **34**, 761–5.

Domingue, G. J., Roberts, J. A., Laucirica, R., Ratner, M. H., Bell, D. P., Suarez, G. M., Kallenius, G. & Svenson, S. (1985). Pathogenic significance of P-fimbriated *Escherichia coli* in urinary tract infections. *Journal of Urology*, **133**, 983–9.

Donnenberg, M. S. & Welch, R. A. (1996). Virulence determinants of uropathogenic *Escherichia coli*. In *Urinary Tract Infections: Molecular Pathogenesis to Clinical Management*. eds. H. L. T. Mobley & J. W. Warren. pp. 135–74. Washington DC: ASM Press.

Dowling, K., Roberts, J. A. & Kaack, M. B. (1987). P-fimbriated *Escherichia coli* urinary tract infection: a clinical correlation. *Southern Medical Journal*, **80**, 1533–6.

Duguid, J. P., Clegg, S. & Wilson, M. I. (1979). The fimbrial and non-fimbrial haemagglutinins of *Escherichia coli*. *Journal of Medical Microbiology*, 12, 213–27.

Duguid, J. P. & Old, D. C. (1980). Adhesive properties of enterobacteriaceae. *Receptor Recognition Series B*, **6**, 187–217.

Dulawa, J., Jann, K., Thomsen, M., Rambausek, M. & Ritz, E. (1988). Tamm–Horsfall glycoprotein interferes with bacterial adherence to human kidney cells. *European Journal of Clinical Investigation*, **18**, 87–91.

Duncan, J. L. (1988). Differential effect of Tamm–Horsfall protein on adherence of *Escherichia coli* to transitional epithelial cells. *Journal of Infectious Diseases*, **158**, 1379–82.

Eisenstein, B. I. & Jones, G. W. (1988). The spectrum of infections and pathogenic mechanisms of *Escherichia coli*. *Advances in Internal Medicine*, 33, 231–52.

Elo, J., Tallgren, L. G., Vaisanen, V., Korhonen, T. K., Svenson, S. B. & Makela, P. H. (1985). Association of P and other fimbriae with clinical pyelonephritis in children. *Scandinavian Journal of Urology and Nephrology*, **19**, 281–4.

Emody, L., Batai, I., Kerenyi, M., Szekely, J. & Polyak, L. (1982). Anti-*Escherichia coli* α-haemolysin in control and patient sera. *Lancet*, **ii**, 986.

Enerback, A., Larsson, A. C., Leffler, H., Lundell, A., de Man, P., Nilsson, B. & Svanborg Eden, C. (1987). Binding to galactose-α1–4-galactose β-containing receptors as potential diagnostic tool in urinary tract infection. *Journal of Clinical Microbiology*, **25**, 407–11.

Evans, D. J., Evans, D. G., Hohne, C., Noble, M. A., Haldane, E. V., Lior, H. & Young, L. S. (1981). Hemolysin and K antigens in relation to serotype and hemagglutination type of *Escherichia coli* isolated from extraintestinal infections. *Journal of Clinical Microbiology*, **13**, 171–8.

Falbo, V., Famiglietti, M. & Caprioli, A. (1992). Gene block encoding production of cytotoxic necrotizing factor 1 and hemolysin in *Escherichia coli* isolates from extraintestinal infections. *Infection and Immunity*, **60**, 2182–7.

Falbo, V., Pace, T., Picci, L., Pizzi, E. & Caprioli, A. (1993). Isolation and nucleotide sequence of the gene encoding cytotoxic necrotizing factor 1 of *Escherichia coli*. *Infection and Immunity*, **61**, 4909–14.

Falkowski, W., Edwards, M. & Schaeffer, A.J. (1986). Inhibitory effect of substituted aromatic hydrocarbons on adherence of *Escherichia coli* to human epithelial cells. *Infection and Immunity*, **52**, 863–6.

Fernandez-Beros, M. E., Kissel, V., Lior, H. & Cabello, F. C. (1990). Virulence-related genes in ColV plasmids of *Escherichia coli* isolated from human blood and intestines. *Journal of Clinical Microbiology*, **28**, 742–6.

Firon, N., Ofek, I. & Sharon, N. (1984). Carbohydrate-binding sites of the mannose-specific fimbrial lectins of enterobacteria. *Infection and Immunity*, **43**, 1088–90.

Fletcher, K. S., Bremer, E. G. & Schwarting, G. A. (1979). P blood group regulation of glycosphingolipid levels in human erythrocytes. *Journal of Biological Chemistry*, **254**, 11196–8.

Fowler, J. E. & Stamey, T. A. (1977). Studies of introital colonization in women with recurrent urinary infections. VII. The role of bacterial adherence. *Journal of Urology*, **117**, 472–6.

Fried, F. A. & Wong, R. J. (1970). Etiology of pyelonephritis: significance of hemolytic *Escherichia coli*. *Journal of Urology*, **103**, 718–21.

Fujita, K., Yamamoto, T., Yokota, T. & Kitagawa, R. (1989). *In vitro* adherence of type 1-fimbriated uropathogenic *Escherichia coli* to human ureteral mucosa. *Infection and Immunity*, **57**, 2574–9.

Funfstuck, R., Tschape, H., Stein, G., Kunath, H., Bergner, M. & Wessel, G. (1986). Virulence properties of *Escherichia coli* strains in patients with chronic pyelonephritis. *Infection*, **14**, 145–50.

Gander, R. M., Thomas, V. L. & Forland, M. (1985). Mannose-resistant hemagglutination and P receptor recognition of uropathogenic *Escherichia coli* isolated from adult patients. *Journal of Infectious Diseases*, **151**, 508–13.

Garg, U. C., Ganguly, N. K., Sharma, S. & Bhatnagar, R. (1987). Antipili antibody affords protection against ascending pyelonephritis in rats: evaluated by renal brush border membrane enzymes. *Biochemistry International*, **14**, 517–24.

Glynn, A. A., Brumfitt, W. & Howard, C. J. (1971). K antigens of *Escherichia coli* and renal involvement in urinary-tract infections. *Lancet*, i, 514–16.

Goetz, M. B. (1989). Priming of polymorphonuclear neutrophilic leukocyte oxidative activity by type 1 pili from *Escherichia coli*. *Journal of Infectious Diseases*, **159**, 533–42.

Goetz, M. B., Kuriyama, S. M. & Silverblatt, F. J. (1987). Phagolysosome formation by polymorphonuclear neutrophilic leukocytes after ingestion of *Escherichia coli* that express type 1 pili. *Journal of Infectious Diseases*, 156, 229–33.

Goldhar, J., Perry, R., Golecki, J. R., Hoschutzky, H., Jann, B. & Jann, K. (1987). Nonfimbrial, mannose-resistant adhesins from uropathogenic *Escherichia coli* O83:K1:H4 and O14:K?:H11. *Infection and Immunity*, **55**, 1837–42.

Goldhar, J., Yavzori, M., Keisari, Y. & Ofek, I. (1991). Phagocytosis of *Escherichia coli* mediated by mannose resistant non-fimbrial haemagglutinin (NFA-1). *Microbial Pathogenesis*, **11**, 171–8.

Goldman, R. C., Joiner, K. & Leive, L. (1984). Serum-resistant mutants of *Escherichia coli* O111 contain increased lipopolysaccharide, lack an O antigen-containing capsule, and cover more of their lipid A core with O antigen. *Journal of Bacteriology*, **159**, 877–82.

Goullet, P. & Picard, B. (1990). Electrophoretic type B_2 of carboxylesterase B for characterisation of highly pathogenic *Escherichia coli* strains from extra-intestinal infections. *Journal of Medical Microbiology*, **33**, 1–6.

Goullet, P. H. & Picard, B. (1986). Highly pathogenic strains of *Escherichia coli* revealed by the distinct electrophoretic patterns of carboxylesterase B. *Journal of General Microbiology*, **132**, 1853–8.

Gower, P. E., Taylor, P. W., Koutsaimanis, K. G. & Roberts, A. P. (1972). Serum bactericidal activity in patients with upper and lower urinary tract infections. *Clinical Sciences*, **43**, 13–22.

Green, C. P. & Thomas, V. L. (1981). Hemagglutination of human type O erythrocytes, hemolysin production, and serogrouping of *Escherichia coli* isolates from patients with acute pyelonephritis, cystitis, and asymptomatic bacteriuria. *Infection and Immunity*, **31**, 309–15.

Grünberg, J., Perry, R., Hoschützky, H., Jann, B., Jann, K. & Goldhar, J. (1988). Nonfimbrial blood group N-specific adhesin (NFA-3) from *Escherichia coli* O20:KX104:H-, causing systemic infection. *FEMS Microbiology Letters*, **56**, 241–6.

Hacker, J. (1992). Role of fimbrial adhesins in the pathogenesis of *Escherichia coli* infections. *Canadian Journal of Microbiology*, **38**, 720–7.

Hacker, J., Bender, L., Ott, M., Wingender, J., Lund, B., Marre, R. & Goebel, W. (1990). Deletions of chromosomal regions coding for fimbriae and hemolysins occur *in vitro* and *in vivo* in various extraintestinal *Escherichia coli* isolates. *Microbial Pathogenesis*, **8**, 213–25.

Hacker, J., Hof, H., Emody, L. & Goebel, W. (1986). Influence of cloned *Escherichia coli* hemolysin genes, S-fimbriae and serum resistance on pathogenicity in different animal models. *Microbial Pathogenesis*, **1**, 533–47.

Hacker, J., Schroter, G., Schrettenbrunner, A., Hughes, C. & Goebel, W. (1983). Hemolytic *Escherichia coli* strains in the human fecal flora as potential urinary pathogens. *Zentralblatt für Bakteriologie und Hygiene A*, **254**, 370–8.

Hagberg, L., Hull, R., Hull, S., Falkow, S., Freter, R. & Svanborg Eden, C. (1983). Contribution of adhesins to bacterial persistence in the mouse urinary tract. *Infection and Immunity*, **40**, 265–72.

Hagberg, L., Jodal, U., Korhonen, T. K., Lidin-Janson, G., Lindberg, U. & Svanborg Eden, C. (1981). Adhesion, hemagglutination, and virulence of *Escherichia coli* causing urinary tract infections. *Infection and Immunity*, **31**, 564–70.

Hagberg, L., Leffler, H. & Svanborg Eden, C. (1985). Non-antibiotic prevention of urinary tract infection. *Infection*, **13**, S196-S200.

Hales, B. A., Beverley-Clarke, H., High, N. J., Jann, K., Perry, R., Goldhar, J. & Boulnois, G. J. (1988). Molecular cloning and characterization of the genes for a non-fimbrial adhesin from *Escherichia coli*. *Microbial Pathogenesis*, **5**, 9–17.

Hanisch, F-G., Hacker, J. & Schroten, H. (1993). Specificity of S fimbriae on recombinant *Escherichia coli*: preferential binding to gangliosides expressing NeuGcα(2–3)Gal and NeuAcα(2–8)NeuAc. *Infection and Immunity*, **61**, 2108–15.

Hanley, J., Salit, I. E. & Hofmann, T. (1985). Immunochemical characterization of P pili from invasive *Escherichia coli*. *Infection and Immunity*, **49**, 581–6.

Hanson, L. A., Ahlstedt, S., Fasth, A., Jodal, U., Kaijser, B., Larrson, P., Lindberg, Lindberg, U., Olling, S., Sohl-Akerlung, A. & Svanborg Eden, C. (1977). Antigens of *Escherichia coli*, human immune response, and the pathogenesis of urinary tract infections. *Journal of Infectious Diseases*, **136**, S144–9.

Harber, M. J., Topley, N. & Asscher, A. W. (1986). Virulence factors of urinary pathogens. *Clinical Sciences*, **70**, 531–8.

Harjai, K., Chhibber, S., Rao Bhau, L. N. & Sharma, S. (1993). Introduction of plasmid carrying incomplete genes for aerobactin production alters virulence of *Escherichia coli* HB101. *Microbial Pathogenesis*, **17**, 261–70.

Hedges, S., Anderson, P., Lidin-Janson, G., De Man, P. & Svanborg, C. (1991). Interleukin-6 response to deliberate colonization of the human urinary tract with Gram-negative bacteria. *Infection and Immunity*, **59**, 421–7.

High, N. J., Hales, B. A., Jann, K. & Boulnois, G. J. (1988). A block of urovirulence genes encoding multiple fimbriae and hemolysin in *Escherichia coli* O4:K12:H⁻. *Infection and Immunity*, 56, 513–17.

Hoschützky, H., Lottspeich, F. & Jann, K. (1989a). Isolation and characterization of the α-galactosyl-1, 4-β-galactosyl-specific adhesin (P adhesin) from fimbriated *Escherichia coli*. *Infection and Immunity*, **57**, 76–81.

Hoschützky, H., Nimmich, W., Lottspeich, F. & Jann, K. (1989b). Isolation and characterization of the non-fimbrial adhesin NFA-4 from uropathogenic *Escherichia coli* O7:K98:H6. *Microbial Pathogenesis*, **6**, 351–9.

Hughes, C., Hacker, J., Duvel, H. & Goebel, W. (1987). Chromosomal deletions and rearrangements cause coordinate loss of hemolysin, fimbriation, and serum resistance in a uropathogenic strain of *Escherichia coli*. *Microbial Pathogenesis*, 2, 227–30.

Hughes, C., Hacker, J., Roberts, A. & Goebel, W. (1983). Hemolysin production as a virulence marker in symptomatic and asymptomatic urinary tract infections caused by *Escherichia coli*. *Infection and Immunity*, **39**, 546–51.

Hughes, C., Phillips, R. & Roberts, A. P. (1982). Serum resistance among *Escherichia coli* strains causing urinary tract infection in relation to O type and the carriage of hemolysin, colicin, and antibiotic resistance determinants. *Infection and Immunity*, **35**, 270–5.

Hull, S. I., Bieler, S. & Hull, R. A. (1988). Restriction fragment length polymorphism and multiple copies of DNA sequences homologous with probes for P-fimbriae and hemolysin genes among uropathogenic *Escherichia coli*. *Canadian Journal of Microbiology*, **34**, 307–11.

Hultgren, S. J., Porter, T. N., Schaeffer, A. J. & Duncan, J. L. (1985). Role of type 1 pili and effects of phase variation on lower urinary tract infections produced by *Escherichia coli*. *Infection and Immunity*, **50**, 370–7.

Ikäheimo, R., Siitonen, A., Kärkkäinen, U. & Helena Mäkelä, P. (1993). Virulence characteristics of *Escherichia coli* in nosocomial urinary tract infection. *Clinical Infectious Diseases*, **16**, 785–91.

Israele, V., Darabi, A. & McCracken, G. Jr. (1987). The role of bacterial virulence factors and Tamm–Horsfall protein in the pathogenesis of *Escherichia coli* urinary tract infection in infants. *American Journal of Diseases of Children*, **141**, 1230–4.

Iwahi, T., Abe, Y., Nakao, M., Imada, A. & Tsuchiya, K. (1983). Role of type 1 fimbriae in the pathogenesis of ascending urinary tract infection induced by *Escherichia coli* in mice. *Infection and Immunity*, **39**, 1307–15.

Iwahi, T., Abe, Y. & Tsuchiya, K. (1982). Virulence of *Escherichia coli* in ascending urinary-tract infection in mice. *Journal of Medical Microbiology*, **15**, 303–16.

Jacobson, S., Carstensen, A., Kallenius, G. & Svenson, S. (1986a). Fluorescence-activated cell analysis of P-fimbriae receptor accessibility on uroepithelial cells of patients with renal scarring. *European Journal of Clinical Microbiology*, **5**, 649–54.

Jacobson, S. H., Kallenius, G., Lins, L. E. & Svenson, S. B. (1986b). P-fimbriae receptors in patients with chronic pyelonephritis. *Journal of Urology*, **139**, 900–3.

Jacobson, S. H., Katouli, M., Tullus, K. & Brauner, A. (1990). Phenotypic differences and characteristics of pyelonephritogenic strains of *Escherichia coli* isolated from children and adults. *Journal of Infection*, **21**, 279–86.

Jacobson, S. H., Lins, L. E., Svenson, S. B. & Kallenius, G. (1985). Lack of correlation of P blood group phenotype and renal scarring. *Kidney International*, **28**, 797–800.

Jacobson, S. H., Östenson, C.-G., Tullus, K. & Brauner, A. (1992). Serum resistance in *Escherichia coli* strains causing acute pyelonephritis and bacteraemia. *APMIS*, **100**, 147–53.

Jacobson, S. H., Tullus, K., Wretlind, B. & Brauner, A. (1988). Aerobactin-mediated uptake of iron by strains of *Escherichia coli* causing acute pyelonephritis and bacteremia. *Journal of Infection*, **16**, 147–52.

Jann, K. & Jann, B. (1983). The K antigens of *Escherichia coli*. *Progress in Allergy*, **33**, 53–79.

Jann, K., Schmidt, G., Blumenstock, E. & Vosbeck, K. (1981). *Escherichia coli* adhesion to *Saccharomyces cerevisiae* and mammalian cells: role of piliation and surface hydrophobicity. *Infection and Immunity*, **32**, 484–9.

Jantausch, B. A., Wiedermann, B. L., Hull, S. I., Nowicki, B., Getson, P. R., Rushton, H. G., Majd, M., Luban, N. L. & Rodriguez, W. J. (1992). *Escherichia coli* virulence factors and ^{99m}Tc-dimercaptosuccinic acid renal scan in children with febrile urinary tract infection. *Pediatric Infectious Diseases Journal*, **11**, 343–9.

Johanson, I., Lindstedt, R. & Svanborg, C. (1992). Roles of the *pap*- and *prs*-encoded adhesins in *Escherichia coli* adherence to human uroepithelial cells. *Infection and Immunity*, **60**, 3416–22.

Johnson, J. R. (1988a). P-fimbriated *E. coli* urinary tract infection [Letter]. *Southern Medical Journal*, **81**, 1070.

Johnson, J. R. (1991a). Virulence factors in *Escherchia coli* urinary tract infection. *Clinical Microbiology Reviews*, **4**, 80–128.

Johnson, J. R. & Berggren, T. (1994a). Pigeon and dove eggwhite protect mice against renal infection due to P fimbriated *Escherichia coli*. *American Journal of Medical Sciences*, **307**, 335–9.

Johnson, J. R., Goullet, P., Picard, B., Moseley, S. L., Roberts, P. L. & Stamm, W. E. (1991b). Association of carboxylesterase B electrophoretic pattern with presence and expression of urovirulence factor determinants and antimicrobial resistance among strains of *Escherichia coli* causing urosepsis. *Infection and Immunity*, **59**, 2311–15.

Johnson, J. R., Moseley, S. L., Roberts, P. L. & Stamm, W. E. (1988b). Aerobactin and other virulence factor genes among strains of *Escherichia coli* causing urosepsis: association with patient characteristics. *Infection and Immunity*, **56**, 405–12.

Johnson, J. R., Ørskov, I., Ørskov, F., Goullet, P., Goullet, P., Picard, B., Moseley, S. L., Roberts, P. L. & Stamm, W. E. (1994b). O, K, and H antigens predict virulence factors, carboxylesterase B pattern, antimicrobial resistance, and host compromise among *Escherichia coli* strains causing urosepsis. *Journal of Infectious Diseases*, **169**, 119–26.

Johnson, J. R., Roberts, P. L. & Stamm, W. E. (1987). P-fimbriae and other virulence factors in *Escherichia coli* urosepsis: association with patients' characteristics. *Journal of Infectious Diseases*, **156**, 225–9.

Johnson, J. R. & Ross, A. E. (1993). P$_1$-antigen-containing avian egg whites as inhibitors of P adhesins among wild-type *Escherichia coli* strains from patients with urosepsis. *Infection and Immunity*, **61**, 4902–5.

Johnson, J. R. & Stamm, W. E. (1989). Urinary tract infections in women: diagnosis and therapy. *Annals of Internal Medicine*, **111**, 906–17.

Johnson, J. R., Swanson, J. L. & Neill, M. A. (1992). Avian P1 antigens inhibit agglutination mediated by P fimbriae of uropathogenic *Escherichia coli*. *Infection and Immunity*, **60**, 578–83.

Jonas, D., Schultheis, B., Klas, C., Krammer, P. H. & Bhakdi, S. (1993). Cytocidal effects of *Escherichia coli* hemolysin on human T lymphocytes. *Infection and Immunity*, **61**, 1715–21.

Kaack, M. B., Martin, L. N., Svenson, S. B., Baskin, G., Steele, R. H. & Roberts, J. A. (1993). Protective anti-idiotype antibodies in the primate model of pyelonephritis. *Infection and Immunity*, **61**, 2289–95.

Kaack, M. B., Roberts, J. A., Baskin, G. & Patterson, G. M. (1988). Maternal immunization with P fimbriae for the prevention of neonatal pyelonephritis. *Infection and Immunity*, **56**, 1–6.

Kaijser, B. (1973a). Immunology of *Escherichia coli*: K antigen and its relation to urinary tract infection. *Journal of Infectious Diseases*, **127**, 670–7.

Kaijser, B. (1981). Studies on the K antibody response in rabbits immunized with a pool of five different K antigen-containing *Escherichia coli*. *International Archives of Allergy and Applied Immunology*, **65**, 300–3.

Kaijser, B. (1983a). Peroral immunization of healthy adults with live *Escherichia coli* O4K12 bacteria. *International Archives of Allergy and Applied Immunology*, **70**, 164–8.

Kaijser, B. & Ahlstedt, S. (1977a). Protective capacity of antibodies against *Escherichia coli* O and K antigens. *Infection and Immunity*, **17**, 286–9.

Kaijser, B., Hanson, L. A., Jodal, U., Lidin-Janson, G. & Robbins, J. B. (1977b). Frequency of *E. coli* K antigens in urinary-tract infections in children. *Lancet*, **i**, 663–4.

Kaijser, B., Larsson, P., Nimmich, W. & Soderstrom, T. (1983b). Antibodies of *Escherichia coli* K and O antigens in protection against acute pyelonephritis. *Progress in Allergy*, **33**, 275–88.

Kaijser, B., Larsson, P., Olling, S. & Schneerson, R. (1983c). Protection against acute, ascending pyelonephritis caused by *Escherichia coli* in rats, using isolated capsular antigen conjugated to bovine serum albumin. *Infection and Immunity*, **39**, 142–6.

Kaijser, B. & Olling, S. (1973b). Experimental hematogenous pyelonephritis due to *Escherichia coli* in rabbits: the antibody response and its protective capacity. *Journal of Infectious Diseases*, **128**, 41–9.

Kallenius, G. & Mollby, R. (1979). Adhesion of *Escherichia coli* to human periurethral cells correlated to mannose-resistant agglutination of human erythrocytes. *FEMS Microbiology Letters*, **5**, 295–9.

Kallenius, G., Mollby, R., Svenson, S. B., Helin, I., Hultberg, H., Cedergren, B. & Winberg, J. (1981a). Occurrence of P fimbriated *Escherichia coli* in urinary tract infection. *Lancet*, **ii**, 1369–72.

Kallenius, G., Mollby, R., Svenson, S. B., Winberg, J., Lundblad, A., Svensson, S. & Cedergren, B. (1980a). The P^K antigen as receptor for the haemagglutinin of pyelonephritic *Escherichia coli*. *FEMS Microbiology Letters*, **7**, 297–302.

Kallenius, G., Mollby, R. & Winberg, J. (1980b). *In vitro* adhesion of uropathogenic *Escherichia coli* to human periurethral cells. *Infection and Immunity*, **28**, 972–80.

Kallenius, G., Svenson, S. B., Hultberg, H., Mollby, R., Winberg, J. & Roberts, J. A. (1983). P-fimbriae of pyelonephritogenic *Escherichia coli*: significance for reflux and renal scarring–a hypothesis. *Infection*, **1**, 73–6.

Kallenius, G., Svenson, S. B., Mollby, R., Cedergren, B., Hultberg, H. & Winberg, J. (1981b). Structure of carbohydrate part of receptor on human uroepithelia cells for pyelonephritogenic *Escherichia coli*. *Lancet*, **ii**, 604–6.

Kallenius, G. & Winberg, J. (1978). Bacterial adherence to periurethral epithelial cells in girls prone to urinary-tract infections. *Lancet*, **ii**, 540–3.

Kalmanson, G. M., Harwick, H. J., Turck, M. & Guze, L. B. (1975). Urinary-tract infection: localization and virulence of *Escherichia coli*. *Lancet*, **i**, 134–6.

Kärkkäinen, U., Ikäheimo, R., Katila, M.-L. & Mäntyjärvi, R. (1991). P fimbriation of *Escherichia coli* strains from patients with urosepsis demonstrated by a commercial agglutination test (PF TEST). *Journal of Clinical Microbiology*, **29**, 221–4.

Karr, J. F., Nowicki, B., Truong, L. K., Hull, R. A. & Hull, S. I. (1989). Purified P fimbriae from two cloned gene clusters of a single pyelonephritogenic strain adhere to unique structures in the human kidney. *Infection and Immunity*, **57**, 3594–600.

Karr, J. F., Nowicki, B. J., Truong, L. D., Hull, R. A., Moulds, J. J. & Hull, S. I. (1990). *pap-2*-encoded fimbriae adhere to the P blood group-related glycosphingolipid stage-specific embryonic antigen 4 in the human kidney. *Infection and Immunity*, **58**, 4055–62.

Kaul, A., Martens, M., Nagamani, M., Kumar, D., Lublin, D., Nowicki, S. & Nowicki, B. (1993). Decay accelerating factor (DAF) is the natural receptor for the Dr-fimbriae of uropathogenic *Escherichia coli* in the human endometrium. In 93rd General Meeting, American Society for Microbiology, 16–20 May 1993, Atlanta, p. 57. Washington DC: American Society for Microbiology.

Keith, B. R., Maurer, L., Spears, P. A. & Orndorff, P. E. (1986). Receptor-binding function of type 1 pili effects bladder colonization by a clinical isolate of *Escherichia coli*. *Infection and Immunity*, **53**, 693–6.

Ketyi, I. (1981). Suckling mouse model of urinary tract infections caused by *Escherichia coli*. *Acta Microbiologica Hungarica*, **28**, 393–9.

Ketyi, I., Naumann, G. & Nimmich, W. (1983). Urinary tract infectivity of R strains of *Escherichia coli* carrying various virulence factors. *Acta Microbiologica Hungarica*, 30, 155–61.

Kinane, D. F., Blackwell, C. C., Brettle, R. P., Weir, D. M., Winstanley, F. P. & Elton, R. A. (1982). ABO blood group, secretor state, and susceptibility to recurrent urinary tract infection in women. *British Medical Journal*, **285**, 7–9.

Kiselius, P. V., Schwan, W. R., Amundsen, S. K., Duncan, J. L. & Schaffer, A. J. (1989). *In vivo* expression and variation of *Escherichia coli* type 1 and P pili in the urine of adults with acute urinary tract infections. *Infection and Immunity*, **57**, 1656–62.

Klemm, P. (1985). Fimbrial adhesins of *Escherichia coli*. *Reviews of Infectious Diseases*, **7**, 321–40.

König, B., Schönfeld, W., Scheffer, J. & König, W. (1990). Signal transduction in human platelets and inflammatory mediator release induced by genetically cloned hemolysin-positive and -negative *Escherichia coli* strains. *Infection and Immunity*, **58**, 1591–9.

Korhonen, T. K., Eden, S. & Svanborg Eden, C. (1980). Binding of purified *Escherichia coli* pili to human urinary tract epithelial cells. *FEMS Microbiology Letter*, **7**, 237–40.

Korhonen, T. K., Leffler, H. & Svanborg Eden, C. (1981). Binding specificity of piliated strains of *Escherichia coli* and *Salmonella typhimurium* to epithelial cells, *Saccharomyces cerevisiae* cells, and erythrocytes. *Infection and Immunity*, **32**, 796–804.

Korhonen, T. K., Parkkinen, J., Hacker, J., Finne, J., Pere, A., Rhen, M. & Holthofer, H. (1986a). Binding of *Escherichia coli* S fimbriae to human kidney epithelium. *Infection and Immunity*, **54**, 322–7.

Korhonen, T. K., Vaisanen, V., Saxen, H., Hultberg, H. & Svenson, S. B. (1982). P-antigen-recognizing fimbriae from human uropathogenic *Escherichia coli* strains. *Infection and Immunity*, **37**, 286–91.

Korhonen, T. K., Virkola, R. & Holthofer, H. (1986b). Localization of binding sites for purified *Escherichia coli* P fimbriae in the human kidney. *Infection and Immunity*, **54**, 328–32.

Korhonen, T. K., Virkola, R., Vaisanen-Rhen, V. & Holthofer, H. (1986c). Binding of purified *Escherichia coli* O75X adhesin to frozen sections of human kidney. *FEMS Microbiology Letters*, **35**, 313–18.

Kreft, B., Bohnet, S., Carstensen, O., Hacker, J. & Marre, R. (1993). Differential expression of interleukin-6, intracellular adhesion molecule 1, and major histocompatibility complex class II molecules in renal carcinoma cells stimulated with S fimbriae of uropathogenic *Escherichia coli*. *Infection and Immunity*, **61**, 3060–3.

Kröncke, K.-D., Ørskov, I., Ørskov, F., Jann, B. & Jann, K. (1990). Electron microscopic study of coexpression of adhesive protein capsules and poly-saccharide capsules in *Escherichia coli*. *Infection and Immunity*, **58**, 2710–14.

Kunin, C. M., Hua Hua, T., Krishman, C., Van Arsdale White, L. & Hacker, J. (1993). Isolation of a nicotinamide-requiring clone of *Escherichia coli* O18:K1:H7 from women with acute cystitis: resemblance to strains found in neonatal meningitis. *Clinical Infectious Diseases*, **16**, 412–16.

Kusecek, B., Wloch, H., Mercer, A., Vaisanen, V., Pluschke, G., Korhonen, T. & Achtman, M. (1984). Lipopolysaccharide, capsule, and fimbriae as virulence factors among O1, O7, O16, O18, or O75 and K1, K5, or K100 *Escherichia coli*. *Infection and Immunity*, **43**, 368–79.

Labigne-Roussel, A. & Falkow, S. (1988). Distribution and degree of heterogeneity of the afimbrial-adhesin-encoding operon *(afa)* among uropathogenic *Escherichia coli* isolates. *Infection and Immunity*, **56**, 640–8.

Lafont, J. P., Dho, M., d'Hauteville, H. M., Bree, A. & Sansonetti, P. J. (1987). Presence and expression of aerobactin genes in virulent avian strains of *Escherichia coli*. *Infection and Immunity*, **55**, 193–7.

Leffler, H., Lomberg, H., Gotschlich, E., Hagberg, L., Jodal, U., Korhonen, T., Samuelsson, E., Schoolnik, G. & Svanborg Eden, C. (1982). Chemical and clinical studies on the interaction of *Escherichia coli* with host glycolipid receptors in urinary tract infection. *Scandinavian Journal of Infectious Diseases*, **33**, 46–51.

Leffler, H. & Svanborg Eden, C. (1980). Chemical identification of a glycosphingolipid receptor for *Escherichia coli* attaching to human urinary tract epithelial cells and agglutinating human erythrocytes. *FEMS Microbiology Letters*, **8**, 127–34.

Leffler, H. & Svanborg Eden, C. (1981). Glycolipid receptors for uropathogenic *Escherichia coli* on human erythrocytes and uroepithelial cells. *Infection and Immunity*, 34, 920–9.

LeRoy, D., Expert, D., Razafindratsita, A., Deroussent, A., Cosme, J., Bohuon, C. & Andremont, A. (1992). Activity and specificity of a mouse monoclonal antibody to ferric aerobactin. *Infection and Immunity*, **60**, 768–72.

Leusch, H-G., Drzeniek, Z., Markos-Pusztai, Z. & Wagener, C. (1991). Binding of *Escherichia coli* and *Salmonella* strains to members of the carcinoembryonic antigen family: differential binding inhibition by aromatic α-glycosides of mannose. *Infection and Immunity*, **59**, 2151–7.

Leusch, H.-G., Hefta, S. A., Drzeniek, Z., Hummel K., Markos-Pusztai, Z. & Wagener, C. (1990). *Escherichia coli* of human origin binds to carcinoembryonic antigen (CEA) and non-specific crossreacting antigen (NCA). *FEBS Letters*, **261**, 405–9.

Lichodziejewska, M., Topley, N., Steadman, R., MacKenzie, R. K., Verrier-Jones, K. & Williams, J. D. (1989). Variable expression of P fimbriae in *Escherichia coli* urinary tract infection. *Lancet*, **ii**, 1414–18.

Lindberg, U., Hanson, L. A., Jodal, U., Lidin-Janson, G., Lincoln, K. & Olling, S. (1975). Asymptomatic bacteriuria in school girls. II. Differences in *Escherichia coli* causing asymptomatic and symptomatic bacteriuria. *Acta Paediatrica Scandinavica*, **64**, 432–6.

Linder, H., Engberg, I., Mattsby Baltzer, I., Jann, K. & Svanborg Eden, C. (1988). Induction of inflammation by *Escherichia coli* on the mucosal level: requirement for adherence and endotoxin. *Infection and Immunity*, **56**, 1309–13.

Linder, H., Engberg, I., Van Kooten, C., De Man, P. & Svanborg-Eden, C. (1990). Effects of anti-inflammatory agents on mucosal inflammation induced by infection with Gram-negative bacteria. *Infection and Immunity*, **58**, 2056–60.

Lindstedt, R., Baker, N., Falk, P., Hull, R., Hull, S., Karr, J., Leffler, H., Svanborg Eden, C. & Larson, G. (1989). Binding specificities of wild-type and cloned *Escherichia coli* strains that recognize globo-A. *Infection and Immunity*, **57**, 3389–94.

Lindstedt, R., Larson, G., Falk, P., Jodal, U., Leffler, H. & Svanborg, C. (1991). The receptor repertoire defines the host range for attaching *Escherichia coli* strains that recognize Globo-A. *Infection and Immunity*, **59**, 1086–92.

Linggood, M. A. & Ingram, P. L. (1982). The role of a hemolysin in the virulence of *Escherichia coli* for mice. *Journal of Medical Microbiology*, **15**, 25–30.

Lipsky, B. A. (1989). Urinary tract infections in men. Epidemiology, pathophysiology, diagnosis, and treatment. *Annals of Internal Medicine*, **110**, 138–50.

Ljungh, A. & Wadstrom, T. (1983). Fimbriation of *Escherichia coli* in urinary tract infections. Comparisons between bacteria in the urine and subcultured bacterial isolates. *Current Microbiology*, **8**, 263–8.

Lomberg, H., Cedergren, B., Leffler, H., Nilsson, B., Carlstrom, A. S. & Svanborg Eden, C. (1986). Influence of blood group on the availability of receptors for attachment of uropathogenic *Escherichia coli*. *Infection and Immunity*, **51**, 919–26.

Lomberg, H., Hanson, L. A., Jacobson, B., Jodal, U., Leffler, H. & Svanborg Eden, C. (1983). Correlation of P blood group, vesicoureteral reflux, and bacterial attachment in patients with recurrent pyelonephritis. *New England Journal of Medicine*, **308**, 1189–92.

Lomberg, H., Hellstrom, M., Jodal, U., Leffler, H., Lincoln, K. & Svanborg Eden, C. (1984). Virulence-associated traits in *Escherichia coli* causing first and recurrent episodes of urinary tract infection in children with or without vesicoureteral reflux. *Journal of Infectious Diseases*, **150**, 561–9.

Lomberg, H., Hellstrom, M., Jodal, U., Ørskov, I. & Svanborg Eden, C. (1989a). Properties of *Escherichia coli* in patients with renal scarring. *Journal of Infectious Diseases*, **159**, 579–82.

Lomberg, H., Jodal, U., Svanborg Eden, C., Leffler, H. & Samuelsson, B. (1981). P1 blood group and urinary tract infection. *Lancet*, **i**, 551–2.

Lomberg, H. & Svanborg Edén, C. (1989b). Influence of P blood group phenotype on susceptibility to urinary tract infection. *FEMS Microbiology Immunology*, **47**, 363–70.

Low, D., David, V., Lark, D., Schoolnik, G. & Falkow, S. (1984). Gene clusters governing the production of hemolysin and mannose-resistant hemagglutination are closely linked in *Escherichia coli* serotype O4 and O6 isolates from urinary tract infection. *Infection and Immunity*, **43**, 353–8.

Lund, B., Marklund, B. I., Stromberg, N., Lindberg, F., Karlsson, A. & Normark, S. (1988). Uropathogenic *Escherichia coli* can express serologically identical pili of different receptor binding specificities. *Molecular Microbiology*, **2**, 255–63.

Mabeck, C. E., Ørskov, F. & Ørskov, I. (1971). *Escherichia coli* serotypes and renal involvement in urinary-tract infection. *Lancet*, **i**, 1312–14.

Majd, M., Rushton, H. G., Jantausch, B. & Wiedermann, B. L. (1991). Relationship among vesicoureteral reflux, P-fimbriated *Escherichia coli*, and acute pyelonephritis in children with febrile urinary tract infection. *Journal of Pediatrics*, **119**, 578–85.

Makita, A. & Yamakawa, T. (1964). Biochemistry of organ glycolipids. III. The structures of human kidney cerebroside sulfuric ester, ceramide dihexoside and ceramide trihexoside. *Journal of Biochemistry*, **55**, 365–70.

Marild, S., Wettergren, B., Hellstrom, M., Jodal, U., Lincoln, K., Ørskov, I., Ørskov, F. & Svanborg Eden, C. (1988). Bacterial virulence and inflammatory response in infants with febrile urinary tract infection or screening bacteriuria. *Journal of Pediatrics*, **112**, 348–54.

Marklund, B.-I., Tennent, J. M., Garcia, E., Hamers, A., Baga, M., Lindberg, F., Gaastra, W. & Normark, S. (1992). Horizontal gene transfer of the *Escherichia coli pap* and *prs* pili operons as a mechanism for the development of tissue-specific adhesive properties. *Molecular Microbiology*, **6**, 2225–42.

Marre, R., Hacker, J., Henkel, W. & Goebel, W. (1986). Contribution of cloned virulence factors from uropathogenic *Escherichia coli* strains to nephropathogenicity in an experimental rat pyelonephritis model. *Infection and Immunity*, **54**, 761–7.

Marre, R., Kreft, B. & Hacker, J. (1990). Genetically engineered S and F1C fimbriae differ in their contribution to adherence of *Escherichia coli* to cultured renal tubular cells. *Infection and Immunity*, **58**, 3434–7.

Martensson, E. (1966). Neutral glycolipids of human kidney isolation, identification, and fatty acid composition. *Biochimia et Biophysica Acta*, **116**, 296–308.

Maslow, J. N., Mulligan, M. E., Adams, K. S., Justis, J. C. & Arbeit, R. D. (1993). Bacterial adhesins and host factors: role in the development and outcome of *Escherichia coli* bacteremia. *Clinical Infectious Diseases*, **17**, 89–97.

McCabe, W. R., Kaijser, B., Olling, S., Uwaydah, M. & Hanson, L. A. (1978). *Escherichia coli* in bacteremia: K and O antigens and serum sensitivity of strains from adults and neonates. *Journal of Infectious Diseases*, 138, 33–41.

Mobley, H. L. T., Chippendale, G. R., Tenney, J. H., Hull, R. A. & Warren, J. W. (1987). Expression of type 1 fimbriae may be required for persistence of *Escherichia coli* in the catheterized urinary tract. *Journal of Clinical Microbiology*, **25**, 2253–7.

Mobley, H. L. T., Green, D. M., Trifillis, A. L., Johnson, D. E., Chippendale, G. R., Lockatell, C. V., Jones, B. D. & Warren, J. W. (1990). Pyelonephritogenic *Escherichia coli* and killing of cultured human renal proximal tubular epithelial cells: role of hemolysin in some strains. *Infection and Immunity*, **58**, 1281–9.

Moll, A., Manning, P. A. & Timmis, K. N. (1980). Plasmid-determined resistance to serum bactericidal activity: a major outer membrane protein, the *traT* gene product, is responsible for plasmid-specified serum resistance in *Escherichia coli*. *Infection and Immunity*, **28**, 359–67.

Montenegro, M. A., Bitter-Suermann, D., Timmis, J. K., Aguero, M. E., Cabello, F. C., Sanyal, S. C. & Timmis, K. N. (1985). *traT* gene sequences, serum resistance and pathogenicity-related factors in clinical isolates of *Escherichia coli* and other Gram-negative bacteria. *Journal of General Microbiology*, **131**, 1511–21.

Montgomerie, J. Z. (1978). Factors affecting virulence in *Escherichia coli* urinary tract infections. *Journal of Infectious Diseases*, **137**, 645–7.

Montgomerie, J. Z., Bindereif, A., Nielands, J. B., Kalmanson, J. M. & Guze, L. B. (1984). Association of hydroxamate siderophore (aerobactin) with *Escherichia coli* isolated from patients with bacteremia. *Infection and Immunity*, **46**, 835–8.

Mulholland, S. G., Mooreville, M. & Parsons, C. L. (1984). Urinary tract infections and P blood group antigens. *Urology*, **24**, 232–5.

Neeser, J. R., Koellreutter, B. & Wuersch, P. (1986). Oligomannoside-type glycopeptides inhibiting adhesion of *Escherichia coli* strains mediated by type 1 pili: preparation of potent inhibitors from plant glycoproteins. *Infection and Immunity*, **52**, 428–36.

Nicholson, A. M. & Glynn, A. A. (1975). Investigation of the effect of K antigen in *Escherichia coli* urinary tract infections by use of a mouse model. *British Journal of Experimental Pathology*, **56**, 549–53.

Nicolle, L. E., Muir, P., Harding, G. K. M. & Norris, M. (1988). Localization of urinary tract infection in elderly, institutionalized women with asymptomatic bacteriuria. *Journal of Infectious Diseases*, **157**, 65–70.

Nilius, A. M. & Savage, D. C. (1984). Serum resistance encoded by colicin V plasmids in *Escherichia coli* and its relationship to the plasmid transfer system. *Infection and Immunity*, **43**, 947–53.

Nowicki, B., Holthofer, H. & Saraneva, T. (1986). Location of adhesion sites for P fimbriated and for O75X-positive *Escherichia coli* in the human kidney. *Microbial Pathogenesis*, **1**, 169–80.

Nowicki, B., Labigne, A., Moseley, S., Hull, R., Hull, S. & Moulds, J. (1990). The Dr hemagglutinin, afimbrial adhesins AFA-I and AFA-III, and F1845 fimbriae of uropathogenic and diarrhea-associated *Escherichia coli* belong to a family of hemagglutinins with Dr receptor recognition. *Infection and Immunity*, **58**, 279–81.

Nowicki, B., Moulds, J., Hull, R. & Hull, S. (1988). A hemagglutinin of uropathogenic *Escherichia coli* recognizes the Dr blood group antigen. *Infection and Immunity*, **56**, 1057–60.

Nowicki, B., Rhen, M., Vaisanen-Rhen, V., Pere, A. & Korhonen, T. K. (1985a). Fractionation of a bacterial cell population by adsorption to erythrocytes and yeast cells. *FEMS Microbiology Letters*, **26**, 35–40.

Nowicki, B., Rhen, M., Vaisanen-Rhen, V., Pere, A. & Korhonen, T. K. (1985b). Kinetics of phase variation between S and type-1 fimbriae of *Escherichia coli*. *FEMS Microbiology Letters*, **28**, 237–42.

Nowicki, B., Svanborg Eden, C., Hull, R. & Hull, S. (1989). Molecular analysis and epidemiology of the Dr hemagglutinin of uropathogenic *Escherichia coli*. *Infection and Immunity*, **57**, 446–51.

O'Hanley, P., Lalonde, G. & Ji, G. (1991). α-Hemolysin contributes to the pathogenicity of piliated digalactoside-binding *Escherichia coli* in the kidney: efficacy of an α-hemolysin vaccine in preventing renal injury in the BALB/c mouse model of pyelonephritis. *Infection and Immunity*, **59**, 1153–61.

O'Hanley, P., Lark, D., Falkow, S. & Schoolnik, G. (1985a). Molecular basis of *Escherichia coli* colonization of the upper urinary tract in BALB/c mice. *Journal of Clinical Investigation*, **75**, 347–60.

O'Hanley, P., Lark, D., Normark, S., Falkow, S. & Schoolnik, G. K. (1983). Mannose-sensitive and Gal–Gal binding *Escherichia coli* pili from recombinant strains. *Journal of Experimental Medicine*, **158**, 1713–9.

O'Hanley, P., Low, D., Romero, I., Lark, D., Vosti, K., Falkow, S. & Schoolnik, G. (1985b). Gal–Gal binding and hemolysin phenotypes and genotypes associated with uropathogenic *Escherichia coli*. *New England Journal of Medicine*, **7**, 414–20.

O'Hanley, P., Marcus, R., Hyeon Baek, K., Denich, K. & Ji, G. E. (1993). Genetic conservation of *hlyA* determinants and serological conservation of HlyA: basis for developing a broadly cross-reactive subunit *Escherichia coli* α-hemolysin vaccine. *Infection and Immunity*, **61**, 1091–7.

Ofek, I., Goldhar, J., Eshdat, Y. & Sharon, N. (1982). The importance of mannose-specific adhesins (lectins) in infections caused by *Escherichia coli*. Scandinavian *Journal of Infectious Diseases*, **33**, 61–7.

Ofek, I., Mirelman, D. & Sharon, N. (1977). Adherence of *Escherichia coli* to human mucosal cells mediated by mannose receptors. *Nature*, **265**, 623–5.

Ofek, I., Mosek, A. & Sharon, N. (1981). Mannose-specific adherence of *Escherichia coli* freshly excreted in the urine of patients with urinary tract infections, and of isolates subcultured from the infected urine. *Infection and Immunity*, **34**, 708–11.

Ofek, I., Rest, R. F. & Sharon, N. (1992). Nonopsonic phagocytosis of microorganisms: phagocytes use several molecular mechanisms to recognize, bind, and eventually kill microorganisms. *ASM News*, **58**, 429–35.

Öhman, L., Hed, J. & Stendahl, O. (1982). Interaction between human polymorphonuclear leukocytes and two different strains of type 1 fimbriae-bearing *Escherichia coli*. *Journal of Infectious Diseases*, **146**, 751–7.

Olling, S., Hanson, L. A., Holmgren, J., Jodal, U., Lincoln, K. & Lindberg, U. (1973). The bactericidal effect of normal human serum on *E. coli* strains from normals and from patients with urinary tract infections. *Infection*, **1**, 24–8.

Opal, S., Cross, A. & Gemski, P. (1982). K antigen and serum sensitivity of rough *Escherichia coli*. *Infection and Immunity*, **37**, 956–60.

Opal, S. M., Cross, A. S., Gemski, P. & Lyhte, L. W. (1990). Aerobactin and α-hemolysin as virulence determinants in *Escherichia coli* isolated from human blood, urine, and stool. *Journal of Infectious Diseases*, **161**, 794–6.

Orino, K. & Naiki, M. (1990). Two kinds of P-fimbrial variants of uropathogenic *Escherichia coli* recognizing Forssman glycosphingolipid. *Microbiology Immunology*, **34**, 607–15.

Ørskov, F. (1978). Virulence factors of the bacterial cell surface. *Journal of Infectious Diseases*, **137**, 630–3.

Ørskov, F. & Ørskov, I. (1983a). Summary of a workshop on the clone concept in the epidemiology, taxonomy, and evolution of the entero-bacteriaceae and other bacteria. *Journal of Infectious Diseases*, **148**, 346–57.

Ørskov, I. & Ørskov, F. (1983b). Serology and *Escherichia coli* fimbriae. *Progress in Allergy*, **33**, 80–105.

Ørskov, I. & Ørskov, F. (1985). *Escherichia coli* in extra-intestinal infections. *Journal of Hygiene, Cambridge*, **95**, 551–75.

Ørskov, I., Ørskov, F. & Birch-Andersen, A. (1980). Comparison of *Escherichia coli* fimbrial antigen F7 with type 1 fimbriae. *Infection and Immunity*, **27**, 657–66.

Ørskov, I., Ørskov, F., Birch-Andersen, A., Kanamori, M. & Svanborg Eden, C. (1982). O, K, H and fimbrial antigens in *Escherichia coli* serotypes associated with pyelonephritis and cystitis. *Scandinavian Journal of Infectious Diseases*, **33**, 18–25.

Ørskov, I., Svanborg Eden, C. & Ørskov, F. (1988). Aerobactin production of serotyped *Escherichia coli* from urinary tract infections. *Medical Microbiology and Immunology (Berlin)*, **177**, 9–14.

Österberg, E., Hallander, H. O., Kallner, A., Lundin, A., Svensson, S. B. & Aberg, H. (1990). Female urinary tract infection in primary health care: bacteriological and clinical characteristics. *Scandinavian Journal of Infectious Diseases*, **22**, 477–84.

Ott, M., Bender, L., Blum, G., Schmittroth, M., Achtman, M., Tschäpe, H. & Hacker, J. (1991). Virulence patterns and long-range genetic mapping of extraintestinal *Escherichia coli* K1, K5, and K100 isolates: use of pulsed-field gel electrophoresis. *Infection and Immunity*, **59**, 2664–72.

Ott, M., Hacker, J., Schmoll, T., Jarchau, T., Korhonen, T. K. & Goebel, W. (1986). Analysis of the genetic determinants coding for the S-fimbrial adhesin (*sfa*) in different *Escherichia coli* strains causing meningitis or urinary tract infections. *Infection and Immunity*, **54**, 646–53.

Otto, G., Sandberg, T., Marklund, B.-I., Ulleryd, P. & Svanborg, C. (1993). Virulence factors and *pap* genotype in *Escherichia coli* isolates from women with acute pyelonephritis, with or without bacteremia. *Clinical Infectious Diseases*, **17**, 448–56.

Parkkinen, J., Finne, J., Achtman, M., Vaisanen, V. & Korhonen, T. K. (1983). *Escherichia coli* strains binding neuraminyl α2–3 galactosides. *Biochemical and Biophysical Research Commununications*, **111**, 456–61.

Parkkinen, J., Ristimaki, A. & Westerlund, B. (1989). Binding of *Escherichia coli* S fimbriae to cultured human endothelial cells. *Infection and Immunity*, **57**, 2256–9.

Parkkinen, J., Virkola, R. & Korhonen, T. K. (1988). Identification of factors in human urine that inhibit the binding of *Escherichia coli* adhesins. *Infection and Immunity*, **56**, 2623–30.

Pecha, B., Low, D. & O'Hanley, P. (1989). Gal–Gal pili vaccines prevent pyelonephritis by piliated *Escherichia coli* in a murine model: single-component Gal–Gal pili vaccines prevent pyelonephritis by homologous and heterologous piliated *E. coli* strains. *Journal of Clinical Investigation*, **83**, 2102–8.

Pere, A., Nowicki, B., Saxen, H., Siitonen, A. & Korhonen, T. K. (1987). Expression of P, type-1 and type 1C fimbriae of *Escherichia coli* in the urine of patients with acute urinary tract infection. *Journal of Infectious Diseases*, 156, 567–74.

Pere, A., Selander, R. K. & Korhonen, T. K. (1988). Characterization of P fimbriae on O1, O7, O75, rough, and nontypable strains of *Escherichia coli*. *Infection and Immunity*, **56**, 1288–94.

Pere, A., Vaisanen-Rhen, V., Rhen, M., Tenhunen, J. & Korhonen, T. K. (1986). Analysis of P fimbriae on *Escherichia coli* O2, O4, and O6 strains by immunoprecipitation. *Infection and Immunity*, **51**, 618–25.

Phillips, I., Eykyn, S., King, A., Grandsden, W. R., Rowe, B., Frost, J. A. & Gross, R. J. (1988). Epidemic multiresistant *Escherichia coli* infection in West Lambeth health district. *Lancet*, i, 1038–41.

Picard, B., Picard-Pasquier, N., Krishnamoorthy, R. & Goullet, P. (1991). Characterization of highly virulent *Escherichia coli* strains by ribosomal DNA restriction fragment length polymorphism. *FEMS Microbiology Letters*, **82**, 183–8.

Plos, K., Carter, T., Hull, S., Hull, R. & Svanborg Eden, C. (1990). Frequency and organization of *pap* homologous DNA in relation to clinical origin of uropathogenic *Escherichia coli*. *Journal of Infectious Diseases*, **161**, 518–24.

Reid, G. & Sobel, J. D. (1987). Bacterial adherence in the pathogenesis of urinary tract infection: a review. *Reviews of Infectious Diseases*, **9**, 470–87.

Reinhart, H. H., Obedeanu, N. & Sobel, J. D. (1990). Quantitation of Tamm–Horsfall protein binding to uropathogenic *Escherichia coli* and lectins. *Journal of Infectious Diseases*, **162**, 1335–40.

Rhen, M., Klemm, P. & Korhonen, T. K. (1986). Identification of two new hemagglutinins of *Eschrichia coli*, N-acetyl-D-glucosamine-specific fimbriae and a blood group M-specific agglutinin, by cloning the corresponding genes in *Escherichia coli* K-12. *Journal of Bacteriology*, **168**, 1234–42.

Riegman, N., Kusters, R., van Veggel, H., Bergmans, H., van Bergen en Henegouwen, P., Hacker, J. & van Die, I. (1990). F1C fimbriae of a uropathogenic *Escherichia coli* strain: genetic and functional organization of the *foc* gene cluster and identification of minor subunits. *Journal of Bacteriology*, **172**, 1114–20.

Robbins, J. B., McCracken, G. H., Gotschlich, E. C., Ørskov, F., Ørskov, I. & Hanson, L. A. (1974). *Escherichia coli* K1 capsular polysaccharide associated with neonatal meningitis. *New England Journal of Medicine*, **22**, 1216–20.

Roberts, J. A. (1986). Pyelonephritis, cortical abscess, and perinephric abscess. *Urologic Clinics of North America*, **13**, 637–45.

Roberts, J. A., Hardaway, K., Kaack, B., Fussell, E. N. & Baskin, G. (1984a). Prevention of pyelonephritis by immunization with P-fimbriae. *Journal of Urology*, **131**, 602–7.

Roberts, J. A., Kaack, B., Kallenius, G., Mollby, R., Winberg, J. & Svenson, S. B. (1984b). Receptors for pyelonephritogenic *Escherichia coli* in primates. *Journal of Urology*, **131**, 163–8.

Roberts, J. A., Marklund, B.-I., Ilver, D., Kaack, M. B., Baskin, G., Mollby, R., Winberg, J. & Normark, S. (1993). The α-Gal-1–4-β-Gal specific tip adhesin of *E. coli* P-fimbriae is needed for pyelonephritis to occur in the normal urinary tract: fulfillment of 'molecular' Koch's postulates. In *33rd ICAAC*, 17–20 October 1993, New Orleans, Washington DC: American Society for Microbiology.

Roberts, M., Wooldridge, K. G., Gavine, H., Iravati Kuswandi, S. & Williams, P. H. (1989). Inhibition of biological activities of the aerobactin receptor protein in rough strains of *Escherichia coli* by polyclonal antiserum raised against native protein. *Journal of General Microbiology*, **135**, 2387–98.

Rodriguez-Ortega, M., Ofek, I. & Sharon, N. (1987). Membrane glycoproteins of human polymorphonuclear leukocytes that act as receptors for mannose-specific *Escherichia coli*. *Infection and Immunity*, **55**, 968–73.

Rydberg, J. & Helin, I. (1991). A simple reliable agglutination test for screening P-fimbriated *Escherichia coli* in children with urinary tract infections gives valuable clinical information. *Scandinavian Journal of Infectious Diseases*, **23**, 573–5.

Salit, I. E., Hanley, J., Clubb, L. & Fanning, S. (1988a). The human antibody response to uropathogenic *Escherichia coli*: a review. *Canadian Journal of Microbiology*, **34**, 312–18.

Salit, I. E., Hanley, J., Clubb, L. & Fanning, S. (1988b). Detection of pilus subunits (pilins) and filaments by using anti-P pilin antisera. *Infection and Immunity*, **56**, 2330–5.

Salmon, J. E., Kapur, S. & Kimberly, R. P. (1987). Opsonin-independent ligation of Fc receptors: the 3G8-bearing receptors on neutrophils mediate the phagocytosis of concanavalin A-treated erythrocytes and nonopsonized *Escherichia coli*. *Journal of Experimental Medicine*, **166**, 1798–813.

Sandberg, T., Kaijser, B., Lidin-Janson, G., Lincoln, K., Ørskov, F., Ørskov, I., Stokland, E. & Svanborg Eden, C. (1988). Virulence of *Escherichia coli* in relation to host factors in women with symptomatic urinary tract infection. *Journal of Clinical Microbiology*, **25**, 1471–6.

Sauter, S. L., Rutherford, S. M., Wagener, C., Shively, J. E. & Hefta, S. A. (1991). Binding of nonspecific cross-reacting antigen, a granulocyte membrane glycoprotein, to *Escherichia coli* expressing type 1 fimbriae. *Infection and Immunity*, **59**, 2485–93.

Schaeffer, A. J., Jones, J. M. & Dunn, J. K. (1981). Association of *in vitro Escherichia coli* adherence to vaginal and buccal epithelial cells with susceptibility of women to recurrent urinary-tract infections. *New England Journal of Medicine*, **304**, 1062–6.

Schaeffer, A. J., Jones, J. M., Falkowski, W. S., Duncan, J. L., Chmiel, J. S. & Plotkin, B. J. (1982). Variable adherence of uropathogenic *Escherichia coli* to epithelial cells from women with recurrent urinary tract infection. *Journal of Urology*, **128**, 1227–30.

Schaeffer, A. J., Schwan, W. R., Hultgren, S. J. & Duncan, J. L. (1987). Relationship of type 1 pilus expression in *Escherichia coli* to ascending urinary tract infection in mice. *Infection and Immunity*, **55**, 373–80.

Schmidt, M. A., O'Hanley, P., Lark, D. & Schoolnik, G. K. (1988). Synthetic peptides corresponding to protective epitopes of *Escherichia coli* digalactoside-binding pilin prevent infection in a murine pyelonephritis model. *Proceedings of the National Academy of Science*, **85**, 1247–51.

Schönian, G., Sokolowkska-Köhler, W., Rollmann, R., Schubert, A., Gräser, Y. & Presber, W. (1992). Determination of S fimbriae among *Escherichia coli* strains from extraintestinal infections by colony hybridization and dot enzyme immunoassay. *Zentralblatt für Bakteriologie A*, **276**, 273–9.

Schoolnik, G. K. (1989). How *Escherichia coli* infects the urinary tract. *New England Journal Medicine*, **320**, 804–5.

Seetharama, S., Cavalieri, S. J. & Snyder, I. S. (1988). Immune response to *Escherichia coli* α-hemolysin in patients. *Journal of Clinical Microbiology*, **26**, 850–6.

Senior, D., Baker, N., Cedergren, B., Falk, P., Larson, G., Lindstedt, R. & Svanborg Eden, C. (1988). Globo-A- a new receptor specificity for attaching *Escherichia coli*. *FEBS Letters*, **237**, 123–7.

Sheinfeld, J., Schaeffer, A. J., Cordon-Cardo, C., Rogatko, A. & Fair, W. R. (1989). Association of the Lewis blood-group phenotype with recurrent urinary tract infections in women. *New England Journal of Medicine*, **320**, 773–7.

Siitonen, A. (1992). *Escherichia coli* in fecal flora of healthy adults: serotypes, P and type 1C fimbriae, non-P mannose-resistant adhesins, and hemolytic activity. *Journal of Infectious Diseases*, **166**, 1058–65.

Silver, R. P., Aaronson, W., Vann, W. F. (1988). The K1 capsular polysaccharide of *Escherichia coli*. *Reviews of Infectious Diseases*, **10**, 282–6.

Silver, R. P., Finn, C. W., Vann, W. F., Aaronson, W., Schneerson, R., Kretschmer, P. J. & Garon, C. F. (1981). Molecular cloning of the K1 capsular polysaccharide genes of *E. coli*. *Nature*, **289**, 696–98.

Silverblatt, F. J. & Cohen, S. (1979). Antipili antibody affords protection against experimental ascending pyelonephritis. *Journal of Clinical Investigation*, **64**, 333–6.

Silverblatt, F. J., Weinstein, R. & Rene, P. (1982). Protection against experimental pyelonephritis by antibodies to pili. *Scandinavian Journal of Infectious Diseases*, *Supplement*, **33**, 79–82.

Sjostedt, S. (1946). Pathogenicity of certain serological types of *E. coli*; their mouse toxicity, hemolytic power, capacity for skin necrosis, and resistance to phagocytosis and bactericidal faculties of human blood. *Acta Pathologica et Microbiologica Scandinavica*, **63**, 1–130.

Smith, H. W. (1963). The haemolysins of *Escherichia coli*. *Journal of Pathology and Bacteriology*, **85**, 197–211.

Smith, H. W. & Huggins, M. B. (1980). The association of the O18, K1 and H7 antigens and the ColV plasmid of a strain of *Escherichia coli* with its virulence and immunogenicity. *Journal of General Microbiology*, **121**, 387–400.

Smith, H. W. & Huggins, M. B. (1985). The toxic role of α-haemolysin in the pathogenesis of experimental *Escherichia coli* infection in mice. *Journal of General Microbiology*, **131**, 395–403.

Sobota, A. E. & Apicella, L. L. (1991). Reduction in the anti-adherence activity of Tamm–Horsfall protein with increasing concentration of calcium. *Urological Research*, **19**, 177–180.

Sokurenko, E. V., Courtney, H. S., Abraham, S. N., Klemm, P. & Hasty, D. L. (1992). Functional heterogeneity of type 1 fimbriae of *Escherichia coli*. *Infection and Immunity*, **60**, 4709–19.

Stamm, W. E., Hooton, T. M., Johnson, J. R., Johnson, C., Stapleton, A., Roberts, P. L. & Fihn, S. D.. (1989). Urinary tract infections: from pathogenesis to treatment. *Journal of Infectious Diseases*, **159**, 400–8.

Stapleton, A., Moseley S. & Stamm, W. E. (1991). Urovirulence determinants in *Escherichia coli* isolates causing first episode and recurrent cystitis in women. *Journal of Infectious Diseases*, **163**, 773–9.

Stapleton, A., Nudelman, E., Clausen, H., Hakomori, S. & Stamm, W. E. (1992). Binding of uropathogenic *Escherichia coli* R45 to glycolipids extracted from vaginal epithelial cells is dependent on histo-blood group secretor status. *Journal of Clinical Investigation*, **90**, 965–72.

Stenqvist, K., Lidin-Janson, G., Sandberg, T. & Svanborg Eden, C. (1989). Bacterial adhesion as an indicator of renal involvement in bacteriuria of pregnancy. *Scandinavian Journal of Infectious Diseases*, **21**, 193–9.

Stenqvist, K., Sandberg, T., Lidin-Janson, G., Ørskov, F., Ørskov, I. & Svanborg Eden, C. (1987). Virulence factors of *Escherichia coli* in urinary isolates from pregnant women. *Journal of Infectious Diseases*, **156**, 870–7.

Strömberg, N., Marklund, B.-I., Lund, B., Ilver, D., Hamers, A., Gaastra, W., Karlsson, K.-A. & Normark, S. (1990). Host-specificity of uropathogenic *Escherichia coli* depends on differences in binding specificity to Galα 1–4Gal-containing isoreceptors. *EMBO Journal*, **9**, 2001–10.

Strömberg, N., Nyholm, P.-G., Pascher, I. & Normark, S. (1991). Saccharide orientation at the cell surface affects glycolipid receptor function. *Proceedings of the National Academy of Sciences, USA*, **88**, 9340–4.

Svanborg Eden, C. (1986). Bacterial adherence in urinary tract infections caused by *Escherichia coli*. *Scandinavian Journal of Urology and Nephrology*, **20**, 81–8.

Svanborg Eden, C. & De Man, P. (1987). Bacterial virulence in urinary tract infection. *Infectious Disease Clinincs of North America*, **1**, 731–50.

Svanborg Eden, C., Eriksson, B. & Hanson, L. A. (1977). Adhesion of *Escherichia coli* to human uroepithelia cells *in vitro*. *Infection and Immunity*, **18**, 767–74.

Svanborg Eden, C., Eriksson, B., Hanson, L. A., Jodal, U., Kaijser, B., Lidin Janson, G., Lindberg, U. & Olling, S. (1978a). Adhesion to normal human uroepithelial cells of *Escherichia coli* from children with various forms of urinary tract infection. *Journal of Pediatrics*, **93**, 398–403.

Svanborg Eden, C., Freter, R., Hagberg, L., Hull, R., Hull, S., Leffler, H. & Schoolnik, G. (1982). Inhibition of experimental ascending urinary tract infection by an epithelial cell-surface receptor analogue. *Nature*, **298**, 560–2.

Svanborg Eden, C. & Hansson, H. A. (1978b). *Escherichia coli* pili as possible mediators of attachment to human urinary tract epithelial cells. *Infection and Immunity*, **21**, 229–37.

Svanborg Eden, C., Jodal, U., Hanson, L. A., Lindberg, U. & Akerlund, A. S. (1976). Variable adherence to normal human urinary-tract epithelial cells of *Escherichia coli* strains associated with various forms of urinary tract infection. *Lancet*, **ii**, 490–2.

Svenson, S. B., Hultberg, H., Kallenius, G., Korhonen, T. K., Mollby, R. & Winberg, J. (1983). P-fimbriae of pyelonephritogenic *Escherichia coli*: identification and chemical characterization of receptors. *Infection*, **11**, 61–67.

Svenson, S. B., Kallenius, G., Mollby, R., Hultberg, H. & Winberg, J. (1982). Rapid identification of P-fimbriated *Escherichia coli* by a receptor-specific particle agglutination test. *Infection*, **10**, 209–214.

Swanson, T. N., Bilge, S. S., Nowicki, B. & Moseley, S. L. (1991). Molecular structure of the Dr adhesin: nucleotide sequence and mapping of receptor-binding domain by use of fusion constructs. *Infection and Immunity*, **59**, 261–8.

Swenson, D. L., Bukanov, N. O., Berg, D. E. & Welch, R. A. (1996). Two pathogenicity islands in urpathogenic *Escherichia coli* J96: cosmid cloning and sample sequencing. *Infection and Immunity*, **64**, 3736–43.

Tambic, T., Oberiter, V., Delmis, J. & Tambic, A. (1992). Diagnostic value of a P-fimbriation test in determining duration of therapy in children with urinary tract infections. *Clinical Theurapeutics*, **14**, 667–71.

Taylor, P. W. (1976). Immunochemical investigations on lipopolysaccharides and acidic polysaccharides from serum-sensitive and serum-resistant strains of *Escherichia coli* isolated from urinary-tract infections. *Journal of Medical Microbiology*, **9**, 405–21.

Taylor, P. W. (1983). Bactericidal and bacteriolytic activity of serum against gram-negative bacteria. *Microbiological Reviews*, **47**, 46–83.

Timmis, K. N., Boulnois, G. J., Bitter-Suermann, D. & Cabello, F. C. (1985). Surface components of *Escherichia coli* that mediate resistance to the bactericidal activities of serum and phagocytes. *Current Topics in Microbiology and Immunology*, **118**, 197–218.

Tippet, P., Andrews, P. W., Knowles, B. B., Solter, D. & Goodfellow, P. N. (1986). Red cell antigens P (globoside) and Luke: identification by monoclonal antibodies defining the murine stage specific embryonic antigens-3 and -4 (SSEA-3 and -4). *Vox Sanguinis*, **51**, 53–6.

Tomisawa, S., Kogure, T., Kuroume, T., Leffler, H., Lomberg, H., Shimabukoro, N., Terao, K. & Svanborg Eden, C. (1989). P blood group and proneness to urinary tract infection in Japanese children. *Scandinavian Journal of Infectious Diseases*, **21**, 403–8.

Topley, N., Steadman, R., Mackenzie, R., Knowlden, J. M. & Williams, J. D. (1989). Type 1 fimbriate strains of *Escherichia coli* initiate renal parenchymal scarring. *Kidney International*, **36**, 609–16.

Tullus, K., Brauner, A., Fryklund, B., Munkhammar, T., Rabsch, W., Reissbrodt, R. & Burman, L. G. (1992). Host factors *versus* virulence-associated bacterial characteristics in neonatal and infantile bacteraemia and meningitis caused by *Escherichia coli*. *Journal of Medical Microbiology*, **36**, 203–8.

Tullus, K., Fryklund, B., Berglund, B., Kallenius, G. & Burman, L. G. (1988). Influence of age on faecal carriage of P-fimbriated *Escherichia coli* and other gram-negative bacteria in hospitalized neonates. *Journal of Hospital Infection*, **11**, 349–56.

Tullus, K., Horlin, K., Svenson, S. B. & Kallenius, G. (1984). Epidemic outbreaks of acute pyelonephritis caused by nosocomial spread of P fimbriated *Escherichia coli* in children. *Journal of Infectious Diseases*, **150**, 728–36.

Tullus, K., Jacobson, S. H., Katouli, M. & Brauner, A. (1991). Relative importance of eight virulence characteristics of pyelonephritogenic *Escherichia coli* strains assessed by multivariate statistical analysis. *Journal of Urology*, **146**, 1153–5.

Turck, M., Petersdorf, R. G. & Fournier, M. R. (1962). The epidemiology of non-enteric *Escherichia coli* infections: prevalence of serological groups. *Journal of Clinical Investigation*, **41**, 1760–5.

Vahlne, G. (1945). Occurrence of Bact. coli under normal and pathological conditions, with special reference to the antigenic aspects. *Acta Pathologica et Microbiologica Scandinavica*, **63**, 1–127.

Vaisanen, V., Elo, J., Tallgren, L. G., Siitonen, A., Makela, P. H., Svanborg Eden, C., Kallenius, G., Svenson, S. B., Hultberg, H. & Korhonen, T. (1981). Mannose-resistant haemagglutination and P antigen recognition are characteristics of *Escherichia coli* causing pyelonephritis. *Lancet*, **ii**, 1366–9.

Vaisanen-Rhen, V. (1984a). Fimbria-like hemagglutinin of *Escherichia coli* O75 strains. *Infection and Immunity*, **46**, 401–7.

Vaisanen-Rhen, V., Elo, J., Vaisanen, E., Siitonen, A., Ørskov, I., Ørskov, F., Svenson, S. B., Makela, P. H. & Korhonen, T. (1984b). P-fimbriated clones among uropathogenic *Escherichia coli* strains. *Infection and Immunity*, **43**, 149–55.

Vaisanen-Rhen, V., Korhonen, T. K. & Finne, J. (1983). Novel cell-binding activity specific for *N*-acetyl-D-glucosamine in an *Escherichia coli* strain. *Science*, **159**, 233–6.

Van den Bosch, J. F., de Graaff, J. & MacLaren, D. M. (1979). Virulence of *Escherichia coli* in experimental hematogenous pyelonephritis in mice. *Infection and Immunity*, **25**, 68–74.

Van den Bosch, J. F., Postma, P., Koopman, P. A. R., de Graff, J. & MacLaren, D. M. (1982). Virulence of urinary and faecal *Escherichia coli* in relation to serotype, haemolysin and haemagglutination. *Journal of Hygiene, Cambridge*, **88**, 567–77.

Van den Bosch, J. F., Verboom-Sohmer, U., Postma, P., de Graaff, J. & MacLaren, D. M. (1980). Mannose-sensitive and mannose-resistant adherence to human uroepithelial cells and urinary virulence of *Escherichia coli*. *Infection and Immunity*, **29**, 226–33.

Van Die, I., Hoekstra, W. & Bergmans, H. (1987). Analysis of the primary structure of P-fimbrillins of uropathogenic *Escherichia coli*. *Microbial Pathogenesis*, **3**, 149–54.

Van Die, I., van Megen, I., Zuidweg, E., Hoekstra, W., de Ree, H., Van den Bosch, H. & Bergmans, H. (1986). Functional relationship among the gene clusters encoding $F7_1$, $F7_2$, F9, and F11 fimbriae of human uropathogenic *Escherichia coli*. *Journal of Bacteriology*, **167**, 407–10.

Van Dijk, W. C., Verbrugh, H. A., Peters, R., van der Tol, M. E., Petersin, P. K. & Verhoef, J. (1978). *Escherichia coli* K antigen in relation to serum-induced lysis and phagocytosis. *Journal of Medical Microbiology*, **10**, 123–30.

Van Dijk, W. C., Verbrugh, H. A., van der Tol, M. E., Peters, R. & Verhoef, J. (1979). Role of *Escherichia coli* K capsular antigens during complement activation, C3 fixation, and opsonization. *Infection and Immunity*, **25**, 603–9.

Vermeulen, C., Cross, A., Byrne, W. R. & Zollinger, W. (1988). Quantitative relationship between capsular content and killing of K1-encapsulated *Escherichia coli*. *Infection and Immunity*, **56**, 2723–30.

Verweij-van Vught, A. M. J. J., Van den Bosch, J. F., Namavar, F., Sparrius, M. & MacLaren, D. M. (1983). K antigens of *Escherichia coli* and virulence in urinary tract infection: studies in a mouse model. *Journal of Medical Microbiology*, **16**, 147–55.

Virkola, R. (1987). Binding characteristics of *Escherichia coli* type 1 fimbriae in the human kidney. *FEMS Microbiology Letters*, **40**, 257–62.

Virkola, R., Parkkinen, J., Hacker, J. & Korhonen, T. K. (1993). Sialyloligosaccharide chains of laminin as an extracellular matrix target for S fimbriae of *Escherichia coli*. *Infection and Immunity*, **61**, 4480–4.

Virkola, R., Westerlund, B., Holthofer, H., Parkkinen, J., Kekomaki, M. & Korhonen, T. K. (1988). Binding characteristics of *Escherichia coli* adhesins in human urinary bladder. *Infection and Immunity*, **56**, 2615–22.

Waalwijk, C., MacLaren, DM. & de Graaf, J. (1983). In vivo function of hemolysin in the nephropathogenicity of *Escherichia coli*. *Infection and Immunity*, **42**, 245–9.

Waters, V. L. & Crosa, J. H. (1991). Colicin V virulence plasmids. *Microbiological Reviews*, **55**, 437–50.

Weiser, J. N. & Gotschlich, E. C. (1991). Outer membrane protein A (OmpA) contributes to serum resistance and pathogenicity of *Escherichia coli* K-1. *Infection and Immunity*, **59**, 2252–8.

Welch, R. A. (1991). Pore-forming cytolysins of Gram-negative bacteria. *Molecular Microbiology*, **5**, 521–8.

Westerlund, B., Kuusela, P., Risteli, J., Risteli, L., Vartio, T., Rauvala, H., Virkola, R. & Korhonen, T. K. (1989). The O75X adhesin of uropathogenic *Escherichia coli* is a type IV collagen-binding protein. *Molecular Microbiology*, **3**, 329–37.

Westerlund, B., Siitonen, A., Elo, J., Williams, P. H., Korhonen, T. K. & Makela, P. H. (1988). Properties of *Escherichia coli* isolates from urinary tract infections in boys. *Journal of Infectious Diseases*, **158**, 996–1002.

Williams, P. H. (1979). Novel iron uptake system specified by ColV plasmids: an important component in the virulence of invasive strains of *Escherichia coli*. *Infection and Immunity*, **26**, 925–32.

Williams, P. H. & Warner, P. J. (1980). ColV plasmid-mediated, colicin V-independent iron uptake system of invasive strains of *Escherichia coli*. *Infection and Immunity*, **29**, 11–16.

Wold, A. E., Caugant, D. A., Lidin-Janson, G., de Man, P. & Svanborg, C. (1992). Resident colonic *Escherichia coli* strains frequently display uropathogenic characteristics. *Journal of Infectious Diseases*, **165**, 46–52.

Wold, A. E., Mestecky, J., Tomana, M., Kobata, A., Ohbayashi, H., Endo, T. & Svanborg Eden, C. (1990). Secretory immunoglobulin A carries oligosaccharide receptors for *Escherichia coli* type 1 fimbrial lectin. *Infection and Immunity*, **58**, 3073–7.

Wold, A. E., Thorssen, M., Hull, S. & Svanborg Eden, C. (1988). Attachment of *Escherichia coli* via mannose- or Galα1–4Galβ-containing receptors to human colonic epithelial cells. *Infection and Immunity*, **56**, 2531–7.

Yamamoto, T., Fujita, K. & Yokota, T. (1990). Adherence characteristics to human small intestinal mucosa of *Escherichia coli* isolated from patients with diarrhea or urinary tract infections. *Journal of Infectious Diseases*, **162**, 896–908.

Zingler, G., Blum, G., Falkenhagen, U., Ørskov, I., Ørskov, F., Hacker, J. &

Ott, M. (1993). Clonal differentiation of uropathogenic *Escherichia coli* isolates of serotype O6:K5 by fimbrial antigen typing and DNA long-range mapping techniques. *Medical Microbiology and Immunology*, **182**, 13–24.

Zingler, G., Ott, M., Blum, G., Falkenhagen, U., Naumann, G., Sokolowska-Köhler & W. Hacker, J. (1992). Clonal analysis of *Escherichia coli* serotype O6 strains from urinary tract infections. *Microbial Pathogenesis*, **12**, 299–310.

Zingler, G., Schmidt, F., Ørskov, I., Ørskov, F., Falktenhagen, U. & Naumann, G. (1990). K-antigen identification, hemolysin production, and hemagglutination types of *Escherichia coli* O6 strains isolated from patients with urinary tract infections. *Zentralblatt fur Bakteriologie und Hygiene A*, **274**, 372–81.

Part four

Responses to infection

19

Cellular activation by uropathogenic *Escherichia coli*

R. STEADMAN and N. TOPLEY

The vast majority of urinary tract infections are due to strains of *Escherichia coli* that have a unique ability to colonise the urinary tract and initiate covert (asymptomatic) and symptomatic infections. During the last 30 years the 'theory of special pathogenicity' has become firmly established to account for the virulence of *E. coli* in the urinary tract (Johnson, 1991; and see Chapter 18).

It has become evident that the process of bacterial attachment to the periurethral, bladder and kidney mucosa, and the interaction of *E. coli* with phagocytic cells attracted to these sites in the course of inflammatory reactions may be crucial to the outcome of the process of infection. Since it is clear that urinary tract infection represents a heterogeneous group of conditions, an understanding of the processes of inflammation at particular sites is essential for an understanding of the extent and progress of tissue damage in the urinary tract.

Three well-recognised barriers protect the host from infection by micro-organisms: (i) the mechanical barrier provided by the skin and mucosa, (ii) the barrier provided by a range of non-specific cidal substances, such as complement, present in body fluids, and (iii) the action of circulating and tissue-localised phagocytic cells. Mononuclear and polymorphonuclear phagocytes (neutrophils) circulate in the peripheral blood and migrate through the endothelium of the microvasculature to sites of infection and inflammation. This migration is directed by chemotactic agents released by a variety of cells at the endothelium and subendothelial interstitium, and is facilitated by the increased expression of adhesion molecules on the migrating and local cell populations. Infiltrating phagocytic cells actively ingest micro-organisms and other foreign particles and have potent antimicrobial systems that kill and digest the internalised particles. Phagocytic cells also have the capacity to elaborate mechanisms for the control and co-ordination of the inflammatory response, a property particularly exemplified by macrophages, which synthesise a wide variety of inflammatory mediators and cytokines.

It has become increasingly apparent that, in addition to the central role of leucocytes in inflammation, mucosal surfaces participate directly in the control of inflammatory processes. In this respect, epithelial cells that line the bowel and respiratory tract, and mesothelial cells that line the pleural and peritoneal spaces contribute to the control of inflammation by the secretion of cytokines and expression of adhesion molecules that are important in the recruitment and margination of leucocytes (Madara, 1990; Goodman *et al.*, 1992; Topley *et al.*, 1993). Thus, the activation and control of the inflammatory processes in response to infection are a complex, but co-ordinated, series of events that involve tissue cells as well as circulating and tissue-resident phagocytes. The goal of this cascade is to eliminate the infecting organism and maintain tissue integrity. However, the results of uncontrolled inflammation may be physical and functional damage to the surrounding tissues.

Inflammatory events in the urinary tract

Infections of the lower and upper urinary tract may be acute or chronic. Although the vast majority are caused by a single bacterial species, *E. coli*, the outcome in terms of symptoms and tissue damage may vary. This has led to a search for the bacterial virulence markers responsible for, or associated with, these conditions and also for the possible host factors that predispose to infections of the urinary tract.

Symptomatic infection, cystitis or acute pyelonephritis, of the anatomically normal urinary tract does not usually result in long-term tissue damage. Both conditions result in the activation of inflammatory events, characterised, in the case of cystitis, by local symptoms, such as frequency of micturition and dysuria and, in acute pyelonephritis, by systemic markers of inflammation, including raised body temperature, increased concentrations of acute phase proteins and raised erythrocyte sedimentation rate. These events are accompanied by the migration of large numbers of leucocytes into the urine (pyuria). The acute inflammatory process is sufficient to eradicate infection without damage to host tissues, and there is no proven relationship between acute pyelonephritis and the development of renal scarring.

Reflux of urine from the bladder to the kidney (vesico–ureteric reflux) in the presence of urinary tract infection or ureteric abnormalities also results in acute inflammatory activation in the kidney. In these conditions the repeated episodes of infection and inflammation are associated with renal parenchymal tissue damage and lead to the scarring characteristic of chronic pyelonephritis. The crucial initiating event in this scarring process appears, from clinical observations and animal experiments, to be the result of a single episode of acute inflammation in the neonatal kidney. Animal models suggest that reduction of inflammation by the prevention of neutrophil infiltration is sufficient to inhibit the development of renal scarring (Glauser *et al.*, 1982; Slotki & Asscher, 1982; Meylan *et al.*, 1989).

A group of individuals has been described, in whom urinary tract infection is not accompanied by symptoms. The individuals remain asymptomatic even in the presence of significant and, in some cases, long-standing bacteriuria. If their urinary tract is normal, there is no evidence that they are susceptible to renal scarring. Though covert bacteriuria can be associated with renal scarring, there is no evidence for a causative relationship (Asscher, 1980).

The activation of the inflammatory process in the urinary tract appears to have a common mechanism in the generation of signals by the urothelium, resulting in the recruitment of leucocytes from the circulation. The several possible outcomes of this process depend on the host and on the infecting organism. Moreover, it is becoming increasingly apparent that the degree of inflammation contributes to the eventual outcome of the disease process.

Activation of mucosal immunity by *Escherichia coli*

Leucocyte infiltration is characteristic of cystitis, acute pyelonephritis and reflux nephropathy. The mechanisms by which this process is initiated are poorly understood. The activation of mucosal cells by *E. coli* has been studied *in vivo* and *in vitro* and it has been demonstrated that *E. coli* can stimulate the release of cytokines (Figure 19.1) from cultured bladder and kidney uroepithelial cell lines (Agace *et al.*, 1993a,b). Inoculation of *E. coli* into the bladder of human volunteers results in increased concentrations of interleukin-6 (IL-6) in the urine (Hedges *et al.*, 1991, 1992a,b), but the response does not depend on the fimbrial phenotype of the infecting strain. More recently it has been shown that the urinary concentration of interleukin-8 (IL-8), a potent chemokine for neutrophils, is raised after infection and that the fimbrial phenotype expressed by the infecting strains determines the extent of the response

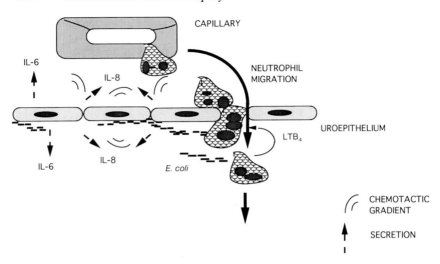

Fig. 19.1. Suggested 'cytokine' network that operates during the activation of mucosal immunity in the lower urinary tract.

(Agace *et al.*, 1993a,b). Local synthesis of IL-8 may be the mechanism by which neutrophils are attracted to the site of infection and thus it may be at least partly responsible for the characteristic pyuria associated with UTI. These observations parallel those made of the peritoneal cavity, in which IL-8 secretion by mesothelial cells is pivotal in the basolateral apical transmigration of leucocytes in response to infection (Topley *et al.*, 1993).

In many inflammatory conditions IL-6 levels are raised. This cytokine is associated with the stimulation of acute phase proteins, but the significance of its local generation in the urinary tract is unclear. In other systems, secretion of IL-6 appears to represent a response to inflammation, rather than its initiation, and it may act as an anti-inflammatory molecule that controls the synthesis of pro-inflammatory cytokines by other cell types (Andreka *et al.*, 1989; Schindler *et al.*, 1990). It is not surprising, therefore, that there is no correlation between urinary IL-6 levels and the magnitude of leucocyte infiltration (Linder *et al.*, 1991).

The degree of uroepithelial cell activation, as judged by IL-6 and IL-8 synthesis and neutrophil influx, is related to the expression of type-1 and P-fimbriae by *E. coli* (Agace *et al.*, 1993a,b). The secretion of IL-8 correlates directly with the degree of neutrophil influx. This suggests that uroepithelial secretion of IL-8 may be important in the recruitment of neutrophils and the subsequent presence of these cells in the urine, which is characteristic of acute symptomatic urinary tract infection.

The mechanism by which *E. coli* activates uroepithelial cells to stimulate the synthesis of IL-6 and IL-8 remains to be fully identified, but it is clear that a direct interaction between pathogen and uroepithelium, mediated by fimbriae, is one of the mechanisms of activation. Cytokine synthesis also occurs in the absence of a direct interaction, which suggests that soluble stimuli, possibly lipopolysaccharide or haemolysin, can also activate uroepithelial cells. Intercellular adhesion molecule-1 is of central importance in the trafficking of leucocytes to sites of inflammation (Rothlein & Wegner 1992) and it has been shown with cultured uroepithelial cells that lipopolysaccharide directly activates leucocyte clustering on the cell surface (Wille *et al*., 1992; Elgavish 1993).

The importance of host reactivity to lipopolysaccharide for mucosal immunity has also been investigated with inbred C3H/HeJ and C3H/HeN lipopolysaccharide-responder and non-responder mice (Hagberg *et al*., 1985; Shahin *et al*., 1987; Svanborg-Eden *et al*., 1988). The results suggest that, after infection with defined *E. coli* strains, responder mice, with the Lps_n, Lps_n phenotype, have a rapid influx of neutrophils into the bladder, which results in clearance of the infection. In non-responder mice with the Lps_d, Lps_d phenotype there is no such influx of neutrophils and the infection persists. This indicates that the responder phenotype is important for the mucosal clearance of Gram-negative infections and suggests that the interaction and activation of inflammatory processes at the uroepithelium are important in the outcome of infection. So far there is no evidence to suggest that such a mechanism operates in human infection, but the subject deserves further study.

Host factors and inflammation

The importance of host resistance in the unique susceptibility of certain groups of individuals to urinary tract infection is clear from epidemiological studies. This has led to the search for host characteristics, apart from anatomical abnormalities, that predispose to such infections. These include the blood group, secretor status and urine secretory immunoglobulin A (IgA) concentrations (Kinane *et al*., 1982; Lomberg *et al*., 1986; Sheinfeld *et al*., 1989; Floege *et al*., 1990).

On the basis of C-reactive protein concentration, erythrocyte sedimentation rate and body temperature, it has been suggested that non-secretors, who do not secrete blood group antigens into their body fluids, have a significantly higher inflammatory response during renal infection compared with secretors. An over-representation of non-secretors in a group of patients with scarring has been observed (Jacobsen & Lomberg, 1990) and it was concluded that the susceptibility of such individuals to renal scarring may be related to enhanced inflammatory activation in the renal parenchyma (Lomberg *et al.*, 1992).

These observations suggest that the absence of secreted blood group antigens from the environment of mucosal surfaces, in this case the uroepithelium, may lead to its increased susceptibility to attachment, colonisation and activation by *E. coli*. It is interesting that the increased activation in non-secretors appears to be independent of the expression of P-fimbriae (Lomberg *et al.*, 1992). This supports information about the prevalence of the P_1 phenotype among those susceptible to renal scarring. These data also provide evidence that *E. coli* strains that cause renal scarring are different from those responsible for other forms of urinary tract infection (Lomberg *et al.*, 1983, 1984, 1986). Similarly, in animal models of renal scarring, type-1-fimbriate *E. coli*, which cause the highest degree of leucocyte activation *in vitro*, also produce the largest renal scars (Topley *et al.*, 1989). On the other hand, P-fimbriate and non-fimbriate *E. coli* did not activate leucocytes *in vitro* and did not produce significant renal scarring.

Leucocyte activation by *Escherichia coli*

The binding of opsonised and, in some cases, non-opsonised bacteria to leucocytes can result in a series of responses aimed at killing and eliminating the micro-organism. The most rapid of these responses is the activation of the respiratory burst, a process primarily responsible for the bactericidal activity of leucocytes (Weiss, 1989). This results in a rapid increase in the consumption of molecular oxygen that is used by a membrane-bound reduced nicotinamide adenine dinucleotide phosphate (NADPH) oxidase present in leucocytes to generate superoxide anions and other bactericidal oxygen radicals (Jones *et al.*, 1993). After phagocytosis, ingested bacteria are killed in phagosomes by the combined action of these reactive oxygen species and potent lysosomal proteases and hydrolases.

Activation of the respiratory burst by a variety of stimuli, including bacteria, has been extensively studied (Öhman *et al.*, 1982; Svanborg-Eden *et al.*, 1984), often by the measurement of phagocyte chemiluminescence, which reflects the magnitude of the respiratory burst (Figure 19.2).

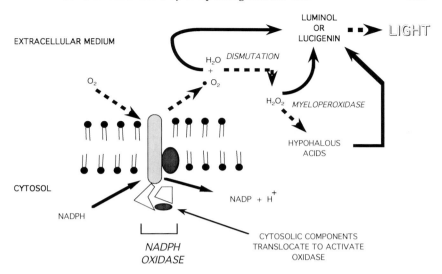

Fig. 19.2. Respiratory burst activation in leucocytes involves the break-down of molecular oxygen by a membrane-bound oxidase to form the superoxid radical $.O_2$. The oxidase is active only when fully assembled with components that are translocated from the cytoplasm. The super-oxide anion may be converted non-enzymatically, or by the action of superoxide dismutase, to H_2O_2, which in turn is converted into potent antibacterial hypohalous acids by the action of myeloperoxidase. Any of these highly reactive metabolites will react with luminescent reagents, such as luminol or lucigenin, to generate light which can be used as a measure of the respiratory burst.

In the case of *E. coli*, type-1-fimbriate organisms have usually been used. Non-opsonised type-1-fimbriate *E. coli* bind to and activate leucocytes (Silverblatt *et al.*, 1979; Blumenstock & Jann, 1982; Goetz, 1987, 1989) and activation can be reproduced with purified type-1 fimbriae, which supports the importance of fimbriae in the activation process (Goetz, 1989).

Neutrophil degranulation in response to Escherichia coli

The interaction of type-1-fimbriate *E coli* with neutrophils also results in the triggering of lysosomal granule exocytosis (Steadman *et al.*, 1988). This interaction may be thought of as being primarily involved in the intracellular killing and digestion of ingested organisms, but, in addition, reactive oxygen products and the contents of the lysosomal granules released extracellularly also increase the potential for damage to

Table 19.1. *The lysosomal granule contents of the human neutrophil*

Primary (Azurophil)	Secondary (Specific)	Gelatinase
Myeloperoxidase	Collagenase	Gelatinase
Elastase	Gelatinase	Acetyltransferase
Cathepsins (incl. cathepsin G)	Lysosyme (?)	
Proteinase-3	Sialidase	
Azurocidin	Heparanase	
α1-Antitrypsin	Histaminase	
Glycerophosphatases	Lysosyme	
Defensins	Plasminogen activator	
Bactericidal permeability	β2-microglobulin	
increasing protein		
α-mannosidase	Lactoferrin	
N-acetyl-β-glucosaminidase	Transcobalamin	
Sialidase		
β-glucuronidase		
Heparin-binding protein		
Ubiquitin		

surrounding tissues (Steadman *et al.*, 1988; Topley *et al.*, 1989; Weiss, 1989).

Neutrophils contain at least three different types of lysosomal granule, characterised by morphology and differences in enzyme content (Table 19.1). Primary (azurophilic) granules contain a variety of hydrolases and proteases, including elastase and cathepsin G. Human neutrophil elastase is a potent serine protease with broad substrate specificity against most extracellular matrix proteins (Weiss, 1989; Heck *et al.*, 1990; Steadman *et al.*, 1993). Other antibacterial proteins present in primary granules are lysozyme, bactericidal permeability increasing protein (BPI) and other antimicrobial cationic proteins, including the low-molecular-weight defensins. Myeloperoxidase (MPO), which converts the hydrogen peroxide produced by superoxide dismutase into antibacterial hypohalous acids, is also present in these granules (Weiss, 1989). Secondary granules contain collagenase and gelatinase and other proteins, such as lactoferrin and transcobalamin, but their role in inflammation is unclear. Tertiary granules appear mainly to be gelatinase stores. They share with secondary granules a role in the up-regulation of plasma membrane-associated adhesion proteins, such as CD11b/CD18, and receptors for matrix proteins, such as laminin, collagen and fibronectin. These proteins are inserted in the inner face of the granule membranes and are translocated to the cell surface when the granules fuse with the plasma membrane to release their contents. The activation of the respiratory burst and the comprehensive exocytosis of all types of lysosomal granules result from the binding of type-1-fimbriate strains of *E. coli* (Steadman *et al.*, 1988; Topley *et al.*, 1989). Non-fimbriate strains or strains of other fimbrial type, do not activate a respiratory burst and lead to the release of secondary and tertiary granules independently of primary granules.

There is a correlation between the size and severity of scarring in response to *E. coli in vivo* and the release of superoxide and proteases from neutrophils incubated with the same strains *in vitro* (Topley *et al.*, 1989). Many of the proteolytic enzymes released from activated neutrophils are also associated with tissue damage in a variety of other inflammatory   diseases,   such   as   rheumatoid   arthritis   and glomerulonephritis.

Neutrophil activation with phenotypically modified Escherichia coli

Since type-1-fimbriate *E. coli* are potent activators of the respiratory burst and of leucocyte degranulation, the ability of a variety of *E. coli* strains, grown under various conditions, to modulate fimbrial expression and to activate neutrophil chemiluminescence has been investigated. Since only strains that expressed this adhesin significantly activated the respiratory burst, the importance of type-1 fimbriae was confirmed. Non-fimbriate strains and those that expressed only P-fimbriae did not activate neutrophils (Topley *et al.*, 1989) (Figure 19.3).

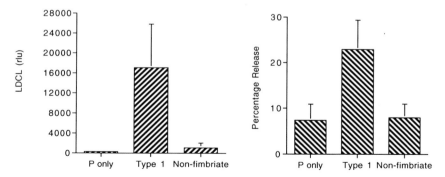

Fig. 19.3. Activation of the human neutrophil respiratory and neutral protease release burst by uropathogenic strains of *Escherichia coli* of different fimbrial phenotypes. LDCL, luminol-dependent chemiluminescence.

Binding *of* Escherichia coli *to leucocyte surface proteins*

A number of glycoproteins have been isolated from leucocyte membranes that bind type-1 fimbriae in a mannoseinhibitable manner (Rodrigues-Ortega *et al.*, 1987; Gabarah *et al.*, 1991). These include the leucocyte integrin chains CD11a, CD11b, CD11c and CD18. It is clear, however, that Fc receptor expression is also important for the binding of type-1 fimbriae, but not for the binding of strains that bear other fimbriae (Fine *et al.*, 1980; Wright & Jong, 1986; Salmon *et al.*, 1987). It may well be that these receptors are targeted by type-1-fimbriate *E. coli* simply because they are glycoproteins rich in mannoside residues. On the other hand, the binding of non-type-1-fimbriate organisms seems to depend only on the presence on the neutrophil surface of the leucocyte integrin CD11b/CD18 (CR3) and the complement receptor CR1 (CD35) (Steadman *et al.*, 1991); such binding is not inhibited by mannose and the mechanism of this interaction has yet to be elucidated. Human macrophages also bind type-1-fimbriate *E. coli* in a mannose-dependent manner (Boner *et al.*, 1989).

Surface charge and hydrophobicity

Polysaccharide capsules expressed by strains of *E. coli* inhibit phagocytosis (Øhman *et al.*, 1982) and abolish the capacity of the organisms to trigger neutrophil activation (Steadman *et al.*, 1990a,b). It has, therefore, been suggested that physico-chemical factors, such as net surface charge or surface hydrophobicity, may affect the response of inflammatory cells to *E. coli* (Stendahl *et al.*, 1981; Öhman *et al.*, 1982). Although type-1 fimbriae are hydrophobic structures, there is no correlation between the relative surface hydrophobicity of *E. coli* and neutrophil activation (Steadman *et al.*, 1989). Electrostatic forces have, however, been shown to play an important role in the selective uptake of charged particles by phagocytes and in controlling intercellular contact (Papdimitriou, 1982; Mutsaers & Papdimitriou, 1988). The cationic amino-acid homopolymer poly (L-lysine) [(Lyes)$_n$ neutralises cell surface negative charges and facilitates the activation of leucocytes in several systems (Shier *et al.*, 1984; Pugliese *et al.*, 1987,1989). Furthermore, neutralisation of membrane charge with poly-cations augments the phagocytosis of Gram-positive organisms (Peterson *et al.*, 1984). Poly (L-lysine) also enhances the neutrophil response to strains of *E. coli* that do not express type-1 fimbriae, including strains that express only P-fimbriae. However, responses that depend on type-1 fimbriae are inhibited by similar amounts of PLL. Since these effects were observed with all strains tested, it seems reasonable to regard them as independent of other differences in outer membrane or capsule composition. The effect of PLL was also reversed by the polyanion heparin, which suggests that the effect was related solely to changes in net surface charge, rather than to specific irreversible changes in the neutrophil membrane (Steadman *et al.*, 1990a). While type-1-fimbriate *E. coli* activate neutrophils specifically, non-specific activation that depends on neutralisation of neutrophil surface charges may result from activation by non-fimbriate organisms or organisms that express fimbriae with a different adhesin specificity.

α-Haemolysin

Many pathogenic strains of *E. coli* cause lysis of erythrocytes by the production of haemolysins. This may be useful for the sequestration of iron, which is essential for bacterial growth (see Chapter 12). Indeed, in animal models, production of haemolysin is associated with pathogenicity. Three different haemolysins have been isolated from *E. coli*. The α-haemolysin is the only truly secreted protein of *E. coli*, while the β-haemolysin, which is antigenically distinct from α-haemolysin, remains cell associated. The λ-haemolysin is produced by *E. coli* mutants that are resistant to nalidixic acid (Smith, 1963; Watton & Smith, 1969). Apart from erythrocytes, mouse fibroblasts and human leucocytes are also lysed by α-haemolysin with kinetics similar to those of erythrocyte lysis (Cavalieri & Snyder, 1982a,b,c). There appears to be a rank order of leucocyte susceptibility to α-haemolysin: monocytes are the most susceptible and lymphocytes are less so. At non-lytic concentrations, α-haemolysin reduces neutrophil phagocytosis and chemotaxis, while at the same time the respiratory burst is activated with resultant generation of potentially toxic oxygen radicals (Cavalieri & Snyder, 1982b,c). The *E. coli* haemolysins are considered in detail in Chapter 11.

In addition to its cytolytic activity, α-haemolysin stimulates arachidonic acid mobilisation and activates the leucocyte 5-lipoxygenase pathway (Scheffer *et al.*, 1985; König *et al.*, 1986). This results in the generation of leukotrienes, many of which possess potent biological properties. Leukotriene synthesis has been demonstrated *in vivo* during experimental *E. coli* infection, and probably involves co-operation between leucocytes and the vascular endothelium (Grimminger *et al.*, 1990). Cloned *E. coli* strains and plasmid-transformed strains have been used to study the effect of α-haemolysin production on the stimulation of human and rat leucocytes. Uropathogenic *E. coli* generate leukotriene B$_4$ (LTB$_4$) production by human neutrophils and monocytes in a dose- and time-dependent manner (Steadman *et al.*, 1990b). The neutrophil response does not, however, depend on the fimbrial type, nor is it associated with an increasing haemolytic potential of the stimulating strains, but the monocyte response correlates strongly with the haemolytic activity of the strains.

While α-haemolysin is generated during exponential growth of *E. coli* (Springer & Goebel, 1980), fimbriae are optimally expressed in the stationary phase (Eisenstein, 1981). Adjustment of the growth conditions for the optimal suppression or enhancement of fimbrial expression makes no difference to the ability of *E. coli* to activate 5-lipoxygenase activity in neutrophils. This suggests that haemolytic activity is quantitatively related to activation of the 5-lipoxygenase pathway of monocytes, but not that of neutrophils. Since non-haemolytic strains, strains that lack type-1 fimbriae and those in the stationary phase generate immuno-reactive LTB$_4$ from neutrophils, it seems likely that a mechanism independent of type-1 fimbrial adherence or α-haemolysin is also involved in 5-lipoxygenase activation by these organisms. The nature of this mechanism is unknown.

The role of cytokines in the amplification of neutrophil activation

Activation of neutrophils by IgG-coated particles via the Fc receptor (Fitzharris *et al.*, 1987) and by zymosan, via complement receptor type 3 (CD11b/CD18)(Williams *et al.*, 1985, 1986), results in independently regulated effector responses. In addition, complement activation and Fc receptor functions that lead to monocyte and macrophage phagocytosis of opsonised *E. coli* are enhanced as a result of cell binding to the extracellular matrix.

The inflammatory cytokine tumour necrosis factor-α (TNF-α) increases the expression of the CD11/CD18 family of adhesion proteins and CR1 (CD35) on neutrophils (Berger *et al.*, 1988). We have used TNF-α to differentiate between responses to *E. coli* strains that express particular adhesins and found that augmentation of neutrophil responses was highly selective (Petersen *et al.*, 1990; Steadman *et al.*, 1990c), but the intracellular mechanism of stimulation by TNF-α has not so far been elucidated. Recombinant human TNF-α selectively augments neutrophil responses to uropathogenic strains of *E. coli* that do not express type-1 fimbriae (Steadman *et al.*, 1991). In many cases the generation of LTB_4 increases in a synergistic fashion from undetectable levels. In addition, the release of vitamin B_{12}-binding protein from the secondary granule is increased additively above control levels. This suggests that a specific cell surface/bacterium interaction is augmented in neutrophils after pre-treatment with TNF-α, and that the response is selective. This augmentation is not inhibited by the increase in capsule expression when these strains are grown in Vogel Bonner's modified medium. After pre-treatment with TNF-α, however, the response of neutrophil LTB_4 to encapsulated strains is augmented, which emphasises the potential of this cytokine for selective amplification of the inflammatory response. Pre-treatment with TNF-α does not augment neutrophil activation by type-1-fimbriate strains at concentrations that augment responses to strains that do not express these fimbriae. These amounts of TNF-α are also optimal for the augmentation of neutrophil responses to zymosan (Petersen *et al.*, 1990; Steadman *et al.*, 1990c).

Lipopolysaccharide

Lipopolysaccharide (LPS) is a component of the outer membrane of Gram-negative bacteria (see Chapter 5). The lipid A moiety of LPS is a potent toxin that is released during bacterial cell death, including during infection. It is an extremely effective activator of host defence mechanisms, resulting in the release of inflammatory mediators, including prostaglandins and cytokines, and complement activation (Westphal *et al.*, 1982; Jann & Jann, 1985). These properties of lipid A may be mediated independently by different parts of the molecule and both its lipid side chain and its carbohydrate backbone may be involved (Matsuura *et al.*, 1986). The stimulation of responses via the classical complement pathway has been ascribed to lipid A, while those via the alternative pathway may be activated by the polysaccharide side chains. The specific interaction of LPS with inflammatory cells is mediated by the binding of LPS and its serum binding protein to CD14 on the leucocyte surface. The latter is a GPI-linked 50-kDa glycoprotein. Blocking antibodies to CD14 inhibit the LPS-dependent release of cytokines from macrophages and reduce the up-regulation of neutrophil CR3-dependent adhesion that results from LPS treatment. The signalling mechanisms resulting from this interaction have not been identified.

Phase variation and cellular activation

An array of antigenic structures is expressed by *E. coli in vivo* and *in vitro*. Phase variation is one process by which expression of surface structures is rapidly and independently changed. The interaction of *E. coli* with phagocytic cells, particularly *in vivo*, is therefore likely to be a highly complex process. For this reason, much of the experimental work on the activation of phagocytic cells by *E. coli* has been designed to ensure that the organisms are of a specific phenotype.

Modulation of bacterial structure

Rapid variations may take place in the expression of surface structures in bacterial populations (Swaney *et al.*, 1977; Ørskov *et al.*, 1979; Swansen & Barrera, 1983). These phenomena include, for example, phase variation due to changes at the level of DNA transcription, and form variation due to post-transcriptional changes. Phase variation results in the modification of structural protein synthesis, such as expression of fimbriae, while form variation results in alterations in non-protein components, such as capsular polysaccharide antigens. The precise mechanisms by which these processes are regulated remain to be identified, but it is evident that they take place *in vivo*(Nowicki *et al.*, 1984; Lichodziejewska *et al.*, 1989). Thus, the proportion of P-fimbriate bacteria present in infected urine is subject to constant change that may affect the way in which organisms are recognised and handled by the host.

Phase variation in the type-1 fimbriation of *E. coli* was described by Brinton (1959) and was characterised by Swaney *et al.* (1977). All the members of an *E. coli* population contained the genetic information for type-1 fimbriae, but only part of the population expressed these structures at any time and the number of fimbriae per cell was also subject to considerable variation. It was concluded that two mechanisms were operative, true phase variation resulting from tight control of gene expression and phenotypic variation ('qualitative regulation'). Both mechanisms were completely separate from true mutation, since all the variants contained the genetic information to produce fimbriae. The two processes are not, however, mutually exclusive, because both are affected by environmental influences, including temperature, growth phase and medium composition, such as culture in liquid versus solid medium. The genetic basis of phase variation is complex. Eisenstein (1981), using a gene fusion technique, demonstrated that the expression of a fused *lac/pil* operon system oscillated, suggesting that the phase variation between fimbriate and non-fimbriate states was under transcriptional control. This oscillation appeared to be an all-or-none phenomenon, between the expressed and the non-expressed state of the gene. The calculated transition rates between type-1-fimbriate and non-fimbriate expression, and *vice versa*, were 1/1000 bacteria per generation and 3/1000 bacteria per generation, respectively. Eisenstein (1981) postulated that phase variation was likely to be an important mechanism in the pathogenicity of *E. coli*. Abraham *et al.* (1985) confirmed that this oscillation of type-1 fimbrial synthesis occurs at the transcriptional level and that, for a single laboratory strain of *E. coli* (K-12), the switch from 'on' to 'off' is due to the inversion of a specific segment of genomic DNA.

Phase variation has also been shown to occur with other *E. coli* fimbrial types (Rhen *et al.*, 1983). It has been demonstrated, with the pyelonephritogenic *E. coli* strain KS71 that had previously been shown to contain four different fimbrial antigens, that rapid phase variation takes place between alternate fimbrial antigens (Nowicki *et al.*, 1984, 1985). These workers concluded that this phase variation is more rapid than that previously described for the flagella of *Salmonella* spp. Kinetic and functional analysis of this rapid phase variation showed that the different fimbrial types occurred mainly on separate bacterial cells and that the rate of change between fimbrial types or between fimbrial and non-fimbrial phases could be as rapid as 1.6/100 bacteria per generation (Nowicki *et al.*, 1984, 1985).

It is quite clear that modulation of surface expression of fimbriae occurs in response to changes in growth conditions. Our experiments on modulation by growth in broth, as against solid media, resulted in different patterns of fimbrial expression in genotypically identical *E. coli* strains. These changes resulted in significant differences in the ability of *E. coli* to activate the respiratory burst, degranulation and to initiate renal scarring in an animal chronic pyelonephritis model (Topley *et al.*, 1989). These results, when taken together with observations by Lichodziejewska *et al.* (1989) and those of Nowicki *et al.* (1984), which show that phase variation occurs *in vivo*, strongly suggest that this may be an important determinant of the degree of cell activation by *E. coli* strains.

The consequences *in vivo* of leucocyte activation by *Escherichia coli*

The induction of renal parenchymal scars by *E. coli* depends directly on the expression of type-1 fimbriae. Neutrophil activation is essential for the initiation of the tissue damage that precedes the formation of the scars characteristic of chronic pyelonephritis (Bille & Glauser, 1982; Slotki & Asscher, 1982; Meylan *et al.*, 1989; Topley *et al.*, 1989). In an animal model of chronic pyelonephritis, there is a very close correlation between the ability of strains of *E. coli* to activate the neutrophil respiratory burst and lysosomal exocytosis, and the degree of scarring produced (Figure 19.4). In the absence of scarring there is, however, an extensive inflammatory infiltrate in response to non-fimbriate or P-fimbriate organisms. Thus, neutrophil recruitment alone, even in the damaged kidney, is not sufficient to activate the scarring process and the inflammation associated with these non-fimbriate or P-fimbriate organisms does not initiate renal scarring.

In acute pyelonephritis, *E. coli* colonises the upper urinary tract as part of an ascending infection and, we have noted above, the inflammatory response is probably initiated by mucosal activation. It is well established that *E. coli* strains that express P-fimbriae are associated with this form of urinary tract infection (Lomberg *et al.*, 1983). This condition in adults is not, however, associated with renal scarring (Lomberg *et al.*, 1984, 1986, 1989; Topley *et al.*, 1989). This appears to indicate that activation of

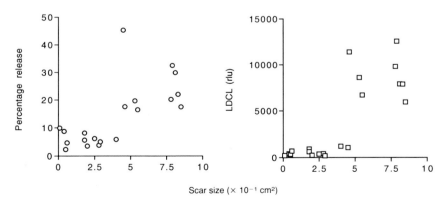

Fig. 19.4. Correlation of scar size in a model of chronic pyelonephritis with neutrophil neutral protease release and chemiluminescence *in vitro* in response to the same *Escherichia coli* strains. LDCL, luminol-dependent chemiluminescence.

inflammation by these organisms alone is insufficient to initiate the scarring. The organisms responsible for scar formation are genotypically distinct from those that cause acute pyelonephritis in the unobstructed urinary tract (Lomberg *et al.*, 1984, 1989; Johnson, 1991). This suggests that the factors responsible for activation of the degree of inflammation required to initiate the scarring process are distinct from those that enable *E. coli* to activate inflammation in the normal urinary tract and/or that the degree of activation is modulated by other host factors.

Organisms that do not express type-1 adhesins *in vitro* do not initiate a respiratory burst and do not stimulate the release of the potentially tissue-damaging contents of primary granules (Steadman *et al.*, 1988; Topley *et al.*, 1989). Neutrophil proteases from the primary granule cleave extracellular matrix molecules and generate fragments with potent biological properties (Senior *et al.*, 1989; Steadman *et al.*, 1993). In this way, the inflammatory process may be amplified by the generation of chemotactic proteolytic products. The interaction of neutrophils with type-1-fimbriate organisms would, therefore, initiate and amplify tissue destruction by a mechanism that is not activated by the interaction with non-type-1 fimbriate strains. Thus, the potential of a particular strain of *E. coli* to cause tissue damage and renal scarring may be linked directly to its ability to stimulate comprehensive neutrophil activation.

Once tissue damage has been initiated, the interaction of infiltrating monocyte/macrophages and activated neutrophils with the damaged tissues is important in the development of scarring and stimulation of collagen synthesis by renal cortical cells. Macrophages express several surface receptors for the binding and phagocytosis of opsonised and non-opsonised micro-organisms (Speert, 1992). In addition to their roles as phagocytic cells, however, activated macrophages exert a controlling influence on many other cell types. Thus, while they have an antibacterial repertoire similar to that of neutrophils, macrophages also release a large variety of cytokines, growth factors, complement components and other inflammatory mediators (Auger & Ross, 1992). Some of these are chemotactic for neutrophils and other monocytic cells. Others contribute to and control tissue remodelling by the induction of fibroblast proliferation and biosynthetic activity. There is, however, little information about the role of monocytes in the development or progress of renal scarring in response to *E. coli*.

Leucocytes may be selectively activated by a variety of *E. coli* virulence factors. Isolated bacterial products affect neutrophil adhesion, chemotaxis and activation. The response of neutrophils to intact bacteria is complex. Variation in the response of neutrophils following interaction with *E. coli in vitro* may be directly related to the degree of tissue damage that different strains are capable of causing *in vivo*. In addition, anatomical and functional changes of the urinary tract predispose the host to particular types of infection. Clinical observations support the notion that renal scarring occurs in children with vesico-ureteric reflux as a result of *E. coli* that gain access to the kidney through ruptured renal pelvic epithelium, but which do not necessarily express the virulence factors associated with colonisation of the lower tract (Smellie *et al.*, 1975, 1981). Although leucocyte infiltration occurs in response to kidney infection with all *E. coli* strains, it is only those that express type-1 fimbriae that are able to generate renal scars (Topley *et al.*, 1989), which suggests that the degree of activation of inflammation is crucial to the outcome of infection. This is supported by the observations in humans, namely that parameters of inflammation, such as C-reactive protein, erythrocyte sedimentation rate and temperature, are higher in patients susceptible to renal scarring than in those who are not (Lomberg *et al.*, 1992).

In animal models, scarring is initiated within 24 hours of infection and depends on neutrophil infiltration (Glauser *et al.*, 1982; Meylan *et al.*, 1989; Topley *et al.*, 1989). The release of neutrophil elastase is probably responsible for the tissue damage that precedes the scarring process (Steadman *et al.*, 1988; Topley *et al.*, 1989). Whether bacterial factors also affect the monocyte/macrophage, lymphocyte, epithelium, fibroblast or other renal cell responses during the scarring process remains to be determined. However, it has recently been shown, with a murine model of ascending pyelonephritis, that many cytokines and growth factor messenger RNA are produced locally in the kidney. This suggests that *E. coli* infection in the kidney can activate many of the cell populations that participate in the inflammatory process (Rugo *et al.*, 1992).

Conclusions

An attempt has been made to identify the mechanisms by which *E. coli* activates host cells and to examine the potential pathogenicity of these processes during various forms of UTI. Future research must focus on defining in greater detail how these interactions affect the initiation, establishment and severity of infection.

Recent interest in the ability of *E. coli* to activate mucosal immunity *in vivo* and *in vitro* provides evidence that the interaction between the uroepithelium and *E. coli* is not merely a process of passive adherence, but that cellular activation, such as cytokine release and up-regulation of adhesion molecule expression, occurs during this event. This leads to the hypothesis that the activation of non-phagocytic cells may be an important initial pivotal stage in determining whether infection becomes established or cleared, as well as in determining the severity of the subsequent leucocyte-mediated inflammatory process. It will be of interest to determine *in vivo* and *in vitro* the mechanisms of this activation process and the extent to which different pathogenic *E. coli* strains activate the epithelia of the lower and upper tract. Such investigations will provide many interesting avenues for future research.

Acknowledgements

We should like to acknowledge all those involved, both past and present, in urinary tract infection research in the Kidney Research Unit Foundation (KRUF), particularly Sir William Asscher, Dr Ruth Mackenzie, Susan Chick, the late Dr Mike Harber, Dr Ian Slotki, David Jenner, Janice Knowlden, Dr Monika Lichodziejewska, Dr Michelle James-Ellison, Dr Kate Verrier-Jones and Professor John Williams, all of whom have contributed significantly to our knowledge in this field. We would also like to thank Professor John Williams for his helpful comments and Cheryl Patterson for her help in preparing the manuscript. The authors are supported by the Kidney Research Unit for Wales Foundation, The National Kidney Research Foundation and the Medical Research Council.

References

Abraham, J. M., Freitag, C. S., Clements, J. R. & Eisenstein, B. I. (1985). An invertible element of DNA controls phase variation of type 1 fimbriae *Escherichia coli. Proceedings of the National Academy of Sciences, USA*, **82**, 5724–7.
Abraham, S. N., Sun, D., Dale, J. B. & Beachey, E. H. (1988). Conservation of the D-mannose adhesion protein among type 1 fimbriated members of the family enterobacteriaceae. *Nature*, **336**, 682–4.
Agace, W., Hedges, S., Andersson, U., Andersson, J., Ceska, M. & Svanborg, C. (1993a). Selective cytokine production by epithelial cells following exposure to *Escherichia coli.Infection and Immunity*, **61**, 602–9.
Agace, W. W., Hedges, S. R., Ceska, M. & Svanborg, C. (1993b). Interleukin-8 and the neutrophil response to mucosal Gram-negative infection. *Journal of Clinical Investigation*, **92**, 780–5.
Andreka, D., Le, J. & Vilcek, J. (1989). IL-6 inhibits lipopolysaccharide-induced tumor necrosis factor production in cultured human monocytes, U937 cells, and in mice. *Journal of Immunology*, **143**, 3517–23.

Asscher, A. W. (1980). *The Challenge of Urinary Tract Infections*, pp. 52–73. London: Academic Press.

Auger, M. J. & Ross, J. A. (1991). The biology of macrophage. In *The Macrophage*, eds. C. D. Lewis & J. O'D. McGee, pp. 1–74. Oxford: Oxford University Press.

Berger, M., Watzler, E. M. & Wallis, R. S. (1988). Tumour necrosis factor is the major monocyte product that increases complement receptor expression on mature human neutrophils. *Blood*, **71**, 151–8.

Bille, J. & Glauser, M. P. (1982). Protection against chronic pyelonephritis in rats by suppression of acute suppuration; effect of colchicine and neutropenia. *Journal of Infectious Diseases*, **146**, 220–6.

Blumenstock, E. & Jann, K. (1982). Adhesion of piliated *Escherichia coli* strains to phagocytes; differences between bacteria with mannose-sensitive pili and those with mannose-resistant pili. *Infection and Immunity*, **35**, 264–9.

Boner, G., Maashilkar, A. M., Rodrigues-Ortega, M. & Sharon, N. (1989). Lectin-mediated non-opsonic phagocytosis of type 1 *Escherichia coli* by human peritoneal macrophages of uremic patients treated by peritoneal dialysis. *Journal of Leukocyte Biology*, **46**, 239–45.

Brinton, C. C. (1959). Non-flagellar appendages of bacteria. *Nature*, **183**, 782–6.

Brinton, C. C. (1965). The structure, function, synthesis and genetic control of bacterial pili and a molecular model for DNA and RNA transport in Gram-negative bacteria. *Transactions of the New York Academy of Sciences*, **27**, 1003–54.

Cavalieri, S. J. & Snyder, I. S. (1982a). Cytotoxic activity of partially purified *Escherichia coli* alpha hemolysin. *Journal of Medical Microbiology*, **15**, 11–21.

Cavalieri, S. J. & Snyder, I. S. (1982b). Effect of *Escherichia coli* alpha hemolysin on human peripheral leukocyte function *in vitro*. *Infection and Immunity*, **37**, 966–74.

Cavalieri, S. J. & Snyder, I. S. (1982c). Effect of *Escherichia coli* alpha hemolysin on human peripheral leukocyte viability *in vitro*. *Infection and Immunity*, **36**, 455–61.

Duguid, J. P. & Old, D. C. (1980). Adhesive properties of Enterobacteriaceae. In *Bacterial Adherence*, ed. E. H. Beachey, pp. 185–217. London: Chapman & Hall.

Eisentein, B. I. (1981). Phase variation in *Escherichia coli* is under transcriptional control. *Science*, **214**, 337–9.

Elgavish, A. (1993). Effects of *Escherichia coli* and *E. coli* lipopolysaccharide on the function of human ureteral epithelial cells cultured in serum-free medium. *Infection and Immunity*, **61**, 3304–12.

Fine, D. P., Harper, B. L., Carpenter, E. D., Davis, C. P., Cavallo, T. & Kukian, J. C. (1980). Complement-independent adherence of *Escherichia coli* to complement receptors *in vitro*. *Journal of Clinical Investigation*, **66**, 465–72.

Fitzharris, P., Cromwell, R., Moqhel, R., Hartnell, A., Walsh, G. M., Harvey, C. & Kay, A. B. (1987). Leukotriene B4 generation by human neutrophils following IgG-dependent stimulation. *Immunology*, **61**, 449–55.

Floege, J., Böddeker, M., Stolte, H. & Hock, H. M. (1990). Urinary IgA secretory IgA and secretory component in women with recurrent urinary tract infections. *Nephron*, **56**, 50–5

Gabarah, A., Gahmberg, C. G., Ofek, I., Jacobi, U. & Sharon, N. (1991). Identification of the leukocyte adhesion molecules CD11 and CD 18 as receptors for type-1-fimbriated (mannose-specific) *Escherichia coli*. *Infection and Immunity*, **59**, 4524–30.

Glauser, M. P., Lyons, J. M. & Braude, A. I. (1982). Prevention of chronic experimental pylonephritis by suppression of acute suppuration. *Journal of Clinical Investigation*, **61**, 403–7.

Goetz, M. B. (1987). Phagolysosome formation by polymorphonuclear neutrophilic leukocytes after ingestion of *Escherichia coli* that express type 1 pili. *Journal of Infectious Diseases*, **156**, 229–33.

Goetz, M. B. (1989). Priming of polymorphonuclear neutrophilic leukocyte oxidative activity by type 1 pili from *Escherichia coli*. *Journal of Infectious Diseases*, **159**, 533–42.

Goodman, R. B., Wood, R. G., Martin, T. R., Hanson-Painton, O. & Kinasewitz, G. T. (1992) Cytokine-stimulated human mesothelial cells produce chemotactic activity for neutrophils including NAP-1/IL-8. *Journal of Immunology*, **148**, 457–65.

Grimminger, F., Thomas, M., Obernitz, R., Walmrath, D., Bhakdi, S. & Seeger, W. (1990) Inflammatory lipid mediator generation elicited by viable haemolysin forming *Escherichia coli* in lung vasculature. *Journal of Experimental Medicine*, **172**, 1115–25.

Hacker, J., Hughes, C., Hof, H. & Goebel, W. (1983). Cloned hemolysin genes from *Escherichia coli* that cause urinary tract infection determine different levels of toxicity in mice. *Infection and Immunity*, **42**, 57–63.

Hagberg, L., Briles, D. E. & Svanborg Eden, C. (1985). Evidence for separate genetic defects in C3H/HeJ and C3HeB/FeJ mice, that affect susceptibility to Gram-negative infections. *Journal of Immunology*, **134**, 4118–22.

Hanson, M. S. & Brinton, C. C. (1988). Identification and characterisation of *Escherichia coli* type 1 tip adhesion protein. *Nature*, **332**, 265–8.

Harber, M. J., Topley, N. & Asscher, A. W. (1986). Virulence factors of urinary pathogens. *Clinical Science*, **70**, 531–8.

Heck, L. W., Blackburn, W. D., Irwin, M. H. & Abrahamson, D. R. (1990). Degradation of basement membrane laminin by human neutrophil elastase and cathepsin G. *American Journal of Pathology*, **136**, 1267–74

Hedges, S., Andersson, P., Lindin-Janson, G., De Man, P. & Svanborg, C. (1991). Interleukin-6 response to deliberate colonisation of the urinary tract with Gram negative bacteria. *Infection and Immunity*, **59**, 421–7.

Hedges, S., Stenqvist, K., Lindin-Janson, G., Martinell, J., Sandberg, T. & Svanborg, C. (1992a). Comparison of urine and serum concentrations of interleukin-6 in women with acute pyelonephritis or asymptomatic bacteriuria. *Journal of Infectious Diseases*, **166**, 653–6.

Hedges, S., Svensson, M. & Svanborg, C. (1992b). Interleukin-6 response of epithelial cell lines to bacterial stimulation *in vitro*. *Infection and Immunity*, **60**, 1295–301.

Hughes, C., Hacker, J., Roberts, A. & Goebel, W. (1983). Hemolysin production as a virulence marker in symptomatic and asymptomatic urinary tract infections caused by *Escherichia coli*. *Infection and Immunity*, **39**, 546–51.

Hultgren, S. J., Lindberg, F., Magnusson, G., Kihlberg, J., Tennent, J. & Normark, S. (1989). The Pap G adhesin of uropathogenic *Escherichia coli* contains separate regions for receptor binding and for the incorporation into the pilus. *Proceedings of the National Academy Sciences, USA*, **86**, 4357–61.

Jacobson, S. H. & Lomberg, H. (1990). Over-representation of blood group non-secretors in adults with renal scarring. *Scandinavian Journal of Urology and Nephrology*, **24**, 145–50.

Jann, K. & Jann, B. (1985). Cell surface components and virulence: *Escherichia coli* O and K antigens in relation to virulence and pathogenicity. In *The Virulence of Escherichia coli; Reviews and Methods*, ed. M. Sussman, pp. 157–76. London: Academic Press.

Johnson, J. R. (1991). Virulence factors in *Escherichia coli* urinary tract infection. *Clinical Microbiology Reviews*, **4**, 80–128.

Jones, O. T. G., Jones, S. A., Hancock, J. T. & Topley, N. (1993). Composition and organisation of the NADPH oxidase of phagocytes and other cells. *Biochemical Society Transactions*, **21**, 343–6.

Kinane, D. F., Blackwell, C. C., Brettle, R. P., Weir, D. M. & Winstanteg, F. P. (1982). ABO blood group, secretor status and susceptibility to urinary tract infection. *British Medical Journal*, **3**, 7–9.

Klemm, P. (1984). The fimA gene encoding the type 1 fimbrial subunit of *Escherichia coli*. *European Journal of Biochemistry*, **143**, 395–9.

Klemm, P. & Christiansen, G. (1987). Three *fim* genes required for the regulation of length and mediation of adhesion of *Escherichia coli* type 1 fimbriae. *Molecular and General Genetics*, **208**, 439–45.

König, B., König, W., Scheffer, J., Hacker, J. & Goebel, W. (1986). Role of *Escherichia coli* alpha hemolysin and bacterial adherence in infection: requirement for release of inflammatory mediators from granulocytes and mast cells. *Infection and Immunity*, **54**, 886–92.

Lichodziejewska, M., Topley, N., Steadman, R., Mackenzie, R. K., Verrier-Jones, K. & Williams, J. D. (1989) Variable expression of P-fimbriae in *Escherichia coli* urinary tract infection. *Lancet*, **i**, 1414–18.

Lindberg, F. P., Lund, B., Johannsson, L. & Normark, S. (1987). Localisation of the receptor binding protein adhesin at the tip of the bacterial pilus. *Nature*, **328**, 84–7.

Lindberg, F. P., Lund, B. & Normark, S. (1984). Genes of pyelonephritogenic *Escherichia coli* required for digalactoside specific agglutination of human cells. *EMBO Journal*, **3**, 1167–73.

Linder, H., Engberg, I., Hoschutzky, H., Mattsby-Baltzer, I. & Svanborg, C. (1991). Adhesin-dependent activation of mucosal interleukin-6 production. *Infection and Immunity*, **59**, 4357–62.

Lomberg, H., Hanson, L. A., Jacobsson, B., Jodal, U., Leffler, H. & Svanborg-Eden, C. (1983). Correlation of p blood group, vesico-ureteric reflux and bacterial attachment in patients with recurrent pyelonephritis. *New England Journal of Medicine*, **308**, 1189–92.

Lomberg, H., Hellström, M., Jodal, U., Leffler, H., Lincoln, K. & Svanborg-Eden, C. (1984). Virulence associated strains of *Escherichia coli* causing recurrent episodes of urinary tract infection in children with or without vesico-ureteric reflux. *Journal of Infectious Diseases*, **150**, 561–9.

Lomberg, H., Hellström, M., Jodal, U. & Svanborg Edén, C. (1986). Renal scarring and non attaching bacteria. *Lancet*, **ii**, 1341.

Lomberg, H., Hellström, M., Jodal, U., Ørskov, I. & Svanborg-Edén, C. (1989). Properties of *Escherichia coli* in patients with renal scarring. *Journal of Infectious Diseases*, **159**, 579 82.

Lomberg, H., Jodal, U., Leffler, H., De Man, P. & Svanborg, C. (1992). Blood group non-secretors have an increased inflammatory response to urinary tract infection. *Scandinavian Journal of Infectious Diseases*, **24**, 77–83.

Madara, J. L. (1990). Pathobiology of the intestinal epithelial barrier. *American Journal of Pathology*, **137**, 1273–81.

Matsuura, M., Kojuma, Y., Hamma, J. Y., Kumazawa, Y., Yamamoto, A., Kiso, M. & Hasegawa, A. (1986). Effects of backbone structures and sterospecificities of lipid A subunit analogues on their biological activities. *Journal of Biochemistry*, **99**, 1377–84.

Meylan, P. R., Markert, M., Bille, J. & Glauser, M. P. (1989). Relationship between neutrophil-mediated oxidative injury during acute experimental pyelonephritis and chronic renal scarring. *Infection and Immunity*, **57**, 2196–202.

Mutsaers, S. E. & Papdimitriou, J. M. (1988). Surface charge of macrophages and their interaction with charged particles. *Journal of Leukocyte Biology*, **44**, 17–26.

Nowicki, B., Rhen, M., Väisänen-Rhen, V., Pere, A. & Korhonen, T. K. (1984). Immunofluorescence study of fimbrial phase variation in *Escherichia coli*KS71. *Journal of Bacteriology*, **160**, 691–5.

Nowicki, B., Rhen, M., Väisänen-Rhen, V., Pere, A. & Korhonen, T. K. (1985). Kinetics of phase variation between S and type 1 fimbriae of *Escherichia coli*. *FEMS Microbiology Letters*, **28**, 237–42.

Öhman, L., Hed, J. & Stendahl, O. (1982). Interactions between human polymorphonuclear leukocytes and two different strains of type 1 fimbriae bearing *Escherichia coli*. *Journal of Infectious Diseases*, **146**, 751–7.

Ørskov, F., Ørskov, I., Sutton, A., Schneerson, R., Lindt, W., Egan, W., Hoff, G. E. & Robbins, J. B. (1979). Form variation in *Escherichia coli*K1: determined by acetylation of the capsular polysaccharide. *Journal of Experimental Medicine*, **149**, 669–85.

Papadimitriou, J. M. (1982). An assessment of the surface charge of single resident and exudate macrophages and multinucleate giant cells. *Journal of Pathology*, **138**, 17–24.

Petersen, M., Steadman, R., Matthews, N. & Williams, J. D. (1990). Zymosan induced leukotriene B4 generation by human neutrophils is augmented by rhTNFa but not chemotactic peptide. *Immunology*, **70**, 75–81.

Peterson, P. K., Gekker, G., Shapiro, R., Freiberg, M. & Keane, W. F. (1984). Polyamino acid enhancement of bacterial phagocytosis by human polymorphonuclear leukocytes and peritoneal macrophages. *Infection and Immunity*, **43**, 561–6.

Pugliesi, F., Mené, P., Anania, M. C. & Linotti, G. A. (1989). Neutralisation of the anionic sites of cultured rat mesangial cells by poly-L-lysine. *Kidney International*, **35**, 817–23.

Pugliesi, F., Singh, A. K., Kasinath, B. S. & Lewis, E. J. (1987). Glomerular epithelial cell polyanion neutralisation is associated with enhanced prostanoid production. *Kidney International*, **32**, 57–61.

Rhen, M., Mäkelä, P. H. & Korhonen, T. K. (1983). P fimbriae of *Escherichia coli* are subject to phase variation. *FEMS Microbiology Letters*, **19**, 267–71.

Rodrigues-Ortega, M., Ofek, I. & Sharon, N. (1987). Membrane glycoproteins of human polymorphonuclear leukocytes that act as receptors for mannose-specific *Escherichia coli*. *Infection and Immunity*, **55**, 968–73.

Rothlein, R. & Wegner, C. (1992). Role of intercellular adhesion molecule-1 in the inflammatory response. *Kidney International*, **41**, 617–9.

Rugo, H. S., O'Hanley, P., Bishop, A. G., Pearce, M. K., Abrams, J. S., Howard, M. & O'Garra, A. (1992). Local cytokine production in a murine model of *Escherichia coli* pyelonephritis. *Journal of Clinical Investigation*, **89**, 1032–9.

Salmon, J. E., Kapur, S. & Kimberley, R. P. (1987). Opsonin-independent ligation of Fc γ-receptors. The 3G8 receptors on neutrophils mediate the phagocytosis of concanavalin A-treated erythrocytes and non-opsonised *Escherichia coli*. *Journal of Experimental Medicine*, **166**, 1798–813.

Scheffer, J., König, W., Hacker, J. & Goebel, W. (1985). Bacterial adherence and hemolysin production from *Escherichia coli* involves histamine and leukotriene release from various cells. *Infection and Immunity*, **50**, 271–8.

Schindler, R., Mancilla, J., Enders, S., Ghorbani, R., Clark, S. C. & Dinarello, C. A. (1990). Correlations in the production of interleukin-6, IL-1 and TNFα in human blood mononuclear cells: IL-6 suppresses IL-1 and TNF. *Blood*, **75**, 40–7.

Senior, R. M., Hinek, A., Griffin, G. L., Pipolo, D. J., Crouch, E. C. & Mecham, R. P. (1989). Neutrophils show chemotaxis to type IV collagen and its 7S domain and contain a 67kD type IV collagen binding protein with lectin properties. *American Journal of Respiratory Cell Molecular Biology*, **1**, 479–87.

Shahin, R. D., Engberg, I., Hagberg, L. & Svanborg Eden, C. (1987). Neutrophil recruitment and bacterial clearance correlated with LPS responsiveness in local Gram-negative infection. *Journal of Immunology*, **138**, 3475–80.

Sheinfeld, J., Schaeffer, A. J., Corolon, C., Rogatko, A. & Fair, W. R. (1989). Association of the Lewis blood group phenotype with recurrent urinary tract infection in women. *New England Journal of Medicine*, **320**, 773–7.

Shier, V. T., Dubordieu, D. & Durbin, J. P. (1984). Polycations as prostaglandin synthesis inducers. Stimulation of arachidonic acid release and prostaglandin synthesis in cultured fibroblasts by poly-L-lysine and other synthetic polycations. *Biochimica et Biophysica Acta*, **793**, 238–50.

Silverblatt, F. J., Dreyer, J. S. & Shauer, S. (1979). Effect of pili on susceptibility of *Escherichia coli* to phagocytosis. *Infection and Immunity*, **24**, 218–23.

Slotki, I. N. & Asscher, A. W. (1982). Prevention of scarring in experimental pyelonephritis in the rat by early antibiotic therapy. *Nephron*, **30**, 262–8.

Smellie, J. M., Edwards, D., Hunter, N., Normand, I. C. S. & Prescod, N. (1975). Vesico–ureteric reflux and renal scarring. *Kidney Internatinal*, **8**, Supplement 4, S65–72.

Smellie, J. M., Edwards, D., Normand, I. C. S. & Prescod, N. (1981). Effect of vesico–ureteric reflux on renal growth in children with urinary tract infection. *Archives of Diseases of Children*, **56**, 593–600.

Smith, H. W. (1963). The haemolysins of *Escherichia coli*. *Journal of Pathology and Bacteriology*, **85**, 197–211.

Speert, D. P. (1980). Macrophages in bacterial infection. In *The Macrophage*, eds. C. D. Lewis & J. O'D. McGee, pp. 215–64. Oxford: Oxford University Press.

Springer, W. & Goebel, B. (1980). Synthesis and secretion of hemolysin by *Escherichia coli*. *Journal of Bacteriology*, **144**, 53–9.

Steadman, R., Irwin, M. H., St John, P. L., Blackburn, W. D., Heck, L. W. & Abrahamson, D. R. (1993). Laminin cleavage by activated human neutrophils yields proteolytic fragments with selective migratory properties. *Journal of Leukocyte Biology*, **53**, 354–65.

Steadman, R., Knowlden, J. M., Lichodziejewska, M. & Williams, J. D. (1990a). The influence of net surface charge on the interaction of uropathogenic *Escherichia coli* with human neutrophils. *Biochimica et Biophysica Acta*, **1053**, 37–42.

Steadman, R., Matthews, N., Lichodziejewska, M. & Williams, J. D. (1991). Human neutrophil responses to pathogenic *Escherichia coli* are receptor specific and selectively augmented by recombinant human TNFa. *Journal of Infectious Diseases*, **163**, 1033–9.

Steadman, R., Petersen, M. M., Topley, N., Williams, D., Matthews, N., Spur, B. & Williams, J. D. (1990c). Differential augmentation by recombinant human tumour necrosis factor α of neutrophil responses to particulate zymosan and glucan. *Journal of Immunology*, **144**, 2712–18.

Steadman, R., Topley, N., Jenner, D. E., Davies, M. & Williams, J. D. (1988). Type 1 fimbriate *Escherichia coli* stimulates a unique pattern of degranulation by human polymorphonuclear leukocytes. *Infection and Immunity*, **56**, 815–22.

Steadman, R., Topley, N., Knowlden, J. M., Mackenzie, R. K. & Williams, J. D. (1989). The assessment of relative surface hydrophobicity as a factor involved in the activation of human polymorphonuclear leukocytes by uropathogenic strains of *Escherichia coli*. *Biochimica et Biophysica Acta*, **1013**, 21–7.

Steadman, R., Topley, N., Knowlden, J., Spur, B. & Williams, J. D. (1990b). Leukotriene B_4 generation by human monocytes and neutrophils stimulated by uropathogenic strains of *Escherichia coli*. *Biochimica et Biophysica Acta*, **1052**, 264–72.

Stendahl, O., Dahlgren, C., Edebo, M. & Øhman, L. (1981). Recognition mechanisms in mammalian phagocytosis. *Monographs of Allergy*, **17**, 12–27.

Svanborg-Eden, C., Bjorksten, L. M., Hull, R., Hull, S., Magnusson, K. E., Leffler, H. & Moldavano, Z. (1984). Influence of adhesins on the interaction of *Escherichia coli* with human phagocytes. *Infection and Immunity*, **44**, 672–80.

Svanborg Eden, C., Shahin, R. & Briles, D. E. (1988). Host resistance to mucosal Gram-negative infection: susceptibility of lipopolysaccharide nonresponder mice. *Journal of Immunology*, **140**, 3180–5.

Swaney, L. M., Ying-Peng, L., Chuen-Mo, T., Cheng-Chin, T., Ippen-Ihler, K. & Brinton, C. C. (1977). Isolation and characterisation of *Escherichia coli*phase variants and mutants deficient in type 1 pilus production. *Journal of Bacteriology*, **130**, 495–505.

Swansen, J. & Barrera, O. (1983). Conococcal pilus subunits size heterogeneity correlates with transitions in colony piliation phenotype, not with changes in colony morphology. *Journal of Experimental Medicine*, **158**, 1459–72.

Topley, N., Mackenzie, R., Jörres, A., Coles, G. A., Davies, M. & Williams, J. D. (1993). Cytokine networks in CAPD: interactions of resident cells during inflammation in the peritoneal cavity. *Peritoneal Dialysis International*, **13**, S282–5.

Topley, N., Steadman, R., Mackenzie, R. K., Knowlden, J. M. & Williams, J. D. (1989). Type 1 fimbriate strains of *Escherichia coli* initiate renal parenchymal scarring. *Kidney International*, **36**, 609–16.

Watton, S. J. & Smith, D. H. (1969). New haemolysin produced by *Escherichia coli*. *Journal of Bacteriology*, **98**, 304–305.

Weiss, S. (1989). Tissue destruction by neutrophils. *New England Journal of Medicine*, **320**, 365–76.

Westphal, O., Jann, K. & Himmelspach, K. (1982). Chemistry and immunochemistry of bacterial lipopolysaccharides as cell wall antigens and endotoxins. *Progress in Allergy*, **3**, 9–39.

Wille, J. J., Park, J. & Elgavish, A. (1992). Effects of growth factors, hormones, bacterial lipopolysaccharides and lipotechoic acids on the clonal growth of normal ureteral epithelial cells in serum free culture. *Journal of Cellular Physiology*, 150, 52–8.

Williams, J. D., Lee, T. H., Lewis, R. A. & Austen, K. F. (1985). Intracellular retention of the 5-lipoxygenase pathway product leukotriene B4 by human neutrophils activated with unopsonized zymosan. *Journal of Immunology*, **134**, 2624–30.

Williams, J. D., Topley, N., Alobaidi, H. M. & Harber, M. J. (1986). Activation of human polymorphonuclear leukocytes by particulate zymosan is related to both its major carbohydrate components: glucan and mannan. *Immunology*, **58**, 117–24.

Wright, S. D. & Jong, M. T. C. (1986). Adhesion-promoting receptors on human macrophages recognise *Escherichia coli* by binding to lipopolysaccharide. *Journal of Experimental Medicine*, **164**, 1876–88.

20

Immune responses to *Escherichia coli*

J. W. GRAY

Infection and colonisation by *Escherichia coli* is associated with a variety of host immune responses that are of broad significance for an understanding of the host–microbe interaction. Thus, production of a given antibody is evidence that the corresponding antigen is expressed *in vivo* and that it may be involved in pathogenesis. Similarly, knowledge of the immune response may point to immunological approaches to the treatment of infections and the development of vaccines. Since *E. coli* is a major pathogen of neonates, infants and young animals, an understanding of these immune mechanisms offers potential strategies for the protection of those at risk.

Many so-called natural antibodies are thought to result from exposure to microbial antigens. Given the universality of exposure to *E. coli*, this may be the origin of natural antibodies, including the A, B, H(O) blood group antibodies. Other natural antibodies, including anti-galactosyl antibody, have been implicated in the pathogenesis of certain autoimmune diseases.

Detection of immune responses can be used in the diagnosis of infection. Thus, demonstration of an antibody response has been used to identify the site of infection within the urinary tract and retrospective evidence of infection with Vero cytotoxin-producing *E. coli* can be obtained from patients with haemolytic uraemic syndrome.

The close relationship between *E. coli* and other Enterobacteriaceae suggests that the immune responses to these organisms may have much in common.

The antigens of *Escherichia coli*

The cell envelope of *E. coli* is a complex structure that contains various antigens and virulence factors. The antigens occur in many different combinations that may be shared with other members of the Enterobacteriaceae. Since the majority of *E. coli* occur as distinct clones, it can be predicted that isolates identified by the same serological determinants are likely to express other traits, such as adhesins, haemolysin or toxin production.

Lipopolysaccharide

The structure of lipopolysaccharide (LPS) has been comprehensively described (Bayston & Cohen, 1990). Briefly, LPS comprises three well-defined parts: (i) the serotype-specific O-side-chain polysaccharide, of which over 160 different types have been identified in *E. coli*, (ii) the core oligosaccharide which is less variable, and of which only six or seven variations exist amongst the Enterobacteriaceae, and (iii) lipid A, the most conserved structure, which is responsible for the toxic properties of LPS. The O-side-chain is the most immunogenic region of LPS, and gives rise to the production of specific anti-O-antibodies that confer a high degree of protection. Lipopolysaccharide has been implicated in the pathogenesis of a variety of clinical syndromes, the most familiar of which is septic shock (see Chapter 5).

Capsule

Many strains of *E. coli* produce polysaccharide capsules that are important virulence factors that enable the bacteria to evade or resist non-specific host defences during the early phase of infection (Van Dijk *et al.*, 1981; see Chapter 4). Specific anti-K-antibodies are necessary for optimal opsonisation of K-antigen-bearing strains. K-antigens, particularly K1, have relatively low immunogenicity, because they share partial identity with certain host structures (Silver *et al.*, 1988).

Fimbriae

There is a clear correlation between bacterial adhesion and pathogenesis (Krogfelt, 1991). Up to 70 per cent of wild-type *E. coli* express mannose-sensitive type-1 fimbriae. Fimbriae such as K88, K99 and colonisation factor antigen (CFA) are associated with diarrhoeal diseases, and S-fimbriae with neonatal meningitis. Uropathogenic *E. coli* are particularly associated with P-fimbriae and a heterogeneous group of mannose-resistant fimbriae including S-, G- and M-fimbriae that mediate attachment to epithelial cells.

Outer-membrane proteins

The outer-membrane proteins (OMPs) of *E. coli* are well characterised, and include epitopes they have in common with other Enterobacteriaceae. Cross-reacting OMPs include porin protein, the heat-modifiable protein (Hm) and Braun's lipoprotein (BLp) (Henriksen & Maeland, 1987, 1990).

Enterobacterial common antigen

The enterobacterial common antigen (ECA) is a family-specific glycophospholipid antigen located in the outer leaflet of the outer membrane (Kuhn *et al.*, 1988). Interest in the immune response to ECA was stimulated by the prospect of a single antigen-based serological diagnostic test for infection with all members of the Enterobacteriaceae, and by the possibility that immunisation with ECA might confer broad cross-protection. The importance of ECA in pathogenicity is uncertain, but anti-ECA antibodies are protective in some situations (Domingue *et al.*, 1970).

Lipoprotein

Lipoprotein is a component of the innermost layer of the Gram-negative bacterial cell wall that is chemically and antigenically similar amongst the Enterobacteriaceae. It has excited attention for the same reasons as ECA. Detectable antibody is rare in healthy individuals, but only a small and variable proportion of infected patients respond to this antigen (Griffiths *et al.*, 1977).

α-Haemolysin

This is a cytolytic protein toxin secreted by most haemolytic strains of *E. coli* (see Chapter 11). Production of α-haemolysin is an important virulence factor and anti-α-haemolysin antibody titres correlate closely with the degree of invasiveness of infection (Emödy *et al.*, 1982).

Immunity to *Escherichia coli* in infants

Soon after birth, neonates are exposed to many potentially pathogenic micro-organisms. Most newborn and very young infants are able to cope with these organisms with the support of passive and active specific immunity and various non-specific defence mechanisms.

During the first few days of life, *E. coli* appears in the faeces of most neonates and later infants are continually exposed to different serotypes, some of which, such as *E. coli* K1 or enteropathogenic *E. coli*, possess particular virulence attributes (Hanson *et al.*, 1983; see Chapter 3). Some of these serotypes appear to colonise more efficiently than others. Since exposure of mothers and infants to *E. coli* is almost universal, the mechanisms that protect the infant from *E. coli* infection have been widely studied. An understanding of immunity to *E. coli* infection is important, not only because of the importance of *E. coli* as a pathogen, but also because it can serve as a paradigm for immunity to other infections.

Immunity conferred by breast feeding

Breast feeding protects infants from a number of infections, including *E. coli* diarrhoea (Cruz *et al.*, 1988) and urinary tract infection (Pisacane *et al.*, 1992). A variety of defence factors is probably important in breast-fed infants, but the precise role of each has not been defined. Colostrum and milk contain a number of non-specific antimicrobial substances (Boesman-Finkelstein & Finkelstein, 1982), such as lactoferrin, which sequesters iron so as to deprive gut-associated bacteria of the free iron necessary for proliferation, and lysozyme, which hydrolyses glycosidic bonds in peptidoglycan. Various glycolipids, glycoproteins and free oligosaccharides may inhibit binding of *E. coli* and its enterotoxins to receptors (Holmgren *et al.*, 1981). Colostrum contains high levels of secretory immunoglobulin A (sIgA), and between 0.5 and 1 g of IgA per day may be transferred to the neonate. Small amounts of IgM and IgG are also present in early milk. After a few days, the concentration of immunoglobulin in breast milk decreases ten-fold and then remains relatively constant throughout the rest of lactation (Carlsson *et al.*, 1976). The disproportionately high amount of sIgA in breast milk, and the weak correlation between milk and serum levels have been attributed to local antibody production by plasma cells in breast tissue under lactogenic hormonal influence. Breast milk antibodies are directed against numerous *E. coli* antigens, including a wide variety of O- and K-antigens and various adhesins, including antigens not expressed by the commensal strains carried by the mother.

Breast-fed infants harbour fewer bacterial strains than artificially fed infants, which may, to some extent, simply reflect lower exposure to bacteria. Follow-up of mothers and their infants has shown that the latter can become colonised with O- and K-types of *E. coli* in spite of the presence of antibody to these antigens in the maternal milk and serum (Gothefors *et al.*, 1976; Carlsson *et al.*, 1982). Indeed, in artificial colonisation experiments, breast-fed infants may actually be colonised more frequently than formula-fed infants, possibly because the presence of sIgA favours type-1-fimbriated strains with greater adherence potential (Lodinovà-Zàdníkovà *et al.*, 1991). Another possible effect of antibodies is that they select for rough mutants with reduced virulence (Gothefors *et al.*, 1976). Daily administration of human colostrum also reduces the incidence of diarrhoea in non-breast-fed hospitalised infants (Cruz *et al.*, 1988). However, administration of bovine milk immunoglobulin concentrate from cows hyperimmunised with the major *E. coli* serotypes did not affect the incidence of diarrhoeal disease in bottle-fed children (Brunser *et al.*, 1992).

The avidity of the milk sIgA antibodies for *E. coli* antigens is quite high, and they are believed to be efficient neutralising antibodies that protect the infant from the effects of endotoxin in the bowel. There is, however, considerable variation in avidity between individuals (Sennhauser *et al.*, 1989) and, in particular, sIgA avidity in Pakistani mothers has been shown to be significantly lower than in Swedish women (Robertson *et al.*, 1988). A satisfactory explanation for this observation has not been proposed.

The effect of breast milk antibodies may be more long-lasting than simply the provision of passive immunity. *In vitro* and *in vivo* experimental observations have provided evidence that anti-idiotypic antibodies in breast milk may stimulate sIgA production in neonates, but this has not been confirmed (Avananzini *et al.*, 1992).

Secretory antibody production by infants

Production of sIgA in saliva has generally been measured several hours after breast feeding, when residual maternal antibody in the infants mouth should be minimal. Infants appear to be able to respond to microbial exposure with significant sIgA production at about six to seven days of age. By six weeks of age the response to local antigens is probably the main source of antibody in both breast-fed and formula-fed infants (Stephens, 1986). Production of secretory IgM may, at least to some extent, compensate for the lack of sIgA in early life (Mellander *et al.*, 1984). Typically, the IgA response of the child is rather slow to mature, and may not reach adult levels until at least five years of age (Gleeson *et al.*, 1987). There is, however, evidence to suggest that the age and rate of sIgA production depends on exposure to the organism. Firstly, antibody levels tend to be higher in formula-fed infants exposed to a larger number of bacteria than those who are breast-fed (Hanson *et al.*, 1990). Secondly, heavy microbial exposure in developing countries is associated with an earlier antibody response of greater magnitude (Mellander *et al.*, 1985). Further evidence that neonates can produce antibody comes from the demonstration of anti-*E. coli* antibodies in infants from immunoglobulin-deficient mothers (Hahn-Zoric *et al.*, 1992).

Serum antibodies in infants

In the absence of intrauterine infection, the newborn usually has little or no serum IgA or IgM, but high levels of IgG of maternal origin are present. The infant begins to produce IgM and IgA, and later IgG, against *E. coli* antigens, but this takes a few months to become established (Hanson *et al.*, 1990). Serum antibody may appear earlier in formula-fed infants (Ogura, 1987). By the age of seven to nine months, the avidity of serum IgG in the infant reaches that of transplacentally acquired IgG, but serum antibody titres are usually low. Artificial colonisation experiments generally only lead to production of local antibodies, without a systemic response (Lodinovà-Zàdníkovà *et al.*, 1991). Serum antibodies do not appear to protect against gastro-intestinal colonisation, but may be important in neutralising endotoxin that originates in the bowel.

Young infants with elevated C-reactive protein (CRP) concentrations have serum IgG anti-*E. coli* O-antibodies of significantly lower avidity than those in whom the CRP concentration is in the normal range (Hanson *et al.*, 1990). Serum anti-K1 antibody protects experimental rats from septicaemia due to orally administered *E. coli* (Hanson *et al.*, 1990) and other serum antibodies probably also prevent tissue invasion by intestinal *E. coli*.

The origin of natural antibodies

Normal sera contain a variety of natural antibodies, many of which are thought to be of heterogenetic microbial origin. The classical natural antibodies are the A, B and H(O) erythrocyte agglutinins. In contrast to other blood group systems, most notably rhesus (Rh), anti-A and anti-B isohaemagglutinins are always present in the sera of individuals who lack the corresponding antigen (Wiener, 1951). Human blood group A and B isoantibodies were at one time assumed to be inherited by pairs of linked genes, each representing a blood group antigen and its complementary antibody. According to the immunogenic hypothesis, the ability to produce antibody is inherited but isoantibodies can only be demonstrated when the antibody-producing mechanism has been exposed to exogenous cross-reactive or homologous antigens.

Natural antibodies are most intensely haemagglutinating at low temperatures, and increased thermal agitation at higher temperatures tends to cause dissociation of the less than perfect antigen–antibody complexes. In addition, most infants do not synthesise anti-A and anti-B agglutinins until three to six months after birth. Evidence that supports the role of bacteria in stimulating natural antibody production comes from the presence of substances with A, B and H(O) specificity amongst enteric bacteria and from immunisation studies of fowl and of humans with bacteria with blood-group-active substances. The role of microbes in the origin of blood group isoantibodies has been extensively reviewed by Springer (1971).

It is probable that, in some of the early work on blood group antigenic activity in bacteria, the growth media were contaminated with blood-group-active substances. However, Schiff (1934) reported that *Shigella* grown in fully defined media possess substances with a close serological relationship to natural blood group antigens. Other Gram-negative enteric bacteria, including *E. coli*, were subsequently shown to be serologically related to human blood group antigens. Thus, Springer *et al.* (1961) found that 137 of 282 clinical isolates of Gram-negative bacteria had A, B, H(O) blood group activity, including 64 of 135 strains of *E. coli*. About ten per cent of blood-group-active bacteria appeared to be about as powerful inhibitors of haemagglutination as the human blood-group-specific glycoproteins present in secretions. However, the strains used in this study had been isolated from a variety of sites and may not, therefore, accurately reflect the blood group activity of the intestinal flora.

Most bacterial strains have one predominant activity, of which H(O) or B have been found to be the commonest specificities. Certain blood group specificities are serotype dependent, for example *E. coli* O86 shows high B activity and lower A activity, while *E. coli* O127 and O128 have high H(O) activity. However, there is not always a strict correspondence between blood group specificity and O-antigen specificity. Moreover, bacteria that cross-react with their respective O-antisera do not necessarily share the same blood group activity.

Serological relationships between Gram-negative enteric bacteria and human blood group antigens have led to the hypothesis that constant immunisation against the intestinal flora leads to the production of anti-blood group A or B agglutinins. Springer (1971) showed that anti-human blood group B agglutinins were present in the majority of ordinary White Leghorn chicks by the age of 30 days, whereas such antibodies were undetectable in germ-free chicks after 60 days. Moreover, germ-free fowl, mono-contaminated by feeding *E. coli* O86, formed potent anti-human blood group B antibodies within 25 days. Whilst these studies provided evidence of formation of natural anti-blood-group antibodies in birds, the relevance of these findings to humans was questioned. It was subsequently shown that humans of all ages over one week may form isoantibodies in response to the ingestion or inhalation of blood-group-active *E. coli* O86.

Further evidence for the microbial origin of natural haemagglutinins has been provided by chemical studies of bacterial and blood group antigens (Springer, 1971). The specificity of blood group A, B and H(O) glycoproteins is associated with oligosaccharide subunits composed of D-galactose, L-fucose, N-acetyl-D-glucosamine and N-acetyl-D-galactosamine. These sugars have been found in the LPS of a number of blood-group-active bacteria. The terminal residue has been identified as most important in determining serological specificity. While attempts to correlate the blood group activities of bacteria with the chemistry of their O-antigens have to take into account the possible effects of the procedures used in their isolation, general agreement has been found between the nature of the carbohydrate building blocks and the observed blood group activity of bacteria. Whilst no significant activity in bacteria has been reported when the monosaccharide responsible for the major part of a given activity is absent from the O-antigen, the converse is not necessarily the case, presumably because the sugars must be linked in a particular sequence or orientation in order to be antigenic.

Human isoantibodies A and B, therefore, appear to be readily elicited by the widely distributed blood-group-active antigens of microbes *via* physiological routes, provided that the genetically determined apparatus of the host is responsive. However, individuals may also be exposed to blood-group-active substances in other ways, for example in foods. Therefore, these studies are consistent with, but cannot confirm, the hypothesis that naturally occurring antibodies are actually of microbial origin.

Since A, B and H(O) blood group antigens frequently occur in bacteria, it is conceivable that blood group agglutinins may have a protective effect against infection with blood-group-active bacteria. In rabbits immunised with human blood-group-B-specific substance, serum bactericidal and isoagglutinin titres rose 60-fold (Muschel & Osawa, 1959). Whilst the decrease in anti-blood-group antibodies after absorption with *E. coli* O86 or blood-group-B erythrocytes approached 100 per cent, removal of *E. coli* O86-stimulated antibodies and bactericidal activity by absorption with blood-group B erythrocytes was barely significant. This emphasises the limited significance of the B-reactive grouping in relation to the entire antigenic mosaic of the bacterium. Growth of blood group-active bacteria is temporarily inhibited when they are grown with heat-inactivated hyperimmune sera of corresponding blood group antibody specificity, while sera from neonates with blood group B possess anti-*E. coli* O86 activity. Clinical studies suggest that the blood group has minimal influence on susceptibility to infection with *E. coli*. Wittels & Lichtman (1986) reported that individuals of blood groups B and AB were over-represented amongst patients with *E. coli* septicaemia. Blood group does not, however, appear to be important in determining susceptibility to diarrhoea due to enterotoxigenic *E. coli* (Van Loon *et al.*, 1991).

The role of bacterial components in the production of naturally occurring antibodies in other blood group systems has also been studied (Savalonis *et al.*, 1988). Some strains of *E. coli* O125:B15 possess Kell-like activity. Significant Rh, M or N activity has not been reported, which is consistent with the rare occurrence of these agglutinins without deliberate stimulation.

Anti-galactosyl antibody (anti-Gal) is another natural antibody present in large amounts in normal human sera (Galili *et al.*, 1988), contributing as much as one per cent of circulating IgG. It is the only natural IgG antibody found in high titres in normal individuals. Anti-gal shows specificity for the carbohydrate epitope galactosyl-α-(1→3)-galactosyl [Gal-α(1→3)-Gal], and appears to be involved in the destruction of normal senescent and some pathological erythrocytes. The antigen appears to be present in a cryptic form on young erythrocytes, but is exposed *de novo* on the senescent erythrocyte population, labelling these cells for phagocytosis. Anti-Gal binds to a variety of bacteria, including *E. coli*, which suggests that constant production of anti-Gal is the result of on-going stimulation by intestinal bacteria that express Gal-$\alpha(1\rightarrow3)$-Gal. While it would seem, therefore, that senescent erythrocytes can provide the stimulus for anti-Gal production, no increase in anti-Gal is seen in haematological disorders where there is an increased proportion of cells binding anti-Gal.

In many bacteria the Gal-$\alpha(1\rightarrow3)$-Gal epitopes are present in the carbohydrate side chains of LPS but, in others, including *E. coli* O86, the epitopes appear to be expressed elsewhere, possibly in the capsule or the cell wall glycoprotein. In blood group A or O individuals, affinity-chromatography-purified anti-Gal contained antibody clones that also interacted with Gal-$\alpha(1\rightarrow3)$-Fuc-$\alpha(1\rightarrow2)$-Gal, the blood group B antigenic epitope. More than 85 per cent of anti-B antibodies have been found to bind to Gal-$\alpha(1\rightarrow3)$-Gal and Gal-$\alpha(1\rightarrow3)$-Fuc-$\alpha(1\rightarrow2)$-Gal residues. Thus, anti-Gal may account for most of the so-called anti-blood group-B activity.

An increased titre of anti-Gal has been reported in a number of infectious and autoimmune diseases, including Chagas' disease, American cutaneous leishmaniasis, auto-immune thyroiditis, Henoch–Schoenlein purpura and some patients with rheumatoid arthritis. Binding of anti-Gal to trypsin-treated human thyroid cells has been reported, which suggests that there are cryptic Gal-$\alpha(1\rightarrow3)$-Gal structures on other human tissues. Thus, the sharing of antigens between cryptic epitopes on human tissues and immunogenic glycosidic structures on bacterial cell walls may lead to the initiation of autoimmune processes in tissues where these cryptic structures are exposed as the result of pathological processes. Fragmented *E. coli* O86 has been shown to adhere to normal fibroblasts and to HeLa cells, and subsequently to mediate the binding of anti-Gal to the surface of these cells. Adhesion of bacteria *in vivo* may occur in the same way, resulting in an anti-Gal-mediated reaction against such cells. Another mechanism by which bacteria may precipitate anti-Gal binding to host cells has been proposed. Bacteria that express Gal-$\alpha(1\rightarrow3)$-Gal epitopes have been shown to possess the enzyme $\alpha(1\rightarrow3)$-galactosyl transferase, and it has been suggested that this enzyme may be able to generate Gal-$\alpha(1\rightarrow3)$-Gal structures on human cells.

The antibody response to infection with *Escherichia coli*

The nature of exposure to *E. coli* ranges from superficial gastro-intestinal colonisation to pathological systemic infection. The range of the resulting immune responses is equally wide.

Antibodies against Escherichia coli *in healthy individuals*

The prevalence and titres of naturally occurring anti-*E. coli* antibodies in populations vary considerably, depending on factors such as the assay used, the timing of collection of the sera, the population examined and the *E. coli* strain used as the antigen.

In germ-free rats artificially colonised with *E. coli* O6:K13, a secretory antibody response dominated by IgA and a strong serum antibody response has been demonstrated, with an evolving response pattern to different antigens. Serum anti-LPS IgG and IgM appeared within one week and a response of lower magnitude to type-1 fimbriae appeared one to three weeks later, while antibody to β-galactosidase, an internal antigen, appeared only after five to ten weeks (Wold *et al.*, 1989). Artificial colonisation of human infants has been shown to elicit a strong local secretory antibody response, but no detectable serum antibody response (Lodinovà-Zàdníkovà *et al.*, 1991). Prolonged follow-up of adults has shown that carriage strains of *E. coli* and other enteric bacteria vary over time (Robinet, 1962). However, antibody levels against different serotypes tend to remain fairly constant and appear to be characteristic of the host, rather than reflecting changes in the gastro-intestinal flora. There is no evidence that the presence of antibody protects against efficient colonisation by the homologous strain.

Naturally occurring anti-*E. coli* antibodies are IgM and predominantly directed against O-specific LPS side chains, and typically antibodies to a large number of serotypes can be detected. Antibodies to LPS core components are also predominantly IgM and can be detected in low titres by enzyme-linked immunosorbant assay (ELISA) or immunofluorence techniques in most healthy individuals aged more than three years (Law & Marks, 1985; Nys *et al.*, 1988). Neutropenic patients may be deficient in such antibodies, which may in part explain their susceptibility to septicaemia with Gram-negative bacteria.

A low level of anti-ECA antibodies is present in most normal human sera (Malkamäki, 1981). The pattern of occurrence of such antibodies tends to parallel that of anti-O-antibodies, with a rise in titre in early childhood, especially after the age of six months, followed by a decline in later life. Titres have been reported to be higher in females, and may reflect the higher incidence of urinary tract infection in women. Low levels of antibodies to OMPs (Griffiths *et al.*, 1985) and other antigens such as a-haemolysin (Emödy *et al.*, 1982; Seetharama *et al.*, 1988) are also found in most healthy sera.

Naturally occurring anti-O-antibodies in bile, mainly IgM and IgA, are rather less frequent than in serum, and appear to be substantially derived from local sources (Hansen & Jackson, 1990).

The antibody response in Escherichia coli *urinary tract infection*

Uropathogenic *E. coli* are characterised by a set of virulence attributes, including certain O-types, capsular antigens, haemolysin, aerobactin, resistance to killing by normal human sera and the presence of specific adhesins. The serological response to urinary tract infection has been well characterised (Salit *et al.*, 1988).

In animals, healing of acute *E. coli* urinary tract infection is associated with the development of an immune response and subsequent resistance to the infecting strain (Salit *et al.*, 1988). During the course of infection, the major immunoglobulin synthesised in the kidney and bladder is IgG. Secretory IgA is also produced within the pyelonephritic kidney, but only very small amounts are produced by the infected bladder. In vaccination studies antibodies to O-, K- and P-antigens have been shown to protect against ascending infection.

Approximately 90 per cent of human patients with acute pyelonephritis develop a significant rise in antibody titre, compared with only about five per cent of patients with uncomplicated cystitis (Salit *et al.*, 1988). The predominant antibody is directed against the O-antigen and is mainly of the IgM class. In patients with recurrences, IgG is formed, presumably because of previous immune stimulation. The most striking elevation of antibody is found in pyelonephritis, and the lowest levels after cystitis, however there is an overlap in antibody levels between the two conditions and antibody titres in asymptomatic bacteriuria may be as high as in acute pyelonephritis (Mattsby-Baltzer *et al.*, 1981). Presence of type-specific antibody does not appear to protect against pyelonephritis. Persistence of infection in the kidney and acquisition of new infections have been shown to occur in spite of high titres of O-specific antibody to the infecting organism. Elevated levels of antibody to lipid A, as compared with healthy controls, have been demonstrated in patients with all degrees of urinary tract infection.

Information about the occurrence and protective efficacy of anti-P-fimbrial antibodies is conflicting. Weak serum anti-P-fimbrial antibody has been demonstrated in up to 85 per cent of patients with acute pyelonephritis (Agata *et al.*, 1989; Kanai *et al.*, 1990). Some workers have been able to detect urinary anti-fimbrial antibody, whereas others have not. Patients with cystitis have very low levels of anti-P-antibodies, and titres do not increase during convalescence. P-fimbriae are immunologically heterogeneous and, in general, monoclonal antibodies exhibit only minimal, if any, intertype cross-reactivity, or are F-type specific (Johnson, 1991). *In vitro*, anti-P-antibodies often fail to block adherence even when mediated by the homologous P-fimbriated strain. However anti-P-antibodies appear to protect animals against renal infection with homologous and possibly heterologous P-fimbriated strains (Klemm, 1985; Kaack *et al.*, 1988).

Capsular antigens, especially K1, are poor immunogens, and serum antibody is rarely found in patients with pyelonephritis. However anti-capsular immunity is protective in animal models of UTI (Kaijser *et al.*, 1983).

Elevated titres of serum antibody against OMPs can be detected in patients with UTI, as compared with healthy controls. Patients with acute pyelonephritis show a significant increase in titre during convalescence (Nicolle *et al.*, 1989), although this has not been confirmed by others (Salit *et al.*, 1988). There is little information about the antibody response to ECA in UTI, but these antibodies have been shown to protect rabbits against retrograde and haematogenous challenge with *Proteus mirabilis* (Domingue *et al.*, 1970). Elevated titres of serum anti-a-haemolysin have been found in patients with UTI, levels correlating with the invasiveness of infection (Seetharama *et al.*, 1988).

Detection of antibody-coated bacteria may be useful in localising UTI in certain groups of patients, but the technique has never achieved widespread acceptance. The major difficulty is establishing an end-point. The antibody that is detected is thought to be IgG produced locally in renal tissue and directed primarily against O-antigens (Stamm, 1983).

The antibody response to Escherichia coli *septicaemia*

After natural infection the antibody response is directed chiefly against LPS (McCabe *et al.*, 1972). Patients may respond differently to different LPS epitopes and their responses are a function of the structure of the particular LPS that elicits the response. In general, the antibody response is directed primarily against specific O-determinants and in the acute phase it is mainly a T-cell-independent IgM response (McCabe *et al.*, 1972). High levels of antibody to core LPS epitopes are not seen, although a greater response may be seen where the infecting strain has a rough or part-rough phenotype. About one-third to a half of patients with septicaemia have a detectable, though usually modest, antibody response to core determinants, while a fivefold to sevenfold increase in anti-O-antibodies can usually be demonstrated. (Cross *et al.*, 1989).

O-specific antibodies increase serum bactericidal activity and accelerate clearance of homologous bacteria or LPS from the bloodstream. Tumour necrosis factor (TNF) and consequently interleukin-6 (IL-6) production induced by homologous challenge are decreased, and anti-O-antibodies also protect against development of the Shwartzman reaction. It is thought that anti-core antibodies are at best only weakly opsonic and are believed to act principally as antitoxins, binding to and neutralising the biologically active LPS core. Reports are conflicting about whether core antibodies protect against development of the Shwartzman reaction (Baumgartner *et al.*, 1990).

In patients with Gram-negative septicaemia O-side-chain antibodies afford a high degree of strain-specific protection, while antibodies to core determinants appear to offer protection that extends to heterologous and homologous strains. Early work *in vitro* suggested that core antibodies were broadly cross-reactive. However the core region of LPS shows a degree of structural heterogeneity, which raises theoretical doubts about these early observations, given that antigen–antibody reactions are generally highly specific (Ziegler, 1988). Subsequent studies with monoclonal antibodies to investigate cross-reactivity have not resolved the issue. Conflicting results were obtained that appear to depend on variables such as the physical state of the bacteria or the LPS used for the assay, the assay method and the specificity of the antibody (Shenep *et al.*, 1987). Moreover, it is uncertain whether antibody can gain access to core target sites in smooth strains (Gigliotti & Shenep, 1985). The immunological reactivity of Gram-negative bacteria with antisera to rough mutants is most readily apparent in the early exponential phase of bacterial growth. This suggests that immunodeterminants shared with rough mutants may be more accessible in smooth bacteria during the early phase of bacterial growth. It has also been proposed that serum factors may be able to unmask core glycolipid antigenic sites on the LPS of smooth strains (Chedid *et al.*, 1968) but other workers have been unable to confirm this. There remains significant doubt, therefore, as to whether the apparent protection afforded by core antibodies is due to a specific immunological mechanism at all.

The apparent ability of naturally occurring anti-core antibodies to protect against the shock and death associated with Gram-negative septicaemia, and the *in vitro* evidence for cross-reactivity have excited considerable interest in these antibodies as a means for the prevention and treatment of Gram-negative septic shock (Overbeek & Veringa, 1990; Young *et al.*, 1991). Polyclonal antisera against rough mutant bacteria were found to protect against the toxic sequelae of endotoxin in various experimental animal models. Active immunisation of experimental animals with polysaccharide-deficient strains, such as the J5 mutant of *E. coli* O111 or *Salmonella minnesota* R595, can evoke increases of antibody of tenfold or greater. Some studies found that these antibodies conferred broad cross-protection, although others were unable to confirm this and cited differences in the challenge dose or the strain or species of animal used as possible explanations. Vaccination of healthy humans with *E. coli* J5 gives a response rate of 60 to 80 per cent (Schwartzer *et al.*, 1988; Baumgartner *et al.*, 1991). Post-immunisation sera from these individuals have been shown to protect mice challenged with homologous and heterologous Gram-negative bacteria. However, the antibody response is transient and not enhanced by revaccination, probably because the antigens are T-cell-independent and elicit an immune response with little or no immunological memory. Passive immunisation with polyclonal anti-J5 antisera was effective in decreasing mortality in patients with septic shock and in reducing the incidence of shock when administered prophylactically to patients at high risk of Gram-negative septicaemia (Young *et al.*, 1991; Zanetti *et al.*, 1991). However, the differences in many of the studies only just reached statistical significance and the outcome could not be convincingly correlated with the level of anti-core antibodies, which raised further doubts about the origin of the protection. IgM is important in protective immunity but it is difficult to isolate and purify. This delayed the commercial availability of antisera for proper evaluation in large clinical trials. These difficulties were overcome by the preparation of monoclonal antibodies (MAbs), one of which, a human IgM MAb (centoxin, HA-A1; Centocor), was available in the United Kingdom for a short time. The results of trials of MAbs have been extensively reviewed (Zanetti *et al.*, 1991). Briefly, when administered to patients with Gram-negative septicaemia, MAbs were found significantly to reduce the incidence of shock and death. However, detailed analysis and comparison of studies revealed conflicting results and there is some doubt about the comparability of the test and control groups. Moreover, a Phase III trial of centoxin in the United States of America was abandoned, and the drug voluntarily withdrawn, when it was found that the possible beneficial effects of centoxin in Gram-negative bacteraemia were offset by adverse effects in patients with other causes of septic shock (Horton, 1993).

Most *E. coli* strains associated with invasive infections are encapsulated and specific anti-capsular antibodies are required for their efficient opsonisation. During infection, most individuals develop anti-O-antibodies but antibodies to K-antigens are less common, though they afford a far greater protective effect than anti-O-antibodies (Kaijser & Ahlstedt, 1977; Overbeek & Veringa, 1990).

Patients with *E. coli* septicaemia may respond to various other epitopes, including ECA (McCabe *et al.*, 1972), a-haemolysin (Seetharama *et al.*, 1988) and various OMPs (Henriksen & Maeland, 1987, 1990). In general, there is no correlation between the magnitude of the antibody response to LPS and these other antigens, nor have any of these antibodies usually been reported to affect the development or outcome of septicaemia in humans. Evidence of a protective function for anti-OMP antibodies has, however, come from experimental salmonellosis in mice (Kuusi *et al.*, 1979). Western blotting of sera from patients with *E. coli* septicaemia has demonstrated an antibody response to various OMPs (Henriksen & Maeland, 1987). Absorption of sera with live intact organisms suggests that BLp is the predominant cell-surface-located antigen. Further evidence for its accessibility as an antigenic target comes from the observation that specific BLp reactivity can be detected in virtually all sera positive in a crude OMP ELISA (Henriksen & Maeland, 1990).

The antibody response in enteric Escherichia coli *infections*

Vero-cytotoxin-producing Escherichia coli

Vero cytotoxin-producing *E. coli* (VTEC) are an important cause of diarrhoea in some geographical settings, and can cause two life-threatening complications, haemorrhagic colitis and haemolytic-uraemic syndrome (HUS). At least two Vero cytotoxins, VT1 and VT2, are associated with disease in humans and VTEC isolates may produce either or both of these toxins (Karmali, 1989). Antibodies to bacterial components and to Vero cytotoxins can be detected in infections with VTEC;

such antibodies are either not found, or found in low titres, in healthy individuals (Chart *et al.*, 1989; Kishore *et al.*, 1992). The main immune response in VTEC infection is an IgM response to O157 LPS, and detection of such antibodies is useful in providing evidence of infection where faecal VTEC or Vero cytotoxin cannot be demonstrated (Chart *et al.*, 1989). Patients do not appear to produce IgG antibodies but about half produce serum IgA antibody, which in some cases may be the only marker of infection (Chart & Rowe, 1992). Sera from patients with non-O157 VTEC infections may react with O157 LPS by ELISA and in immunoblots, which suggests that more than one LPS epitope is important (Kishore *et al.*, 1992). Information about the duration of the immune response is limited, but antibody has usually been found to disappear in two to three months (Bitzan *et al.*, 1991; Kishore *et al.*, 1992).

Antibodies to both VT1 and VT2 can be detected by ELISA (Rowe *et al.*, 1993). Most patients with *E. coli* O157:H7 infection develop an antibody response to VT2 but only about half develop a response to VT1.

Vero cytotoxin is generally considered to be central to the pathogenesis of HUS (Karmali, 1989). However, complement-fixing IgG and IgM antibodies that lyse cultured umbilical vein endothelial cells have been reported in the sera of patients with HUS, suggesting that anti-endothelial-cell antibodies may be involved in the pathogenesis of vascular injury (Leung *et al.*, 1988).

Enterotoxin-producing Escherichia coli

In humans enterotoxin-producing *E. coli* (ETEC) are a major cause of infant diarrhoea in developing countries and the commonest cause of travellers' diarrhoea. They are also of major importance as a cause of diarrhoea in young livestock (Gross, 1991). The diarrhoea is due to production of heat-labile enterotoxin (LT) and/or heat-stable enterotoxins (ST). The latter are poorly antigenic. In order to cause diarrhoea, ETEC must also adhere to the small intestinal mucosa and various fimbrial antigens, including K88 in porcine strains, F41 in bovine strains and various CFAs in human strains, have been described. Most patients with diarrhoea due to LT-producing ETEC can be shown to develop a serum and local antibody response to LT, CFA and LPS, which confers homologous immunity, while asymptomatic acquisition of the organism is generally not associated with an immune response (Stoll *et al.*, 1986). In paired samples from convalescents, an eightfold to ninefold rise in anti-CFA and a fourfold rise in anti-LT can be demonstrated (Clemens *et al.*, 1990). Immunity appears to be primarily directed towards CFA-type fimbrial antigens, and heterologous protection is not conferred where the only common antigen is LT (Levine *et al.*, 1979). Antibodies to LT and CFA appear to afford synergistic protection from diarrhoea while, for ETEC that carry several adhesins, antibodies directed against several adhesins are more effective than antibodies against a single adhesin (Duchet-Suchaux, 1988). Anti-LT activity appears to be primarily directed against the B-subunit of the toxin, but it has been shown that LT can also be neutralised by specific monoclonal anti-A-antibodies. Serum anti-CFA and anti-LT-antibody titres have been reported to be similar in patients and controls, indicating that these antibodies do not protect against LT-ETEC diarrhoea. However, bovine milk immunoglobulin concentrate has successfully been used to protect volunteers challenged with ETEC O78:H11. Fimbrial vaccines (K88, K99, 987P) are routinely given parenterally to pregnant cattle, sheep and pigs in order to protect suckling neonates. These vaccines result in a high-level humoral immune response, but secretory mucosal antibodies are not produced. High titres of antibody are, however, achieved in colostrum and milk, which protects the offspring (Moon *et al.*, 1988). In spite of initial concerns, these vaccines have been used for more than ten years without evidence of the emergence of new or previously low-prevalence fimbrial types (Moon & Bunn, 1993). Trials of CFA-type fimbrial vaccines in humans have had some success in protecting against ETEC diarrhoea (Czerkinsky *et al.*, 1993). Diarrhoea in humans due to experimental challenge of volunteers with ETEC O78:H11 can also be prevented by passive immunisation with bovine milk immunoglobulin concentrate (Tacket *et al.*, 1988).

Enteroinvasive Escherichia coli

Enteroinvasive *E. coli* (EIEC) cause dysentery similar to shigellosis by an invasive mechanism that depends on the presence of certain OMPs (Gross, 1991). In animal models the intestinal sIgA response is the principal component of the immune response and is probably the basis of immunity to reinfection. Serogroup-specific antibodies appear to be highly protective but other antigens, such as a plasmid-encoded protein antigen, appear to be much less important for protective immunity (O'Hanley & Cantey, 1981; Ketyi & Pal, 1987).

Enteropathogenic Escherichia coli

Infantile enteritis due to enteropathogenic *E. coli* (EPEC) is a particularly important cause of diarrhoea in developing countries (Gross, 1991). The diarrhoea appears to be due to the capacity of EPEC to adhere and efface the microvillous surface structure of intestinal epithelial cells. In many strains localised adhesion is associated with the presence of a plasmid-encoded 94-kDa OMP, EPEC adherence factor (EAF). It has been shown by immunoblotting that recipients of EAF-positive strains develop both serum and breast milk antibody to this protein. The antibodies have been shown to inhibit bacterial attachment *in vitro*, and to protect individuals from diarrhoea after challenge with EAF-positive strains. However an antiserum raised to a HEp-2 adhesin did not react with the EAF of all EPEC, indicating some interstrain antigenic variation (Chart *et al.*, 1988).

An EPEC-type strain of *E. coli* O15, RDEC-1, that is pathogenic for rabbits expresses a fimbrial adhesin, AF/R1. This is used as a naturally occurring animal model of human EPEC infection (Boedeker *et al.*, 1988). Specific anti-AF/R1 fimbrial antibody and anti-O15 antibody can be demonstrated after infection. Anti-O15 appears to afford better protection than anti-fimbrial antibody, which is consistent with observations *in vitro* that AF/R1 is an accessory virulence factor (Wolf *et al.*, 1988).

Cell-mediated immunity in *Escherichia coli* infections

While the humoral response to *E. coli* infection has been extensively studied, aspects of cell-mediated immunity have received far less attention. Evidence that cell-mediated immunity may be important in defence against *E. coli* infection first came from studies of lung infection. Most subsequent work, which has been reviewed by Ahlstedt *et al.* (1983), has addressed the possible role of cell-mediated immunity in causing renal damage in urinary tract infection. Briefly, suppression of cell-mediated immunity was found in children with acute pyelonephritis, and no significant lymphoblastogenic responses to *E. coli* antigens have been recorded. Suppression of cell-mediated immunity reactions may moderate the inflammatory reaction in the infected kidney and so decrease renal damage, but there is little or no evidence that cell-mediated immunity mechanisms protect against renal infections (Miller *et al.*, 1986).

References

Agata, N., Ohta, M., Miyazawa, H., Mori, M., Kido, N. & Kato, N. (1989). Serological response to P-fimbriae of *Escherichia coli* in patients with urinary tract infections. *European Journal of Clinical Microbiology and Infectious Diseases*, **8**, 156–9.

Ahlstedt, S., Hagberg, M., Jodal, U. & Mårild, S. (1983). Cell-mediated immune parameters in children with pyelonephritis caused by *Escherichia coli*. *Progress in Allergy*, **33**, 289–97.

Avananzini, M. A., Plebani, A., Monafo, V., Pasinetti, G., Teani, M., Colombo, A., Mellander, L., Carlsson, B., Hanson, L. A., Ugazio, A. G. & Burgio, G. R. (1992). A comparison of secretory antibodies in breast-fed and formula-fed infants over the first six months of life. *Acta Paediatrica Scandinavica*, **81**, 296–301.

Baumgartner, J. D., Heumann, D., Calandra, T. & Glauser, M. P. (1991). Antibodies to lipopolysaccharides after immunization with rough mutant *Escherichia coli* J5. *Journal of Infectious Diseases*, **163**, 769–72.

Baumgartner, J. D., Heumann, D., Gerain, J., Weinbreck, P., Grau, G. E. & Glauser, M. P. (1990). Association between protective efficacy of anti-lipopolysaccharide (LPS) antibodies and suppression of LPS-induced tumour necrosis factor alpha and interleukin 6. Comparison of O side chain-specific antibodies with core LPS antibodies. *Journal of Experimental Medicine*, **171**, 889–96.

Bayston, K. F. & Cohen, J. (1990). Bacterial endotoxin and current concepts in the diagnosis and treatment of endotoxaemia. *Journal of Medical Microbiology*, **31**, 73–83.

Bitzan, M., Moebius, E., Ludwig, K., Müller-Wiefel, D. E., Heesemann, J. & Karch, H. (1991). High incidence of serum antibodies to *Escherichia coli* O157 lipopolysaccharide in children with hemolytic-uremic syndrome. *Journal of Pediatrics*, **119**, 380–5.

Boedeker, E. C. (1988). Intestinal infection with *Escherichia coli* strain RDEC-1 in the rabbit: pathogenesis and host immune responses. In *Mucosal Immunity and Infections at Mucosal Surfaces*, eds. W. Strober, M. E. Lamm, J. R. McGhee & S. P. James, pp. 355–72. New York: Oxford University Press.

Boesman-Finkelstein, M. & Finkelstein, R. A. (1982). Sequential purification of lactoferrin, lysozyme and secretory immunoglobulin A from human milk. *FEBS Letters*, **144**, 1–5.

Brunser, O., Espinoza, J., Figueroa, G., Araya, M., Spencer, E., Hilpert, H., Link-Amster, H. & Brussow, H. (1992). Field trial of an infant formula containing anti-rotavirus and anti-*Escherichia coli* milk antibodies from hyperimmunised cows. *Journal of Pediatric Gastroenterology and Nutrition*, **15**, 63–72.

Carlsson, B., Gothefors, L., Ahlstedt, S., Hanson, L. Å. & Winberg, J. (1976). Studies of *Escherichia coli* O antigen specific antibodies in human milk, maternal serum and cord blood. *Acta Paediatrica Scandinavica*, **65**, 216–24.

Carlsson, B., Kaijser, B., Ahlstedt, S., Gotherfors, L. & Hanson, L. Å. (1982). Antibodies against *Escherichia coli* capsular (K) antigens in human milk and serum. *Acta Paediatrica Scandinavica*, **71**, 313–18.

Chart, H. & Rowe, B. (1992). Improved detection of infection by *Escherichia coli* O157 in patients with haemolytic uraemic syndrome by means of IgA antibodies to lipopolysaccharide. *Journal of Infection*, **24**, 257–61.

Chart, H., Scotland, S. M. & Rowe, B. (1989). Serum antibodies to *Escherichia coli* serotype O157:H7 in patients with hemolytic uremic syndrome. *Journal of Clinical Microbiology*, **27**, 285–90.

Chart, H., Scotland, S. M., Willshaw, G. A. & Rowe, B. (1988). HEp-2 adhesion and the expression of a 94 kDa outer-membrane protein by strains of *Escherichia coli* belonging to enteropathogenic serogroups. *Journal of General Microbiology*, **134**, 1315–21.

Chedid, L., Parant, M., Parant, F. & Boyer, F. (1968). A proposed mechanism for natural immunity to enterobacterial pathogens. *Journal of Immunology*, **100**, 292–301.

Clemens, J. D., Svennerholm, A. M., Harris, J. R., Huda, S., Rao, M., Neogy, P. K., Khan, M. R., Ansaruzzaman, M., Rahaman, S., Ahmed, F., Sack, D. A., Kay, B., Van Loom, F. & Holmgren, J. (1990). Seroepidemiologic evaluation of anti-toxic and anti-colonization factor immunity against infections by LT-producing *Escherichia coli* in rural Bangladesh. *Journal of Infectious Diseases*, **162**, 448–53.

Cravioto, A., Tello, A., Villafán, H., Ruiz, J., del Vedovo, S. & Neeser, J.-R. (1991). Inhibition of localized adhesion of enteropathogenic *Escherichia coli* to HEp-2 cells by immunoglobulin and oligosaccharide fractions of human colostrum and breast milk. *Journal of Infectious Diseases*, **163**, 1247–55.

Cross, A. S., Sidberry, H. & Sadoff, J. C. (1989). The human antibody response during natural bacteremic infection with Gram-negative bacilli against lipopolysaccharide core determinants. *Journal of Infectious Diseases*, **160**, 225–36.

Cruz, J. R., Gil, L., Cano, F., Caceres, P. & Pareja, G. (1988). Breast milk anti-*Escherichia coli* heat-labile toxin IgA antibodies protect against toxin-induced infantile diarrhoea. *Acta Paediatrica Scandinavica*, **77**, 658–62.

Czerkinsky, C., Svennerholm, A. M. & Holmgren, J. (1993). Induction and assessment of immunity at enteromucosal surfaces in humans: implications for vaccine development. *Clinical Infectious Diseases*, **16**, Supplement 2, S106–16.

Domingue, G., Salhi, A., Rountree, C. & Little, W. (1970). Prevention of experimental hematogenous and retrograde pyelonephritis by antibodies against enterobacterial common antigen. *Infection and Immunity*, **2**, 175–82.

Duchet-Suchaux, M. (1988). Protective antigens against enterotoxigenic *Escherichia coli* O101:K99,F41 in the infant mouse diarrhea model. *Infection and Immunity*, **56**, 1364–70.

Emödy, L., Batai, I. Jr., Kerényi, M. & Székely, J. Jr. (1982). α-haemolysin may have a pathogenic role in extra-intestinal manifestations of infections. *Lancet*, **2**, 986.

Galili, U., Mandrell, R. E., Hamadeh, R. M., Shohet, S. B. & Griffiss, J. M. (1988). Interaction between human natural anti-α-galatosyl immunoglobulin G and bacteria of the human flora. *Infection and Immunity*, **56**, 1730–7.

Gigliotti, F. & Shenep, J. L. (1985). Failure of monoclonal antibodies to core glycolipid to bind intact smooth strains of *Escherichia coli*. *Journal of Infectious Diseases*, **151**, 1005–11.

Gleeson, M., Cripps, A. W., Clancy, R. L., Wlodarczyk, J. H., Dobson, A. J. & Hensley, M. J. (1987). The development of IgA-specific antibodies to *Escherichia coli* O antigen in children. *Scandinavian Journal of Immunology*, **26**, 639–43.

Gothefors, L., Carlsson, B., Ahlstedt, S., Hanson, L. A. & Winberg, J. (1976). Influence of maternal gut flora and colostral and cord serum antibodies on presence of *Escherichia coli* in faeces of the newborn infant. *Acta Paediatrica Scandinavica*, **65**, 225–32.

Griffiths, E., Stevenson, P., Thorpe, R. & Chart, H. (1985). Naturally-occurring antibodies in human sera that react with the iron-regulated outer membrane proteins of *Escherichia coli*. *Infection and Immunity*, **47**, 808–13.

Griffiths, E. K., Yoonessi, S. & Neter, E. (1977). Antibody response to enterobacterial lipoprotein of patients with varied infections due to Enterobacteriaceae. *Proceedings of the Society for Experimental Biology and Medicine*, **154**, 246–9.

Gross, R. J. (1991). The pathogenesis of *Escherichia coli* diarrhoea. *Reviews in Medical Microbiology*, **2**, 37–44.

Hahn-Zoric, M., Carlsson, B., Bjorkander, J., Osterhaus, A. D., Mellander, L. & Hanson, L. A. (1992). Presence of non-maternal antibodies in newborns of mothers with antibody deficiencies. *Pediatric Research*, **32**, 150–4.

Hansen, P. G. & Jackson, G. D. (1990). The occurrence and sources of natural antibody in human bile and serum against the O antigens of two *Escherichia coli* serotypes. *Scandinavian Journal of Immunology*, **32**, 537–44.

Hanson, L. Å., Ashraf, R., Cruz, J. R., Hahn-Zoric, M., Jalil, F., Nave, F., Reimer, M., Zaman, S. & Carlsson, B. (1990). Immunity related to exposition and bacterial colonization of the infant. *Acta Paediatrica Scandinavica*, Supplement, **365**, 38–45.

Hanson, L. Å., Söderström, T., Brinton, C., Carlsson, B., Larsson, P., Mellander, L. & Svanborg Eden, C. (1983) Neonatal colonization with *Escherichia coli* and the ontogeny of the antibody response. *Progress in Allergy*, **33**, 40–52.

Henriksen, A. Z. & Maeland, J. A. (1987). Serum antibodies to outer membrane proteins of *Escherichia coli* in healthy persons and patients with bacteremia. *Journal of Clinical Microbiology*, **25**, 2181–8.

Henriksen, A. Z. & Maeland, J. A. (1990). Antibody response to defined domains on enterobacterial outer membrane proteins in healthy persons and patients with bacteraemia. *APMIS*, **98**, 163–72.

Holmgren, J., Svennerholm, A.-M. & Åhrén, C. (1981). Nonimmunoglobulin fraction of human milk inhibits bacterial adhesion (haemagglutination) and enterotoxin binding of *Escherichia coli* and *Vibrio cholerae*. *Infection and Immunity*, **33**, 136–41.

Horton, R. (1993). Voluntary suspension of centoxin. *Lancet*, **341**, 298.

Johnson, J. (1991). Virulence factors in *Escherichia coli* urinary tract infection. *Clinical Microbiology Reviews*, **4**, 80–128.

Kaack, M. B., Roberts, J. A., Baskin, G. & Patterson, G. M. (1988). Maternal immunization with P fimbriae for the prevention of neonatal pyelonephritis. *Infection and Immunity*, **56**, 1–6.

Kaijser, B. & Ahlstedt, S. (1977). Protective capacity of antibodies against *Escherichia coli* O and K antigens. *Infection and Immunity*, **17**, 286–9.

Kaijser, B., Larsson, P., Olling, S. & Schneerson, R. (1983). Protection against acute, ascending pyelonephritis caused by *Escherichia coli* in rats, using isolated capsular antigen conjugated to bovine serum albumin. *Infection and Immunity*, **39**, 142–6.

Kanai, S., Mikake, K., Agata, N., Ohta, M. & Kato, N. (1990). Antibody response to P-fimbriae of *Escherichia coli* in patients with genitourinary tract infections. *Hinyokika Kiyo*, **36**, 1–6.

Karmali, M. A. (1989). Infection by verocytotoxin-producing *Escherichia coli*. *Clinical Microbiology Reviews*, **2**, 15–38.

Ketyi, I. & Pal, T. (1987). Protective value of the plasmid-coded outer membrane protein of enteroinvasive *Escherichia coli*. *Acta Microbiologica Hungarica*, **34**, 165–71.

Kishore, K., Rattan, A., Bagga, A., Srivastava, R. N., Nath, N. M. & Shriniwas. (1992). Serum antibodies to verotoxin-producing *Escherichia coli* (VTEC) strains in patients with haemolytic uraemic syndrome. *Journal of Medical Microbiology*, **37**, 364–7.

Klemm, P. (1985). Fimbrial adhesins of *Escherichia coli*. *Reviews of Infectious Diseases*, **7**, 321–40.

Krogfelt, K. A. (1991). Bacterial adhesion: genetics, biogenesis, and role in pathogenesis of fimbrial adhesins of *Escherichia coli*. *Reviews of Infectious Diseases*, **13**, 721–35.

Kuhn, H.-M., Dieter, U. M. & Mayer, H. (1988). ECA, the enterobacterial common antigen. *FEMS Microbiology Reviews*, **54**, 195–222.

Kuusi, N., Nurminen, M., Saxen, H., Valtonen, M. & Mäkelä, P. H. (1979). Immunization with major outer membrane proteins in experimental salmonellosis of mice. *Infection and Immunity*, **25**, 857–62.

Law, B. J. & Marks, M. I. (1985). Age-related prevalence of human serum IgG and IgM antibody to the core glycolipid of *Escherichia coli* strain J5, as measured by ELISA. *Journal of Infectious Diseases*, **6**, 988–94.

Leung, D. Y. M., Moake, J. L., Havens, P. L., Kim, M. & Pober, J. S. (1988). Lytic anti-endothelial cell antibodies in haemolytic-uraemic syndrome. *Lancet*, **2**, 183–6.

Levine, M. M., Nalin, D. R., Hoover, D. L., Bergquist, E. J., Hornick, B. & Young, C. R. (1979). Immunity to enterotoxigenic *Escherichia coli*. *Infection and Immunity*, **23**, 729–36.

Lodinovà-Zàdníkovà, R., Slavíkovà, M., Tlaskalovà-Hohenovà, H., Adlerberth, I., Hanson, L. Å., Wold, A., Carlsson, B., Svanborg, C. & Mellander, L. (1991). The antibody response in breast-fed and non-breast-fed infants after artificial colonization of the intestine with *Escherichia coli* O83. *Pediatric Research*, **29**, 396–9.

Malkamäki, M. (1981). Antibodies to enterobacterial common antigen: standardisation of the passive hemagglutination test and levels in normal human sera. *Journal of Clinical Microbiology*, **13**, 1074–9.

Mattsby-Baltzer, I., Claesson, I., Hanson, L. Å., Jodal, U., Kauser, B., Lindberg, U. & Peterson, H. (1981). Antibodies to lipid A during urinary tract infection. *Journal of Infectious Diseases*, **144**, 319–28.

McCabe, W. R., Kreger, B. E. & Johns, M. (1972). Type-specific and cross-reactive antibodies in Gram-negative bacteremia. *New England Journal of Medicine*, **287**, 261–7.

Mellander, L., Carlsson, B. & Hanson, L. Å. (1984). Appearance of secretory IgM and IgA antibodies to *Escherichia coli* in saliva during early infancy and childhood. *Journal of Pediatrics*, **104**, 564–8.

Mellander, L., Carlsson, B., Jalil, F., Söderström, T. & Hanson, L.Å.(1985). Secretory IgA antibody response against *Escherichia coli* antigens in infants in relation to exposure. *Journal of Pediatrics*, **107**, 430–3.

Miller, T. E., Findon, G., Cawley, S. & Clarke, I. (1986). Cellular basis of host defence in pyelonephritis. II. Acute infection. *British Journal of Experimental Pathology*, **67**, 191–200.

Moon, H. W. & Bunn, T. O. (1993). Vaccines for preventing enterotoxigenic *Escherichia coli* infections in farm animals. *Vaccine*, **11**, 213–20.

Moon, H. W., Rogers, D. G. & Rose, R. (1988). Effects of an orally administered live *Escherichia coli* pilus vaccine on duration of lacteal immunity to enterotoxigenic *Escherichia coli* in swine. *American Journal of Veterinary Research*, **49**, 2068–71.

Muschel, L. H. & Osawa, E. (1959). Human blood group substance B and *Escherichia coli* O86. *Proceedings of the Society for Experimental Biology*, **101**, 614–17.

Nicolle, L. E., Brunka, J., Ujack, E. & Bryan, L. (1989). Antibodies to major outer membrane proteins of *Escherichia coli* in urinary tract infection in the elderly. *Journal of Infectious Diseases*, **160**, 627–33.

Nys, M., Joassin, L., Somzee, A. & Demonty, J. (1988). Enzyme-linked immunosorbent assay for immunoglobulin G subclass antibodies specific for enterobacterial Re core glycolipid in healthy individuals and in patients infected by Gram-negative bacteria. *Journal of Clinical Microbiology*, **26**, 857–62.

Ogura, H. (1987). Serum antibodies to *Escherichia coli* in breast-fed and bottle-fed infants. *Acta Medica Okayama*, **41**, 161–3.

O'Hanley, P. D. & Cantey, J. R. (1981). Immune response of the ileum to invasive *Escherichia coli* diarrhoeal disease in rabbits. *Infection and Immunity*, **31**, 316–22.

Overbeek, B. P. & Veringa, E. M. (1990). Role of antibodies and antibiotics in aerobic Gram-negative septicemia: possible synergism between antimicrobial treatment and immunotherapy. *Reviews of Infectious Diseases*, **13**, 751–60.

Pisacane, A., Graziano, L., Mazzarella, G., Scarpellino, B. & Zona, G. (1992). Breast-feeding and urinary tract infection. *Journal of Pediatrics*, **120**, 87–9.

Robertson, D. M., Carlsson, B., Coffman, K., Hahn-Zoric, M., Jalil, F., Jones, C. & Hanson, L. Å. (1988). Avidity of IgA antibody to *Escherichia coli* polysaccharide and diphtheria toxin in breast milk from Swedish and Pakistani mothers. *Scandinavian Journal of Immunology*, **28**, 783–9.

Robinet, H. G. (1962). Relationship of host antibody to fluctuations of *Escherichia coli* serotypes in the human intestine. *Journal of Bacteriology*, **84**, 896–901.

Rowe, P. C., Orrbine, E., Lior, H., Wells, G. A., McLaine, P. N. & the CPKDRC co-investigators. (1993). A prospective study of exposure to verotoxin-producing *Escherichia coli* among Canadian children with haemolytic uraemic syndrome. *Epidemiology and Infection*, **110**, 1–7.

Salit, I., Hanley, J., Clubb, L. & Fanning, S. (1988). The human antibody response to uropathogenic *Escherichia coli*: a review. *Canadian Journal of Microbiology*, **34**, 312–18.

Savalonis, J. M., Kalish, R. I., Cummings, E. A., Ryan, R. W. & Aloisi, R. (1988). Kell blood group activity of Gram-negative bacteria. *Transfusion*, **28**, 229–32.

Schiff, F. (1934). Zur kenntuis der blutantigene des shigabazillus. *Zeitschrift für Immunitätsforschung*, **82**, 46–52.

Schwartzer, T. A., Alcid, D. V., Numsuwan, V. & Gocke, D. J. (1988). Characterization of the human antibody response to an *Escherichia coli* O111:B4 (J5) vaccine. *Journal of Infectious Diseases*, **158**, 1135–6.

Seetharama, S., Cavalieri, S. J. & Snyder, I. S. (1988). Immune response to *Escherichia coli* alpha-hemolysin in patients. *Journal of Clinical Microbiology*, **26**, 850–56.

Sennhauser, F. H., MacDonald, R. A., Robertson, D. M. & Hosking, C. S. (1989). Comparison of concentration and avidity of specific antibodies to *E. coli* in breast milk and serum. *Immunology*, **66**, 394–7.

Shenep, J. L., Gigliotti, F., Davis, D. S. & Hildner, W. K. (1987). Reactivity of antibodies to core glycolipid with Gram-negative bacteria. *Reviews of Infectious Diseases*, **9** Supplement 5, S639–43.

Silver, R. P., Aaronson, W. & Vann, W. F. (1988). The K1 capsular polysaccharide of *Escherichia coli*. *Reviews of Infectious Diseases*, **10**, Supplement 2, S282–6.

Springer, G. F. (1971). Blood-group and Forssman antigenic determinants shared between microbes and mammalian cells. *Progress in Immunology*, **15**, 9–77.

Springer, G. F., Williamson, P. & Brandes, W. C. (1961). Blood group activity of Gram-negative bacteria. *Journal of Experimental Medicine*, **113**, 1077–93.

Stamm, W. E. (1983). Localization of urinary tract infections. In *Urinary Infection. Insights and Prospects*, eds. B. François & P. Perrin, pp. 47–56. London: Butterworths.

Stephens, S. (1986). Development of secretory immunity in breast fed and bottle fed infants. *Archives of Disease in Childhood*, **61**, 263–9.

Stoll, B. J., Svennerholm, A. M., Gotherfors, L., Barua, D., Huda, S. & Holmgren, J. (1986). Local and systemic antibody responses to naturally acquired enterotoxigenic *Escherichia coli* diarrhoea in an endemic area. *Journal of Infectious Diseases*, **153**, 527–34.

Tacket, C. O., Losonsky, G., Link, H., Hoang, Y., Guesry, P., Hilpert, H. & Levine, M. M. (1988). Protection by milk immunoglobulin concentrate against oral challenge with enterotoxigenic *Escherichia coli*. *New England Journal of Medicine*, **318**, 1240–3.

Van Dijk, W. C., Verbrugh, H. A., Van Erne-Van Der Tol, M. E., Peters, R. & Verhoef, J. (1981). *Escherichia coli* antibodies in opsonisation and protection against infection. *Journal of Medical Microbiology*, **14**, 381–9.

Van Loon, F. P. L., Clemens, J. D., Sack, D. A., Rao, M. R., Ahmed, F., Chowdhury, S., Harris, J. R., Ali, M., Chakraborty, J., Khan, M. R., Neogy, P. K., Svennerholm, A. M. & Holmgren, J. (1991). ABO blood groups and the risk of diarrhea due to enterotoxigenic *Escherichia coli*. *Journal of Infectious Diseases*, **163**, 1243–6.

Wiener, A. S. (1951). Origin of naturally occurring hemagglutinins and hemolysins: a review. *Journal of Immunology*, **66**, 287–95.

Wittels, E. G. & Lichtman, H. C. (1986). Blood group incidence and *Escherichia coli* bacterial sepsis. *Transfusion*, **26**, 533–5.

Wold, A. E., Dahlgren, U. I. H., Hanson, L. Å., Mattsby-Baltzer, I. & Midvetdt, T. (1989). Difference between bacterial and food antigens in mucosal immunogenicity. *Infection and Immunity*, **57**, 2666–73.

Wolf, M. K., Andrews, G. P., Fritz, D. L., Sjogren, R. W. Jr., Boedeker, E. C. (1988). Characterization of the plasmid from *Escherichia coli* RDEC-1 that mediates expression of adhesin AF/R1 and evidence that AF/R1 pili promote but are not essential for enteropathogenic disease. *Infection and Immunity*, **56**, 1846–57.

Young, L. S., Proctor, R. A., Beutler, B., McCabe, W. R. & Sheagren, J. N. (1991). University of California/Davis Interdepartmental Conference on Gram-negative septicemia. *Reviews of Infectious Diseases*, **13**, 666–87.

Zanetti, G., Glauser, M. P. & Baumgartner, J.-D. (1991). Use of immunoglobulins in prevention and treatment of infection in critically ill patients: review and critique. *Reviews of Infectious Diseases*, **13**, 985–92.

Ziegler, E. J. (1988). Protective antibody to endotoxin core: the emperor's new clothes? *Journal of Infectious Diseases*, **158**, 286–90.

21

Vaccines against enterotoxigenic *Escherichia coli*

A.-M. SVENNERHOLM and J. HOLMGREN

Enterotoxigenic *Escherichia coli* (ETEC) are the commonest cause of diarrhoea in children in developing countries (Black, 1993). It has been estimated that at least 650 million episodes of ETEC diarrhoea occur annually in Africa, Asia and Latin America, resulting in almost 800,000 deaths (Black, 1986, 1993). ETEC are found at low frequency in the industrialised world, but they affect travellers from these regions to developing countries (Black, 1990). Indeed, it has been suggested that almost half of the 18–20 million international travellers at risk develop diarrhoea, one-third to half of which is due to ETEC (Black, 1990). Although the symptoms of travellers' diarrhoea are usually relatively mild, the disease is one of the main health problems for international travellers (Steffen, 1986). It is also well established that ETEC is a common worldwide cause of fatal diarrhoea in newborn piglets and calves (Moon & Bunn, 1993).

Enterotoxigenic *E. coli* cause disease by colonising the small intestine and producing a heat-labile (LT) and/or a heat-stable (ST) enterotoxin that cause fluid and electrolyte secretion in the bowel (Guerrant, 1985). The illness caused by these organisms ranges from a mild diarrhoea without dehydration to a severe cholera-like disease (Black, 1986). In the first five years of life, many children in the developing world suffer as many as seven or eight bouts of diarrhoea annually, and up to four of these are caused by ETEC (Black, 1993). It has also been suggested that it is these repeated episodes of diarrhoea, rather than lack of food, that are a major cause of malnutrition (Mata, 1980). Thus, any intervention that can even partially reduce mortality and morbidity due to ETEC would be of great significance to public health and may also have a beneficial effect on the nutritional status of children in developing countries.

In spite of the serious health problems caused by ETEC, as yet there is

Table 21.1. *Postulated annual reduction in the number of cases of disease due to* enterotoxigenic Escherichia coli *(ETEC) produced by vaccines with different protective efficiencies*

	Reduction in number of cases ($\times 10^3$)		
	Vaccine[a] protective efficacy (per cent)		
	40	60	80
Residents in developing countries			
Diarrhoea	200,000	300,000	400,000
Mortality	150	230	300
International travellers			
Diarrhoea	800	1,200	1,600

[a] Assumed coverage: developing countries 50 per cent; travellers 80 per cent.

no effective ETEC vaccine for use in humans. Even a vaccine with relatively modest protective efficacy would probably have an enormous impact, by reducing the several hundred million episodes of diarrhoea and the several hundred thousand deaths annually in children in the developing world (Table 21.1). Such a vaccine would also play an important role in improving the health of travellers, particularly those to Latin America, Asia and Africa (Table 21.1). Against this background, intensive efforts have been made for many years to develop an effective ETEC vaccine for use in humans.

Numerous vaccines are available for immunoprophylaxis against veterinary ETEC diarrhoea. Thirty-two different ETEC vaccines were licensed in 1992 for use in various animal species in the United States of America (Moon & Bunn, 1993). Most of these are based on the principle of immunising the pregnant sow or cow, for the induction of specific breast milk antibodies that can protect suckling neonates against diarrhoea in the period from birth to weaning.

Can an effective ETEC vaccine for humans be developed?

The marked decrease with age in the incidence of ETEC diarrhoea in children in developing countries (Black, 1986) and the reduced disease-to-infection ratio during the first five years of life in areas where ETEC are highly endemic strongly suggest that protective immunity develops after repeated, naturally occurring ETEC infections (Cravioto *et al.*, 1988; López-Vidal *et al.*, 1990). This decrease is not due to age-related host factors, since adults from industrialised countries experience high rates of ETEC diarrhoea when visiting areas where ETEC are endemic (Black, 1990). Observations of North American volunteers also support the notion that protective immunity develops against ETEC. Thus, an initial infection with virulent ETEC organisms provides significant protection against diarrhoea after challenge with the homologous strain (Levine *et al.*, 1979; Levine, 1990).

Further strong evidence for the potential of inducing protective immunity against ETEC disease in humans comes from a large field trial in 1985 to 1988 of an orally administered B subunit plus whole cell cholera vaccine in Bangladesh (Clemens *et al.*, 1988). The B subunit component of the vaccine cross-reacts immunologically with *E. coli* LT and provides significant, though short-lived, protection against diarrhoea due to LT-producing ETEC. In particular, ETEC infections associated with severe life-threatening dehydration were reduced by 86 per cent in the first few months after immunisation with the vaccine. In a subsequent study, the same vaccine was shown to afford highly significant protection against *E. coli* LT disease in Finnish travellers to Morocco for a limited vacation period (Peltola *et al.*, 1991). Protection against LT-producing *E. coli* was 60 per cent and that against mixed infections, in which ETEC was combined with any other pathogen, was 71 per cent.

The evidence presented above is consistent with the notion that it should be possible to develop an effective ETEC vaccine for use in humans. In order to design an immunogen with broad protective potential in various populations and countries, it is necessary to take account of new insights into the pathogenesis and immunity of ETEC disease and identification of the protective antigens involved.

Mechanisms of disese and immunity in ETEC infections

Enterotoxins and antitoxic immunity

The most important virulence factors in ETEC are plasmid encoded and include various colonisation factors as well as the LT and ST enterotoxins. The relative importance of the different *E. coli* enterotoxins can be determined from epidemiological surveys, which show that about one-third of all clinical ETEC isolates produce LT, one-third produce ST and one-third produce both enterotoxins. *Escherichia coli* LT is similar in structure and function to cholera toxin (CT) in that it consists of a toxic A subunit attached to five B subunits that mediate binding to cell membrane receptors. The A and B LT subunits both cross-react immunologically with the corresponding CT subunits, but both toxins have specific A- and B-subunit epitopes (Guerrant, 1985; Holmgren & Svennerholm, 1992). The immune response against LT is directed mainly against the B subunit of the molecule but antibodies against the A subunit of LT can also neutralise LT (Svennerholm *et al.*, 1986a). In this LT differs from CT, in that antibodies against the A subunit of CT are inefficient at neutralising the toxin.

The only heat-stable enterotoxin produced by human ETEC strains is the methanol-soluble STa, while porcine ETEC may produce either or both of STa and methanol-insoluble heat-stable enterotoxin, STb (Rao, 1985). STa is a small polypeptide that consists of only 18 (porcine STp) or 19 (human STh) amino-acids and stimulates guanylate cyclase activity in intestinal epithelial cells. While LT is a strong immunogen, STa is not immunogenic unless coupled, either chemically or by recombinant technology, to a carrier protein (Frantz & Robertson, 1981; Svennerholm *et al.*, 1986). For this reason STa released during infection does not induce an antibody response. It remains unknown whether immunity to ST can be induced by immunogenic ST-conjugates to provide significant protection in humans against disease due to *E. coli* that produce this toxin.

Colonisation factors and antibacterial immunity

An important prerequisite for ETEC to cause disease is colonisation of the intestine to allow the production of enterotoxin in close proximity to enterocytes. Colonisation usually depends on receptor–ligand and bacterium–host cell interactions specific for the species, the phenotype and the epithelial cell type of the host. All ETEC appear to possess distinct fimbrial, fibrillar or non-fimbrial protein attachment factors, the so-called colonisation factors.

Epidemiological studies in several countries have shown that up to 50–80 per cent of all clinical ETEC isolates express one of the following three distinct colonisation factor antigens (CFA): CFA/I, CFA/II or CFA/IV (Gothefors *et al.*, 1985; López-Vidal *et al.*, 1990; Binsztein *et al.*, 1991; Wolf *et al.*, 1993; Sommerfelt *et al.*, 1996). While CFA/I is a homogeneous protein, CFA/II consists of the three coli surface antigens CS1, CS2 and CS3; CS3 is usually expressed alone or together with either CS1 or CS2 (Evans & Evans, 1989; Gaastra & Svennerholm, 1996). Similarly, CFA/IV consists of CS4, CS5 and CS6. The latter is not a fimbrial antigen but is usually expressed with the fimbrial proteins CS4 or CS5. A number of additional putative colonisation factors (PCF) have recently been described, including PCFO159, PCFO166, CS7, CS17 and CFA/III but they are found only at low frequency. Thus, in a recent study in Argentina, it was found that only 23 per cent of ETEC strains negative for CFA/I, CFA/II and CFA/IV expressed any of the above PCF (Viboud *et al.*, 1993). Similarly, in retrospective studies in Central Africa, Burma and Peru, these factors were found on only 18–27 per cent of clinical ETEC isolates (McConnell *et al.*, 1991). In a rabbit non-ligated intestine model (RITARD), most CFA and PCF, that is CFA/I, CFA/II, CFA/III, CFA/IV, PCFO159, CS7 and CS17, promote colonisation of the rabbit intestine by ETEC, which suggests that they are true colonisation factors (Åhrén & Svennerholm, 1985; Svennerholm *et al.*, 1990, 1992). Other potential colonisation factors of *E. coli*, for example PCFO20 and PCFO2230, have been described but their roles have yet to be established (Darfeuille-Michaud *et al.*, 1986; Viboud *et al.*, 1993).

Antibacterial immunity to ETEC can, to a great extent, be ascribed to local bowel immunity to the various colonisation factors, but mucosal antibodies against O-antigens may also play a role in protection against ETEC of the homologous O-serogroup. However, the wide diversity of human ETEC O-serogroups (Black, 1986) limits the role of lipopolysaccharides (LPS) as protective antigens. In animals, anti-CFA antibodies are very effective in providing passive protection against ETEC that express homologous CFA. In experimental infections with CFA-positive *E. coli*, anti-CFA antibodies act synergistically with anti-LT antibodies in affording protection (Åhrén & Svennerholm, 1982). An initial infection with CFA-positive organisms in the RITARD model protects only against subsequent infection with ETEC that express homologous CFA or CS factors (Åhrén & Svennerholm, 1985; Svennerholm *et al.*, 1990). Synergy between antitoxic and anti-CFA immunity has also been demonstrated with the aid of this model (Åhrén & Svennerholm, 1985).

Candidate vaccines

On the basis of information about the key ETEC antigens and the major immune mechanisms that operate in ETEC infections, we concluded that an effective ETEC vaccine should ideally evoke both anti-colonisation and antitoxic immune responses. This means that the vaccine should contain most of the prevalent CFA and CS factors in combination with a suitable LT or LT/ST toxoid. Since neither the bacteria nor the toxins they produce are invasive, the aim should be to induce specific local bowel secretory immunoglobulin A (sIgA) antibody production against the CFAs and enterotoxin. Such mucosal immune responses are more effectively evoked by oral than by parenteral administration of antigens. An ideal ETEC vaccine should, therefore, be given by mouth and should contain a combination of bacterial-cell-derived and toxin-derived antigens. A number of different candidate oral ETEC vaccines that consist of CFAs and toxin antigens, either alone or in combination, have recently been developed (Table 21.2). The various approaches to the development of such vaccines will be described below.

Purified fimbrial vaccines

The most important bacterial antigens to be included in ETEC vaccines are CFAs with a high prevalence on ETEC strains in various geographical areas. These are CFA/I, CFA/II and CFA/IV and probably a few others. Such a vaccine might consist of purified fimbriae alone or in combination with a suitable enterotoxoid. Purified CFA are, however, relatively expensive to prepare and, in addition, isolated CFAs are very sensitive to proteolytic degradation in the human gastro-intestinal tract (Evans *et al.*, 1984; Levine *et al.*, 1986). Thus, very few human volunteers, even after oral immunisation as many as six times with high doses of purified CFA/I, responded with mucosal or serum antibody and none was protected against challenge with ETEC that express CFA/I (Evans *et al.* 1984). Similarly, a significant anti-CFA antibody response in the intestine was not detected in volunteers given multiple doses of purified CFA/II even after neutralisation of gastric acidity (Levine *et al.*, 1986). However, when the purified fimbriae were administered directly into the small intestine through a gastro-intestinal tube, most volunteers developed significant rises in intestinal sIgA antibodies against CFA/II. This suggests that purified CFAs are very sensitive to proteolytic degradation and that a special delivery system may be necessary. This is supported by

Table 21.2. *Candidate enterotoxigenic* Escherichia coli *(ETEC) vaccines*

	Disadvantages	Reference
Inactivated vaccines		
Purified colonisation factors	Unstable in gastro-intestinal secretions	Evans *et al.* (1984) Levine *et al.* (1986)
Enterotoxoids (CTB, LTB, CTB–ST and LTB–ST)	Suitable ST toxoid not available; LT toxoids have restricted coverage	Clemens *et al.* (1988) Peltola *et al.* (1991) Aitken & Hirst (1993) Svennerholm *et al.* (1988) Sanchez *et al.* (1988)
Formalin-inactivated *E. coli* that express colonisation factors and enterotoxoid	Mixture of substances	Svennerholm *et al.* (1989) Åhrén *et al.* (1993) Wennerås *et al.* (1992)
Colicin-E2-inactivated ETEC	Restricted coverage; inactivation reproducible?	Evans *et al.* (1988)
Live vaccines		
Colonisation-factor-positive attenuated ETEC	Simultaneous administration of several strains necessary	Levine (1990) Levine *et al.* (1986)
Attenuated heterologous strains that express colonisation factors	Poor colonisation factor expression	Yamamoto *et al.* (1985) Giron *et al.* (1995)

CTB, cholera toxin subunit B; LTB, heat-labile enterotoxin B subunit; ST, heat-stable enterotoxin.

the observation that even neutralised gastric juice reduces the immunogenicity of purified ETEC fimbriae (Schmidt *et al.*, 1985). In an attempt to determine how CFAs may be protected against degradation in the stomach, studies of humans have recently been carried out in which purified CFA are incorporated into biodegradable polymer microspheres (Reid *et al.*, 1993) but the results have not been very encouraging. Although high doses of purified CFA/II were given to volunteers on four occasions, significant protection was not induced against subsequent challenge with CFA/II-positive ETEC (protective efficacy 30 per cent; $p = 0.11$) (Tacket *et al.*, 1994)

Enterotoxoids

Identification of the subunit structure of LT and its immunological relatedness to CT and demonstration of the roles of the various subunits in toxicity and immunogenicity have indicated that purified cholera or LT B subunits (CTB or LTB) are suitable toxoid candidates for the induction of anti-LT immunity. Furthermore, LTB and CTB are particularly well suited as oral immunogens, because they are stable in the intestinal milieu and are capable of binding to the intestinal epithelium, including the M cells of Peyer's patches (Neutra & Kraehenbuhl, 1992). These properties are important for stimulating mucosal immunity and local immunological memory.

Clinical trials have shown that CTB may afford significant protection against *E. coli* LT disease (Clemens *et al.*, 1988; Peltola *et al.*, 1991) and, in animals, CTB was as efficient as LTB in inducing protection against experimental ETEC infection (Holmgren & Svennerholm, 1992). However, LTB-specific epitopes have been identified (Holmgren & Svennerholm, 1979) and monoclonal antibodies have been produced that react strongly with LTB but not with CTB and that are able to neutralise *E. coli* LT in tissue culture (Svennerholm *et al.*, 1986). It cannot, be excluded, therefore, that an LT toxoid may be slightly more effective than CTB in inducing protective anti-LT immunity. On the other hand, no strain as yet available produces large quantities of LTB, as is the case for CTB. Thus, a recombinant *Vibrio cholerae* strain has been constructed, by deletion of the gene for the toxic A subunit, which overproduces CTB (Sanchez & Holmgren, 1989). Very simple methods have been developed that allow purification of several grams of purified recombinant CTB (rCTB) from a 1000-litre fermenter culture of this strain (Holmgren *et al.*, 1994). Such rCTB is, at present, probably the most readily available toxoid component for an ETEC vaccine. However, in an attempt to prepare a more LT-like enterotoxoid, the structural gene for CTB has been genetically modified to encode B subunits that also contain LTB-specific epitopes (Lebens *et al.*, 1996).

The significance of anti-ST immunity for protection against ST-producing *E. coli* remains undefined. By coupling *E. coli* STa to various carrier proteins, such as bovine serum albumin, CTB or CFA by means of various chemical reagents, conjugates have been prepared that give rise to ST-neutralising antibodies (Frantz & Robertson, 1981; Svennerholm *et al.*, 1986). Furthermore, chimeric proteins that consist of *E. coli* ST coupled to CTB by recombinant techniques have also been effective in inducing an immune response against ST (Aitken & Hirst, 1993). All of these chemical and recombinant ST-conjugates have, however, retained ST toxic activity. Though it has been possible to prepare non-toxic ST peptides, by protein synthesis or recombinant methods (Sanchez *et al.*, 1988; Svennerholm *et al.*, 1988), immunisation with such peptides coupled to various carrier proteins has, in most cases, failed to induce ST-neutralising antibodies. Even though it may be possible to prepare a non-toxic ST-conjugate that can elicit high levels of ST-neutralising antibodies, it is doubtful whether such a toxoid can play an important role in an ETEC vaccine. Because of the very small size of the ST molecule, very large amounts of specific antibodies will be necessary to provide for neutralisation. Furthermore, since previous studies have shown that the cholera B subunit can protect against strains that produce only LT as well as those that produce LT and ST, an ST toxoid would probably only have an important role in protecting against *E. coli* strains that produce ST alone.

Inactivated CFA–ETEC vaccines

Another approach to the construction of inactivated ETEC vaccines is to prepare killed ETEC organisms that express on their surface in an immunogenic form the most important CFAs and to combine these with an appropriate toxoid. Such a vaccine, with the potential for providing broad protective coverage against ETEC diseases in different countries, has been developed in collaboration with the National Bacteriological Laboratory in Sweden (SBL). This vaccine contains inactivated *E. coli* that express the most prevalent CFA fimbriae in immunogenic form, that is CFA/I and the various subcomponents of CFA/II and CFA/IV (CS1–CS5), and O-antigens commonly associated with ETEC in combination with CTB. The bacteria were inactivated by mild treatment with formalin at various temperatures for several days. This resulted in complete killing of the bacteria without significant loss of antigenicity by the various antigens (Svennerholm *et al.*, 1989). Indeed, it was possible to show, with a very sensitive CFA inhibition enzyme-linked immunosorbent assay (ELISA) (López-Vidal & Svennerholm, 1990), that the bacteria retained 50–100 per cent of their CFA antigenicity after inactivation. Furthermore, the CFA-antigens of the inactivated bacteria were stable, even after incubation for several hours in human gastro-intestinal secretions (Svennerholm *et al.*, 1989). This suggests that formalin-treated fimbriae are more resistant to proteolysis compared to native CFAs (Evans *et al.*, 1984; Levine *et al.*, 1986).

An alternative method for the inactivation of ETEC without damage to their protein antigens has been developed (Evans *et al.*, 1988). This involves treatment of *E. coli* with colicin E2, which enters the bacterial cell by way of receptors on sensitive strains. Oral immunisation with ETEC killed by colicin E2 induces an intestinal IgA antibody response against LT and CFA. Some protection was also observed against *E. coli* that express homologous and heterologous CFA. However, the extent to which colicin E2 treatment can be relied upon to inactivate various *E. coli* strains reproducibly for use in human vaccines remains to be established.

Live vaccines

Live bacteria that express the major CFAs and produce enterotoxoid have also been considered as candidate ETEC vaccines. They multiply in the bowel and may, therefore, give sustained antigen stimulation to the local intestinal immune system. An example of such a vaccine that has been tested in human volunteers for mucosal immunogenicity and protective efficacy is a non-toxigenic mutant *E. coli* strain that expresses CS1- and CS3 antigens. Volunteers fed a relatively high dose of these organisms developed significant intestinal sIgA responses against CS1 and CS3. Immunisation with a single dose of this mutant strain afforded protection with 75 per cent efficacy, against challenge with a toxigenic *E. coli* strain of heterologous serotype that expressed CS1 and CS3. However, 15 per cent of the volunteers developed some diarrhoea after infection with this toxin-negative mutant, so making it unsuitable as a vaccine strain (Levine, 1990). Such a strain probably only has the potential to protect against ETEC that express CFA/II, but these are relatively uncommon in most parts of the world. Against this background, attempts have been made to develop safe live vaccines that express on their surface the most prevalent CFAs in an immunogenic form and that produce an enterotoxoid, such as LTB (Levine, 1990).

Various colonisation factors, such as CFA/I, CFA/II and CFA/IV, are not normally expressed on the same strain and it has not yet been possible to clone successfully the genes for different CFA into the same host for stable surface expression. Therefore, live vaccines must be based, at least for the time being, on a mixture of several different strains, with the possibility of overgrowth of one the vaccine strains, with suppression of the others. Moreover, there is the risk that live vaccines may revert to toxicity by taking up toxin-encoding plasmids, and then probably to produce only relatively low levels of enterotoxoid during growth *in vivo*.

Another approach that has been used to produce a live ETEC vaccine has been to introduce CFA-encoding plasmids into heterologous bacteria, such as attenuated salmonellas, which, because of their invasive properties, can reside in the bowel for long periods. It has, for example, been possible to express CFA/I fimbriae on the surface of the Ty21a typhoid vaccine strain (Yamamoto *et al.*, 1985) and on an Aro⁻ *S. typhi* mutant (Hone *et al.*, 1988). However, since such attenuated typhoid strains are relatively poor intestinal immunogens, of which multiple doses are required to elicit significant protective immunity (Ferreccio *et al.*, 1989), they are probably not ideal vectors for heterologous mucosal antigens. A new generation of attenuated *S. typhi* strains that are immunogenic when administered as a single dose have recently been developed. Cloned genes for the expression of CFA/I and CS3 have been introduced on stable plasmids into such a *S. typhi* strain (CVD 908) and a high level of co-expression of the two fimbriae was achieved (Girón *et al.*, 1995).

Other attenuated bacterial strains, such as of *Shigella* or *Vibrio cholerae*, have also been considered as live vectors for the expression of CFA. Thus, expression of CFA/I and CS3 fimbriae in an attenuated *Sh. flexnerii* 2a live vaccine candidate has been reported (Noriega *et al.*, 1994). A problem with these various approaches appears to be the introduction of several CFA and CS factors together with CTB into the same host organism. Furthermore, heterologous live vectors will not provide any immunity against *E. coli* O-antigens.

Clinical trials of inactivated CTB–CFA ETEC vaccines

The types of ETEC vaccines that have been most extensively studied consist of various combinations of formalin-inactivated CFA-carrying ETEC in combination with B subunit 'toxoid'. A prototype of such an ETEC vaccine consisted of a mixture of killed CFA/I-, CS1-, CS2- and CS3-positive *E. coli* and CTB. The CTB, included in the whole cell cholera vaccine, was added to the killed *E. coli*, which consisted of a selection of the common ETEC O-serogroups, namely O6, O78 and O139, that expressed the various fimbriae in high concentrations (Table 21.3).

The safety and immunogenicity of this prototype CTB–CFA ETEC vaccine in adult Swedish volunteers have been studied extensively. In

Table 21.3. *IgA immune responses of Swedish volunteers to oral CTB–CFA enterotoxigenic* Escherichia coli *vaccines*

	Frequency (per cent) of significant responders		
	Prototype CTB–CFA vaccine		rCTB–CFA vaccine
	Intestinal lavage[a]	Blood ASC[b]	Blood ASC[c]
CFA/I	9/11 (82)	18/21 (86)	21/25 (84)
CS1+CS3	9/11 (82)	19/21 (90)	20/26 (77)
CS2	8/11 (73)	N.T.	9/11 (82)
CS4	N.T.	N.T.	18/26 (69)
CS5	N.T.	N.T.	23/25 (92)
CTB	10/11 (91)	21/21 (100)	26/26 (100)

[a] Data from Åhrén *et al.* (1993).
[b] Data from Wennerås *et al.* (1992).
[c] Jertborn, Åhrén, & Svennerholm, unpublished.
ASC, antibody-secreting cells; CFA, colonisation factor antigen; CS, coli-surface associated antigen; CTB, cholera toxin subunit B; N.T., not tested.

particular, the capacity of the vaccine to induce a local intestinal mucosal sIgA antibody response has been evaluated. Specific IgA antibodies in intestinal lavage fluid (Åhrén *et al.*, 1993) and mucosa-derived antibody-secreting cells (ASC) in peripheral blood (Wennerås *et al.*, 1992) were studied by analysing immune responses against the various CFA expressed by the vaccine strains and CTB. The potential of the vaccine to give rise to a mucosal T-cell response was also evaluated (Wennerås *et al.*, 1994). The vaccine, which contained 10^{11} formalin-killed *E. coli* and 1 mg of CTB, was given orally, in a bicarbonate-buffered solution, to about 100 volunteers, who received two or three doses at two-week intervals.

Surveillance for side-effects showed that the vaccine was safe and did not give rise to significant side-effects (Åhrén *et al.*, 1993; Wennerås *et al.*, 1992). Specific immune responses in intestinal lavage fluids were determined by measuring specific IgA titres by ELISA as a proportion of total IgA in specimens collected before and after each immunisation. Significant IgA antibody responses were observed against CFA/I, CFA/II and CTB in a majority of those vaccinated (Table 21.3). In most cases maximum intestinal antibody responses were obtained after only two doses of vaccine but in some volunteers there was a decrease, particularly in the CFA response, after the third dose as compared with that after the

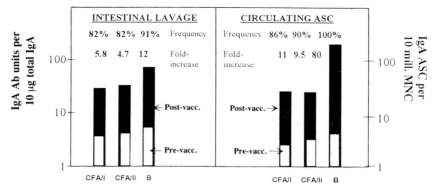

Fig. 21.1. Immunoglobulin A (IgA) responses in intestinal lavage fluid associated with IgA-antibody-secreting cells (ASC). Rises after oral immunisation with the prototype B subunit CFA–ETEC vaccine. CFA, colonisation factor antigen; ETEC, entrotoxigenic *Escherichia coli*, MNC, mononuclear cells.

second dose (Åhrén *et al.*, 1993). It is interesting that the frequencies of the intestinal antitoxin and anti-CFA responses were comparable with those previously observed to occur in adult Bangladeshis convalescing from diarrhoea induced by CFA-positive *E. coli* (Stoll *et al.*, 1986).

This prototype ETEC vaccine also gave rise, in 85–100 per cent of the volunteers, to significant increases in peripheral blood ASC with specificities for CFA/I, CFA/II and CTB (Wennerås *et al.*, 1992). The responses were predominantly in IgA-producing cells but high frequencies of IgM ASC responses against CFA and of IgG ASC responses to CTB were also seen. Since the number of CFA–ASC did not increase after administration of a third dose of vaccine, these results support the conclusion that two oral doses of vaccine are probably sufficient to induce an optimal CFA-specific immune response. The frequencies and magnitudes of significant IgA immune responses in intestinal lavage fluid and of peripheral blood lymphocyte IgA responses were comparable for the different CFAs and CTB (Figure 21.1). These results support the notion that circulating ASC responses may reflect specific local IgA responses in the intestine.

Since the prototype ETEC vaccine gave rise to CFA-specific ASC in the circulation, we determined whether the vaccine could also give rise to vaccine-specific T-cells in the blood of adult Swedish volunteers (Wennerås *et al.*, 1992). The results showed that after one to three oral doses of vaccine, stimulation of blood mononuclear cells *in vitro* with CFA/I or CFA/II resulted in significant, though modest, proliferative responses that were accounted for mainly by CD4 T-cells and to a lesser extent by CD8 T-cells. Furthermore, a majority of the immunised volunteers had circulating T-cells capable of producing large amounts of λ-interferon after exposure to either of the CFA *in vitro*. This suggests that the vaccine is able to induce the migration of specific mucosal T-cell immunocytes from the intestine into the bloodstream and that a simple approach *in vitro* to assess mucosa-derived T-cell responses against oral ETEC vaccines may be to determine λ-interferon production by peripheral blood T-cells after stimulation by specific antigen.

Though bacteria that express CFA induce significant local immune responses in the intestine, these organisms in the prototype vaccine were relatively inefficient at eliciting specific serum antibody against the various CFAs (Åhrén *et al.*, 1993). The CTB component, on the other hand, induced serum antibody responses comparable in frequency and magnitude to those in intestinal lavage fluid. Furthermore, while ASC responses against CFA were predominantly in IgA- and IgM-producing cells, and almost absent in IgG-producing cells, significant antitoxic ASC responses were seen only in IgA and IgG cells (Wennerås *et al.*, 1992). These differences may be due to the relatively small size of the CTB molecule. This is only a few nanometers in diameter and may easily be taken up from the bowel by intestinal mucosal cells and presented to the systemic immune system. By comparison, CFA-fimbriated *E. coli* are large (*c.* 2 µm x 5 µm) and may only be presented to the mucosa-associated lymphoid tissue.

The modest ability of the CFA-fimbriated bacteria to induce a serum antibody response may complicate evaluation of the CTB–CFA ETEC vaccine in extended Phase I and II trials, particularly in children in endemic areas. Thus, determination of mucosal immune responses, either as specific IgA antibodies in intestinal lavage fluid or as mucosa-derived T- or B-cells in peripheral blood (which requires 20–30 ml of whole blood per specimen), cannot readily be used in children. There is, therefore, a need to devise other methods to evaluate the immune responses against ETEC vaccines, which can be applied to large groups of volunteers, including children.

An oral recombinant CTB–CFA ETEC vaccine

Encouraging results in various trials with the prototype ETEC vaccine in adult Swedish volunteers has led to a more definitive formulation for the ETEC vaccine by SBL, Stockholm, Sweden. This vaccine contains recombinant CTB (rCTB; Sanchez & Holmgren, 1989) and five different *E. coli* strains that express CFA/I and the various subcomponents of CFA/II and CFA/IV. Based on results from several epidemiological studies of virulence factors in ETEC in various geographical areas, this vaccine has a potential protective coverage of some 80–85 per cent.

This rCTB–CFA ETEC vaccine has recently been evaluated for safety and immunogenicity in various Phase I and Phase II trials in Sweden, the United States of America, Egypt and Bangladesh. So far, more than 400 adult or school-age children volunteers have received one or two oral doses of the vaccine. The studies have all shown that the vaccine elicits a mucosal immune response and that it does not give rise to any significant side-effects. The rCTB–CFA vaccine gives rise to comparable frequencies of ASC responses against CFA/I, CFA/II and CTB as the prototype vaccine in Swedish volunteers (Table 21.3). In most instances, the vaccine, which contains bacteria that express CS4 and CS5, also evokes ASC responses against these colonisation factors (Jertborn *et al.*, 1997). The magnitude of ASC responses against the various CFA is comparable to, or higher than, that induced by the prototype ETEC vaccine. Similarly, the rCTB–CFA ETEC vaccine appears to be less efficient in inducing a serum immune response as compared with a mucosal immune response against the different CFAs.

Preliminary results of the phase I trials of the rCTB–CFA ETEC vaccine in Egypt (Savarino *et al.*, 1997) and in Bangladesh (Qadri *et al.*, 1997) suggest that it gives rise to comparable frequencies and magnitudes of ASC responses in the Egyptian, Bangladeshi and Swedish volunteers (Jertborn *et al.*, 1997). Studies are also in progress in Bangladesh to compare ASC responses, in peripheral blood and in the intestine, induced by the vaccine and clinical ETEC disease.

In an attempt to develop a simple alternative approach to the measurement of intestinal immune responses, stool specimens were collected from some of the vaccines to evaluate the possibility of measuring specific IgA antibody responses in extracts of faeces. The results suggest that assay of anti-CFA antibodies in faeces (Li *et al.*, 1992) can be used instead of measurement of immune responses in intestinal lavage fluid. However, measurements of immune responses in stools are less sensitive as compared with measurements in intestinal lavage fluids (Åhrén *et al.*, to be published).

Studies of protective efficacy

The promising results obtained from the studies of the rCTB–CFA ETEC vaccine, in progress in various countries, have encouraged the planning of several Phase III trials of the vaccine in children in endemic areas and in travellers to these areas. The ETEC vaccine and placebo will first be tested in a double-blind trial for its ability to protect European travellers on short Nile cruises. This trial was initiated by Steffen and his colleagues in 1996. If this study confirms that the vaccine is safe and affords protective immunity in adults, it will be tested in children in various countries where the incidence of ETEC diarrhoea is high. If Phase I and Phase II trials in progress confirm that the vaccine is safe and immunogenic in children in Egypt, Phase III trials will be carried out.

Further development of ETEC vaccines

The results of recent epidemiological studies, and others that are still in progress, suggest that some of the most prevalent PCF should be included in an ETEC vaccine to increase its protective coverage. Thus, for example, CS17 has been found in moderate frequencies on clinical ETEC isolates in certain areas (McConnell *et al.*, 1991; Sommerfelt *et al.*, 1996), but these fimbriae only been observed in low frequencies on ETEC in Argentina (Viboud *et al.*, 1993).

Another possible means of increasing the protective coverage of an ETEC vaccine may be to add structures or epitopes that can induce antibodies that react with several different CFAs and PCFs. Though the various human ETEC fimbriae do not cross-react immunologically, as judged by immunodiffusion or slide agglutination tests with antisera or monoclonal antibodies against whole intact fimbriae, it has been shown that some anti-CFA antibodies bind not only to the homologous but also to certain heterologous CFA subunits (McConnell *et al.*, 1989). As a result of the highly conserved amino-terminal regions of the subunit proteins of many of the CFA (de Graaf & Gaastra, 1994; Gaastra & Svennerholm, 1996), the existence of cross-reactive epitopes, at least in these regions, has been suggested (Cassels *et al.*, 1992; Rudin & Svennerholm, 1994). It has also been shown by animal studies that certain CFAs can prime and boost immune responses against heterologous fimbriae with related amino-terminal regions (Rudin & Svennerholm, 1994). Moreover, monoclonal antibodies raised against isolated CFA subunits have been found to cross-react immunologically *in vitro* with several different CFAs (Rudin *et al.*, 1994). One of these monoclonal antibodies reacts with a synthetic peptide that consists of the 25 amino-terminal amino-acids of CFA/I. These cross-reactive monoclonal antibodies inhibit the binding of ETEC that express homologous and heterologous CFA for human enterocytes, and they confer passive protection in animals against challenge with ETEC that express other CFAs (Rudin *et al.*, 1996).

These results support the existence of epitopes that are common to several CFA, either in their amino-terminal region, or in other sequences of the CFA subunit protein. Recently such a linear epitope, IDLLQ, was identified at the amino-terminal end of CFA/I. A monoclonal antibody with specificity for this epitope inhibited binding to human enterocytes of ETEC that express CFA/I or CS4 (Rudin *et al.*, 1995; Rudin & Svennerholm, 1996). Work is in progress to determine whether it is possible to synthesise peptides that contain this epitope. It is hoped that such epitopes may increase the protective range of an ETEC vaccine containing only a few CFA. Another possible means of inducing cross-protective CFA immunity may be to provide CFA subunits in isolated form, or to express them at high concentration on the surface of living or inactivated *E. coli*.

Acknowledgements

Financial support for the various studies on CTB–CFA ETEC vaccines was provided by the Swedish Medical Research Council, the Swedish Agency for Research Co-operation with Developing Countries and the World Health Organisation. The fruitful collaboration in various trials of the CTB–CFA ETEC vaccine of Drs Marianne Jertborn, Christina Åhrén, Christine Wennerås (Göteborg, Sweden), Stephen Severino and colleagues (Cairo, Egypt) and Firdausi Qadri and colleagues (ICDDR,B, Bangladesh) is gratefully acknowledged.

References

Åhrén, C. & Svennerholm, A.-M. (1982). Synergistic protective effect of antibodies against *Escherichia coli* enterotoxin and colonization factor antigens. *Infection and Immunity*, **38**, 74–9.

Åhrén, C. & Svennerholm, A.-M. (1985). Experimental enterotoxin-induced *Escherichia coli*diarrhoea and protection induced by previous infection with bacteria of the same adhesin or enterotoxin type. *Infection and Immunity*, **50**, 255–61.

Åhrén, C., Wennerås, C., Holmgren, J. & Svennerholm, A.-M. (1993). Intestinal antibody response after oral immunization with a prototype enterotoxigenic *Escherichia coli* vaccine. *Vaccine*, **11**, 929–34.

Aitken, R. & Hirst, T. R. (1993). Recombinant enterotoxins as vaccines against *Escherichia coli*-mediated diarrhoea. *Vaccine*, **11**, 227–33.

Binsztein, N., Jouve, M. J., Viboud, G. I., Lopez-Moral, L., Rivas, M., Ørskov, I., Åhrén, C. & Svennerholm, A.-M. (1991). Colonization factors of enterotoxigenic *Escherichia coli* in children with diarrhoea in Argentina. *Journal of Clinical Microbiology*, **29**, 1893–8.

Black, R. E. (1986). The epidemiology of cholera and enterotoxigenic *E. coli* diarrhoeal disease. In *Development of Vaccines and Drugs against Diarrhoea*, eds. J. Holmgren, A. Lindberg & R. Möllby, pp. 23–32. Lund: Studentlitteratur.

Black, R. E. (1990). Epidemiology of traveller's diarrhoea and relative importance of various pathogens. *Reviews of Infectious Diseases*, **12**, S73-S79.

Black, R. E. (1993). Epidemiology of diarrhoeal disease: implications for control by vaccines. *Vaccine*, **11**, 100–6.

Black, R. E., Brown, K. H. & Becker, S. (1984). Effects of diarrhea associated with specific enteropathogens in the growth of children in Bangladesh. *Pediatrics*, **73**, 799–805.

Cassels, F. J., Deal, C. D., Reid, R. H., Jarboe, D. L., Nauss, J. L., Carter, J. M. & Boedeker, E. C. (1992). Analysis of *Escherichia coli* colonization factor antigen I linear B-cell epitopes, as determined by primate responses, following protein sequence verification. *Infection and Immunity*, **60**, 2174–81.

Clemens, J., Sack, D. A., Harris, J. R., Chakraborty, J., Neogy, P. K., Stanton, B. F., Huda, N., Khan, M. U., Kay B. A., Khan, M. R., Ansaruzzaman, N., Yunus, A., Rao M.R., Svennerholm, A.-M. & Holmgren, J. (1988). Cross-protection by B subunit-whole cell cholera vaccine against diarrhoea associated with heat-labile toxin-producing enterotoxigenic *Escherichia coli*: results of a large-scale field trial. *Journal of Infectious Diseases*, **158**, 372–7.

Cravioto, A., Reyes, R. E., Ortega, R., Fernandéz, G., Hernandez, R. & López, D. (1988). Prospective study of diarrhoea diseases in a cohort of rural Mexican children: incidence and isolated pathogens during the first two years of life. *Epidemiology and Infection*, **101**, 123–34.

Darfeuille-Michaud, A., Forestier, C., Joly, B. & Cluzel, R. (1986). Identification of a nonfimbrial adhesive factor of an enterotoxigenic *Escherichia coli* strain. *Infection and Immunity*, **52**, 468–75.

Evans, D. G., Evans Jr, D. J., Opekun, A. R. & Graham, D. Y. (1988). Non-replicating oral whole cell vaccine protective against enterotoxigenic *Escherichia coli* (ETEC) diarrhoea: stimulation of anti-CFA (CFA/I) and anti-enterotoxin (anti-LT) intestinal IgA and protection against challenge with ETEC belonging to heterologous serotypes. *FEMS Microbiology and Immunology*, **47**, 117–26.

Evans, D. G., Graham, D. Y., Evans, D. J. Jr. & Opekun, A. (1984). Administration of purified colonization factor antigens (CFA/I, CFA/II) of enterotoxigenic *Escherichia coli* to volunteers. *Gastroenterology*, **87**, 934–40.

Evans, D. J. & Evans, D. G. (1989). Determinants of microbial attachment and their genetic control. In *Enteric Infection. Mechanisms, Manifestations and Management*, eds. M. J. G. Farthing, & G. T. Keusch, pp. 31–40. London: Chapman & Hall.

Ferreccio, C., Levine, M. M., Rodriguez, H., Contreras, R., Chilean Typhoid Committee. (1989). Comparative efficacy of two, three or four doses of Ty21a live oral typhoid vaccine in enteric-coated capsules. A field trial in an endemic area. *Journal of Infectious Diseases*, **159**, 766–9.

Frantz, J. C. & Robertson, D. C. (1981). Immunological properties of *Escherichia coli* heat-stable enterotoxins: development of a radio-immunoassay specific for heat-stable enterotoxins with suckling mouse activity. *Infection and Immunity*, **33**, 193–8.

Gaastra, W. & Svennerholm, A.-M. (1996). Colonisation factors of human enterotoxigenic *Escherichia coli*. *Trends in Microbiology*, in press.

Girón, J. A., Xu, J.-G., González, C. R., Hone, D. M., Kaper, J. B. & Levine, M. M. (1995). Simultaneous expression of CFA/I and CS3 colonization factor antigens of enterotoxigenic *Escherichia coli* by DaroC, DaroD *Salmonella typhi* vaccine strain CVD 908. *Vaccine*, **13**, 939–46.

Gothefors, L., Åhrén, C., Stoll, B., Barua, D. K., Ørskov, F., Salek, M. A. & Svennerholm, A.-M. (1985). Presence of colonization factor antigens on fresh isolates of fecal *Escherichia coli*: a prospective study. *Journal of Infectious Diseases*, **152**, 1128–33.

de Graaf, F. K. & Gaastra, W. (1994). Fimbriae of enterotoxigenic *Escherichia coli*. In *Fimbriae: Adhesion, Genetics, Biogenesis and Vaccines*, ed. P. Klemm, pp. 53–84. Kent: CRC Press.

Guerrant, R. L. (1985). Microbial toxins and diarrhoeal disease: introduction and overview. In *Microbial Toxins and Diarrhoeal Disease*, eds. D. Evered, & J. Whelan, pp. 1–13. London: Pitman.

Holmgren, J., Osek, J. & Svennerholm, A.-M. (1994). Protective oral cholera vaccine based on combination of cholera toxin B subunit and inactivated cholera vibrios. In Vibrio cholerae and *Cholera: Molecular to Global Perspectives*, eds. I. K. Wachsmuth, P. A. Blake, Ø. Olsvik, pp. 415–24. Washington DC: American Society for Microbiology.

Holmgren, J. & Svennerholm, A.-M. (1979). Immunological cross-reactivity between *Escherichia coli* heat-labile enterotoxins and cholera toxin A and B subunits. *Current Microbiology*, **19**, 255–8.

Holmgren, J. & Svennerholm, A.-M. (1992). Bacterial enteric infections and vaccine development. *Gastroenterology Clinics of North America*, **21**, 283–302.

Hone, D., Attridge, S., Van den Bosch, L., & Hackett, J. (1988). A chromosomal integration system for stabilization of heterologous genes in Salmonella-based vaccine strains. *Microbial Pathogenesis*, **5**, 407–12.

Jertborn, M., Åhrén, C., Holmgren, J. & Svennerholm, A.-M. (1995). Safety and immunogenicity of an oral inactivated enterotoxigenic *Escherichia coli* vaccine, submitted for publication.

Lebens, M., Shahabi, V., Houze, T., Lindblad, M. & Holmgren, J. (1996). Synthesis of hybrid molecules between heat-labile enterotoxin and cholera B subunits: potential for use in a broad spectrum vaccine, *Infection and Immunity*, **64**, 2144–50.

Levine, M. M. (1990). Vaccines against enterotoxigenic *Escherichia coli* infections. In *New Generation Vaccines*, eds. G. Woodrow, & M. M. Levine, pp. 649–60. New York: Marcel Dekker.

Levine, M. M., Morris, J. G., Losonsky, G., Boedeker, E. & Rowe, B. (1986). Fimbriae (pili) adhesins as vaccines. In *Protein-Carbohydrate Interactions in Biological Systems*, eds. D. L. Lark, S. Normark, B. E. Uhlin & H. Wolf-Watz, pp. 143–5. London: Academic Press.

Levine, M. M., Nalin, D. R., Hoover, D. L., Bergquist, E. J., Hormick, R. B. & Young, C. R. (1979). Immunity to enterotoxigenic *Escherichia coli*. *Infection and Immunity*, **23**, 729–36.

Li, A., Pal, T., Forsum, U. & Lindberg, A. (1992). Safety and immunogenicity of the live oral auxotrophic *Shigella flexneri* SFL124 in volunteers. *Vaccine*, **10**, 395–404.

López-Vidal, Y., Calva, J. J., Trujillo, A., De León, A. P., Ramos, A., Svennerholm, A.-M. & Ruiz-Palacios, G. (1990). Enterotoxins and adhesins of enterotoxigenic *Escherichia coli*: are they risk factors for acute diarrhoea in the community? *Journal of Infectious Diseases*, **162**, 442–7.

López-Vidal, Y. & Svennerholm, A.-M. (1990). Monoclonal antibodies against the different subcomponents of CFA/II of enterotoxigenic *Escherichia coli* and their use in diagnostic tests. *Journal of Clinical Microbiology*, **28**, 1906–12.

Mata, L. (1980). Diarrhoeal disease: a leading world health problem. In *Cholera and Related Diarrhoeas*, pp. 1–14. Basel: Karger.

McConnell, M. M., Chart, H. & Rowe, B. (1989). Antigenic homology within human enterotoxigenic *Escherichia coli* fimbrial colonization factor antigens CS1, CS2, CS4 and CS17. *FEMS Microbiology Letters*, **61**, 105–8.

McConnell, M. M., Hibbard, M. L., Penny, M. E., Scollond, S. M., Chaesty, T. & Rowe, B. (1991). Surveys of human enterotoxigenic *Escherichia coli* from three different geographical areas for possible colonization factors. *Epidemiology and Infection*, **106**, 477–84.

Moon, H. & Bunn, T. O. (1993). Vaccines for preventing enterotoxigenic *Escherichia coli* infections in farm animals. *Vaccine*, **11**, 213–20.

Neutra, M. R. & Kraehenbuhl, J.-P. (1992). Transepithelial transport and mucosal defence I: the role of M cells. Elsevier Science Publishers 2, 134–8.

Noriega, F. R., Wang, J. Y., Losonsky, G., Maneval, D. R., Hone, D. M. & Levine, M. M. (1994). Construction and characterization of attenuation Δ*aroA* Δ*virG Shigella flexneri* 2a strain CVD 1203, a prototype live oral vaccine. *Infection and Immunity*, **62**, 5168–72.

Peltola, H., Siitonen, A., Kyrönseppä, H., Simula, I., Mattila, L., Oksanen, P., Kataja, M. J. & Cadoz, M. (1991). Prevention of travellers' diarrhoea by oral B-subunit/whole cell cholera vaccine. *Lancet*, **338**, 1285–9.

Qadri, F., Wennerås, C., Bardhan, P. K., Hossain, J., Albert, M. J., Sack, R. B. & Svennerholm, A.-M. (1997). B cell responses to enterotoxigenic Escherichia coli (ETEC) in vaccines and patients after oral immunization and infection, in preparation.

Rao, M. C. (1985). Toxins which activate guanylate cyclase: heat-stable enterotoxins. In *Microbial Toxins and Diarrhoeal Disease*, eds. D. Evered, & J. Whelan, pp. 74–93. London: Pitman.

Reid, R. H., Boedeker, E. C., McQueen, C. E., Davis, D., Tseng, L.-Y.,

Kodak, J., Sau, K., Wilhelmsen, C. L., Nellore, R., Dalal, P. & Bhagat, H. R. (1993). Preclinic evaluation of microencapsulated CFA/II oral vaccine against enterotoxigenic *E. coli*. *Vaccine*, **11**, 159–67.

Rudin, A., McConnell, M. M. & Svennerholm, A.-M. (1994). Monoclonal antibodies against enterotoxigenic *Escherichia coli* colonization factor antigen I (CFA/I) that cross-react immunologically with heterologous CFAs. *Infection and Immunity*, **62**, 4339–46.

Rudin, A., Olbe, L. & Svennerholm, A.-M. (1996). Monoclonal antibodies against fimbrial subunits of colonisation factor antigen I (CFA/I) inhibit binding to human enterocytes and protect against enterotoxigenic *Escherichia coli* expressing heterologous colonisation factors. *Microbial Pathogenesis*, **20**, 35–45.

Rudin, A. & Svennerholm, A.-M. (1994). Colonization factor antigens (CFAs) sof enterotoxigenic *Escherichia coli* can prime and boost immune responses against heterologous CFAs. *Microbial Pathogenesis*, **16**, 131–9.

Rudin, A. & Svennerholm, A.-M. (1996) Identification of a cross-reactive continuous B-cell epitope in enterotoxigenic *Escherichia coli* colonization factor antigen I. *Infection and Immunity*, in press.

Sack, R. B. (1986). Treatment and prevention of travelers' diarrhea. In *Development of Vaccines and Drugs against Diarrhea*, eds. J. Holmgren, A. Lindberg, & R. Möllby, pp. 289–301. Lund: Studentlitteratur.

Sanchez, J. & Holmgren, J. (1989). Recombinant system for overexpression of cholera toxin B subunit in *Vibrio cholerae* as a basis for vaccine development. *Proceedings of the National Academy of Sciences, USA*, **86**, 481–5.

Sanchez, J., Svennerholm, A.-M. & Holmgren, J. (1988). Genetic fusion of a non-toxic heat-stable enterotoxin-related decapeptide antigen to cholera toxin B-subunit. *FEBS Letters*, **241**, 110–4.

Savarino, S. J., Brown, F. M., Hall, E., Bassily, S., Youssef, F., Wierzba, T., Peruski, L., El-Masry, N. A., Safwat, M., Rao, M., Bourgeouis, A. L., Jertborn, M., Svennerholm, A.-M., Lee, J. J. & Clemens, J. D. (1997). Safety and immunogenicity of an oral, killed, enterotoxigenic *Escherichia coli*-cholera toxin B subunit vaccine in Egyptian adults, in preparation.

Schmidt, M., Kelley, E. P., Tseng, L. Y. & Boedeker, E. C. (1985). Towards an oral *E. coli* pilus vaccine for travelers' diarrhea: susceptibility to proteolytic digestion. *Gastroenterology*, **82**, 1575.

Sommerfelt, H., Steinsland, H., Grewal, H. M. S., Viboud, G. I., Bhandari, N., Gaastra, W., Svennerholm, A.-M. & Bhan, K. (1996). Colonisation factors of enterotoxigenic *Escherichia coli* isolated from children in North India. *Journal of Infectious Diseases*, in press.

Spira, W. N., Sack, R. B. & Froelich, J. L. (1981). Simple adult rabbit model for *Vibrio cholerae* and enterotoxigenic *Escherichia coli* diarrhoea. *Infection and Immunity*, **32**, 739–47.

Steffen, R. (1986). Epidemiological studies of traveller's diarrhoea, severe gastrointestinal infections and cholera. *Reviews of Infectious Diseases*, **8**, 122–30.

Stoll, B. J., Svennerholm, A.-M., Gothefors, L., Barua, D., Huda, S. & Holmgren, J. (1986). Local and systemic antibody responses to naturally acquired enterotoxigenic *Escherichia coli* diarrhoea in an endemic area. *Journal of Infectious Diseases*, **153**, 527–34.

Svennerholm, A.-M., Holmgren, J. & Sack, D. A. (1989). Development of oral vaccines against enterotoxigenic *Escherichia coli* diarrhoea. *Vaccine*, **7**, 196–8.

Svennerholm, A.-M., Lindblad, M., Svennerholm, B. & Holmgren, J. (1988). Synthesis of nontoxic, antibody-binding *Escherichia coli* heat-stable enterotoxin (ST_a) peptides. *FEMS Microbiology Letters*, **55**, 23–8.

Svennerholm, A.-M., McConnell, M. M. & Wiklund, G. (1992). Roles of different putative colonization factor antigens in colonization of human enterotoxigenic *Escherichia coli* in rabbits. *Microbial Pathogenesis*, **13**, 381–9.

Svennerholm, A.-M., Wennerås, C., Holmgren, J., McConnell, M. M. & Rowe, B. (1990). Roles of different coli surface antigens of colonization factor antigen II in colonization by and protective immunogenicity of enterotoxigenic *Escherichia coli* in rabbits. *Infection and Immunity*, **58**, 341–6.

Svennerholm, A.-M., Wikström, M., Lindblad, M. & Holmgren, J. (1986a). Monoclonal antibodies to *Escherichia coli* heat-labile enterotoxins: neutralizing activity and differentiation of human and porcine LTs and cholera toxin. *Medical Biology*, **64**, 23–30.

Svennerholm, A.-M., Wikström, M., Lindblad, M. & Holmgren, J. (1986b). Monoclonal antibodies against *E. coli* heat-stable toxin (STa) and their use in diagnostic ST ganglioside GM1-enzyme-linked immunosorbent assay. *Journal of Clinical Microbiology*, **24**, 585–90.

Tacket, C. O., Reid, R. H., Boedecker, D. C., Losonsky, G., Nataro, J. P., Bhagat, H. & Edelman, R. (1994). Enteral immunization and challenge of volunteers given enterotoxigenic *E. coli* CFA/II encapsulated in biodegradable microspheres. *Vaccine*, **14**, 1270–4.

Viboud, G., Binsztein, N., Jouve, M. & Svennerholm, A.-M. (1993a). A new fimbrial putative colonization factor in human enterotoxigenic *Escherichia coli*. *Infection and Immunity*, **61**, 5190–7.

Viboud, G. I., Binsztein, N. & Svennerholm, A.-M. (1993b). Characterization of monoclonal antibodies against putative colonization factors of enterotoxigenic *Escherichia coli* and their use in an epidemiological study. *Journal of Clinical Microbiology*, **31**, 558–64.

Wennerås, C., Svennerholm, A.-M., Åhrén, C. & Czerkinsky, C. (1992). Antibody-secreting cells in human peripheral blood after oral immunization with an inactivated enterotoxigenic *Escherichia coli* vaccine. *Infection and Immunity*, **60**, 2605–11.

Wennerås, C., Svennerholm, A.-M. & Czerkinsky, C. (1994). Vaccine-specific T cells in human peripheral blood after oral immunization with an inactivated enterotoxigenic *Escherichia coli* vaccine. *Infection and Immunity*, **62**, 874–9.

Wolf, M. K., Taylor, D. N., Boedeker, E. C., Hyams, K. C., Maneval, D. R., Levine, M. M., Tamura, K., Wilson, R. A. & Echeverria, P. (1993). Characterization of enterotoxigenic *Escherichia coli* isolated from U.S. troops deployed to the Middle East. *Journal of Clinical Microbiology*, **31**, 851–6.

Yamamoto, T., Tamura, Y. & Yokota, T. (1985). Enteroadhesion fimbriae and enterotoxin of *Esherichia coli*: genetic transfer to a streptomycin-resistant mutant of the *galE* oral-route live vaccine *Salmonella typhi* Ty21a. *Infection and Immunity*, **50**, 925–8.

Index